**P9-CSE-815**

# 32nd ANNUAL EDITION

**1989 - 2020**

## Winning Features:

- Comprehensive & Up-to-Date
- Largest Compilation of Fast-Foods
- Researched & Compiled by Allan Borushek (Dietitian)
- Bonus Diet Guides

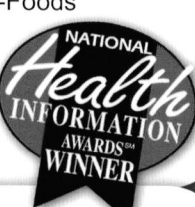

NATIONAL Health INFORMATION AWARDS℠ WINNER

**NATIONAL BEST SELLER**

## ★ PUBLISHING & DISTRIBUTION INFO ★

**10-Week Journal
One Day Per Page**

**COPYRIGHT © 2020 Allan Borushek**

**LARGER PRINT EDITION:**
ISBN 978-1-930448-75-9

**REGULAR EDITION:**
ISBN 978-1-930448-73-5

*DISTRIBUTION & CUSTOM ORDERS:*
**Family Health Publications
419 Main St, Ste 282
Huntington Beach CA 92648
bulkorders@calorieking.com
Phone: (949) 642 8500**

**Online Orders:**
**1-9 Books**: Amazon, Barnes & Noble
**10+ Books:**
email: bulkorders@calorieking.com

THE **CALORIE KING**®

# Calorie
# FAT &
# CARBOHYDRATE
# Counter

**ALLAN BORUSHEK**
~DIETITIAN~
"THE CALORIE KING"

Includes
**200**
Fast-Food
Chains

**BONUS
DIET GUIDES
DIABETES
CHOLESTEROL
SODIUM
FIBER
ALCOHOL**

**CalorieKing.com**

# THE CALORIEKING®
## Calorie, Fat & Carbohydrate Counter

| | |
|---|---|
| Alcoholic Drinks with Alcohol Counts | 24 |
| Baking Ingredients | 30 |
| Bars (Breakfast, Granola, Nutrition) | 31 |
| Beverages: Cocoa & Hot Chocolate | 35 |
|    Coffee & Coffee Drinks | 35 |
|    Energy, Protein, Diet Shakes | 38 |
|    Milk (Plain, Flavored, Mixes) | 47 |
|    Nut/Rice/Cereal/Soy Drinks | 49 |
|    Non-Dairy (Soy/Rice/Cereal/Nut) | 49 |
|    Tea & Iced Tea Drinks | 53 |
| Bread & Bread Products, Bagels | 54 |
| Breakfast Cereals | 57 |
| Cakes, Buns, Donuts, Pastries | 62 |
| Candy, Chocolate, Gum | 68 |
| Cheese & Cheese Products/Dips | 76 |
| Chicken, Poultry | 138 |
| Condiments, Salsa, Pickles | 80 |
| Cookies, Crackers | 81 |
| Crispbreads, Matzo | 88 |
| Cream & Creamers | 89 |
| Desserts (Puddings, Gelatin Desserts) | 90 |
| Eggs, Egg Substitutes, Egg Dishes | 91 |
| Fats, Butter, Spreads, Oils, Mayonnaise | 93 |
| Fish, Shellfish | 95 |
| Flours & Grains | 98 |
| Fruit (Fresh/Packaged/Dried/Snacks) | 99 |
| Ice Cream & Frozen Yogurt/Novelties | 103 |
| Meals, Entrees, Sides: | |
|    Canned/Packaged/Frozen | 111 |
| Meats: Beef, Lamb, Pork, Game | 123 |
|    Hot Dogs, Lunch Meats, SPAM | 128 |
|    Sausages, Franks, Hot Dogs | 127 |
| Muffins, Sweet Rolls & Buns | 67 |
| Nuts, Seeds, Peanut & Seed Butter | 130 |
| Pancakes & Waffles | 132 |
| Pasta & Noodles | 133 |
| Pies (Fruit) Pie/Pastry Crusts | 134 |
| Pizza: Ready-To-Eat | 135 |
|    Frozen | 136 |
| Poultry (Chicken, Turkey, Duck, Goose) | 138 |
| Rice & Rice Dishes | 140 |
| Salads | 141 |
| Salad Dressings | 142 |
| Sauces & Gravy | 144 |
| Seasonings, Seasonings & Spices | 147 |
| Snacks (Popcorn, Chips, Pretzels) | 148 |
| Soups | 152 |
| Soy, Tofu, Supplements/Cough Syrup | 156 |
| Sugar, Sweeteners, Honey, Jam | 157 |
| Syrups, Dessert Toppings | 157 |
| Vegetables (Fresh/Frozen/Canned) | 158 |
| Yogurt, Yogurt Drinks & Probiotics | 162 |

*Eating Out:*

| | |
|---|---|
|    Cafeteria, Sandwiches | 165 |
|    Fair/Carnival/Stadium Foods | 166 |
|    Restaurant & International Foods | 168 |
|    Fast Food Chains & Restaurants Index | 175 |
| A-Z Food Index Back | 282 |

## BONUS DIET GUIDES & COUNTERS

| | |
|---|---|
| Alcohol Guide & Counter | 23 - 29 |
| Caffeine Guide & Counter | 37 |
| Diabetes Guide | 16 - 21 |
| Fats & Cholesterol Guide | 259 - 263 |
| Fiber Guide & Counter | 264 - 269 |
| Protein Guide & Counter | 270 - 274 |
| Salt/Sodium Counter with High Blood Pressure Guide | 275 - 281 |
| Weight Control Guide | 2 - 15 |

# Weight Control Tips

### ✅ Eat & Drink Sensibly

- Avoid fad diets. Eat 3 sensible portion-controlled meals daily.
- Limit fats, high-fat foods/snacks and sugar. Eat adequate fresh fruit & vegetables.
- Limit soft drinks, energy drinks, fruit juice and alcohol. Quench your thirst on water. (See Sample Meal Plan ~ Page 11)

### ✅ Exercise Daily

- Aim for at least 30 minutes daily – even in 5-10 minute lots. For motivation, find an exercise buddy, personal trainer or join a gym. *(Extra Notes ~ Page 12)*

### ✅ Reshape Eating Behaviors

- Be aware of eating and shopping behaviors that lead to overeating.
- Also focus on social and emotional situations that may trigger compulsive eating. *(Extra Notes ~ Page 14)*

### ✅ Keep a Food & Exercise Journal

- A journal helps you see exactly what you eat and drink, and how much you exercise. *(Extra Notes ~ Page 15)*
- An excellent motivator and proven weight loss aid. Keeps you honest!

### ✅ Arrange Moral Support

- Gain the support of family and friends.
- Get extra professional help if required, from your doctor, dietitian, psychologist, exercise trainer, or slimming group.
- Beware of family saboteurs who may discourage you from adopting a healthier diet and lifestyle!

---

### 🧑‍⚕️ DOCTOR CHECK-UP

*Ask your doctor to check your blood pressure, blood sugar and blood cholesterol levels.*

---

## HEALTHY WEIGHTS
### ~ MEN & WOMEN ~
#### (Over 18 Years)

Based on weights with least risk of disease or death from heart disease, diabetes, stroke and cancer.

Based on Body Mass Index of 20-25

BMI calculated as: $\dfrac{Weight (kg)}{Height (m)^2}$

| Height (No Shoes) Ft Ins | | Healthy Weight Range (Pounds) |
|---|---|---|
| 4'7" | ~ | 86-108 |
| 4'8" | ~ | 88-110 |
| 4'9" | ~ | 92-114 |
| 4'10" | ~ | 97-121 |
| 4'11" | ~ | 99-123 |
| 5'0" | ~ | 101-127 |
| 5'1" | ~ | 105-132 |
| 5'2" | ~ | 110-136 |
| 5'3" | ~ | 112-140 |
| 5'4" | ~ | 114-145 |
| 5'5" | ~ | 119-149 |
| 5'6" | ~ | 123-156 |
| 5'7" | ~ | 127-158 |
| 5'8" | ~ | 129-162 |
| 5'9" | ~ | 134-167 |
| 5'10" | ~ | 138-173 |
| 5'11" | ~ | 143-178 |
| 6'0" | ~ | 145-182 |
| 6'1" | ~ | 149-187 |
| 6'2" | ~ | 156-193 |
| 6'3" | ~ | 158-198 |
| 6'4" | ~ | 162-202 |
| 6'5" | ~ | 170-211 |
| 6'6" | ~ | 172-215 |
| 6'7" | ~ | 175-220 |

## Body Fat Distribution & Health

Moderate amounts of body fat do not compromise health. However, excess fat above the hips carries a far greater health risk than fat on or below the hips - better to be a 'pear-shape' than an 'apple-shape'.

**Abdominal obesity** greatly increases the risk of developing diabetes, heart disease, high blood fats, hypertension, stroke, sleep apnea, arthritis and some cancers. So-called 'cellulite' carries no extra health risk.

**Waist Circumference** directly reflects the increased health risk of abdominal obesity. Waist size associated with a high health risk:

**Men** ~ Over 40 inches        **Women** ~ Over 35 inches

## Body Mass Index (BMI)

BMI is a general (but not specific) indicator of body fatness. Although BMI alone is not diagnostic, the higher the BMI, the greater the health risk of developing diabetes, high blood pressure and heart disease. BMI does not apply to heavily muscled persons. BMI is used in a different way for children.

*Abdominal obesity greatly increases the risk of ill-health and earlier death.*

**Check Your BMI:** Find your height (no shoes) - look across the row to the weight nearest your own. Then track down to BMI.

| Ht | WEIGHT (LBS) ~ ADULTS | | | | | | | | | | | | | |
|------|-----|-----|-----|-----|-----|-----|-----|-----|-----|-----|-----|-----|-----|-----|
| 5'1" | 100 | 106 | 111 | 116 | 122 | 127 | 132 | 137 | 143 | 148 | 153 | 158 | 185 | 211 |
| 5'2" | 104 | 109 | 115 | 120 | 126 | 131 | 136 | 142 | 147 | 153 | 158 | 164 | 191 | 218 |
| 5'3" | 107 | 113 | 118 | 124 | 130 | 135 | 141 | 146 | 152 | 158 | 163 | 169 | 197 | 225 |
| 5'4" | 110 | 116 | 122 | 128 | 134 | 140 | 145 | 151 | 157 | 163 | 169 | 174 | 204 | 232 |
| 5'5" | 114 | 120 | 126 | 132 | 138 | 144 | 150 | 156 | 162 | 168 | 174 | 180 | 210 | 240 |
| 5'6" | 118 | 124 | 130 | 136 | 142 | 148 | 155 | 161 | 167 | 173 | 179 | 186 | 216 | 247 |
| 5'7" | 121 | 127 | 134 | 140 | 146 | 153 | 159 | 166 | 172 | 178 | 185 | 191 | 223 | 255 |
| 5'8" | 125 | 131 | 138 | 144 | 151 | 158 | 164 | 171 | 177 | 184 | 190 | 197 | 230 | 262 |
| 5'9" | 128 | 135 | 142 | 149 | 155 | 162 | 169 | 176 | 182 | 189 | 196 | 206 | 236 | 270 |
| 5'10" | 132 | 139 | 146 | 153 | 160 | 167 | 174 | 181 | 188 | 195 | 202 | 207 | 243 | 278 |
| 5'11" | 136 | 143 | 150 | 157 | 165 | 172 | 179 | 186 | 193 | 200 | 208 | 215 | 250 | 286 |
| 6'0" | 140 | 147 | 154 | 162 | 169 | 177 | 184 | 191 | 199 | 206 | 213 | 221 | 258 | 294 |
| 6'1" | 144 | 151 | 159 | 166 | 174 | 182 | 189 | 197 | 204 | 212 | 219 | 227 | 265 | 302 |
| 6'2" | 148 | 155 | 163 | 171 | 179 | 186 | 194 | 202 | 210 | 218 | 225 | 233 | 272 | 311 |
| 6'3" | 152 | 160 | 168 | 176 | 184 | 192 | 200 | 208 | 216 | 224 | 232 | 240 | 279 | 319 |
| 6'4" | 156 | 164 | 172 | 180 | 189 | 197 | 205 | 213 | 221 | 230 | 238 | 246 | 287 | 328 |

| BMI | 19 | 20 | 21 | 22 | 23 | 24 | 25 | 26 | 27 | 28 | 29 | 30 | 35 | 40 |

**BMI Classification:**

**BMI Below 19**
Underweight

**BMI 19-24.9**
Healthy Weight
(Low Health Risk)

**BMI 25-29.9**
Overweight
(Moderate Health Risk)

**BMI 30-40**
Obese (High Health Risk)

**BMI Over 40**
Morbid Obesity
(Very High Risk)

Interactive BMI Calculator
www.calorieking.com

# Calories & Weight Loss

## Calories in Food

Calories in food are derived from protein, fat and carbohydrate. Alcohol also provides calories. Vitamins, minerals and water provide no calories.

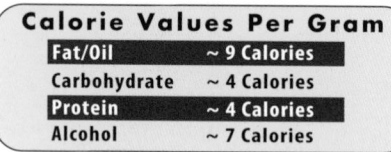

### Calorie Values Per Gram

| Fat/Oil | ~ 9 Calories |
|---|---|
| Carbohydrate | ~ 4 Calories |
| Protein | ~ 4 Calories |
| Alcohol | ~ 7 Calories |

Note that fats have over double the calories of protein and carbohydrate. The higher the fat content of food, the higher the calories.

### Sample Calculation

**QUARTER POUNDER®
WITH CHEESE
has 510 calories
derived from:**

| | | |
|---|---|---|
| 26g Fat (x 9 cals/gram) | = | 234 |
| 40g Carbohyd.(x 4 cals/gram) | = | 160 |
| 29g Protein (x 4 cals/gram) | = | 116 |
| Total Calories | = | 510 |

## Calorie Levels for Weight Loss

Start with a calorie-controlled diet that allows a moderate weight loss of ½ - 1 pound per week. Weight loss is usually much greater in the first few weeks due to extra fluid losses.

Note: It is better to increase exercise rather than lessen food calories too drastically.

### Suggested Calories for Weight Loss

| Women: | Non-active | 1000 - 1200 |
|---|---|---|
| | Active | 1200 - 1500 |
| Men: | Non-active | 1200 - 1500 |
| | Active | 1500 - 1800 |
| Teenagers: | | 1200 - 1800 |

**ChooseMyPlate.gov**

The MyPlate symbol represents the recommended proportion of foods from each food group. It focuses on the importance of making smart food choices in every food group, every day. Daily physical activity is also important. *(More info: www.ChooseMyPlate.gov)*

## Examples of Single Serving Sizes

**Grains (Eat 6 servings per day):**
- 1 slice wholegrain bread (1 oz)
- ½ bun, small bagel or English muffin
- 4 small crackers or 1 tortilla
- 1 oz ready-to-eat wholegrain cereal
- ½ cup cooked cereal, rice or pasta

**Vegetables (Eat 3-5 servings per day):**
- 1 cup raw leafy vegetables
- 1½ cups raw chopped vegetables
- ½ cup cooked vegetables
- ½ - ¾ cup vegetable juice

**Fruit (Eat 3-5 servings per day):**
- 1 medium apple, orange, banana
- ½ cup canned fruit (in own juice)
- ¼ cup dried fruit
- ½ cup fruit juice (unsweetened)
- ¼ medium avocado

**Protein (2-3 servings per day):**
- 2-3 oz (cooked) lean meat/poultry/fish
- 2 eggs or 6 oz tofu or ¼ cup nuts
- 1 cup (cooked) dried beans or chickpeas

**Dairy (2-3 servings per day):**
- 1 cup (8 fl.oz) milk/soy (enriched)/yogurt
- 1½ oz cheese or ½ cup cottage cheese

## Portion Size Counts!

Food portion size is critical to controlling calorie intake for weight control.

Super-sized food servings have become more common when eating out and in the home. This can mean a day's worth of calories being consumed in one meal; or a snack being equivalent to a full meal.

It is easy to underestimate portion size of foods and drinks, and unwittingly consume excess calories – even if the fat content is low or even zero!

To more accurately estimate portion size of different foods, weigh and measure your food with food scales, measuring spoons and cups. Better control of calories will result.

**For a visual idea of portion sizes, visit www.CalorieKing.com** See examples (fries and cola) on this page.

## Allow for Extra Calories in Packaged Food

The actual weight of packaged foods is usually 5-10% more than the label net weight (the minimum legal weight) – and in some cases up to 50% more. However, manufacturers calculate the calories based on the net weight. For actual calories, weigh the product and calculate the extra calories.

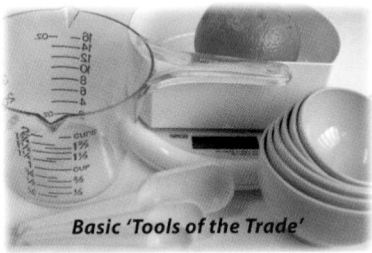

*Basic 'Tools of the Trade'*

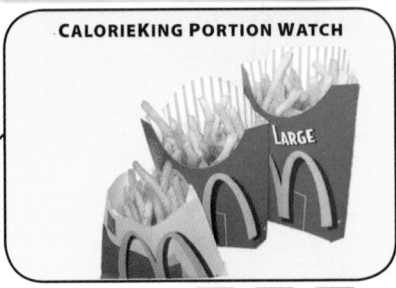

**CALORIEKING PORTION WATCH**

| Fries | Cal | Fat | Carb |
|--------|-----|-----|------|
| Small | 230 | 11 | 29 |
| Medium | 380 | 19 | 48 |
| Large | 500 | 25 | 63 |

**CALORIEKING PORTION WATCH**

| Cola | Cal | Fat | Carb |
|------|-----|-----|------|
| 8 fl.oz Cup | 100 | 0 | 25 |
| 12 fl.oz Can | 150 | 0 | 37 |
| 20 fl.oz Bottle | 250 | 0 | 63 |
| 1 Liter Bottle | 400 | 0 | 100 |
| 2 Liter Bottle | 800 | 0 | 200 |

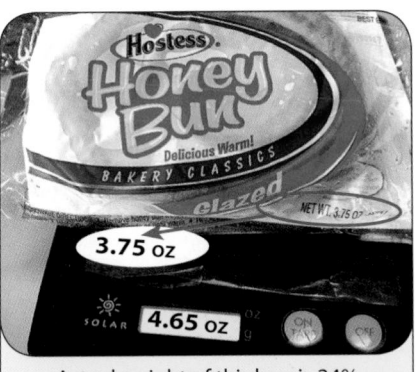

Actual weight of this bun is 24% more than the stated net weight.

# Recommended Fat Intake

## ▶ Fat in the Diet

Fats in the diet are essential for good health. However, too much fat can contribute to obesity and a higher risk of heart disease, high blood pressure, diabetes, gallstone and certain cancers.

Dietary fat and oils have over double the calories of carbohydrates and protein. (Example: Changing from whole-milk to non-fat milk halves the calories.)

| MAXIMUM DESIRABLE FAT INTAKE (DAILY) | |
|---|---|
| **Calories** | **Fat** |
| 1200 cals | 30g fat |
| 1500 cals | 40g fat |
| 1800 cals | 50g fat |
| 2000 cals | 60g fat |
| 2200 cals | 70g fat |
| 2500 cals | 80g fat |
| 3000 cals | 110g fat |

### ZERO GRAMS TRANS FAT

*Don't be fooled by **Zero Grams Trans Fat** boldly displayed on some high-fat snacks. They are still high in fat and calories.*

*Examples: Cheetos 99c pkg ~ 24g fat, 380 cals*
*Lay's Chips (2¾ oz pkg) ~ 27g fat, 430 calories*

0 grams
Trans Fat

## ▶ Beware low-fat foods

It is a mistake to think that eating low-fat or fat-free foods allows you to eat double the quantity. You can end up with even more calories than eating smaller amounts of regular-fat products.

Food products which are fat-free but high in calories include soda drinks, fruit juices, beer, alcoholic spirits, sugar and candy. Bread, rice and pasta also have negligible fat but need to be eaten in controlled amounts.

Ultimately, **it is food portion size as well as total calories that count** whether from fat, carbohydrate or protein. Remember, cows get fat on grass!

*Reduced fat and fat-free foods are not necessarily low calorie. Portion size is still important.*

3 Cookies
**140 Calories**

6 oz Fat-Free Muffin:
**450 calories**

### FOOD LABEL MEANINGS

**FDA Nutrition Claim Definitions**
(All are on a Per Serving Basis)

*Low Calorie:* **40 Calories or less**

*Light or Lite:* **One third fewer calories or, 50% or less fat than regular product**

*Fat-Free:* **Less than half a gram of fat**

*Low-Fat:* **3 grams or less of fat**

*Reduced Fat:* **25% less fat than regular product**

*Fewer or Less Calories:* **At least 25% fewer calories than regular product**

# Tips to Reduce Fat

## ▶ Meats, Poultry, Fish

- **Choose lean cuts** of meat with little marbling. **Trim all visible fat** from meat and remove the skin from poultry. Removal of fat after cooking, is okay (to prevent dryness). Choose 'extra lean' ground beef.
- **Avoid high-fat meat products** such as salami, bacon, sausage and franks.
- **Broil or bake. Avoid frying in oil.** Allow casseroles to cool and skim off surface fat.
- **Avoid fried fish**, frozen fish in batter and canned fish in oil.

## ▶ Fats & Oils

- **Use minimal amounts** of all types of fat and oil. All are high in calories.
- **Choose** 'light' and 'reduced fat' spreads but still use sparingly.
- Use minimal amounts of oil when stir-frying. Use no-stick sprays like Pam.

## ▶ Salad Dressings & Sauces

- **Avoid regular mayonnaise and oil dressings.** Choose 'light', 'reduced fat' or 'fat-free' brands.
- **Choose low-fat or fat-free sauces** (mainly tomato-based). Avoid 'pesto', 'alfredo', 'cheese' and 'creamy' sauces.

## ▶ Milk, Cheese

- **Choose low-fat or nonfat milks and yogurts.** Avoid full-cream milk, cream, Half & Half.
- **Cheese:** Choose fat-free, and low-fat cheese. Part-skim ricotta is still high in fat. Low-fat cottage cheese is a good choice. Cheese substitutes can still be high in fat.

## ▶ Snacks, Cookies, Candy

- **Avoid** high-fat snacks such as potato chips, corn/tortilla chips, cheese puffs, buttered popcorn, chocolate and carob bars.

## ▶ Desserts/Sweets

- **Avoid high-fat desserts**, such as cake, pie, pastries, cheesecake, full-fat puddings.
- **Choose** fresh fruits, fresh fruit salad, canned fruit in water pack, low-fat ice cream. Use low-fat yogurt in place of cream.

## ▶ Fast-Foods & Take-Out

*Check the Fast-Foods Section of this book for actual fat and calorie counts.*

- **Avoid deep-fried foods such as** chicken, french fries and onion rings.
- **Pizzas:** Avoid sausage/pepperoni. Choose vegetarian topping and modest quantity of cheese. Eat a moderate serving. Eat extra salad and fresh fruit.
- **Hamburgers:** Choose medium size, lower fat burgers. Avoid bacon. Have a side salad (with fat-free dressing).
- **Delis:** Choose sandwiches/bread rolls, pitas with low-fat fillings and plain salad. Limit meat/cheese to small portions.
- **Coffees:** Avoid large sizes of latte and frappuccino. Request nonfat milk and no whipped cream. Avoid cookies and pastries.

*Extra Information: www.CalorieKing.com*

---

### FRYING ADDS FAT!

*The greater the surface area of potato exposed to fat or oil, the higher the fat content and calories.*

 **Whole Potato (3 oz)**
**0g Fat** 65 Cals

 **Roasted Potato (3 oz)**
**5g Fat** 155 Cals

 **Fries (Large cut, 3 oz)**
**12g Fat** 220 Cals

 **Fries (Small, 3 oz)**
**15g Fat** 265 Cals

 **Potato Chips (3 oz)**
**30g Fat** 450 Cals

# Carbohydrates ~ Friend or Foe?

## Naturally-Friendly Carbs

- **Carbohydrate foods in their more natural forms** (not overly processed) are essential to good health. They are the main source of fuel for the body, and also provide important vitamins, minerals, antioxidants and fiber – all of which help protect against heart disease, diabetes, hypertension, constipation-related ailments and many other diseases.

- Carbohydrates even help the body produce serotonin, the 'feel good' brain chemical that helps control appetite and overeating. Too little serotonin can lead to mood swings and depression.

## Carbohydrates are found in different forms in food as:

- Sugars in fruit, sugar cane, milk
- Starches in whole grains, legumes, nuts, seeds and vegetables
- Dietary fiber (See Fiber Guide ~ Page 264)

*Glycemic Index & Diabetes ~ Page 21*

| RECOMMENDED CARBOHYDRATE INTAKE | | |
|---|---|---|
| Calories (Daily) | Carbohydrate (Grams) | Percent Carbohydrate Calories |
| 1200 cals | 100-120g | 35-40% |
| 1500 cals | 140-170g | 40-45% |
| 1800 cals | 180-200g | 40-45% |
| 2000 cals | 200-250g | 40-50% |
| 2500 cals | 310-350g | 50-55% |
| 3000 cals | 410-450g | 55-65% |

## How Much Do We Need?

- As shown in the chart, well-balanced diets above 2000 calories contain 50-60% of total calories from carbohydrates.

- At lower calorie levels used for weight control (1200-1500 calories), carbohydrates account for as little as 40% of total calories. This is because protein calories have nutritional priority.

- Carbohydrates & Diabetes ~ *See Page 21*

> **Carbohydrate foods (minimally processed) are essential to good health.**
>
> *Be sure to eat adequate fruit and vegetables (5 - 7 servings) every day.*

## Low-Carbohydrate Diets

- Popular low-carbohydrate diets are extreme in their recommendations to initially cut carb intake to as little as 20 grams per day – the amount in 1 thick slice of bread, or 1 medium apple, or 1 small potato.

- This greatly increases the risk of nutritional deficiencies and compromises health, particularly if fat intake is excessive through fatty meats, high-fat dairy products, and fried foods.

- While overweight Americans do need to reduce carbohydrate intake, it should be done **sensibly as part of reducing portion size and total calories.**

- Simply eating 'low-carb' food products without regard to portion size, calories or fats, will do little to promote weight loss or good health.

- **Low-carb diets (and indeed any diet) only work if total calories are reduced.**

- Refined sugars should be one of the first targets in reducing carb intake.

**FAT MATTERS
CARBS COUNT
BUT CALORIES ARE KING!**

*Extra Info ~ www.CalorieKing.com*

*Sugar-free & lower carb products may still be high in calories and fat.*

- **Excess Sugar:** Many overweight, inactive people consume over 500 calories of refined sugars per day, either self-added or as part of food products. This is equivalent to over 30 level teaspoons – a significant amount in weight control terms. Halving this amount would be reasonable and worthwhile.

**Note: Naturally occurring sugars** in fruits, vegetables and milk are fine when consumed in normal recommended amounts. These foods are also rich in other nutrients.

Refined sugar is referred to as having **'empty calories'**. Sugar supplies calories but negligible nutrients and no fiber.

- **Most sugar in our diet is 'hidden'** in processed foods such as soft drinks, fruit drinks, candy, cookies, cake, jam, sauces, ice cream, desserts, canned foods, and processed breakfast cereals.

For serious weight control, severely limit these foods and substitute healthier higher fiber wholefoods.

**Note:** Be careful not to substitute sugar-rich foods with high-fat foods which might boost calories even more!

- **Be aware that sugar comes in different forms** such as sucrose, glucose, fructose, malt, high-fructose corn syrup, molasses, honey and maple syrup. Check the label.

- **Sugar alcohols** such as sorbitol, mannitol and maltitol are carb-based and have ½ - ¾ the calories of regular sugar. While not counted as sugar on food labels, they do add to the carb count. Excess amounts can cause bloating, gas and diarrhea.

- **Sugar-free sweeteners** make it easy to reduce sugar in drinks and recipes. However, use minimally since research suggests possible ill-effects of some artificial sweeteners on friendly gut microbes. This may increase the risk of glucose intolerance and an increase in appetite.

**Note:** Most recipes can be adapted to contain less sugar with little effect on taste.

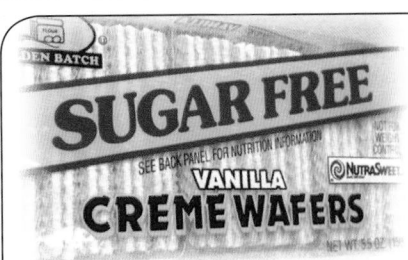

*Sugar-free snacks and foods may be higher in fat and calories than the regular product.*

| Example | ~ Creme Wafers (3): |
|---|---|
| Regular | ~ 115 cals, 6g fat |
| Sugar-Free | ~ 160 cals, 10g fat |

## SUGAR CONTENT OF SOME COMMON FOODS

### Teaspoons of Sugar

| | |
|---|---|
| *Coca Cola* or *Pepsi,* 12 fl.oz | 10 |
| 20 fl.oz size | 17 |
| Iced Tea, sweetened, 12 fl.oz | 8 |
| Chocolate Milk, 12 fl.oz | 6 |
| *Honey Smacks* Cereal, ¾ cup, 1 oz | 4 |
| Popcorn, caramel, 1 cup | 3.5 |
| Chocolate Bar, 1.5 oz | 6 |
| *M&M's* 1.7 oz pkg | 7 |
| Muffin, large, 4 oz | 6 |
| Choc Chip Cookie, 1 oz | 2 |
| Donut, iced | 6 |
| Apple Pie, 1 piece | 7 |
| *Jell-O,* ½ cup | 4.5 |
| Jam, 1 Tbsp, ¾ oz | 2.5 |
| Syrup, maple, 1 Tbsp | 3 |

*Reach for fresh fruit when you want to snack instead of candy or snack products rich in sugar and fat.*

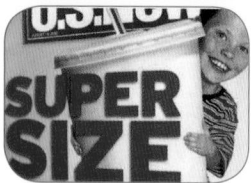

### The XL Generation

Some 15% of American kids and adolescents are overweight; and childhood obesity has doubled over the last 20 years. Diabetes, high blood pressure and high cholesterol are major problem areas for overweight children and adolescents, as are depression, low self-esteem, sleep apnea and bone joint problems.

To address this problem, cooperation is required between kids, parents, schools and government. Weight control is a family and community affair.

*Five Simple Tips To Get Started:*

### ❶ Watch Soda Intake

Limit soda and sugary drinks to one serving on the weekends. Soda should not be an everyday beverage – water should be. When at restaurants or using a soda fountain, choose small servings with ice or choose diet soda instead. Schools should provide water and restrict access to soda as should parents when eating out or in the home!

### ❷ Cut back on Fast-Foods and Eating Out

Many more calories are consumed when you eat out. Healthy meals prepared at home are best for the whole family.

### ❸ Say "No" to Super-Sizing

When meals are upsized, loads more calories are consumed. Choose sensible portion sizes when eating out and at home. Use smaller plates and choose smaller packages.

### ❹ Limit Between-Meal Snacking

Watch out for high-fat and high-calorie snacks – they can have more calories than a meal! Keep your eye on portion sizes and limit salty snack foods and candy to parties and special occasions. Choose fresh fruit, vegetables, nuts and low-fat milk instead.

### ❺ Get Moving ~ Watch Less TV

Kids need at least 60 minutes of physical activity every day. It's critical for their fitness, and greatly lessens the risk of obesity.

Encourage kids to be active out of school hours. Wearing a pedometer can be highly motivational for kids to move more – as can playing dance video games such as *Dance Dance Revolution. Dance Central* (XBox360) and *Wii Fit (Nintendo)* are also excellent fitness motivators.

**Limit TV and non-active computer games** to just one hour per day. Also limit the accompanying snacks! Include exercise in family activities.

*Extra information and tips ~ www.CalorieKing.com*

# Sample Meal Plan ~ 1400 Calories

**For Healthy, Overweight Persons ~ Not for Persons With Any Medical Condition
~ Please Check With Your Doctor & Dietitian ~**

 **Breakfast (approx. 300 cal)**

| | |
|---|---|
| | *1 Small Fruit or ½ oz Dried Fruit* |
| *Plus* | *Cereal: 1½ oz Dry (high fiber)* |
| | *or 1 cup cooked Oatmeal* |
| *Plus* | *½ oz Almonds/Seeds* |
| *Plus* | *Milk (from daily allowance) or Yogurt (low-fat)* |

**Daily Milk Allowance (approx.160 calories)**
*2 cups Non-Fat Milk or 1½ cups Low-fat (1%) Milk
or equivalent Soy Drink, Yogurt, Cheese, Tofu*

**Fat Allowance (140 calories; 15g Fat)**
*4 tsp Fat or 6-8 tsp Diet Margarine or 3 tsp Oil
or 1½ Tbsp Mayonnaise or ½ medium Avocado
or 1½ Tbsp Peanut Butter or 30g Nuts/Seeds*

 **Breakfast ~ Choice 2**

| | |
|---|---|
| | *1 Small Fruit* |
| *Plus* | *2 Eggs (no added fat)* |
| | *or 2 oz Cheese (low-fat)* |
| | *or 4 oz Cottage Cheese (low-fat)* |
| | *or 2 oz Lean/Canadian Bacon* |
| *Plus* | *1 Tomato* |
| *Plus* | *1 Slice Wholegrain Toast* |

 **Between Meals**

*Water, Coffee, Tea, Diet drinks,
Fruit from main meals; Raw Vegetable
Pieces, Milk from Daily Allowance*

 **Lunch (approx. 440 calories)**

| | |
|---|---|
| | *2 slices Wholegrain Bread (2 oz)* |
| | *or 4 Crispbreads/Crackers or 6" Pita* |
| *Plus* | *2 oz lean Meat, Chicken or Turkey* |
| | *or 3½ oz Tuna (in water) or 2½ oz Salmon* |
| | *or 1 oz Cheese or ½ cup (4 oz) Cottage Cheese* |
| | *or ½ cup (4 oz) Ricotta Cheese (low-fat)* |
| | *or ½ cup (4 oz) Fruit Yogurt (low-fat)* |
| | *or ½ cup (4 oz) Bean Salad* |
| *Plus* | *Large Salad (Oil-free dressing)* |
| *Plus* | *1 small Fruit or ½ oz Dried Fruit* |

 **Dinner (approx. 360 calories)**

| | |
|---|---|
| | *Soup (fat-free)* |
| *Plus* | *3 oz lean Meat (cooked weight)* |
| | *or 4 oz Chicken Breast (no skin)* |
| | *or 3 oz Chicken Thigh/Leg (no skin)* |
| | *or 5 oz Fish (grilled, no fat)* |
| | *or ¾ cup (6 oz) Beans (Soy, Kidney, Pinto etc)/Lentils* |
| | *or Low-fat Entree (e.g. Lean Cuisine)* |
| *Plus* | *1 small Potato* |
| | *or ½ cup Rice/Pasta/Sweet Corn* |
| | *or 1 slice Wholegrain Bread* |
| *Plus* | *2-3 servings Vegetables/Salad* |
| *Plus* | *1 small Fruit + Diet Gelatin Dessert* |

# Exercise & Weight Control

- **Persons who exercise regularly lose more weight** and keep it off longer than non-exercisers. Blood glucose control also improves; as do beneficial gut microbes.

- **Exercise also improves general health and well-being.** Mood, confidence and self-esteem are also enhanced.

- **Exercise** is a good way to 'wake up' a sluggish metabolism and burn excess body fat.

- **Aerobic (huff and puff) exercise most days** is great for burning calories and for cardiovascular fitness. But, it is strength training that mainly builds the muscles that burn calories.

- **Strength training is the key to retaining or rebuilding muscles.** As we age, we lose some 6 pounds of muscle per decade. This results in a lower metabolism and fewer calories burnt.

  Muscles are the furnaces that burn calories. The more muscle you have, the more calories burnt – and as a bonus, the more food you can eat.

- **Regular strength training (2-3 times weekly)** can increase our metabolic rate for several days following exercise – with up to an extra 100 calories per day being burnt.

  While 2-3 pounds of muscle may be gained in the first 8-10 weeks, weight from exercised muscles is ok. It is excess fat (particularly abdominal fat) that is a potential health hazard.

- **Body reshaping** is enhanced by gaining muscle and losing fat - even if the scales don't show it.

- **Avoid injury** by beginning with walking, low impact aerobics, or weight-supported exercise (e.g. swimming, cycling). Avoid competitive sports. Allow 2-3 days of recovery between strength training sessions. Get professional advice.

- **How Much?** Start with 10-20 minutes per day and progress to 30-60 minutes per day. Also walk up stairs instead of using elevators. Take a brisk walk at lunch. Use an exercise bike, treadmill or stair machine while watching TV. Walk the dog.

- **How Often?** While aerobic fitness may require only 3-4 sessions weekly, **weight control is a daily event which requires daily exercise to burn calories.** Also add in strength training 2-3 times weekly.

**Note:** Persons on cholesterol-lowering statin drugs may experience muscle pains and weakness (as well as damage to muscle microfibrils). Supplementing with coenzyme Q10, magnesium, selenium, vitamins D and K2, may be beneficial. Check with your healthcare provider.

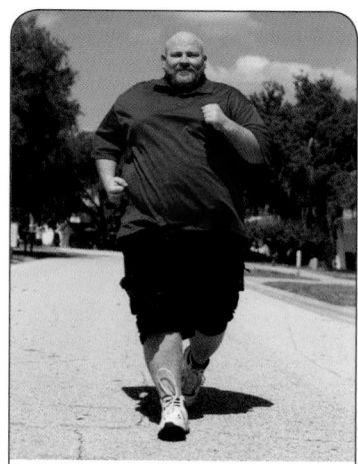

*Brisk walking each day is a safe and effective way to burn calories and keep fit.*
*Try it – you'll like it!*
Be sure to wear sun-protective clothing.

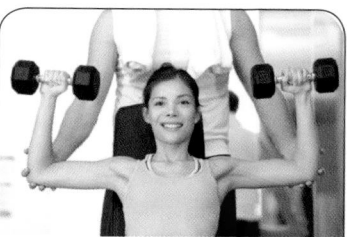

*Strength training is the key to retain or rebuild muscles.*

*Exercized muscles burn extra calories even while you sleep.*

*For extra guidance and motivation, seek a qualified trainer or join a gym.*

# Calories Used in Exercise

Calories Used in Exercise

| LIGHT | MODERATE | HEAVY |
|---|---|---|
| 130 lbs ~ 3 Cals/Min | 130 lbs ~ 5 Cals/Min | 130 lbs ~ 8 Cals/Min |
| 170 lbs ~ 4 Cals/Min | 170 lbs ~ 6 Cals/Min | 170 lbs ~ 10 Cals/Min |
| 220 lbs ~ 5 Cals/Min | 220 lbs ~ 7 Cals/Min | 220 lbs ~ 12 Cals/Min |

**LIGHT**
- Walking, slow
- Cycling, light
- Frisbee playing
- Gardening, light
- Golf, social
- Tennis, doubles
- Housework, cleaning
- Calisthenics, light
- Bowling
- Ping-pong, social
- Ice Skating, light
- Aquarobics, light
- Skate Boarding
- Line/Square Dancing
- Tai Chi, Yoga
- Volleyball

**MODERATE**
- Walking, brisk
- Cycling, moderate
- Swimming, crawl
- Weight-training, light
- Tennis, moderate
- Racquetball, beginners
- Aerobics, light
- Football, touch
- Basketball, Baseball
- Walking Downstairs
- Snow Skiing (downhill)
- Shovelling snow
- Dancing (ballroom)
- Rowing, moderate
- Volleyball, competitive

**HEAVY**
- Walking (power), Jogging
- Cycling (vigorous)
- Swimming, strenuous
- Weight-training, heavy
- Wrestling/Judo, advanced
- Racquetball, advanced
- Tae Bo, Kick Boxing
- Football, training
- Basketball (Pro)
- Climbing Stairs
- Skipping Rope
- Skiing (cross country)
- Aquarobics, advanced
- Dancing (strenuous), Zumba
- Rowing, vigorous
- Martial Arts

Note: Only those sports or activities that are sustained over a period of time (e.g running) qualify for heavy exercise. Stop-start sports such as tennis are considered 'moderate'.

## WALKING PROGRAM

### USE DISTANCE, STEPS OR TIME

| Weeks | Distance | Steps Pedometer | Time |
|---|---|---|---|
| 1-2 | 1 mile | 2000 | 20 mins |
| 3-5 | 1.5 miles | 3000 | 28 mins |
| 6-8 | 2 miles | 3500 | 35 mins |
| 9-10 | 2.5 miles | 4500 | 45 mins |
| 11+ | 3.5 miles | 6000 | 60 mins |

## 10,000 STEPS PER DAY

A pedometer can motivate you to be more active. It clips to your belt or waist band and registers each step.

Alternatively, use a *Fitbit, Garmin* or *Striiv* activity tracker, or your smartphone inbuilt accelerometer.

Aim for 8,000 - 10,000 steps per day, insead of an average of only 3,000 - 4,000 steps.

# Reshaping Eating Behaviors

- Eating is a behavior that is largely controlled by people with whom we live or socialize, places in which we carry out our lives, and our emotions. Become aware of those situations that commonly lead to extra food being eaten.

- We may also be unaware of 'bad' eating habits that can lead to excess calorie intake; e.g. eating quickly, large mouthfuls, eating when tense or bored, finishing a large serving of food when not hungry.

**Tips to help uncover and correct those 'bad' or problem eating habits:**

- **Don't eat while engaged in other activities;** for example, watching TV, reading. Eat only at the table, not at the fridge or while standing.

- **Don't eat quickly.** Chewing slowly allows time to register a feeling of fullness. Don't use fingers, only utensils. Cut food into smaller pieces. Don't load your fork until the previous mouthful is finished.

*Practice saying 'NO' politely but assertively.*

- **Don't purchase problem high calorie foods.** Shop from a set list to prevent impulse buying. Avoid shopping with children.

- **Buy snack foods** in the smallest package. The larger the serving size or package, the more you are likely to eat or drink.

- **Plan meals in advance. Stick to a set menu.**

- **Plan a strategy to avoid uncontrolled eating** and drinking at social events, or when your emotions urge you to binge.

  Rehearse repeatedly in your mind exactly what you will do in such situations. Remind yourself several times each day that you are in charge of your actions and that you can be strong-willed. Seek counseling or coaching on various strategies.

- **Distract yourself** when you feel the urge to snack impulsively. Engage in some activity that will distract you from thinking about food. Examples: go for a walk, brush your teeth, phone a friend.

  If you eat out of boredom, find some new hobby or interest that gets you out of the house. Even enrol in an adult education class.

*Do you use food as an emotional crutch? If so, professional counseling may be helpful.*

**The food journal is the most powerful proven aid for dieters.** Persons who keep a food and exercise journal not only lose more weight, they also keep it off. Here are some of the reasons:

- **Recording your eating and exercise habits** jolts you into realizing just what you do eat and drink each day; and also whether you exercise sufficiently.
- **Helps you identify problem foods** and drinks with excessive calories and fat.
- **Helps identify moods**, situations and events that lead to excessive eating of unwanted calories. You can then plan to overcome or avoid them.
- **Prevents 'calorie amnesia'**, the forgetfulness that leads to rebound weight gain after successful weight loss. Recording puts you back on the right track.
- **Helps you develop greater self-discipline.** You will think twice about overindulging if you have to record it - especially if someone checks your journal regularly. It certainly keeps you honest!
- **Motivates you** to carefully plan your meals and to exercise each day.
- **Serves as a check system** for your doctor, dietitian or counselor to assess your progress and make recommendations.

*Write It Down!*

*"Keeping a journal gives me feedback on exactly what I eat and drink each day.*

*It helps prevent 'calorie amnesia' and reminds me to exercise each day.*

*It's a 'must' for successful weight control!"*

## Easy Ways to Track Your Food & Exercise Calories

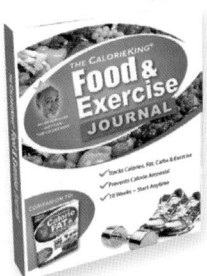

### CalorieKing ~ *Control My Weight*

Make smart food choices wherever you are! Easy to use Available for iPhone, iPad or online.

### Book

10-week journal. One day per page. Weekly Summary page and Progress Checklist.

*Extra Information ~ www.CalorieKing.com*

## What is Diabetes?

Diabetes occurs when the body has difficulty processing glucose sugar in the blood.

- **After digestion**, sugar and starches are changed into **glucose** – the simplest form of sugar vital for body energy and growth.

- Insulin is the hormone which acts like a key that opens the door to body cells and allows glucose to enter.

- **Without enough insulin**, glucose builds up in the blood and passes into the urine. High blood glucose levels lead to frequent urination, extreme thirst, and tiredness.

- **Untreated diabetes increases the risk of damage to nerves and blood vessels.** This, in turn, increases the risk of heart disease, stroke, blindness, kidney damage, foot ulcers and gangrene (with amputation), impotence, Alzheimer's Disease and other prolems.

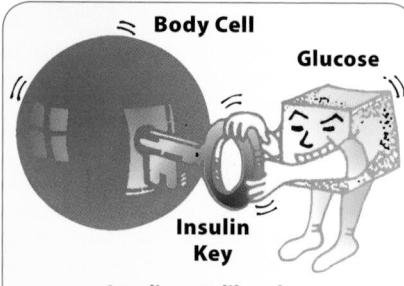

**Body Cell** — **Glucose** — **Insulin Key**

*Insulin acts like a key. It opens the door to body cells and allows glucose to enter.*

**People with type 1 diabetes and some with type 2 have too few or no keys and require insulin injections.**

**Others (primarily type 2) make enough insulin but the body doesn't use it as well as it should – particularly if obese and inactive.**

### SYMPTOMS OF DIABETES

- Frequent urination
- Extreme thirst
- Unusual hunger
- Rapid weight loss
- Extreme fatigue
- Blurred vision
- Skin infections that are slow to heal
- Tingling/numbness in feet

*Note: Diabetes can be present even with no symptoms.*

**DON'T IGNORE DIABETES**

*IT'S A SERIOUS DISEASE!*

### TYPE 2 DIABETES

- Occurs in 90% of diabetes cases
- Occurs mainly in adults - particularly in overweight and inactive persons
- Insulin is produced but body cells resist its action and glucose cannot enter cells
- Usually treated with meal planning and physical activity. Sometimes requires medication (pills or insulin)

### TYPE 1 DIABETES

- Occurs in 10% of diabetes cases
- Usually in children and young adults
- Pancreas produces little or no insulin. Daily insulin injections (or use of an insulin pump) are necessary, as well as:
  - matching pre-meal insulin to the amount of carbohydrate eaten
  - weight control and regular physical activity

### GESTATIONAL DIABETES

- Occurs in some women during pregnancy. It usually disappears after the baby's birth.
- Women who have had gestational diabetes still have a high risk of developing type 2 diabetes within 5 to 10 years. One in 3 do.
- Requires weight control, a healthy lifestyle and regular medical checks during and after pregnancy.

## Are You At Risk for Diabetes?

### *Pre-Diabetes ~ An Early Warning!*

Pre-diabetes means your blood glucose levels are higher than normal, but not high enough to be called diabetes.

**If you have pre-diabetes, you have a higher risk for getting diabetes later on.**

The good news is that you can start taking steps to prevent diabetes by making healthy lifestyle changes – such as losing weight if overweight, and being more physically active.

### *WHAT'S YOUR RISK?*

**Find out if you're at risk for diabetes by answering the following questions:**

- ☐ I have been told I have pre-diabetes
- ☐ I have a family history of diabetes
- ☐ I am African American, Latino American, Asian American, Native American or a Pacific Islander
- ☐ I have had gestational diabetes (diabetes during pregnancy)
- ☐ I am over age 45
- ☐ I am overweight
- ☐ My waist is larger than: 35 inches (for a woman) or 40 inches (for a man)
- ☐ I get little or no physical activity
- ☐ My blood pressure is higher than 130 over 85
- ☐ My HDL (good cholesterol) is too low
- ☐ My triglycerides (blood fats) are too high

### ✓ CHECK YOUR RESULT

- If you've put a check mark in two or more of the boxes, you may be more likely to develop type 2 diabetes.
- Talk with your healthcare provider to see if you should have a blood test for diabetes.

---

### BLOOD GLUCOSE CLASSIFICATION OF DIABETES

| | |
|---|---|
| **Normal:** | **Below 100 mg/dl*** |
| **Pre-Diabetes:** | **100-125 mg/dl*** |
| **Diabetes:** | **Over 125 mg/dl*** |

**(*Fasting Blood Glucose)**

### *KNOW YOUR BGL*

*(Blood Glucose Level)*
*Everyone over the age of 45 should have a blood glucose test every three years.*

## Importance of Weight Control

- **Type 2 diabetes** is more common in people who are overweight.
- **Being overweight** means that your insulin doesn't work as well to control blood glucose levels.
- **Losing just 10 to 20 pounds** can help you better manage your diabetes and lower your risk for heart disease.

**Keys to weight control include:**

- Follow a healthy eating plan
- Control food portions.
- Be physically active every day. Track your daily activity.
- Keep food records ~ *See Page 15*
- Get the support of family and friends.
- **Work with a registered dietitian** who can help you reach a weight that's ideal for you.

### *KEEP MOVING!*

*Every day, do at least 30 minutes of moderate intensity exercise. (even in 5-minute sets)*

*It's the key to improving insulin action. Add muscle strength training 3-4 times a week to double the benefits.*

# Diabetes Guide ~ (Cont)

## Managing Diabetes

Don't battle diabetes alone. Establish a partnership with your doctor, dietitian, certified diabetes educator, and pharmacist.

### Extra Support:
- *American Association of Diabetes Educators*
- *American Diabetes Association*
- *BeyondType1.org*
- *Joslin Diabetes Center*
- *Juvenile Diabetes Research Foundation*
- *National Diabetes Education Program*

### Tips to keep blood glucose within safe limits:

- **Control your food intake.** Know what and when you will eat. Seek referral to a dietitian for expert advice.

- **Exercise regularly.** It assists weight control and can improve sensitivity of body cells to insulin. Plan physical activity into your daily routine.

- **Monitor your blood glucose** at home and work with a blood glucose meter. It will help you become familiar with your blood glucose patterns, and the effects of food, activity and medication.

- **Take insulin or oral medication as prescribed.** If on insulin, know what action to take if hypoglycemia (low blood glucose) occurs. Also educate your family and friends.

## Be Heart Smart ~ Know Your ABCs

If you have diabetes, you are at a higher risk for heart attack and stroke than someone without diabetes. But you can fight back!

### Be smart about your heart!

Take control of the ABCs of diabetes and live a long and healthy life. Talk to your healthcare provider about your ABC targets.

**Ⓐ is for A1C**
The A1C (A-one-C) test – short for hemoglobin A1C. It reflects your average blood glucose (sugar) over the last 3 months.
**Suggested Target: Below 7%**

**Ⓑ is for Blood Pressure**
High blood pressure makes your heart work too hard.
**Suggested Target: Below 130/80**

**Ⓒ is for Cholesterol**
Bad cholesterol, or LDL, can build up and clog your arteries. **Suggested Target: Below 100**

*Blood glucose meters and insulin pumps can greatly improve control of diabetes*

**BLOOD GLUCOSE METERS (EXAMPLES)**

**INSULIN PUMPS (EXAMPLES)**

Roche Accu-Chek    Medtronic MiniMed

Be Smart About Your **Heart**
Control the ABCs of **Diabetes**
➤ A1C
➤ Blood Pressure
➤ Cholesterol

*National Diabetes Education Program*

---

**Be smart about your heart!**
*Take control of the ABC's of diabetes and live a long and healthy life.*

*Talk to your healthcare provider about your ABC targets.*

*Take action now to lower your risk for heart attack, stroke and other diabetes problems.*

---

◄ *Note: These targets are suggested by the National Institutes for Health and the American Diabetes Association*

**Guidelines for choosing a healthy diet apply equally to people with or without diabetes.** Eating a wide variety of foods that are mainly low in fat, low in refined sugars, and high in fiber, is recommended.

However, actual food quantities, as well as when you eat, will also influence control of blood glucose. Your dietitian will individualize a meal plan to suit your food preferences, lifestyle and medical status.

### Here are a few tips:

- **Maintain a healthy weight.** If overweight, even a modest weight loss plus daily physical activity can help manage blood glucose in type 2 diabetes.

- **Don't skip meals.** If you take insulin or an oral hypoglycemic agent, regular meals are important.

  **If on insulin**, eat meals at the same time each day. Eat a similar amount of food at each meal. Eating about the same amount of carbohydrate over the day will make best use of insulin and prevent wide variations in blood glucose levels.

- **Know which foods contain carbohydrate;** and learn how to check the *Nutrition Facts Label* on foods. Check the serving size, total fat and total carbohydrate – not just the sugar content. All carbohydrate breaks down to sugars after digestion.

- **Choose wholegrain breads, cereals and pasta.** Eat fresh fruits, vegetables and legumes. These foods contain more fiber and slow the release of glucose into your blood after a meal.

- **Limit foods high in saturated fat, trans fat and cholesterol.** Enjoy fish, soy foods, and other foods rich in omega-3 fats. *(Extra Notes: Page 259)*

- **Limit sugars and foods high in added sugar** particularly if overweight. Small amounts of sugar as part of a meal may occasionally be okay. Check with your dietitian. *(Extra Notes: Page 9)*

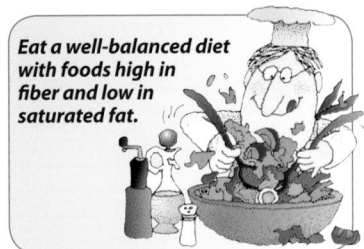

*Eat a well-balanced diet with foods high in fiber and low in saturated fat.*

*A fiber-rich diet assists the growth of friendly gut microbes that can benefit our metabolism, weight and blood glucose levels – as well as hunger, mood and our immune system.*
*(Also see Fiber Guide ~ Page 264)*

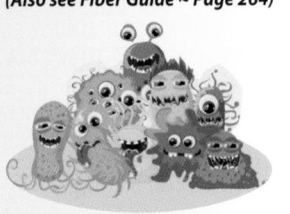

## ALCOHOL TIPS

- **If you drink alcohol, have only moderate amounts:**
  **Men ~ 1-2 drinks/day**
  **Women ~ 1 drink/day**
  For some people, safe drinking will mean no alcoholic drinks at all.
  *(Also see Alcohol Guide ~ Page 23)*

- **Drink along with your food** – especially if you use insulin or diabetes medication pills.

- **Do not omit any carb food** in exchange for an alcoholic drink. However, non-alcoholic beers (12 fl oz) count as one carb exchange.

- **Alcohol increases the risk of hypoglycemia** (low blood sugar) and drug interactions if you take insulin and certain types of diabetes pills.

- **Check with your doctor and dietitian.**

# Diabetes Guide ~ The Plate Method

## The Plate Method – An Easy Way to Eat Healthfully

The plate method is a helpful tool to guide your food choices until you see a dietitian for your own meal plan.

**For a healthy meal:**

- Fill half of your plate with non-starchy vegetables (broccoli, green beans, carrots, cabbage; or mixed salad).
- Fill a quarter of your plate with carbohydrate (wholegrain bread, pasta, potato, brown rice).
- Fill the other quarter of your plate with 3-4 ounces of lean meat, poultry, fish, dried beans, tofu or tempeh.
- Use 1-2 teaspoons of tub margarine or a heart-healthy vegetable oil, or avocado.
- Add a small piece of fruit.

**MAIN MEAL**

Vegetables & Salad Greens

Bread · Starch · Grain

Meat · Protein

**PLUS ONE CHOICE**

**Milk, Fruit, Dessert or other Carb Food**

## How Much Carbohydrate Should You Eat?

A dietitian can best determine how much carbohydrate you need at each of your meals, based on your lifestyle, food preferences, and overall diabetes control.

Until you see a dietitian, aim to keep the amount of carbohydrate you eat the same at each of your meals.

> ### CARB CHOICES MEAL PLAN
> #### One Carb Choice = 15 Grams of Carb
>
> **The amount in:** 1 slice Bread **or** ¾ cup Cereal (unsweetened) **or** 1 small Potato **or** 1 small Fruit

### 🍎 Breakfast
- Eat 2-3 carb choices (30-45 grams)
- Include a lower fat protein source such as egg whites or skim milk.

### 🍎 Lunch and Dinner
- Eat 3-4 carb choices (45-60 grams carb)
- Include fruit and non-starchy vegetables. Choose small portions of lower fat protein foods.

### 🍎 Snacks: If needed, eat 1-2 carb choices (15-30 grams carb).

*Note: Above plan is for adults. Carbohydrate amounts will vary with physical activity level.*

## Carb Type Affects Blood Glucose

The various forms of carbohydrate affect blood glucose levels in different ways. It is difficult to predict the effect of particular foods, sugars, or meals, simply by their carbohydrate content.

Thus the same amount of carbohydrate from different foods may affect blood sugar levels very differently. **Many factors affect the rate of digestion and absorption such as:**

- the type of sugar, starch, and fiber
- the degree of processing and cooking (which increases digestion rate)
- the amount of protein and fat (which slow stomach emptying and digestion).

## Glycemic Index (GI)

**The GI is a method of ranking carbohydrate foods on a scale (0-100)** according to how they affect blood glucose levels. (See next column).

**The higher the GI value**, the greater the food's ability to rapidly raise blood glucose levels; and the more insulin that is needed by the body (not desirable).

**Eating low-GI foods may lead to better control of blood glucose and insulin levels** (which in turn lowers the risk of damage to blood vessels and nerves). The slower digestion of low-GI foods may also help to delay hunger pangs and benefit weight control.

## Cautionary Notes on GI

**Choosing low-GI foods is not a license to eat unlimited amounts.** Calorie restriction and portion control for weight control is of prime importance.

**Also remember**, **low-GI foods are carbohydrate foods** and must still be counted as part of any dietetic carbohydrate plan.

**GI is not meant to be used by itself** without regard to portion size, and other dietary recommendations for healthy eating. Foods are not good or bad on the basis of their GI.

While GI may be a helpful tool for some people with diabetes, what is most important is to control the total amount of carbohydrate that you eat.

## LOWER-GLYCEMIC FOODS

### Slower-Acting Carbohydrates

These foods are more slowly digested and absorbed. They help maintain more even blood glucose levels, as long as excessive amounts are not eaten. Use these foods regularly but still limit portion size for weight control.

*Examples:*

- Dried beans, peas, lentils
- Nuts and seeds
- Wholegrain breads
- Bran cereals, oats
- Sweet corn, barley, quinoa buckwheat
- Wholegrain pasta, basmati rice
- Fresh fruit: apples, avocados, bananas (firm), berries, cherries, grapefruit, grapes, olives, oranges, pears, plums. Fresh juices.
- Vegetables: broccoli, yam, nopales, salad greens
- Milk, yogurt, soy drinks
- Dark chocolate, cacao
- Sugar alcohols (sorbitol, maltitol)

## HIGHER-GLYCEMIC FOODS

### Quicker-Acting Carbohydrates

These foods more rapidly raise blood glucose levels. Eat only in moderation.

- White bread, rice cakes, bagels, croissants, doughnuts
- Low-fiber cereals: Cornflakes, *Rice Krispies, Froot Loops*
- White potatoes, white rice
- Watermelon, ripe bananas, cantaloupe, pineapple
- Soda, sugar-sweetened sports and energy drinks
- Sugar, candy, popcorn (plain)
- Ice cream (low-fat), frozen yogurt

*High-GI fruits and potatoes are still healthy choices when eaten in moderate amounts.*

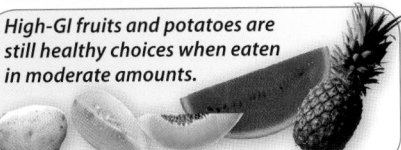

# Notes ♦ Abbreviations ♦ Disclaimer

≫ **Calorie and fat values have been rounded off.**
**Calories** ~ to the nearest 5 or 10 calories.
**Fat** ~ to nearest half gram. **Note:** Trace amounts of fat (less than 0.3 grams) have been treated as zero.

≫ **Carbohydrate figures** in this book are for total carbohydrate, and not **Net Carbs** (which deducts fiber, polydextrose and sugar alcohols from total carbs).

≫ Because manufacturers' figures on labels are rounded off, figures in this book may differ slightly from the label. Serving sizes may also vary.

**C** ~ **Calories**
**F** ~ **Fat (grams)**
**Cb** ~ **Carbohydrate (grams)**

## Abbreviations

tsp = teaspoon
Tbsp or T = Tablespoon
oz = ounce(s)
c = cup
fl.oz = fluid ounce(s)
g = gram(s)
avg = average
pkg = package

## Volume Measures

(All measures are level)
3 tsp = 1 Tbsp
2 Tbsp = 1 fl.oz
½ cup = 4 fl.oz
1 cup = 8 fl.oz
2 cups = 1 Pint
2 Pints = 1 Quart
Note: 8 oz weight is not the same as 8 fl oz volume (space occupied). Dense foods weigh more per set volume. Examples:
1 cup popcorn weighs ½ oz
1 cup milk weighs 8½ oz
1 cup honey weighs 12 oz

## Metric Conversion

½ oz = 14 grams
1 oz = 28.4 grams
2 oz = 57 grams
3½ oz = 100 grams
1 fl.oz = 30 mls
1 cup (8 fl.oz) = 240 mls
33 fl.oz = 1 liter (volume)

---

### IMPORTANT DISCLAIMER

\* The authors and publishers of this book are not physicians and are not licensed to give medical advice. This book is not a substitute for professional advice. Users should consult their medical professional before making any health, medical or other decisions based on the material contained herein.

\* This book is a compilation of original material from other sources intended for educational purposes only. Because food manufacturers constantly change their products, only they are the authoritative source for food's most current nutritional information.

\* Persons using the information herein for any medical purposes, such as matching insulin dosage to carbohydrate intake, should not rely solely on the accuracy of figures herein and should independently check food labels or contact the food manufacturer for the latest data.

### Canadian Readers:

Please note that figures in this book are based on U.S. food products and restaurants. Equivalent Canadian foods may vary and should be checked independently.

### * WARRANTY DISCLAIMER:

THE AUTHOR AND PUBLISHER DISCLAIM ANY LIABILITY ARISING DIRECTLY OR INDIRECTLY FROM THE USE OF THIS BOOK. THE INFORMATION HEREIN IS PROVIDED "AS IS" AND WITHOUT ANY WARRANTY EXPRESSED OR IMPLIED. ALL DIRECT, INDIRECT, SPECIAL, INCIDENTAL, CONSEQUENTIAL OR PUNITIVE DAMAGES ARISING FROM ANY USE OF THIS INFORMATION IS DISCLAIMED AND EXCLUDED.

This information is also provided subject to Family Health Publications' Terms and Conditions found at the website, www.calorieking.com/terms and incorporated herein.

## INFORMATION SOURCES

• U.S. Dept. of Agriculture
• U.S. Food Manufacturers
• Food Industry Boards & Councils
• Author extrapolations

## FEEDBACK WELCOME!

Please contact the author with your queries and suggestions.
feedback@calorieking.com

- **Health Hazards: Excessive alcohol intake** contributes to obesity, high blood pressure, stroke, heart and liver disease, some cancers, and even impotence. **Concentration and short-term memory** are reduced as well as athletic performance.

  **Other alcohol hazards include:** Fetal Alcohol Syndrome, stomach upsets, gut dysbiosis, menstrual and menopausal problems, depression, snoring, sleep problems, work absenteeism, impaired judgement, risky behaviors and social/family problems.

- **Alcohol contributes to obesity** through its high calories and by lessening the body's ability to burn fat. Fat storage is promoted, particularly in the belly – a health danger zone. Alcohol can also stimulate the appetite; and weaken the dieter's resolve!

- **Alcohol is potentially more harmful while dieting:** Blood sugar levels may drop with resultant fatigue and further impairment of concentration, reflexes and driving skills.

*Excess alcohol contributes to obesity, high blood pressure and many other health problems*

### LOWER RISK ALCOHOL LIMITS

 **WOMEN:**
No more than
**1 drink** per day

 **MEN:**
No more than
**2 drinks** per day
(1 drink if over 65 y.o.)

(At least 2 days a week should be alcohol-free)

| 1 DRINK CONTAINS 14 GRAMS ALCOHOL | → 12 fl.oz Regular Beer (5% Alc.) |
| | → OR 14 fl.oz Light Beer (4.2% Alc.) |
| | → OR 5 fl.oz Wine (12% Alc.) |
| | → OR 1½ fl.oz Spirits (80 Proof) |

**Note: You cannot save daily drinks for one occasion. Binge drinking is particularly harmful: 4 drinks for males or 3 drinks for females (within 2 hours).**

For some people, safe drinking means no alcohol at all. Even one drink may impair driving skills, particularly if tired. For women who drink frequently, breast cancer risk is increased by 9% for each drink after the first drink. In men, just 2 drinks a day doubles the risk of cancers of the mouth and throat.

It is advisable not to drink at all if you are:

- pregnant, trying to conceive or breastfeeding
- taking medication or have liver or heart disease (unless approved by your doctor or pharmacist)
- planning to drive, use machinery or play sports
- studying or needing to concentrate
- a child or adolescent

 *Women and adolescents are more prone to alcohol's ill-effects due to their lower body weight, smaller livers and lesser capacity to metabolize alcohol. As we age, our ability to handle alcohol decreases.*

### HOW TO CALCULATE ALCOHOL CONTENT

Percent alcohol on label refers to alcohol volume (ml alcohol/100ml). Note: 100ml = 3½ fl.oz

To convert to grams (weight) of alcohol, multiply the alcohol volume by 0.8 – since 1 ml of alcohol weighs only 0.8 grams.

*EXAMPLE:*
*12 fl.oz Can Beer (5% alcohol)*
5% alc. volume
= 5% of 12 fl.oz = 0.6 fl.oz
= 18ml alcohol (Note: 1 fl.oz = 30ml)
Weight (18ml x 0.8) = 14.4g alcohol

### GOVERNMENT WARNINGS!

(1) According to the Surgeon General, women should not drink alcoholic beverages during pregnancy because of the risk of birth defects.

(2) Consumption of alcoholic beverages impairs your ability to drive a car or operate machinery, and may cause health problems.

### EXTRA INFORMATION
Alcohol & Diabetes ~ See Page 19
Alcohol & The Heart ~ See Page 18
Tips to Avoid Harmful Drinking ~ Page 19

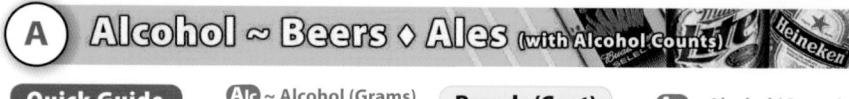
## Quick Guide    Alc ~ Alcohol (Grams)

**Beer:**    Cb ~ Carbohydrate

**Beer Contains Zero Fat:**

| | C | Alc | Cb |
|---|---|---|---|
| **Regular Beer (5% Alc. Vol.):** | | | |
| 7 fl.oz Glass | 80 | 8.5 | 4 |
| 12 fl.oz Bottle/Can/Glass | 140 | 14 | 10 |
| 16 fl.oz/Pint | 185 | 19 | 13 |
| 22 fl.oz Bottle | 260 | 26 | 18 |
| 24 fl.oz Can | 280 | 28 | 20 |
| 32 fl.oz/ ½ Yard | 370 | 38 | 28 |
| 40 fl.oz Bottle | 470 | 47 | 35 |
| 50 fl.oz Football | 590 | 59 | 50 |
| **Light Beer (4.2% Alc. Vol.):** | | | |
| 7 fl.oz Glass | 65 | 7 | 4 |
| 12 fl.oz Bottle/Can/Glass | 110 | 12 | 7 |
| 16 fl.oz/Pint | 145 | 16 | 9 |
| 22 fl.oz Bottle | 200 | 22 | 13 |
| 24 fl.oz Can | 220 | 24 | 14 |
| **Non-Alcoholic Brews:** | | | |
| (Less than 0.5% alcohol by volume) | | | |
| Average all Brands, 12 fl.oz | 70 | 1 | 14 |

## Beer ~ Brands

Note: Figure shown are for the United States except for the states of Utah, Colorado, Kansas and Oklahoma who have certain restrictions limiting the alcohol content to not more than 4% by volume (3.2% by weight).

*Percentage alcohol listed is by volume - not by weight.*
*Per 12 fl.oz Serving*

| | C | Alc | Cb |
|---|---|---|---|
| **Amstel,** Light (3.5%) | 95 | 10 | 5 |
| **Anchor:** Porter (5.6%) | 210 | 15 | 23 |
| Steam (4.9%) | 160 | 14 | 14 |
| **Asahi:** Kuronama (5.3%) | 165 | 14 | 14 |
| Select (4.7%) | 140 | 13 | 11 |
| Super Dry (4.9%) | 150 | 14 | 11 |
| **Bass,** Pale Ale (5.1%) | 155 | 14 | 12 |
| **Beck's:** Original (5%) | 145 | 14 | 11 |
| Premier Light (2.3%) | 65 | 7 | 4 |
| Sapphire (6%) | 160 | 17 | 9 |
| **Big Sky:** Original IPA (6.2%) | 195 | 18 | 17 |
| Moose Drool (5.3%) | 175 | 15 | 16 |
| Scape Goat (4.7%) | 155 | 14 | 14 |
| Trout Slayer Ale ( 4.7%) | 145 | 14 | 12 |
| **Blatz:** Original (4.6%) | 145 | 13 | 13 |
| Light (3.9%) | 110 | 11 | 8 |
| **Blue Moon:** | | | |
| Belgian White (5.4%) | 170 | 15 | 14 |
| Honey Wheat (5.2%) | 155 | 15 | 12 |
| Mango Wheat (5.4%) | 175 | 15 | 16 |
| **Bohemia** (4.73%) | 140 | 14 | 12 |
| **Bud Ice** (5.5%) | 120 | 16 | 4 |

## Brands (Cont)    Alc ~ Alcohol (Grams)

*Per 12 fl.oz Serving*

| | C | Alc | Cb |
|---|---|---|---|
| **Bud Light:** Regular (4.2%) | 110 | 12 | 7 |
| Clamato Chelada (4.2%) | 150 | 12 | 16 |
| Extra Lime (4.2%) | 160 | 12 | 17 |
| Lime (4%) | 115 | 12 | 8 |
| Orange (4.2%) | 145 | 12 | 15 |
| **Budweiser:** Lager (5%) | 145 | 14 | 11 |
| Clamato Chelado (5%) | 185 | 14 | 21 |
| Clamato Picante Chelada (5%) | 200 | 14 | 23 |
| Copper Lager (6.2%) | 195 | 17 | 16 |
| Freedom Reserve (5.4%) | 170 | 15 | 15 |
| Platinum (6%) | 140 | 17 | 5 |
| Select (4.3%) | 100 | 12 | 3 |
| Select 55 (2.4%) | 55 | 7 | 2 |
| **Busch:** Original (4.3%) | 115 | 12 | 7 |
| Ice (5.9%) | 135 | 17 | 4 |
| Light (4.1%) | 95 | 12 | 3 |
| NA (0.4%) | 60 | 1 | 13 |
| **Carlsberg,** Pilsner (5%) | 135 | 14 | 10 |
| **Carta Blanca** (4.6%) | 145 | 13 | 11 |
| **Cerveza,** Aguila (4%) | 125 | 11 | 11 |
| **Colt 45,** Malt Liquor (5.6%) | 155 | 16 | 11 |
| **Coors:** Banquet (5%) | 145 | 14 | 12 |
| Light (4.2%) | 100 | 12 | 5 |
| Non-Alcoholic | 60 | 0 | 12 |
| **Corona:** Extra (4.5%) | 150 | 13 | 13 |
| Light (4.1%) | 100 | 12 | 5 |
| Premier (4%) | 90 | 11 | 11 |
| **Dos Equis XX:** Ambar (4.7%) | 145 | 14 | 12 |
| Lager (4.5%) | 140 | 13 | 11 |
| **Extra Gold** (5%) | 150 | 14 | 12 |
| **Fosters:** Lager (5%) | 145 | 14 | 11 |
| Premium Ale (5.5%) | 160 | 16 | 13 |
| **Genesee:** Beer (4.5%) | 145 | 13 | 13 |
| Light (4%) | 100 | 10 | 4 |
| **George Killian's,** Irish Red (5.4%) | 170 | 16 | 15 |
| **Grolsch:** Premium (5%) | 145 | 14 | 10 |
| **Guinness:** Draught (4%) | 125 | 12 | 10 |
| Extra Stout (6%) | 175 | 17 | 14 |
| Blonde American (5%) | 150 | 14 | 11 |
| Nitro IPA (5.8%), 11.2oz | 155 | 19 | 5 |
| **Hamm's:** Original (4.7%) | 145 | 13 | 12 |
| Special Light (3.9%) | 110 | 12 | 8 |
| **Heineken:** Lager (5%) | 140 | 14 | 10 |
| Special Dark (5%) | 165 | 14 | 15 |
| Premium Light (3.5%) | 100 | 10 | 7 |
| 0.0 (Alchohol-Free) | 75 | 0 | 12 |
| **Hurricane:** Malt Liquor (6%) | 140 | 17 | 4 |
| High Gravity (8.1%) | 185 | 23 | 6 |
| **Icehouse:** Original (5.5%) | 150 | 16 | 10 |
| Light (5%) | 125 | 14 | 7 |
| **Keystone:** Ice (5.9%) | 145 | 17 | 7 |
| Light (4.1%) | 100 | 12 | 5 |

# Alcohol ~ Beers ◊ Ales (with Alcohol Counts) — A

## Brands (Cont) — Alc ~ Alcohol (Grams)

**Beer Contains Zero Fat:**
*Per 12 fl.oz Serving*

| | C | Alc | Cb |
|---|---|---|---|
| King Cobra (6%) | 135 | 17 | 4 |
| Kirin: Ichiban (5%) | 145 | 14 | 11 |
| Light (3.2%) | 95 | 9 | 8 |
| Kokanee (5%) | 145 | 14 | 11 |
| Labatt: Blue (5%) | 135 | 14 | 10 |
| Blue Light (4%) | 110 | 11 | 8 |
| Ultra Light, 52 Calories (2.2%) | 52 | 6 | 2 |
| Landshark, Lager (4.6%) | 150 | 13 | 13 |
| Leinenkugel's: Original (4.7%) | 150 | 13 | 15 |
| Summer Shandy (4.2%) | 135 | 12 | 13 |
| Lone Star: Pale Lager (4.65%) | 135 | 13 | 11 |
| Light (3.85%) | 110 | 11 | 8 |
| Lowenbrau, Original (5%) | 140 | 14 | 12 |
| Magic Hat, #9 (5.1% alc) | 165 | 15 | 15 |
| Magnum, Malt Liquor (5.6%) | 155 | 16 | 11 |
| Michelob: Amber Bock (5.1%) | 150 | 14 | 12 |
| Lager (4.8%) | 160 | 14 | 14 |
| Light (4.1%) | 120 | 12 | 9 |
| Golden Draft Light (4.1%) | 110 | 12 | 7 |
| Ultra Amber (4%) | 95 | 11 | 3 |
| Ultra Light (4.2%) | 95 | 12 | 2.5 |
| Ultra Lime Cactus (4%) | 95 | 11 | 5.5 |
| Ultra Pure Gold (4.1%) | 85 | 12 | 2.5 |
| Mickey's, Malt Liquor (5.6%) | 155 | 16 | 11 |
| Miller: Chill, 100 Calorie (4.2%) | 100 | 12 | 4 |
| Genuine Draft /High Life (4.6%) | 140 | 13 | 12 |
| High Life Light (4.1%) | 110 | 12 | 6 |
| Lite (4.2%) | 95 | 12 | 3 |
| MGD 64 (2.8%) | 65 | 8 | 2.5 |
| **Milwaukee's Best:** | | | |
| Ice (5.9%) | 150 | 17 | 8 |
| Light (4.1%) | 100 | 12 | 3.5 |
| Premium (4.3%) | 130 | 12 | 11 |
| Minnesota's Best, Original (4.9%) | 140 | 14 | 10 |
| Modelo, Especial (4.4%) | 145 | 13 | 14 |
| Molson Canadian: Ice (5.6%) | 170 | 16 | 14 |
| Lager (5%) | 150 | 14 | 12 |
| Light (3.9%) | 120 | 11 | 10 |
| Moosehead, Lager (5%) | 150 | 14 | 11 |
| Natural: Ice (5.9%) | 130 | 17 | 4 |
| Light (4.2%) | 95 | 12 | 3 |
| Negra Modelo (5.4%) | 175 | 15 | 16 |
| Newcastle, Brown Ale (4.7%) | 130 | 13 | 10 |
| O'Douls: Amber (0.4%) | 90 | 1 | 18 |
| Original (0.4%) | 65 | 1 | 13 |
| Old Milwaukee: Lager (4.6%) | 145 | 13 | 13 |
| Light (3.8%) | 110 | 11 | 8 |
| Non-Alcoholic (0.4%) | 60 | 1 | 12 |
| Old Style: Lager (4.7%) | 145 | 13 | 12 |
| Light (4.2%) | 115 | 12 | 7 |
| Pabst: Blue Ribbon (4.7%) | 145 | 13 | 12 |
| Light (3.9%) | 110 | 11 | 8 |

## Cb ~ Carbohydrate

*Per 12 fl.oz Serving Unless Indicated*

| | C | Alc | Cb |
|---|---|---|---|
| Pacifico, Clara (4.4%) | 145 | 13 | 13 |
| Palmier, (4.2%), 11.2 fl.oz | 90 | 11 | 3 |
| Peroni, Nastro Azzurro (5.1%) | 150 | 14 | 12 |
| Piels, Lager (4.3%) | 125 | 12 | 9 |
| Pilsner Urquell, Lager (4.4%) | 155 | 13 | 16 |
| Point: Amber Classic (4.7%) | 160 | 14 | 14 |
| Special Lager (4.7%) | 150 | 14 | 12 |
| Presidente (5%) | 175 | 14 | 5 |
| Redbridge, Lager (4%) | 135 | 10 | 14 |
| Red Dog, Lager (4.8%) | 145 | 14 | 12 |
| Red Hook: ESB (5.8%) | 185 | 16 | 16 |
| India Pale Ale (4.7%) | 190 | 13 | 19 |
| Red Stripe, Jamaican Lager (7%) | 150 | 13 | 14 |
| Redd's: Apple Ale (5%), 12 fl.oz | 165 | 14 | 17 |
| Wicked Hard Ale (8%), av. 10 fl.oz | 230 | 19 | 25 |
| Saint Archer: Blonde (4.8%) | 150 | 14 | 13 |
| Pale Ale (5.5%) | 170 | 16 | 13 |
| Samuel Adams: Boston Lager (5%) | 175 | 14 | 18 |
| Summer Ale, Citrus (5.3%) | 165 | 15 | 15 |
| Sam Adams, Light Lager (4.3%) | 120 | 12 | 8 |
| Sapporo, Prem. Lager (4.9%) | 135 | 14 | 9 |
| Schaefer: Lager (4.6%) | 145 | 13 | 12 |
| Light (3.9%) | 110 | 11 | 8 |
| Schell's: Deer (4.7%) | 145 | 14 | 13 |
| Light (3.5%) | 100 | 10 | 7 |
| Schlitz: Pale Lager (4.6%) | 145 | 13 | 12 |
| Light (3.8%) | 110 | 11 | 8 |
| Schmidt's: Pale Lager (4.6%) | 145 | 13 | 12 |
| Light (3.8%) | 110 | 11 | 8 |
| Sheaf, Stout (5.7%) | 190 | 16 | 19 |
| Shock Top: Belgian White (5.2%) | 165 | 15 | 15 |
| Lemon Shandy (4.2%) | 145 | 12 | 15 |
| Sierra Nevada: Bigfoot (9.6%) | 330 | 28 | 32 |
| Draft Pale Ale (5%) | 155 | 14 | 13 |
| Pale Ale (5.6%) | 175 | 16 | 14 |
| Sol (4.2%) | 130 | 12 | 11 |
| Sparks, Lager (6%) | 250 | 17 | 34 |
| **Steel Reserve:** | | | |
| High Gravity Malt Liquor (8.1%) | 220 | 23 | 15 |
| Steel 6 (6%) | 165 | 17 | 11 |
| Stella Artois, (5%), 11.2 fl.oz | 140 | 14 | 11 |
| Stroh's: Pale Lager (4.6%) | 145 | 13 | 12 |
| Light (3.9%) | 115 | 11 | 7 |
| Tecate: Pale Lager (4.6%) | 140 | 13 | 11 |
| Light (4%) | 110 | 11 | 8 |
| Third Shift, Amber Lager (5.3%) | 185 | 15 | 18 |
| Trader Jose: Premium, 11.2 fl.oz | 145 | 14 | 14 |
| Light (3.8%), 12 fl.oz | 105 | 14 | 8 |
| Victoria Lager (4%) | 135 | 11 | 14 |
| Wild Blue, Lager (8%) | 240 | 23 | 20 |
| Yuengling: Light (3.2%) | 99 | 9 | 9 |
| Traditional Lager (4.5%) | 140 | 13 | 12 |
| ZeigenBock, Amber (4.9%) | 145 | 14 | 11 |

**Alc** ~ Alcohol (Grams)　　**Cb** ~ Carbohydrate

## Ciders ~ Alcoholic/Hard

*Per 12 fl.oz Unless Indicated*

| | C | Alc | Cb |
|---|---|---|---|
| **Ace:** Apple (5%), 12 fl.oz | 145 | 14 | 12 |
| Berry (5%), 12 fl.oz | 155 | 14 | 14 |
| Joker (6.9%), 12 fl.oz | 190 | 19 | 13 |
| Perry (5%), 12 fl.oz | 170 | 14 | 18 |
| Pineapple (5%), 12 fl.oz | 175 | 14 | 19 |
| **Angry Orchard:** Crisp Apple (5%) | 190 | 14 | 25 |
| Green Apple (5.5%), 12 fl.oz | 210 | 14 | 31 |
| Pear (5%), 12 fl.oz | 160 | 14 | 17 |
| Rosé (5.5%), 12 fl.oz | 170 | 16 | 17 |
| **Bold Rock's:** Apple, (4.7%), 12 fl.oz | 140 | 13 | 12 |
| Carolina Draft (4.7%), 12 fl.oz | 145 | 13 | 13 |
| IPA (4.7%), 12 fl.oz | 140 | 13 | 12 |
| Pear (4.7%), 12 fl.oz | 140 | 13 | 12 |
| Premium Dry (6%), 12 fl.oz | 140 | 17 | 6 |
| **Crispin:** Original (5%), 12 fl.oz | 160 | 14 | 15 |
| Blackberry Pear (5%), 12 fl.oz | 170 | 14 | 16 |
| Brut (5.5%), 12 fl.oz | 170 | 16 | 13 |
| Honey Crisp (6.5%), 12 fl.oz | 200 | 18 | 16 |
| Pacific Pear (4.5%), 12 fl.oz | 160 | 13 | 17 |
| Rosé (5%), 12 fl.oz | 160 | 14 | 13 |
| The Saint (6.9%), 12 fl.oz | 230 | 19 | 20 |
| **Hornsby's:** Amber (5.5%) | 180 | 16 | 19 |
| Crisp (5.5%), 12 fl.oz | 190 | 16 | 26 |
| **Johnny Appleseed,** (5.5%) | 210 | 16 | 26 |
| **Magners,** (4.5%) | 125 | 13 | 9 |
| **Michelob,** Ultra Light Cider (4%) | 120 | 10 | 10 |
| **Saint Archer,** Hard Cider (6.1%) | 170 | 17 | 11 |
| **Smith & Forge,** Hard Apple (6%) | 220 | 17 | 26 |
| **Stella Artois Cidre,** (4.5%) | 180 | 13 | 22 |
| **Strongbow:** *Per 11.2 fl.oz* | | | |
| Gold Apple (5%) | 175 | 13 | 19 |
| Original Dry (5%), 12 fl.oz | 145 | 14 | 10 |
| Pear Secco (4.5%) | 135 | 12 | 13 |
| Rosé Apple (5%) | 140 | 13 | 11 |
| **2 Towns Ciderhouse:** | | | |
| Brightcider Apple (6%), 12 fl.oz | 145 | 17 | 7 |
| Ginja Ninja (6%), 12 fl.oz | 145 | 17 | 7 |
| Made Marion (6%), 12 fl.oz | 150 | 17 | 8 |
| Outcider (5%), 12 fl.oz | 155 | 14 | 14 |
| Pacific Pineapple (5%), 12 fl.oz | 150 | 14 | 12 |
| **Woodchuck:** Amber (5%) | 200 | 14 | 21 |
| Granny Smith (5%), 12 fl.oz | 160 | 14 | 11 |
| Pear (4%), 12 fl.oz | 150 | 12 | 18 |
| Raspberry (4%), 12 fl.oz | 170 | 12 | 22 |
| Semi-Dry (5.5%), 12 fl.oz | 160 | 14 | 13 |
| **Wyder's:** Pear (4%), 12 fl.oz | 140 | 11 | 22 |
| Prickly Pineapple (5%), 12 fl.oz | 180 | 14 | 22 |
| Raspberry (4%), 12 fl.oz | 120 | 11 | 17 |
| Reposado (6.9%), 12 fl.oz | 250 | 19 | 30 |

## Quick Guide ~ Table Wines

| *Average all Varieties (11.5% Alc.)* *(Wine Contains Zero Fat)* | C | Alc | Cb |
|---|---|---|---|
| **4 fl.oz,** 1 small wine glass OR ½ large wine glass | 100 | 12 | 3 |
| **6 fl.oz,** (¾ large wine glass) | 145 | 18 | 5 |
| **8 fl.oz,** (1 large wine glass) | 195 | 25 | 7 |
| **½ Carafe/Bottle,** 12 fl.oz | 295 | 37 | 10 |
| **1 Bottle,** 750ml, 25.4 fl.oz | 620 | 78 | 21 |
| **Red Wines:** *Per 4 fl.oz* | | | |
| Burgundy/Cabernet/Merlot, av. | 100 | 11 | 4 |
| **White Wines:** *Per 4 fl.oz* | | | |
| Dry (Chenin; Fume Blanc; Chardonnay) | 95 | 11 | 4 |
| Sparkling, 4 fl.oz | 95 | 11 | 4 |
| Zinfandel Sweet, (Moselle/Sauterne), 4 fl.oz | 85 | 11 | 2 |

## Other Wines

| | C | Alc | Cb |
|---|---|---|---|
| **Champagne:** *Per 4 fl.oz* | | | |
| Average all types, 1 glass | 85 | 11 | 2 |
| with Orange Jce (3:1 orange) | 75 | 8 | 4 |
| with Orange Jce (1:1 orange) | 65 | 5 | 7 |
| **Mulled Wine** (Gluhwein), 4 fl.oz | 180 | 14 | 20 |
| **Non-Alcoholic Wine:** *Less than 0.5% Alcohol* | | | |
| *Ariel:* White varieties, average, 4 fl.oz | 35 | 0.5 | 8 |
| Red varieties, average, 4 fl.oz | 25 | 0.5 | 5 |
| **Flavored/Reduced Alcohol Wine:** | | | |
| *Average All Brands (6% alcohol):* | | | |
| *(Arbor Mist, Wild Vines, Boone's Farm):* | | | |
| 1 small wine glass, 4 fl.oz | 80 | 6 | 10 |
| 1 large wine glass, 8 fl.oz | 160 | 11 | 20 |
| *Skinnygirl,* Red/White, (8.5%), 5 fl.oz | 100 | 10 | 5 |
| **Sake** (Gekkeikan), (16%), 4 fl.oz | 120 | 15 | 5 |
| **Sangria** (Skinnygirl), (4%), 5 fl.oz | 130 | 5 | 23 |

## Dessert Wines

| | C | Alc | Cb |
|---|---|---|---|
| **Madeira** (18%), 2 oz | 85 | 9 | 5 |
| **Marsala** (18%), 2 oz | 110 | 9 | 11 |
| **Port,** Muscatel (18%), 2 oz | 85 | 9 | 5 |
| **Sherry,** (15%), 2 oz: | | | |
| Dry, 1 Sherry glass | 90 | 7 | 7 |
| Sweet/Cream, average | 90 | 7 | 8 |
| **Vermouth** (Martini & Rossi): | | | |
| Extra Dry (18%), 2 oz | 65 | 9 | 2 |
| Martini Rosso (16%), 2 oz | 90 | 8 | 8 |

## Cooking Wines

| | C | Alc | Cb |
|---|---|---|---|
| **Holland House:** | | | |
| **Marsala,** (14%), 2 T., 1 fl.oz | 45 | 4 | 4 |
| **Red/White,** (10%): 2 T., 1 fl.oz | 20 | 2 | 1 |
| 1 cup, 8 fl.oz | 160 | 24 | 8 |
| **Sherry,** (17%), 2 Tbsp, 1 fl.oz | 45 | 5 | 2 |

## Quick Guide · Alc ~ Alcohol (Grams)

**Spirits/Liquors:**
*Includes Bourbon, Brandy, Gin, Rum, Scotch, Tequila, Vodka, Whiskey.*
Note: All spirits with same alcohol proof have similar calories and zero fat.

| *Average All Brands* | C | Alc | Cb |
|---|---|---|---|
| **80 Proof (40% Alcohol by Volume):** | | | |
| 1 fl.oz | 65 | 9.5 | 0 |
| 1.5 fl.oz (1 shot) | 100 | 14 | 0 |
| 3 fl.oz (Double shot) | 195 | 28 | 0 |
| ¹/₂ Bottle, 350 ml (12 fl.oz) | 770 | 113 | 0 |
| 1 Bottle, 700 ml (24 fl.oz) | 1540 | 227 | 0 |
| **86 Proof (43% Alc),** 1.5 fl.oz shot | 105 | 15 | 0 |
| **100 Proof (50% Alc),** 1.5 fl.oz | 125 | 18 | 0 |
| **Shochu (Soju),** av., (25% alc), 2 fl.oz | 65 | 12 | 0 |

### Flavored Spirits

| **Captain Morgan:** *Per 1.5 fl.oz* | | | |
|---|---|---|---|
| **Original** (35%) | 85 | 12 | 0.5 |
| **Black Spiced** (47.3%) | 115 | 14 | 1 |
| **Parrot Bay** (21%), average | 90 | 7.5 | 10 |
| **Silver Spiced** (35%) | 95 | 12 | 2 |
| **Malibu Rum,** Orig./Fruit (21%), 1.5 fl.oz | 80 | 8 | 8 |
| **Southern Comfort** (35%), 1.5 fl.oz | 100 | 13 | 3 |

### Hard Lemonade, Sodas, Seltzers & Tea

| | | | |
|---|---|---|---|
| **Arnold Palmer Spiked,** (5%), 12 fl.oz | 205 | 14 | 28 |
| **Henry's Hard Soda:** | | | |
| Grape (4.2%), 12 fl.oz | 225 | 12 | 35 |
| Lemon Lime/Orange (4.2%) | 190 | 12 | 28 |
| Sparkling Water, av., (4.2%) | 90 | 12 | 2 |
| **Margaritaville:** *Per 12 fl.oz* | | | |
| Lime Margarita (8%) | 310 | 23 | 30 |
| Paradise Punch (8%) | 340 | 23 | 46 |
| **Mike's Hard Lemonade:** | | | |
| Black Cherry (5%), 11.2 fl.oz | 220 | 13 | 33 |
| Lite (5%), 11.2 fl.oz | 150 | 13 | 15 |
| Lemonade (5%), 11.2 fl.oz | 220 | 13 | 33 |
| Lite (5%), 11.2 fl.oz | 100 | 13 | 4 |
| Harder (8%), 16 fl.oz | 395 | 31 | 44 |
| **Not Your Father's Root Beer,** (5.9%), 12 fl.oz | 195 | 17 | 20 |
| **Platform Setzer,** (5%), 11.2 fl.oz | 110 | 13 | 4 |
| **Pura Still,** (4.5%), 11.2 fl.oz | 90 | 12 | 1 |
| **Redd's Wicked,** (8%), av. 10 fl.oz | 230 | 19 | 25 |
| **Bold Rock,** Hard Seltzer (4%), 12 fl.oz | 80 | 11 | 1 |
| **Sparks:** Original (6%), 16 fl.oz | 335 | 23 | 45 |
| Blackberry (8%), 16 fl.oz | 385 | 31 | 44 |
| **Twisted Tea:** Original (5%) | 220 | 14 | 31 |
| Half & Half (5%) | 260 | 14 | 34 |
| **Wild Basin,** (5%), 11.2 fl.oz | 100 | 13 | 1 |
| **Zumbida Mango,** (4.2%), 12 fl.oz | 150 | 12 | 17 |

### Coolers & Premix Cocktails

| **Ready-To-Drink:** | C | Alc | Cb |
|---|---|---|---|
| *Zero Fat Unless Indicated* | | | |
| **Bacardi:** *Per 4 fl.oz* | | | |
| **Party Drinks (Ready To Pour):** | | | |
| Bahama Mama; Mai Tai (10%) | 130 | 9 | 16 |
| Mojito (15%) | 160 | 14 | 16 |
| Rum Island Ice Tea (12.5%) | 150 | 12 | 16 |
| **Bacardi Silver:** *Per 12 fl.oz* | | | |
| Lemonade/Sangria (6%), av. | 270 | 17 | 41 |
| Raz/Strawberry (5%) | 240 | 14 | 36 |
| Mojito (5%) | 240 | 14 | 36 |
| **Bartles & Jaymes:** *Per 11.2 fl.oz* | | | |
| **Malt Based Coolers** (3.2%): | | | |
| Exotic Berry | 195 | 9 | 31 |
| Fuzzy Navel | 215 | 9 | 36 |
| Margarita | 245 | 9 | 43 |
| Pina Colada | 250 | 9 | 45 |
| Pomegranate Raspberry | 205 | 9 | 35 |
| Sangria | 240 | 9 | 40 |
| Strawberry Daiquiri | 205 | 9 | 34 |
| **Captain Morgan's,** | | | |
| Parrot Bay (4.1%), all var. av., 11.2 fl.oz | 210 | 10 | 35 |
| **Chi Chi's:** Long Is. Iced Tea, 4 fl.oz | 145 | 12 | 17 |
| Mexican Mudslide, 4 fl.oz (8g fat) | 240 | 1.5 | 42 |
| Mojito, 4 fl.oz | 160 | 11 | 21 |
| Pina Colada, 4 fl.oz (6g fat) | 240 | 4 | 42 |
| White Russian, 4 fl.oz (7g fat) | 245 | 1.5 | 43 |
| **Daily's,** Frozen Pouches (5%), | | | |
| average all flavors, 10 fl.oz | 285 | 12 | 47 |
| **Jack Daniels,** Country Cocktails (4.8%), | | | |
| average all varieties, 10 fl.oz | 200 | 9 | 30 |
| **Jose Cuervo:** | | | |
| **Margaritas:** | | | |
| Classic Lime (10%), 6 fl.oz | 210 | 14 | 29 |
| Golden (12.7%), 4.7 fl.oz | 170 | 14 | 19 |
| **Seagram's:** | | | |
| **Escapes Coolers** (3.2%): | | | |
| Bahama Mama, 11.2 fl.oz | 200 | 9 | 36 |
| Strawb. Daiquiri, 11.2 fl.oz | 225 | 9 | 41 |
| **Skinnygirl:** | | | |
| Vodka with flavors (30%), 1.5 fl.oz | 75 | 11 | 0 |
| Cocktails (10%), av., 3 fl.oz | 70 | 8 | 4 |
| **Smirnoff:** | | | |
| **Ice** (4.5%): Original, 11.2 fl.oz | 220 | 13 | 33 |
| Mango; Pineapple, av., 11.2 fl.oz | 230 | 13 | 35 |
| **Spiked Sparkling Seltzer,** | | | |
| (4.5%), all flav., 12 fl.oz can | 90 | 13 | 1 |
| **TGI Friday's:** | | | |
| **On The Rocks:** *Per 6 fl.oz* | | | |
| Long Island Ice Tea (15%) | 250 | 21 | 28 |
| Margarita (7.5%) | 185 | 11 | 29 |
| Mudslide (10%) | 365 | 14 | 31 |
| **Blenders** (12.5%), Mudslide, 6 fl.oz | 365 | 18 | 31 |

## Coolers & Premix Cocktails (Cont)

**Ready-To-Drink:** | **C** | **Alc** | **Cb**

**The Club Premix Cocktails:** *Per 3.4 oz Serving (½ can)*

| | C | Alc | Cb |
|---|---|---|---|
| Censored on Beach; Margarita (7.5%) | 105 | 6 | 17 |
| Gin/Vodka Martini (21%), average | 155 | 17 | 0.2 |
| Ice Tea (15%) | 145 | 12 | 17 |
| Manhattan (17%) | 115 | 13 | 5 |
| Mudslide/Pina Colada (10%), average | 200 | 8 | 16 |
| Screwdriver (7.5%) | 95 | 6 | 14 |
| Whiskey Sour (10%) | 95 | 8 | 11 |

### Shooters     **Alc** ~ Alcohol (Grams)

| | | | |
|---|---|---|---|
| Alabama Slammer | 110 | 14 | 2 |
| Amaretto Sour | 120 | 6 | 19 |
| B52 | 145 | 14 | 11 |
| Beam Me Up Scotty | 145 | 13 | 13 |
| Blue Tequila | 160 | 18 | 6 |
| Jager Bomb | 205 | 8 | 30 |
| Jager Bomb, w/ Sugar-Free Red Bull | 155 | 8 | 18 |
| Jell-O Shot: 3 oz, with 1.5 oz Vodka | 180 | 14 | 19 |
| with Diet Jell-O | 110 | 14 | 0 |
| Kamikaze | 75 | 8 | 3 |
| Kool-Aid | 160 | 15 | 14 |
| Orgasm | 100 | 12 | 6 |
| Peppermint Patty | 195 | 8 | 11 |
| Stinger | 170 | 18 | 12 |
| Surfer on Acid | 90 | 7 | 11 |

### Cocktail Mixers ~ Non-Alcoholic

**Bacardi:** *Per 8 fl.oz, Prepared from 2 fl.oz Concentrate*

| | | | |
|---|---|---|---|
| Daiquiris; Rum Runner | 120 | 0 | 32 |
| Margarita | 90 | 0 | 25 |
| Mojito | 110 | 0 | 30 |
| Pina Colada | 170 | 0 | 36 |

**Baja Bob's:** *Per 4 fl.oz*

| | | | |
|---|---|---|---|
| Cranberry Cosmo Martini | 10 | 0 | 2 |
| Pina Colada | 30 | 0 | 4 |

**Jose Cuervo:**

| | | | |
|---|---|---|---|
| Margaritas: Av. all flav., 4 fl.oz | 85 | 0 | 21 |
| Light (Sugar Free), Lime, 4 fl.oz | 5 | 0 | 1 |

**Mr & Mrs T:**

| | | | |
|---|---|---|---|
| Bloody Mary: Original, 5 oz | 30 | 0 | 7 |
| Bold & Spicy, 4 oz | 35 | 0 | 7 |
| Mai Tai | 130 | 0 | 32 |
| Margarita | 100 | 0 | 26 |
| Pina Colada | 170 | 0 | 44 |
| Strawberry Daiquiri | 180 | 0 | 46 |

**TGI Friday's:**

| | | | |
|---|---|---|---|
| Mudslide, 2.3 fl.oz | 110 | 0 | 23 |
| Cosmo; Berrytini, 2 fl.oz | 80 | 0 | 20 |
| Strawb. Daiquiri; Marg., 4 fl.oz | 190 | 0 | 46 |

## Cocktails     **Alc** ~ Alcohol (Grams)

**Made to Standard Recipes (Standard Size):**
(Main Reference: The New American Bartender's Guide)
*Zero Fat Unless Indicated*

| | C | Alc | Cb |
|---|---|---|---|
| Adios Mother F. | 260 | 23 | 23 |
| Bacardi & Coke (with 1.5 oz Bacardi) | 160 | 14 | 17 |
| Bellini, 4.5 fl.oz | 95 | 11 | 7 |
| Bloody Mary (with 1.5 oz Vodka) | 125 | 10 | 7 |
| Blushin' Russian (20g fat) | 405 | 14 | 23 |
| Bourbon & Soda (with 2 oz Bourbon) | 130 | 19 | 0 |
| Brandy Alexander (10g fat) | 300 | 20 | 15 |
| Chupa Naranjas (with 1.5 oz Tequila) | 150 | 16 | 8 |
| Cosmopolitan | 215 | 24 | 12 |
| Daiquiri (w/ 2 oz Rum), av. all types | 140 | 19 | 4 |
| Frozen Daiquiri (with 2 oz Rum): | | | |
| without fruit | 155 | 19 | 6 |
| with fruit (with 1.5 oz Rum) | 145 | 14 | 11 |
| Grasshopper | 260 | 17 | 28 |
| Harvey Wallbanger (2 oz) | 200 | 19 | 17 |
| Highball (1.5 oz Whiskey) | 100 | 14 | 0 |
| Irish Coffee (10g fat) | 205 | 14 | 7 |
| Kahlua Mudslide: with milk (3g fat) | 145 | 11 | 12 |
| with cream (12g fat) | 230 | 11 | 10 |
| Lemon Drop, 4 fl.oz | 130 | 14 | 10 |
| Long Island Iced Tea (with 3 oz Cola) | 270 | 19 | 32 |
| with 3 oz Diet Cola | 235 | 19 | 22 |
| Mai Tai (with 2 oz Rum) | 290 | 24 | 33 |
| Manhattan | 130 | 17 | 5 |
| Margarita | 160 | 18 | 7 |
| Martini: Dry, with 1.5 oz gin | 100 | 14 | 0 |
| Sour Apple, w/ 2 oz Vodka/1 oz Schnapps | 250 | 31 | 10 |
| Mint Julep (with 2½ oz Bourbon) | 180 | 24 | 4 |
| Mojito (with 2 oz rum) | 170 | 19 | 9 |
| Moscow Mule (with 1.5 oz Vodka) | 180 | 14 | 20 |
| Pina Colada (10g fat), 6 oz | 250 | 15 | 18 |
| Red Bull & Vodka (with 1.5 oz vodka) | 210 | 14 | 28 |
| with Sugar Free Red Bull | 105 | 14 | 3 |
| Rum & Coke (with 1.5 oz Rum) | 160 | 14 | 17 |
| Sake Bomb (1.5 oz Sake & 5 oz Beer) | 105 | 12 | 7 |
| Sangria: with 1 oz Fruit Juice, 5 oz | 120 | 12 | 9 |
| with 0.5 oz Brandy, 5.5 oz | 150 | 17 | 9 |
| Screwdriver | 160 | 14 | 15 |
| Sex On The Beach | 235 | 19 | 25 |
| Spritzer (with 3 oz Wine) | 65 | 8 | 2 |
| Tequila Sunrise | 200 | 14 | 25 |
| Tom Collins (with 2 oz Gin) | 210 | 19 | 18 |
| Vodka Soda (with 1.5 oz Vodka) | 100 | 14 | 0 |
| Vodka Tonic (with 1.5 oz Vodka) | 165 | 14 | 18 |
| Whiskey Sour (w/ 2 oz Whiskey) | 155 | 19 | 7 |
| White Russian (10g fat) | 240 | 19 | 7 |

**Non-Alcoholic:**

| | | | |
|---|---|---|---|
| Cinderella | 45 | 0 | 11 |
| Shirley Temple (with 6 oz Ginger Ale) | 140 | 0 | 34 |

## Liqueurs/Cordials  **C** **Alc** **Cb**

*Per 1 fl.oz*

| | C | Alc | Cb |
|---|---|---|---|
| Advocaat (36 Proof; 2g fat) | 85 | 4 | 9 |
| Alizé: Cognac (80 Proof) | 70 | 9 | 2 |
| Gold/Red Passion (32 Proof) | 105 | 4 | 11 |
| Amaretto (56 Proof) | 110 | 7 | 17 |
| Baileys Irish Cream (34 Proof; 4g fat) | 100 | 4 | 8 |
| Benedictine (80 Proof) | 90 | 9 | 5 |
| Chambord (33 Proof) | 105 | 4 | 11 |
| Chartreuse (80 Proof) | 100 | 9 | 9 |
| Cherry Brandy (48 Proof) | 80 | 6 | 9 |
| Coffee Liqueur (53 Proof) | 115 | 7 | 16 |
| Cointreau (80 Proof) | 95 | 9 | 7 |
| Creme de Cacao (54 Proof) | 100 | 6 | 15 |
| Creme de Menthe (72 Proof) | 125 | 9 | 14 |
| Curacao (70 Proof) | 95 | 8 | 6 |
| Drambuie (80 Proof) | 105 | 9 | 9 |
| Frangelico (40 Proof) | 65 | 5 | 12 |
| Galliano (86 Proof) | 100 | 10 | 8 |
| Grand Marnier (80 Proof) | 100 | 9 | 7 |
| (40 Proof) | 85 | 5 | 14 |
| Kirsch (68 Proof) | 80 | 8 | 6 |
| Midori (42 Proof) | 80 | 5 | 11 |
| Ouzo (80 Proof) | 105 | 9 | 11 |
| Pernod (80 Proof) | 75 | 9 | 11 |
| Sambuca (84 Proof) | 100 | 10 | 11 |
| Schnapps (100 Proof) | 115 | 12 | 9 |
| Southern Comfort (70 Proof) | 65 | 8 | 3 |
| Tia Maria (40% Proof) | 90 | 7 | 10 |

## Liqueur Coffee & Hot Drinks

*Per Standard Drink*

| | | | |
|---|---|---|---|
| **Liqueur Coffee:** Av. all types | 200 | 10 | 10 |
| Irish, 1.5 oz Whiskey & 1 oz whip | 205 | 9 | 4 |
| **Hot Toddy,** with 1½ oz liquor, av. all | 170 | 9 | 19 |
| **Mulled Wine** (*Glühwein*), 4 fl.oz, av | 195 | 14 | 25 |

*"The doctor told him to cut down to just one glass a day."*

## TEN TIPS TO AVOID HARMFUL DRINKING

1. **Add up the alcohol** you typically drink each day and on social occasions. How does this compare with 'low risk' amounts? (*See page 23*)

2. **Compare the alcohol content** of different drinks and select the lowest. Request half shots of alcohol in cocktails and mixed drinks. Dilute them and keep topping off with non-alcoholic drinks.

3. **Go easy on 'Light' beers.** At 4% alcohol, on average, they are still high in alcohol compared to regular beer (5% alcohol).

4. **Try low alcohol or non-alcohol alternatives** such as fruit juices and mineral water. Take your own to parties.

5. **Before drinking alcohol,** quench your thirst with water and non-alcoholic drinks – particularly after vigorous exercise or sports.

6. **Slow the rate of drinking.** Chugging or drinking fast is the major cause of illness and death from alcohol poisoning.

7. **Avoid drinking in 'rounds'.**

8. **Have a non-alcoholic 'spacer'** between drinks (e.g. mineral water, orange juice).

9. **Don't drink on an empty stomach.** Food slows the rate of alcohol absorption.

10. **Keep track of the number of drinks** and know when to stop. Stick to a set limit.

*Note: Alcohol can be very dangerous when taken with prescription or street drugs, or when you are very tired.*

***Extra Info: www.CalorieKing.com***

## Cocktail Mixers & Extracts

| | C | Alc | Cb |
|---|---|---|---|
| Angostura Bitters, ¼ tsp | 2 | 0 | 0.5 |
| Grenadine, ½ tsp | 6 | 0 | 2 |
| Lime/Lemon Juice, 2 Tbsp, 1 oz | 10 | 0 | 2 |
| Maraschino Cherry, 1 small | 8 | 0 | 2 |
| Simple Syrup, 1 Tbsp, av. | 50 | 0 | 14 |
| Sweet & Sour Mix, 2 Tbsp, 1 oz | 30 | 0 | 7 |
| Tonic Water, 8 fl.oz | 80 | 0 | 22 |
| **Flavor Extracts** (*McCormick*): | | | |
| Pure Lemon (83%), 1 tsp | 0 | 3.5 | 0 |
| Pure Vanilla (35%), 1tsp | 0 | 1.5 | 0 |

| Baking Ingredients | C | F | Cb |
|---|---|---|---|
| **Almond Flour,** ¼ cup, 1 oz | 160 | 10 | 10 |
| **Almond Paste,** (Marzipan), 2 Tbsp | 170 | 7 | 24 |
| **Apple Pie Filling,** Sweetened, 9.4 oz | 290 | 0 | 69 |
| (Bean Water), ¼ c., 2 oz | 10 | 0 | 2 |
| **Amaranth Flour** (Bob's Red Mill), ¼ cup, 1 oz | 110 | 2 | 20 |
| **Baking Powder:** Regular, 1 tsp | 5 | 0 | 1 |
| Cream of Tartar, 1 tsp | 10 | 0 | 2 |
| Baking Mix (Bisquick): Original, ⅓ cup, 1.5 oz | 160 | 5 | 26 |
| **Batter Mix** (Golden Dipt), All Purpose, ¼ cup | 100 | 0 | 20 |
| **Butter/Margarine,** ½ cup, 4 oz | 800 | 88 | 1 |
| Stick (Land O' Lakes), 0.5 oz | 100 | 11 | 0 |
| **Cacao Butter,** 2 Tbsp, 1 oz | 240 | 28 | 0 |
| **Cacao Powder,** raw: 1 Tbsp, 0.3 oz | 35 | 2 | 3 |
| ¼ cup, 1 oz | 150 | 9 | 11 |
| **Carob Flour,** ½ cup | 115 | 0.5 | 46 |
| **Cassava Flour,** ½ cup, 70g | 260 | 0 | 62 |
| **Chia Seed Protein Powder,** 2 T., 0.5 oz | 25 | 0 | 8 |
| **Chocolate Baking Bars:** Average all Brands | | | |
| Sweet (Baker's): | | | |
| 1 oz portion | 120 | 7 | 16 |
| 4 oz bar | 470 | 28 | 64 |
| Semi-sweet, 1 oz | 140 | 9 | 16 |
| White Baking, 1 oz | 160 | 9 | 16 |
| Unsweetened: 1 oz | 140 | 14 | 8 |
| Grated, 1 cup, 4.5 oz | 660 | 69 | 39 |
| **Chocolate Baking Chips:** Average all Brands | | | |
| Milk Choc./Semi Sweet, 1 oz | 140 | 8 | 18 |
| ½ cup, 3 oz | 420 | 24 | 54 |
| 1 cup, 6 oz | 840 | 48 | 108 |
| Dark, 1 Tbsp, 0.5 oz | 70 | 5 | 3 |
| Mini Kisses (Hershey), 1 piece | 5 | 0.5 | 1 |
| **Cocoa Powder,** unsweetened: | | | |
| 1 Tbsp, 0.2 oz | 15 | 0.5 | 3 |
| ⅓ cup, 1 oz | 60 | 4 | 17 |
| **Coconut,** dried: | | | |
| Sweetened/Flaked: 1 oz | 130 | 8 | 15 |
| ½ cup, 1.3 oz | 195 | 12 | 22 |
| Tsd (Baker's), 1 oz | 170 | 13 | 13 |
| Unsweetened, 1 oz | 190 | 18 | 7 |
| **Coconut Cream/Milk** ~ See Page 89 | | | |
| **Coconut Flour,** 2 Tbsp, 0.5 oz | 60 | 2 | 8 |
| **Coconut Manna** (Nutiva), 1 Tbsp | 100 | 9 | 3 |
| **Cornstarch,** 1 Tbsp | 30 | 0 | 7 |
| **Eggs:** Large (1) | 75 | 5 | 0 |
| Jumbo (1) | 90 | 6 | 0.5 |
| **Egg White:** 1 Egg White | 15 | 0 | 0 |
| ½ cup (4 egg whites), 4 oz | 60 | 0 | 1 |

| Flour: | C | F | Cb |
|---|---|---|---|
| Whole Wheat, 1 cup, 4.2 oz | 400 | 2 | 84 |
| White: 1 Tbsp, 0.3 oz | 25 | 0 | 5.5 |
| 1 cup, 4.2 oz | 400 | 1 | 88 |
| **Flavor Extracts:** Av. all Brands | | | |
| Imitation, 1 tsp | 10 | 0 | 2 |
| Pure Extract, 1 tsp | 10 | 0 | 0.5 |
| Almond; Vanilla, 1 tsp | 10 | 0 | 0.5 |
| **Fruit Pectin:** Swtnd, ¼ tsp | 5 | 0 | 1 |
| Unsweetened, ¼ tsp | 0 | 0 | 0 |
| **Gelatin,** dry, unsweetened, 0.3 oz | 20 | 0 | 0 |
| **Glaze** (Duncan Hines): Choc., 2 T. | 150 | 7 | 21 |
| Vanilla, 2 Tbsp | 140 | 6 | 22 |
| **Hazelnut Meal/Flour,** ¼ cup, 1 oz | 160 | 12 | 8 |
| **Hemp Protein Powder,** ¼ cup, 1.1 oz | 120 | 3 | 10 |
| **Honey,** ½ cup, 6 oz | 515 | 0 | 145 |
| **Lemon/Orange Peel,** ¼ cup | 25 | 0 | 6 |
| **Lighter Bake** (Sunsweet): (Butter & Oil replacement) | | | |
| 1 Tbsp, ½ oz | 35 | 0 | 9 |
| ¼ cup, 2.7 oz | 140 | 0 | 36 |
| **Masa Harina** (Bob's Red Mill), ½ cup, 2 oz | 220 | 2 | 47 |
| **Milk:** Whole, 1 cup, 8 fl.oz | 150 | 8 | 12 |
| 2%, 1 cup, 8 fl.oz | 120 | 5 | 12 |
| 1%, 1 cup, 8 fl.oz | 100 | 2.5 | 12 |
| Fat-Free, 1 cup, 8 fl.oz | 90 | 0.5 | 13 |
| **Oat Flour** (Bob's Red Mill), ⅓ cup, 1.5 oz | 120 | 3 | 26 |
| **Pastry** ~ See Page 134 | | | |
| **Pie Crusts** ~ See Page 134 | | | |
| **Pie Fillings, Fruits** ~ See Page 134 | | | |
| Lemon Creme, ⅓ cup | 130 | 1.5 | 28 |
| Mincemeat, 3.5 oz | 190 | 5 | 45 |
| Pumpkin, 1 cup, 9.3 oz | 270 | 1.5 | 60 |
| **Prune Puree,** ¼ cup, 2.8 oz | 220 | 0 | 55 |
| **Quinoa Flour,** ¼ cup, 1 oz | 110 | 1.5 | 18 |
| **Raisins,** ½ cup, 2.8 oz | 240 | 0.5 | 63 |
| **Rennin,** 0.4 oz pkt | 10 | 0 | 2 |
| **Rice Flour,** ½ cup, 2.8 oz | 290 | 1 | 63 |
| **Soy Milk** ~ See Pages 49-50 | | | |
| **Soy Flour,** (Bob's Red Mill), 100% Whole Ground, ¼ cup, 1 oz | 120 | 6 | 8 |
| **Sprinkles,** all types, 1 tsp | 20 | 1 | 3 |
| **Sugar:** 1 Tbsp, 0.5 oz | 55 | 0 | 14 |
| 1 oz | 110 | 0 | 28 |
| 1 cup, 7 oz | 775 | 0 | 195 |
| 16 oz (1 lb) | 1760 | 0 | 454 |
| **Sweeteners & Sugar Substitutes** ~ See Page 156 | | | |
| **Vinegar,** average all types, 1 oz | 5 | 0 | 1 |
| **Whey,** sweet, dry, 1 oz | 100 | 0.5 | 21 |
| **Yeast:** | | | |
| Active, dry, 0.3 oz pkg | 25 | 0.5 | 3 |
| Bakers, compressed, 1 oz | 30 | 0.5 | 5 |
| Fleischmann's, 0.6 oz pkg | 0 | 0 | 0 |

Note: Actual weight of bars is usually 5-10% more than label Net Weight. Weigh bar and allow extra calories.

## Bars ~ Brands

**C** **F** **Cb**

*Per Bar*

**AdvantEdge** ~ *See EAS*

**Annie's Homegrown:**

| | C | F | Cb |
|---|---|---|---|
| **Gluten Free,** all varieties, 1 oz | 110 | 3 | 20 |

**Organic Chewy Granola Bars:** *Per 0.9 oz Bar*

| | C | F | Cb |
|---|---|---|---|
| Chocolate Chip | 100 | 2.5 | 18 |
| Oatmeal Raisin | 90 | 1.5 | 19 |
| PB Chocolate Chip | 100 | 3.5 | 16 |

**Atkins:**

**Harvest Trail Bars:** *Per 1.34 oz Bar*

| | C | F | Cb |
|---|---|---|---|
| Coconut Almond | 160 | 11 | 16 |
| Dark Chocolate: | | | |
| Peanut Butter | 170 | 13 | 13 |
| Sea Salt Caramel | 180 | 14 | 13 |

**Meal Bars:** *Per 1.7 oz Unless Indicated*

| | C | F | Cb |
|---|---|---|---|
| Allmond Coconut | 200 | 11 | 16 |
| Blueberry Greek Yogurt | 200 | 9 | 21 |
| Choc. Almond Caramel | 190 | 9 | 17 |
| Chocolate Chip Granola | 200 | 9 | 18 |
| Chocolate Peanut Butter, 2 oz | 250 | 14 | 23 |
| Cookies 'n Crème, 1.76 oz | 200 | 11 | 22 |
| Peanut Fudge Granola | 210 | 11 | 16 |
| Vanilla Pecan Crisp | 200 | 0 | 17 |

*Note: Carb figures include 14-15g Fiber & Glycerin*

**Snack Bars:** *Per 1.55 oz Bar Unless Indicated*

| | C | F | Cb |
|---|---|---|---|
| Caramel Chocolate Nut Roll | 190 | 13 | 19 |
| Caramel Chocolate Peanut Nougat | 170 | 11 | 20 |
| Caramel Double Chocolate Crunch | 160 | 9 | 22 |
| Cashew Trail Mix, 1.4 oz | 170 | 11 | 19 |
| Choc. Chip Crisp, 1.23 oz | 140 | 6 | 16 |
| Classic Trail Mix, 1.34 oz | 190 | 15 | 13 |
| Coconut Almond Delight | 200 | 15 | 18 |
| Dark Chocolate Decadence | 150 | 6 | 23 |
| Lemon Bar, Triple Choc., av., 1.4 oz | 160 | 8 | 16 |
| Sweet & Salty Trail Mix, 1.34 oz | 190 | 14 | 15 |

*Note: Snack Bars Carb figures includes 4-15g Sugar Alcohol*

| | C | F | Cb |
|---|---|---|---|
| **Protein Wafer Crisps,** average | 190 | 14 | 9 |

**Balance:**

**Original Bars:**

| | C | F | Cb |
|---|---|---|---|
| Average, 1.8 oz | 200 | 7 | 21 |
| Dark Chocolate var., av., 1.6 oz | 180 | 7 | 22 |

**Duo-licious:** *Per 2 Pieces*

| | C | F | Cb |
|---|---|---|---|
| Choc. C'rml P'nut Nougat, 1.55 oz | 190 | 10 | 22 |
| Choc. Pepeprmint Patty, 1.4 oz | 160 | 4 | 27 |
| Dulce de Leche & Caramel, 1.4 oz | 150 | 5 | 24 |

*Per Bar*

**C** **F** **Cb**

**Cascadian Farms** *(General Mills):*

| | C | F | Cb |
|---|---|---|---|
| **Chewy Granola:** Av. all var., 0.77 oz | 85 | 2 | 16 |
| 1.23 oz Bars: Peanut varieties | 160 | 7 | 22 |
| Chocolate Chip | 140 | 3 | 26 |
| **Crunchy Granola,** av., 2 bars, 1.4 oz | 185 | 8 | 27 |
| **Protein Granola Bars,** av., 1.76 oz | 250 | 15 | 20 |
| **Soft Baked Squares,** av., 1.23 oz | 150 | 5.5 | 23 |

**Clif:**

| | C | F | Cb |
|---|---|---|---|
| **Blueberry Crisp,** 2.4 oz | 250 | 5 | 44 |
| **Builder's,** average, 2.4 oz | 275 | 9 | 30 |
| **Crunch,** average, 1.48 oz | 200 | 9 | 26 |
| **Energy:** Av. all varieties., 2.4 oz | 260 | 6 | 43 |
| Mini size, average, 1.2 oz | 100 | 2.5 | 17 |
| **Fruit Smoothie Filled,** 1.76 oz | 230 | 11 | 29 |
| **Mojo,** average, 1.6 oz | 205 | 10 | 22 |
| **Nut Butter Filled,** av., 1.76 oz | 230 | 11 | 27 |
| **Whey,** P'B & Chocolate, 2 oz | 260 | 13 | 24 |

**Corazonas:**

**Heartbar Oatmeal Squares:** *Per 1.8 oz Bar*

| | C | F | Cb |
|---|---|---|---|
| White Chocolate Macadamia | 200 | 7 | 29 |
| Average other varieties | 185 | 7 | 28 |

**Detour:**

**Lean Muscle:**

| | C | F | Cb |
|---|---|---|---|
| Cookie Dough Caramel Crisp, 3.2 oz | 370 | 12 | 33 |
| P'nut Butter Choc. Crunch, 3.2 oz | 420 | 18 | 33 |

**Lower Sugar,** average all varieties:

| | C | F | Cb |
|---|---|---|---|
| 1.4 oz Bar | 170 | 6 | 16 |
| 2.8 oz Bar | 340 | 13 | 33 |

*Note: Low Sugar Bars Carb figures include 12-28g Sugar Alcohol*

**Simple:**

| | C | F | Cb |
|---|---|---|---|
| Full size, 20g Protein, av., 2 oz | 225 | 7 | 24 |
| Snack size, 10g Protein, av., 1 oz | 110 | 4 | 11 |

| | C | F | Cb |
|---|---|---|---|
| **Smart:** Coconut Almond, 1.3 oz | 150 | 5 | 16 |
| Fruit varieties, 1.3 oz | 130 | 2.5 | 18 |
| Peanut Butter Chocolate, 1.3 oz | 160 | 6 | 16 |

**dotFIT:**

**dotBAR:**

| | C | F | Cb |
|---|---|---|---|
| Double Choc. Brownie, 3.3 oz | 370 | 13 | 38 |
| Peanut Butter Cup, 3.3 oz | 370 | 13 | 38 |

*Note: dotBARS Carb figures includes 21g Sugar Alcohol*

| | C | F | Cb |
|---|---|---|---|
| **dotSTICK,** Iced, all varieties, 2 oz | 190 | 6 | 26 |

*Note: dotSTICK Bars Carb figures includes 8g Sugar Alcohol*

**EAS:**

| | C | F | Cb |
|---|---|---|---|
| **AdvantEDGE,** Protein Bars, average all varieties, 1.76 oz | 190 | 7 | 20 |
| **Extend Bar:** Yogurt, av., 1.4 oz | 150 | 5.5 | 23 |
| Anytime, av. all varieties, 1.4 oz | 150 | 3 | 20 |

*Note: Extend Bars Carb figure includes 3-10g Sugar Alcohol*

## Bars ~ Brands (Cont) | C | F | Cb

*Per Bar*

**Fiber One:**

| | C | F | Cb |
|---|---|---|---|
| 90-Calorie Bar, av., 0.8 oz | 90 | 2 | 17 |
| Chewy: Layered, Dble Choc. Almond, 1.27 oz | 140 | 4 | 25 |
| Oat varieties, average, 1.4 oz | 140 | 4 | 29 |
| Protein: Av. all varieties: 1.2 oz | 140 | 6 | 18 |
| Nut, Chocolate Pretzel, 1.4 oz | 180 | 11 | 15 |

**General Mills:** *Per 1.6 oz Bar*

| | C | F | Cb |
|---|---|---|---|
| Milk 'n Cereal Bar, Honey Nut Cheerios | 160 | 4 | 28 |

**Glucerna:**

**Snack Bars,**

| | C | F | Cb |
|---|---|---|---|
| Peanut/Choc. Chip, av., 1.4 oz | 155 | 5.5 | 20 |

*Note: Carbohydrate figure includes 7g Sugar Alcohol*

| | C | F | Cb |
|---|---|---|---|
| Mini Snack Bar, average, 0.7 oz | 80 | 3.5 | 11 |

*Note: Carbohydrate figure includes 3g Sugar Alcohol*

**Great Value** *(Walmart):*

| | C | F | Cb |
|---|---|---|---|
| Chewy Granola: 90 calorie, 0.8 oz | 90 | 1.5 | 18 |
| Other varieties, 0.8 oz | 100 | 2.5 | 18 |
| Dipped, Peanut Butter, 1.1 oz | 150 | 7 | 20 |
| Protein, average, 1.4 oz | 190 | 12 | 14 |
| Sweet & Salty, Almond, 1.23 oz | 170 | 8 | 20 |
| Crunchy Granola, | | | |
| Oats & Honey, 2 bars, 1.48 oz | 200 | 7 | 29 |
| Fiber, Oats & Chocolate, 1.4 oz | 140 | 4 | 30 |
| Fruit & Grains, Cereal, av., 1.3 oz | 130 | 3 | 25 |

**Health Valley,**

| | C | F | Cb |
|---|---|---|---|
| Multigrain, Cobbler Cereal Bars, average all flavors, 3 oz | 130 | 2.5 | 25 |
| HMR, Benefit Bars, av. all, 1.4 oz | 160 | 5 | 22 |

**Init:** *Per 1.4 oz Bar*

| | C | F | Cb |
|---|---|---|---|
| Dark Choc., average | 180 | 10 | 23 |
| Mixed Nut & Sweet Berries | 180 | 9 | 24 |
| Roasted Nuts & Honey Chipotle | 190 | 13 | 18 |
| Jenny Craig, all var., 1.2 oz | 110 | 3 | 14 |

**Kashi:**

| | C | F | Cb |
|---|---|---|---|
| Cereal Bars, 1.3 oz | 130 | 3 | 25 |
| GoLean, Plant Based Bars, av., 1.6 oz | 195 | 10 | 21 |
| Granola Bars: | | | |
| Chewy, average all varieties, 1.3 oz | 135 | 5 | 23 |
| Chewy Nut Butter, av., 1.23 oz | 150 | 7 | 21 |
| Crunchy, all varieties, 2 bars, 1.4 oz | 175 | 6 | 26 |
| Layered, av. all, 1.1 oz | 125 | 4 | 21 |

**Kellogg's:**

**Nutrigrain** ~ *See page 33*

**Special K** ~ *See page 34*

*Per Bar*

**Kind Bars:** *Per 1.4 oz Bar*

| | C | F | Cb |
|---|---|---|---|
| **Breakfast:** Apple Cinnamon (2) | 210 | 7 | 32 |
| Dark Chocolate Cocoa Protein (2) | 210 | 9 | 26 |
| Honey Oat (2) | 220 | 8 | 33 |
| Orange Cranberry (2) | 200 | 7 | 32 |
| Peanut Butter Dark Chocolate (2) | 220 | 11 | 27 |
| **Fruit & Nut:** Almond & Coconut | 190 | 12 | 21 |
| Blueberry Vanilla & Cashew | 180 | 12 | 19 |
| Fruit & Nut | 200 | 13 | 17 |
| Raspb. Cashew & Chia | 190 | 11 | 21 |
| **Healthy Grain,** av. all varieties, 1.2oz | 145 | 5 | 24 |
| **Nuts & Spices:** Apple Cinnamon | 180 | 12 | 20 |
| Caramel Almond Pumpkin | 200 | 15 | 17 |
| Caramel Alm. Sea Salt | 200 | 16 | 15 |
| Dark Choc. Nuts & Sea Salt | 180 | 15 | 16 |
| Peanut Butter Dark Chocolate | 200 | 13 | 16 |
| **Plus Antioxidants:** Cranberry Almond | 190 | 13 | 18 |
| Pomegranate Blueberry Pistachio | 180 | 11 | 20 |
| **Protein,** average, 1.76 oz | 250 | 17 | 18 |
| **Kind Kids:** | | | |
| Chewy Choc. Chip | 90 | 3 | 16 |
| Chewy Honey Oat | 90 | 2.5 | 16 |
| Chewy Peanut Butter | 100 | 3.5 | 15 |
| **Kudos,** av. all varieties, 0.9 oz | 100 | 3 | 17 |

**Labrada:**

| | C | F | Cb |
|---|---|---|---|
| Cookie Roll, average, 2.8 oz | 315 | 10 | 34 |
| Lean Body Protein Bar: *Per 2.54 oz* | | | |
| Cookie Dough; Fudge Brownie | 290 | 9 | 32 |
| PB Chocolate Chip | 310 | 11 | 32 |
| Lean Body Gold, all var., 2.96 oz | 330 | 8 | 32 |
| Rockin' Roll, Nutty Peanut, 2.47 oz | 290 | 16 | 25 |

**Larabar:**

| | C | F | Cb |
|---|---|---|---|
| Original Fruit & Nut, av. | 200 | 9 | 26 |
| Fruits & Greens, av. | 130 | 3 | 23 |
| Nuts & Seeds, average | 195 | 15 | 13 |

**Lindora Bars:**

**Protein Bars:**

| | C | F | Cb |
|---|---|---|---|
| Caramel Cocoa,1.6 oz | 160 | 5 | 18 |
| Chocolate Mint, 1.45 oz | 150 | 4.5 | 21 |
| Oatmeal Cinn. Raisin, 1.5 oz | 150 | 5 | 19 |
| Peanut Butter Crunch, 1.5 oz | 150 | 5 | 18 |
| Sweet & Salty Crunch. 1.4 oz | 160 | 5 | 21 |
| Zesty Lemon Crunch, 1.5 oz | 160 | 7 | 16 |

**Luna Bars:**

| | C | F | Cb |
|---|---|---|---|
| Regular, av., 1.7 oz | 195 | 7 | 26 |
| Rica, average, 1.4 oz | 165 | 9 | 22 |
| 5G Sugar, average, 1.48 oz | 175 | 9 | 20 |
| Protein, av. all varieties, 1.6 oz | 175 | 5 | 21 |

**Marathon** *(Snickers):*

| | C | F | Cb |
|---|---|---|---|
| **Energy:** Chewy, av. all var., 2 oz | 210 | 8 | 26 |
| Crunchy, Dark Chocolate, 1.6 oz | 150 | 4.5 | 22 |
| **Protein,** average all var., 2.8 oz | 285 | 9 | 40 |

## Bars ~ Brands (Cont)

| | **C** | **F** | **Cb** |
|---|---|---|---|

*Per Bar*

**Mars,** Protein Bar, 2 oz — 200 · 4.5 · 22

**Medifast:**

**Chewy,** all varieties, 1.3 oz — 110 · 3 · 15

**Crunch,** av. all varieties, 1.2 oz — 110 · 3 · 13

*Note: Crunch Bars Carb figure includes 2-3g Sugar Alcohol*

**Maintenance,** Cararmel Nut, 1.5 oz — 170 · 5 · 22

**Met-Rx:**

**Big 100:** *Per 3.52 oz*

| | **C** | **F** | **Cb** |
|---|---|---|---|
| Crispy Apple Pie | 400 | 10 | 48 |
| Chocolate Caramel Coconut | 400 | 10 | 46 |
| Peanut Butter Pretzel | 410 | 12 | 47 |
| Peanut Butter Caramel Crunch | 410 | 13 | 44 |
| Super Cookie Crunch | 410 | 14 | 42 |

**Protein Plus:** Choc. Choc. Chunk, 3 oz — 310 · 10 · 29

Choc. Roasted Peanut w/ Crml, 3oz — 320 · 10 · 33

Peanut Butter Crisp, 3 oz — 310 · 10 · 33

**Mojo Bars** ~ *See Clif*

**Muscle Milk** *(Cytosport):*

**Protein Bars:**

| | **C** | **F** | **Cb** |
|---|---|---|---|
| Almond Cookie Flav.; Choc PB, 2.25 oz | 250 | 9 | 28 |
| B'Day Cake; Cookies 'N Crm, 1.76 oz | 185 | 6 | 23 |
| Blueberry Waffle, 2.18 oz | 230 | 6 | 27 |
| Double Fudge Brownie, 2.22 oz | 240 | 7 | 28 |
| Peanut Butter Cookie, 1.76 oz | 190 | 6 | 22 |

*Note: Protein Bars Carb figures include 6-14g Sugar Alcohol*

**Nature's Path:**

**Chewy Breakfast,** av., 1.2 oz — 140 · 4 · 25

**Love Crunch,** av., 1.1 oz — 150 · 7 · 19

**Superfood,** av., 1.34 oz — 185 · 10 · 20

**Nature Valley:**

**Chewy,** XL Protein, average, 2 oz — 290 · 19 · 21

**Crunchy,** 2 bars, average, 1.5 oz — 190 · 8 · 29

**Nut Crunch,** av. all var, 1.23 oz — 190 · 14 · 14

**Nut Crisp,** average, 0.9 oz — 135 · 9 · 10

**Protein,** all var., 1.4 oz — 190 · 12 · 14

**Sweet & Salty,** average, 1.3 oz — 160 · 7 · 21

**NuGo:**

**Dark,** average all varieties, 1.76 oz — 200 · 6 · 27

**Family:**

| | **C** | **F** | **Cb** |
|---|---|---|---|
| Choc. Banana, 1.76 oz | 190 | 3.5 | 25 |
| Av. other var., 1.76 oz | 170 | 3 | 26 |

**Fiber d'Lish:** Orange Cranb., 1.58 oz — 130 · 3 · 32

Coc. Macaroon; P'nut Choc. Chip, 1.58 oz — 160 · 6 · 28

Average other varieties, 1.58 oz — 135 · 4 · 31

**Gluten Free,** av. all varieties, 1.58 oz — 180 · 4 · 27

**Organic,** all varieties, 1.58 oz — 190 · 5 · 26

**Slim:** Espresso, 1.58 oz — 170 · 5 · 20

Average other varieties — 185 · 5 · 19

*Per Bar*

**NuGo (Cont):**

| | **C** | **F** | **Cb** |
|---|---|---|---|
| **Smarte Carb:** Choc. Black Berry, 1.76 oz | 150 | 3 | 22 |
| Peanut Butter Crunch, 1.76 oz | 160 | 4 | 19 |

*Note: Smarte Carb Carb figures include 12-14 g Sugar Alcohol*

**Stronger:** *Per 2.8 oz Bar*

Cookies 'N Crm; Caramel Pretzel, av. — 290 · 10 · 37

Dark Choc C'rml.; Peanut Cluster, av. — 315 · 13 · 35

**Nutri-Grain** *(Kellogg's):*

**Bakery Delights,**

average, 1.4 oz — 160 · 5 · 27

**Soft Baked B'fast Cereal Bars,**

all varieties, 1.3 oz — 130 · 3.5 · 25

**NutriSystem:**

**Breakfast:** Cinnamon Bun — 150 · 3.5 · 26

Harvest Nut — 160 · 6 · 22

**Lunch:** Choc. P'nut Butter; Trail Mix — 200 · 8 · 24

Double Chocolate Caramel — 180 · 6 · 28

**Snacks:** Dark Chocolate & Sea Salt Nut — 200 · 13 · 16

Average other varieties — 150 · 4 · 23

**Oh Yeah! (ISS):**

**Original:** *Per 3 oz Bar*

Almond Fudge Brownie

| | **C** | **F** | **Cb** |
|---|---|---|---|
| Choc. Caramel Candies | 350 | 17 | 36 |
| Cookie Caramel Crunch | 340 | 13 | 32 |
| Peanut Butter & Caramel | 380 | 19 | 30 |

**Good Grab,** average, 1.6 oz — 190 · 10 · 19

**Optifast:**

**800 Bars:**

| | **C** | **F** | **Cb** |
|---|---|---|---|
| Apple Cinnamon, 1.52 oz | 160 | 4 | 18 |
| Chocolate, 1.65 oz | 160 | 4.5 | 18 |
| Peanut Butter Chocolate, 1.52 oz | 160 | 5 | 18 |

*Note: 800 Bars Carb figures include 1-4g Sugar Alcohol*

**PowerBar:**

**Performance Energy,** average — 230 · 4 · 45

**Plant Protein,** av., 1.76 oz bar — 230 · 13 · 22

**Protein:** Clean Way, average, 2.1 oz — 190 · 5 · 25

*Note: Protein Bars Carb figures include 8g Sugar Alcohol*

Protein Plus, average, 2.1 oz — 205 · 7 · 25

*Note: Protein Plus Bars Carb figures include 16-18g Sugar Alcohol*

**Snack,** average — 230 · 13 · 23

**Power Crunch** *(BNRG):*

**Orig. Protein Bar,** av. all var., 1.4 oz — 205 · 12 · 10

**Power Crunch,** Choklat, av., 0.75 oz — 105 · 6 · 8

**PR:**

**Protein:** Chocolate Mint, 2.1 oz — 200 · 6 · 22

Chocolate Peanut, 1.8 oz — 200 · 7 · 21

Oatmeal Raisin Granola, 1.8 oz — 210 · 7 · 22

**Premier Protein** *(Premier Nutrition):*

**Chocolate Peanut Butter,** 2.54 oz — 290 · 8 · 25

**Dark Chocolate Mint,** 2.54 oz — 280 · 7 · 25

**Yogurt Peanut Crunch,** 2.54 oz — 290 · 8 · 25

Note: Actual weight of bars is usually 5-10% more than label Net Weight. Weigh bar and allow extra calories.

## Bars ~ Brands (Cont)

*Per Bar*

| | **C** | **F** | **Cb** |
|---|---|---|---|
| **Promax:** | | | |
| **Original,** av. all varieties, 2.6 oz | 285 | 6 | 39 |
| **Lower Sugar,** av. all varieties, 2.4 oz | 215 | 7 | 32 |
| *Note: Lower Sugar Carbohydrate figures include 5-6g Sugar Alcohol* | | | |
| **Proti Bars** *(Bariatrix)*, av. all var. | 160 | 5.5 | 16 |
| **PureFit,** av. all varieties, 2 oz | 220 | 7 | 25 |
| **Pure Protein:** | | | |
| **Hi Protein,** average all varieties: | | | |
| 1.76 oz bar | 190 | 5 | 18 |
| 2.1 oz | 195 | 7 | 24 |
| 2.75 oz bar | 300 | 8 | 27 |
| *Note: Carbohydrate figures include 5-8g Sugar Alcohol* | | | |
| **Quaker:** | | | |
| **B'fast Squares:** P'nut Butter, 2.1 oz | 250 | 10 | 35 |
| Other flavors, 2.1 oz | 210 | 4.5 | 41 |
| *Note: Carbohydrate figures include 2-6g Sugar Alcohol* | | | |
| **B'fast Flats:** Banana Honey Nut (3) | 180 | 7 | 27 |
| Av. other varieties (3) | 175 | 6.5 | 28 |
| **Granola Bars:** | | | |
| Chewy: 25% Less Sugar, average, 0.8 oz | 95 | 3 | 17 |
| Big, average all varieties, 1.9 oz | 175 | 6 | 30 |
| Bites, average, 8 pieces | 135 | 5 | 21 |
| Dipps, average, 1.2 oz | 140 | 6 | 22 |
| Snackwich, av., 1.4 oz | 165 | 6 | 29 |
| Yogurt, all varieties, 1.2 oz | 150 | 4.5 | 25 |
| **Quest Bar:** | | | |
| **Hero:** Choc. Caramel Pecan, 2.1 oz | 200 | 11 | 27 |
| Average other varieties, 2.1 oz | 175 | 8 | 30 |
| *Note: Carbohydrate figure include 1-4g Sugar Alcohol* | | | |
| **Protein,,** av., 2.1 oz | 195 | 9 | 22 |
| *Note: Carbohydrate figures includs 1-6g Sugar Alcohol* | | | |
| **RX Bar:** | | | |
| **Protein:** av., 1.83 oz | 210 | 9 | 24 |
| Kids, av., 1.16oz | 130 | 6 | 15 |
| **Skratch Bars:** | | | |
| **Anytime Energy:** *Per 1.76 oz Bar* | | | |
| Cherries & Pistachios; Ginger & Miso | 210 | 10 | 27 |
| Chocolate Chips & Almonds | 200 | 8 | 30 |
| **Slim-Fast:** | | | |
| **Bake Shop Bars,** average all, 1.6 oz | 180 | 6.5 | 17 |
| *Note: Carb includes 12g Sugar Alcohol + 5g Fibre* | | | |
| **Keto:** Bars, av., 1.48 oz | 190 | 14 | 15 |
| *Note: Carb includes 12g Sugar Alcohol + 9g Fibre* | | | |
| Fat Bomb, P'But Butter, 1 cup | 90 | 9 | 6 |
| **Snickers,** Protein Bar, 1.8 oz | 200 | 7 | 18 |
| **Solo,** Gi, average all varieties 1.8 oz | 200 | 7 | 26 |

*Per Bar*

| | **C** | **F** | **Cb** |
|---|---|---|---|
| **Special K:** | | | |
| **Chewy Snack Bars,** | | | |
| av. all varieties, 0.88 oz | 100 | 2 | 19 |
| **Nourish:** | | | |
| Bites, all varieties, 6 pieces | 180 | 9 | 20 |
| Chewy Nut Bars, av. all var., 1.3 oz | 170 | 10 | 16 |
| **Protein Snack,** av. all var., 1.23 oz | 155 | 7 | 17 |
| **Supreme Protein:** | | | |
| **High Protein:** | | | |
| Caramel Nut Chocolate, 3.4 oz | 390 | 15 | 26 |
| PB Crunch, 3 oz | 390 | 18 | 26 |
| PB Jelly, 3.4 oz | 390 | 15 | 35 |
| *Note: Carbohydrate figures include 14-15g Sugar alcohol* | | | |
| **thinkThin:** *Per Bar* | | | |
| **High Protein:** Av. all flavors, 1.94 oz | 230 | 9 | 28 |
| *Note: Carbohydrate figure includes 5-22g Sugar Alcohol* | | | |
| **Prot. & Fiber,** average all var., 1.4 oz | 150 | 5 | 20 |
| **Prot & Superfruit,** av. all varieties | 244 | 9 | 32 |
| **Protein Nut,** average all var., 1.4 oz | 190 | 12 | 16 |
| **Tiger's Milk:** | | | |
| Protein Rich, 1.2 oz | 140 | 5 | 19 |
| Peanut Butter Crunch, 1.2 oz | 150 | 6 | 18 |
| King Size, average all varieties, 2 oz | 225 | 9 | 28 |
| **Trader Joe's:** | | | |
| **Chewy Coated Granola Bars, 6-Packs:** | | | |
| Chocolate Chip, 1.3 oz | 150 | 4 | 26 |
| Raises the Bar, av., 1.2 oz | 140 | 4 | 23 |
| **Fruit Bars:** Fig 1.5 oz | 120 | 2 | 24 |
| Average other varieties, 1.5 oz | 140 | 2.5 | 27 |
| **Granola Bars, 6-packs:** | | | |
| Fiberful, average,1.2 oz | 125 | 5 | 21 |
| Trail Mix, 1.3 oz | 150 | 5 | 23 |
| **Hemp Seed Bar,** 0.9 oz | 120 | 7 | 11 |
| **Tri-O-Plex** *(Chef Jay's):* | | | |
| **High Protein,** | | | |
| Ban. Walnut, 4.2 oz | 405 | 14 | 40 |
| **Duo,** Bursting Peanut Butter | 395 | 17 | 35 |
| **Vega:** | | | |
| **Protein Bars:** Choc. P'Nut Butter, 2.5 oz | 290 | 10 | 27 |
| Sport, Choc. P'nut Butter, 2.1 oz | 260 | 11 | 27 |
| Snack Bar, Choc. Caramel, 1.6 oz | 1280 | 8 | 21 |
| **Wickedly Prime:** *Per 1.4 oz Bar* | | | |
| Banana Nut | 180 | 11 | 21 |
| Cashews & Cranberry | 170 | 9 | 24 |
| Cherry Nut Crunch | 190 | 14 | 15 |
| Nuts & Sea Salt | 200 | 16 | 14 |
| Peanut & Almond | 200 | 15 | 14 |
| **Zone Perfect:** | | | |
| **High Protein Bars,** average, 2 oz | 235 | 9 | 22 |
| **Nutrition Bars:** | | | |
| Chocolate Peanut Butter, 1.76 oz | 210 | 7 | 24 |
| Dark Choc. Almond, 1.58 oz | 190 | 6 | 22 |
| Salted Caramel Brownie, 1.58 oz | 200 | 9 | 19 |

## Cocoa & Hot Chocolate    C   F   Cb

**Cocoa:**

| | C | F | Cb |
|---|---|---|---|
| Small (8 fl.oz): | | | |
|   with Whole Milk | 205 | 8.5 | 22 |
|   with Nonfat Milk | 145 | 1 | 23 |
| Tall (12 fl.oz): with Whole Milk | 280 | 12 | 26 |
|   with Nonfat Milk | 185 | 1 | 28 |
| **Hot Chocolate:** | | | |
| Small (8 fl.oz): with Whole Milk | 180 | 7 | 26 |
|   with Nonfat Milk | 140 | 2 | 27 |
| Tall (12 fl.oz): with Whole Milk | 260 | 10 | 36 |
|   with Nonfat Milk | 190 | 2 | 37 |
| **Cinnabon,** Mochalatta Chill, 16 oz | 420 | 17 | 63 |
| **Swiss Miss,** Mixes, av., 1 packet | 120 | 2.5 | 22 |

## Cocoa - Chocolate Mixes

*Add extra cals/fat/carbohydrate for milk*
**Carnation Breakfast Drinks** ~ *See Page 38*

| | C | F | Cb |
|---|---|---|---|
| **Carnation:** *Per 3 Tbsp* | | | |
| Malted Milk: Original | 90 | 2 | 15 |
|   Chocolate | 90 | 1 | 18 |
| **Ghirardelli:** | | | |
| **Premium Hot Cocoa:** Caramel, 0.8 oz | 90 | 1 | 20 |
|   Chocolate Mocha, 3 Tbsp | 120 | 1.5 | 29 |
|   Double Chocolate, 3 Tbsp | 120 | 1.5 | 30 |
| **Hershey's,** Cocoa, | | | |
|   Natural, unsweetened, | | | |
|   1 Tbsp, 0.2 oz | 10 | 0.5 | 3 |
| **Land O Lakes:** | | | |
| Arctic White Cocoa, 1.3 oz | 160 | 6 | 26 |
| Other varieties, 1.3 oz | 140 | 3.5 | 26 |
| **Nestle:** *Per Per Single Serve Envelope* | | | |
| Chocolate Caramel | 100 | 3 | 19 |
| Dark Chocolate | 100 | 3 | 19 |
| Rich Milk Chocolate: | | | |
|   Regular | 80 | 3 | 14 |
|   Fat Free | 20 | 0 | 4 |
|   No Sugar Added Fat Free | 20 | 0 | 5 |
| **Nesquik Powder:** *Per 2 Tbsp* | | | |
| Chocolate; Strawberry | 50 | 0.5 | 12 |
| Chocolate No Added Sugar | 35 | 1 | 7 |
| **Ovaltine,** All Natural Cocoa Mixes, | | | |
|   average all varieties, 2 Tbsp | 40 | 0 | 10 |
| **Swiss Miss:** *Per Single Serve Envelope* | | | |
| **Breakfast Blends:** Great Start | 60 | 1 | 11 |
|   Pick Me Up | 110 | 2 | 23 |
| **Classics, Milk Chocolate:** | | | |
|   Hot Cocoa Mix | 90 | 2 | 16 |
|   No Added Sugar | 60 | 1 | 11 |
|   with Marshmallow | 90 | 2 | 16 |
|   Rich Chocolate | 120 | 2 | 23 |

## Instant Coffee    C   F   Cb

| | C | F | Cb |
|---|---|---|---|
| **Powder/Granules:** *Regular or Decaffeinated,* | | | |
|   1 level tsp | 2 | 0 | 0.5 |
|   1 rounded tsp | 4 | 0 | 1 |
| **Ground,** 3 tsp | 7 | 0 | 2 |
| **Brewed/Percolated,** 1 cup, 8 fl.oz | 4 | 0 | 1 |
| **Coffee with Milk/Cream/Creamers:** *Per 8 oz Cup* | | | |
| **Black:** | 4 | 0 | 1 |
|   with Whole Milk: Dash, 1 Tbsp | 15 | 0.5 | 2 |
|     2 Tbsp, 1 fl.oz | 25 | 1 | 2.5 |
|   with 2% Milk, 2 Tbsp | 20 | 0.5 | 2.5 |
|   with 1% Milk, 2 Tbsp | 20 | 0.5 | 2.5 |
|   with Fat Free Milk, 2 Tbsp | 15 | 0 | 2.5 |
|   with Soy Milk: 1 Tbsp | 10 | 0 | 1.5 |
|     2 Tbsp, 1 oz | 15 | 0.5 | 2 |
|   with Half & Half: 2 Tbsp | 50 | 3 | 3 |
|     1/4 cup, 2 fl.oz | 90 | 6 | 4 |
|   with Cream (light coffee), 2 Tbsp | 65 | 6 | 2 |
|     with Coffee Mate: Liquid, reg., 1 T. | 20 | 1 | 3 |
|     Liquid Fat Free, 1 Tbsp | 25 | 0 | 2 |
|     Powder, 1 heaping tsp | 15 | 1 | 2 |
| **Sugar ~ Add Extra:** 1 heaping tsp | 25 | 0 | 6 |
|   Single portion, 1 package | 25 | 0 | 6 |
| **Sweeteners,** *(Equal/Splenda/Sweet N Low),* | | | |
|   Powder, 1 package | 0 | 0 | 0 |

## Flavored Coffee Mixes

| | C | F | Cb |
|---|---|---|---|
| **Chicory:** | | | |
| Instant Coffee, 1 tsp | 5 | 0 | 1 |
| Coffee Essence, 1 tsp | 15 | 0 | 4 |
| **Caffé D'Vita:** | | | |
| Hot Cocoa, 1 oz | 110 | 1.5 | 24 |
| Hot Cocoa, Sugar Free, 0.5 oz | 70 | 4.5 | 7 |
| **General Foods International:** | | | |
| Average all varieties, 0.5 oz | 60 | 3 | 10 |
| Sugar-free, av. all varieties, 1 tsp | 30 | 2.5 | 2 |
| Cappuccino Coolers, all varieties, 0.5 oz | 60 | 0 | 15 |
| **Hills Bros:** *Per 3 Tbsp, 1 oz* | | | |
| **Cappuccino:** French Vanilla | 120 | 4.5 | 19 |
|   Chocolate Hazelnut | 110 | 3.5 | 19 |
|   Classic Cappuccino | 120 | 5 | 17 |
|   Dark Chocolate | 110 | 4 | 19 |
|   Mocha Mint | 120 | 4 | 20 |
| **Nescafe,** Memento, 1 stick, | | | |
|   average all varieties | 100 | 2.5 | 19 |
| **Starbucks,** VIA, Iced Coffee, | | | |
|   all varieties, 1 stick/packet | 100 | 0 | 24 |

## Coffee Shops/Restaurants

*Per 8 fl.oz Cup (Unless Indicated)*

| | C | F | Cb |
|---|---|---|---|
| **Coffee,** Regular/Percolated/Filtered | 5 | 0 | 0 |
| **Americano Drip Coffee,** 1 cup | 7.5 | 0 | 1 |
| **Cafe Au Lait:** 1 cup, 8 fl.oz | 60 | 3.5 | 5 |
| Nonfat Milk, 1 cup, 8 fl.oz | 35 | 0 | 5 |
| **Caffe Latté:** | | | |
| 8 fl.oz cup: with Whole Milk | 110 | 6 | 9 |
| with 2% Milk | 100 | 3.5 | 9 |
| with Nonfat Milk | 70 | 0 | 10 |
| 12 fl.oz: with Whole Milk | 180 | 9 | 14 |
| with Nonfat Milk | 100 | 0 | 15 |
| 16 fl.oz: with Whole Milk | 220 | 11 | 18 |
| with Nonfat Milk | 130 | 0 | 19 |
| **Cafe Mocha (Mochaccino):** 8 fl.oz | 150 | 6 | 20 |
| 12 fl.oz | 230 | 9 | 31 |
| 16 fl.oz | 290 | 12 | 41 |
| **Cappuccino:** | | | |
| 8 fl.oz cup: with Whole Milk | 90 | 3.5 | 7 |
| with 2% Milk | 80 | 3 | 8 |
| with Nonfat Milk | 50 | 0 | 8 |
| 12 fl.oz: with Whole Milk | 110 | 6 | 9 |
| with 2% Milk | 90 | 3.5 | 9 |
| with Nonfat Milk | 60 | 0 | 9 |
| 16 fl.oz: with Whole Milk | 140 | 7 | 11 |
| with 2% Milk | 120 | 3.5 | 11 |
| with Nonfat Milk | 80 | 0 | 12 |
| **Mocha:** *With Cream* | | | |
| 8 fl.oz: with Whole Milk | 200 | 11 | 22 |
| with Nonfat Milk | 160 | 6 | 22 |
| 12 fl.oz: Whole Milk | 290 | 15 | 33 |
| with Nonfat Milk | 230 | 8 | 34 |
| **Iced Mocha:** *Without Cream* | | | |
| 12 fl.oz: with Whole Milk | 170 | 6 | 26 |
| with Nonfat Milk | 130 | 2 | 27 |
| **Espresso:** Single (Solo), 1 fl.oz | 5 | 0 | 1 |
| Double (Doppio), 2 fl.oz | 10 | 0 | 2 |
| **Espresso con Panna,** | | | |
| (w/ dollop wh. cream), solo, 1 fl.oz | 30 | 2.5 | 2 |
| **Espresso Macchiato,** solo, 1 fl.oz | 5 | 0 | 1 |
| **Frappuccino:** Tall, 12 fl.oz | 180 | 2.5 | 37 |
| Grande, 16 fl.oz | 240 | 3 | 48 |
| **Frappuccino Mocha:** | | | |
| (with Cream): Tall, 12 fl.oz | 280 | 11 | 43 |
| Grande, 16 fl.oz | 380 | 15 | 57 |
| **Iced Latte,** Similar to Caffe Latte | | | |

McCafe (McDonald's) ~ *See Fast Food, Page 216*
Starbucks ~ *See Fast-Foods Section , Page 243*

## Coffee Substitute Mixes  C  F  Cb

**Roasted Cereal Beverages ~** *(No Caffeine)*

| | C | F | Cb |
|---|---|---|---|
| **Cafix,** Instant Beverage, 1 tsp | 5 | 0 | 1 |
| **Kaffree Roma,** Instant Beverage, 1 tsp | 10 | 0 | 2 |
| **Teeccino,** Herbal Coffees, 1 tsp | 10 | 0 | 2 |

## Irish & Liqueur Coffees

| | C | F | Cb |
|---|---|---|---|
| **Irish Coffee,** without sugar | 175 | 10 | 0 |
| **Liqueur Coffee,** with cream, | | | |
| all varieties, av., 1 fl.oz | 100 | 5 | 7 |

## Coffee Extras

| | C | F | Cb |
|---|---|---|---|
| Chocolate (Cocoa) Topping, $\frac{1}{2}$ tsp | 5 | 0 | 1 |
| Flavored Syrups: Regular, 2 Tbsp | 80 | 0 | 20 |
| Sugar-free, 2 Tbsp | 0 | 0 | 0 |
| Half & Half Cream: 2 Tbsp | 40 | 3.5 | 1 |
| Single serve pkg, $\frac{3}{8}$ fl.oz | 15 | 1.5 | 0.5 |
| Light whipped cream, 2 Tbsp | 15 | 1.5 | 1 |
| Marshmallows, miniature (2) | 5 | 0 | 1 |
| **Sugar:** | | | |
| 1 single portion package | 20 | 0 | 5 |
| 1 level tsp | 15 | 0 | 4 |
| 1 heaping tsp | 25 | 0 | 6 |
| *Equal/Splenda/Sweet 'N Low* | 0 | 0 | 0 |

## Coffee Shop ~ Cakes, Cookies

| | C | F | Cb |
|---|---|---|---|
| **Cookies:** | | | |
| Biscotti, 1 oz | 140 | 6.5 | 18 |
| Chocolate Chip, 3 oz | 350 | 15 | 54 |
| Oatmeal Raisin, 3 oz | 350 | 12 | 56 |
| Peanut Butter, 3 oz | 410 | 25 | 39 |
| White Choc. Macadamia, 3.33 oz | 420 | 20 | 55 |
| **Cakes/Pastries:** | | | |
| Almond Croissant, 5 oz | 620 | 35 | 67 |
| Apple Danish, 5 oz | 450 | 18 | 67 |
| Banana Walnut, 4.5 oz | 410 | 17 | 60 |
| Brownie, 3 oz | 390 | 24 | 42 |
| Bundt, Chocolate, 4 oz | 440 | 21 | 61 |
| Carrot Cake, 4 oz | 400 | 22 | 45 |
| Chocolate Cake, 5 oz | 530 | 28 | 65 |
| Crumble Coffee Cake, 4.5 oz | 500 | 25 | 65 |
| Cupcake, 3 oz | 330 | 16 | 43 |
| Pound Cake, av., 3 oz | 330 | 17 | 40 |
| **Cinnamon Roll,** 6 oz | 500 | 15 | 83 |
| **Donuts:** | | | |
| Sugared, 1.8 oz | 220 | 11 | 27 |
| Glazed, 2 oz | 250 | 12 | 34 |
| **Pretzel,** large, 4 oz | 290 | 5 | 52 |

Starbucks Bakery Items ~ *See Page 244*

## READY TO DRINK COFFEE  Ⓒ Ⓕ Ⓒ

### Bottled & Chilled:
**Califia Farms:** *With Almond Milk*

| | C | F | Cb |
|---|---|---|---|
| Cold Brew Coffee, av., 10.5 fl.oz | 115 | 4.5 | 18 |
| **Dunkin Donuts:** | | | |
| Iced Coffee, av., 13.7 fl.oz | 290 | 6 | 47 |
| **International Delight:** | | | |
| **Iced,** all flavors, 8 fl.oz | 150 | 2.5 | 29 |
| **Light varieties,** 8 fl.oz | 90 | 2.5 | 14 |
| **Kahlua,** Cappuccino Shake, 10.5 fl.oz | 130 | 2 | 24 |
| **Starbucks:** | | | |
| **Cold Brew:** *Per 11 fl.oz* | | | |
| Regular | 50 | 0 | 13 |
| Unsweetened | 15 | 0 | 3 |
| Cocoa & Honey, w/ Cream | 150 | 5 | 24 |
| Vanilla & Fig, w/ Cream | 150 | 4 | 24 |
| **Doubleshot Energy:** *Per 15 fl.oz Can* | | | |
| Coffee Drink | 210 | 2.5 | 36 |
| Hazelnut Drink | 210 | 3 | 31 |
| Mocha/Vanilla Drink | 205 | 2.5 | 34 |
| White Chocolate Drink | 210 | 3 | 31 |
| **Doubleshot Espresso:** *Per 6.5 fl.oz Can* | | | |
| Espresso & Cream | 140 | 6 | 18 |
| Espresso & Cream Light | 70 | 4 | 5 |
| **Frappuccino Coffee Drink:** *Per 9.5 fl.oz Bottle* | | | |
| Mocha | 180 | 3 | 33 |
| Light Mocha | 100 | 3 | 12 |
| Vanilla | 200 | 3 | 37 |
| **Iced Coffee:** *Per 11 fl.oz Bottle* | | | |
| Coffee: with Milk, sweetened | 110 | 0.5 | 23 |
| Light, sweetened | 50 | 0 | 11 |
| Caramel; Vanilla, swtnd, av. | 110 | 0.5 | 23 |
| Vanilla | 120 | 0.5 | 22 |
| **Iced Espresso Classics (Chilled):** *Per 8 fl.oz Bottle* | | | |
| Caffe Mocha | 140 | 2.5 | 23 |
| Caramel Macchiato; Van. Latte | 130 | 2.5 | 21 |
| **Skinny,** Caramel Macchiato, Van. Latte | 70 | 0 | 10 |

**Starbucks Refreshers** ~ *See Page 40*

**TruMoo:**

| **Coffee Milk:** | C | F | Cb |
|---|---|---|---|
| Low-Fat (1%), 8 fl.oz | 130 | 2.5 | 20 |
| Fat-Free, 8 fl.oz | 110 | 0 | 20 |

### Tips to Reduce the Calories in Your Coffee Drinks:
- Request non-fat milk in place of whole or 2% milk
- Downsize to 8 fl.oz or 12 fl.oz
- Avoid cream on frappuccinos
- Replace sugar with *Equal, Splenda, Stevia* or *Sweet 'N Low*
- Avoid syrup add-ons

## CAFFEINE COUNTER

Moderate caffeine intake is not harmful to healthy adults. However, frequent large amounts (over 350mg/day) may cause dependency ('caffeinism') and adversely affect health. **To be safe, limit caffeine to 200mg/day.** Avoid if pregnant, breastfeeding, a child under 8, have sleep problems, an overactive bladder or heart arrhythmia.

| | Caffeine (mg) |
|---|---|
| **Coffee: Instant:** Weak, 1 level teaspoon | 30 |
| Medium, 1 rounded teaspoon | 60 |
| Strong, 1 heaping teaspoon | 100 |
| **Decaffeinated**, 1 rounded teaspoon | 2 |
| **Bags (Folgers)**, 1 bag (6-8 cups) | 115 |
| **Ground**, 1 Tbsp, 0.2 oz | 60 |
| **Bottled (Ready-To-Drink)**, 9.5 fl.oz | 70 |
| **Coffee Shop:** Brewed, 8 fl.oz | 110-150 |
| **Cappuccino/Latte:** 1 cup, 8 fl.oz | 75 |
| Tall, 12 fl.oz | 110 |
| Large, 16 fl.oz | 150 |
| **Decappuccino**, decaffeinated | 5 |
| **Espresso:** Regular/Single/Solo | 75 |
| Double/Doppio | 150 |
| Iced Coffee w/o Milk, 12 fl.oz | 140 |
| Latte, 1 cup, 8 fl.oz | 75 |
| Mocha, 1 cup, 8 fl.oz | 90 |
| Hot Chocolate, 8 fl.oz | 15 |
| **Black Tea:** Weak, 1 cup | 20 |
| Medium Strength, 1 cup | 40 |
| Strong, 1 cup | 70 |
| Decaffeinated Tea, 1 cup | 0-5 |
| Herbal Tea, 1 cup | 0 |
| **Green Tea**, 1 cup | 20 |
| **Iced Tea**, tall glass/can, 12 fl.oz | 20-30 |
| **Soft Drinks:** *Per 12 fl.oz Can* | |
| *Coca-Cola; Pepsi (Regular/Diet)* | 35 |
| *Diet Coke; TAB; RC Cola (Regular)* | 45 |
| *Dr. Pepper; Sunkist Orange* | 40 |
| *Pepsi One; Mountain Dew; Mellow Yellow; Surge* | 55 |
| *Pepsi Max (Regular/Diet) Sun Drop (Reg/Diet)* | 70 |
| *7-Up, Fanta, Sprite, Fresca, Diet Rite Cola* | 0 |
| **Energy Drinks (with added caffeine):** | |
| *(AMP, Adrenaline Rush, Full Throttle Monster, No Fear, Red Bull, Rockstar)* | |
| **Average all brands:** 8 fl.oz | 80 |
| 16 fl.oz | 160 |
| **NOS Energy**, 16 fl.oz | 260 |
| **Chocolate Bars:** Milk Chocolate, 2 oz | 20 |
| Dark Chocolate, 2 oz | 30 |
| **Choc Chip Cookies**, 2 medium, 2 oz | 6 |
| **Chocolate Syrup**, 2 Tbsp, 1.4 oz | 5 |
| **Guarana**, *GNC*, 1 tablet | 90 |
| **Medicinals:** *Excedrin Extra/Migraine*, 1 tab. | 65 |
| *Jet Alert/NoDoz*, 1 tablet | 200 |
| *Stay Awake (Walgreens)*, *Vivarin*, 1 tab. | 200 |

| Energy/Protein Drinks | C | F | Cb |
|---|---|---|---|
| **365** *(Wholefoods)*: | | | |
| Energy Shots, all flav., 2 fl.oz | 25 | 0 | 6 |
| **5-hour Energy,** 2 fl.oz | 4 | 0 | 1 |
| **A.B.B.** | | | |
| **Beyond The Gym:** | | | |
| Amino Force, Watermelon, 22 fl.oz | 25 | 0 | 5 |
| Ripped Force, Fruit Punch, 18 fl.oz | 90 | 0 | 23 |
| **Post Work Out:** | | | |
| Max Recovery, Fruit Punch, 18 fl.oz | 390 | 0.5 | 60 |
| Pure Pro: 35, Van. Smoothie, 12 fl.oz | 170 | 0.5 | 5 |
| 50, Milk Chocolate | 260 | 4.5 | 7 |
| XXL, Strawb. Banana, 22 fl.oz | 910 | 1 | 180 |
| **Pre Work Out:** | | | |
| Speed Shot, Grape, 8.5 fl.oz | 5 | 0 | 1 |
| Speed Stack: Fruit Punch, 18 fl.oz | 5 | 0 | 1 |
| Pumped, Blue Raspb., 22 fl.oz | 30 | 0 | 8 |
| **AdvantEDGE** *(EAS)*, | | | |
| **Powders:** Milk Chocolate, 0.77 oz | 70 | 0 | 2 |
| Lean 15 Protein, 1 oz | 90 | 0.5 | 8 |
| Vegan Soy, Choc., 0.77 oz | 180 | 2 | 20 |
| **RTD:** Shakes, av., 11 fl.oz | 130 | 1 | 6 |
| Carb Control, Cold Brew Coffee, 11 fl.oz | 100 | 2.5 | 3 |
| **All Sport:** Zero, 20 fl.oz | 0 | 0 | 0 |
| Hydration, Blue Raz, 20 fl.oz | 150 | 0 | 40 |
| Zero, 20 fl.oz | 0 | 0 | 0 |
| **AMP** ~ *See Mtn Dew AMP* | | | |
| **Arizona:** | | | |
| **Caution Extreme Performance:** *Per 11.5 fl.oz* | | | |
| Original; Fruit Punch, average | 140 | 0 | 36 |
| **RX Energy,** Herbal Tonic, 16 fl.oz | 180 | 0 | 46 |
| **Shots,** average, 2 fl.oz | 5 | 0 | 1 |
| **Atkins,** Energy Shakes, av., 11 fl.oz | 155 | 9 | 4 |
| **Bariatrix:** *Per 8.45 fl.oz Bottle* | | | |
| **Proti Anytime,** RTD Shakes, av. | 100 | 4 | 4 |
| **Meal Repl. Powder,** all, 2.36 oz | 250 | 3.5 | 21 |
| **Bawls Guarana,** av.,16 fl.oz can | 95 | 0 | 23 |
| **Blue Sky,** Blue Energy Drink, 16 fl.oz | 240 | 0 | 58 |
| **BodyArmor,** SuperDrinks, 16 fl.oz | 140 | 0 | 36 |
| **Bolthouse,** Breakfast Smoothies, | | | |
| Peach/Strawb. Parfait, average | 190 | 2.5 | 35 |
| **Protein Plus:** Choc.; Mango, av. | 205 | 2 | 31 |
| Vanilla Bean | 170 | 3 | 21 |
| **Boost** *(Nestle)*: | | | |
| **Original,** all flavors, 8 fl.oz | 240 | 4 | 41 |
| **CalorieSmart,** all flav., 8 fl.oz | 180 | 7 | 16 |
| **Glucose Control,** all flavors, 8 fl.oz | 190 | 7 | 16 |
| **High Protein,** all flav, 8 fl.oz | 240 | 6 | 28 |
| **Max 30g Prot. Shake,** Rich Choc., 11 fl.oz | 160 | 2 | 7 |
| **Plus,** all flavors, 8 fl.oz | 360 | 14 | 45 |

| | C | F | Cb |
|---|---|---|---|
| **Carnation:** | | | |
| **B'Fast Essentials, Powder:** | | | |
| Av. all flav., 1 env., 1.3 oz | 130 | 1 | 27 |
| Light Start, av. , 0.7 oz | 60 | 0.5 | 12 |
| **Ready To Drink:** Reg., all flav., 8 fl.oz | 240 | 4 | 41 |
| High Protein, average, 8 fl.oz | 220 | 6 | 28 |
| **CeraSport:** EX1 Powder, 2.1 oz | 20 | 0 | 5 |
| Endurance Powder, Van., 1.5 oz pkt | 150 | 0 | 30 |
| Plus Powder, Strawb. Flavor, 1.09 oz | 120 | 0 | 30 |
| Ready To Drink, Citrus, 8.5 fl.oz | 40 | 0 | 10 |
| **Champion Lyte,** Sports Drink, 8 fl.oz | 0 | 0 | 0 |
| **Clif:** Protein Mix, Chocolate, 1.6 oz | 160 | 0 | 31 |
| Shot, Energy Gel, av., 1.2 oz pkt | 100 | 0 | 24 |
| **Coca Cola Energy:** Reg., 8.45 fl.oz | 105 | 0 | 26 |
| No Sugar Added, 8.45 fl.oz | 3 | 0 | 1.5 |
| **Cocaine,** av all, 12 fl.oz can | 90 | 0 | 23 |
| **Core Power:** | | | |
| **26g,** av. all flavors, 14 fl.oz | 170 | 4.5 | 6 |
| **Elite,** 42g, av. all flav., 14 fl.oz | 240 | 3.5 | 11 |
| **Curves,** Prot. Drink, Choc.; Van., 1 oz | 120 | 2 | 11 |
| **EAS** ~ *See AdvantEdge & Myoplex* | | | |
| **Ensure:** *Per Bottle* | | | |
| **Original,** av. all flavors, 8 fl.oz | 220 | 6 | 32 |
| **Clear,** all flavors, 10 fl.oz | 180 | 0 | 37 |
| **Enlive,** av. all flavors, 8 fl.oz | 350 | 11 | 44 |
| **High Protein,** all flav., 8 fl.oz | 160 | 2 | 19 |
| **Max Protein,** all flavors, 8 fl.oz | 150 | 1.5 | 6 |
| **Plus,** av. all flavors, 8 fl.oz | 350 | 11 | 50 |
| **Enterex:** Original, powder, 2 oz | 250 | 9 | 34 |
| Diabetic, all flavors, 8 fl.oz | 220 | 8 | 25 |
| Plus, all flavors, 8 fl.oz | 350 | 11 | 50 |
| Renal, all flavors, 8 fl.oz | 480 | 20 | 56 |
| Total, all flavors, 8 fl.oz e | 220 | 9 | 9 |
| **Enu,** Compl.Nutrit. Shakes, 8.4 fl.oz | 340 | 13 | 39 |
| **Fruit₂O (Veryfine):** Classic 20 fl.oz | 0 | 0 | 0 |
| Sparkling, 20 fl.oz | 0 | 0 | 1 |
| **Full Throttle:** *Per 16 fl.oz* | | | |
| **Energy:** Citrus; Blue Agave | 220 | 0 | 58 |
| Orange | 220 | 0 | 52 |
| **Fuze:** | | | |
| **Fusions:** Berry Punch, 8 fl.oz | 80 | 0 | 21 |
| Strawb. Lemonade, 8 fl.oz | 100 | 0 | 26 |
| **Gatorade G Series:** | | | |
| **Endurance Formula,** all flav., 12 fl.oz | 90 | 0 | 22 |
| **Thirst Quencher:** All flav, 20 fl.oz | 140 | 0 | 36 |
| G2, 12 fl.oz | 30 | 0 | 8 |
| Zero (no sugar), 20 fl.oz | 5 | 0 | 1 |
| **Prime,** Sports Fuel, 4 fl.oz | 100 | 0 | 25 |
| **Recover,** Protein Shakes, 11.2 fl.oz | 280 | 1 | 46 |
| **Whey Protein Powder:** | | | |
| Chocolate, ⅓ cup, 1.1 oz | 120 | 2 | 6 |
| Other Flavors, ⅓ cup, 1 oz | 110 | 1.5 | 4 |
| **Genisoy,** Prot. Pdr, Choc.; Van., 1.3 oz | 125 | 0 | 18 |

| Glaceau: | C | F | Cb |
|---|---|---|---|
| **Vitaminwater,** av. all flav., 20 fl.oz | 120 | 0 | 33 |
| **Glucerna:** Shakes, all flavors, 8 fl.oz | 180 | 9 | 16 |
| Hunger Smart Shakes, av., 8 fl.oz | 180 | 8 | 15 |
| Snack Shake, all flavors, 8 fl.oz | 140 | 5 | 19 |
| **GNC:** | | | |
| **Pro Performance:** | | | |
| Amplified, Mass XXX, all flav., 4 sc. | 750 | 6 | 124 |
| AMP, RTD, Wheybolic 40, Vanilla, 14 fl.oz | 190 | 1.5 | 6 |
| **Total Lean Shakes:** 25, av., 1 scoop | 200 | 3 | 19 |
| Burn, all flavors, 14 fl.oz | 170 | 0.5 | 11 |
| Classic, all flavors, 1 scoop | 175 | 2 | 30 |
| **Guru:** | | | |
| **Org. Energy Drink:** Regular, 8 oz can | 80 | 0 | 21 |
| Lite, 12 oz can | 10 | 0 | 2 |
| **Herbalife:** Nutritional Shakes, 0.9 oz | 90 | 1 | 13 |
| with 8 fl.oz non-fat milk | 170 | 1 | 26 |
| **Hormel:** Med Pass Shakes, 8 fl.oz | 480 | 19 | 58 |
| Mighty Shakes, Frozen, 6 fl.oz | 330 | 10 | 50 |
| Vital Quisine, 500 Shake, average | 520 | 21 | 60 |
| **Hype:** *Per 8.5 fl.oz* | | | |
| **After Dark** | 130 | 0 | 30 |
| **Enlite** | 25 | 0 | 4 |
| **MFP,** | 110 | 0 | 25 |
| **Mohito** | 120 | 0 | 28 |
| **Twisted,** Tropical Punch | 100 | 0 | 24 |
| **Up,** Ice Berry Max | 120 | 0 | 28 |
| **Shot,** 3.5 fl.oz | 35 | 0 | 8.5 |
| **Jarrow:** | | | |
| **Whey Protein:** Unflav., 0.8 oz | 90 | 2 | 1 |
| Flavors, average, 1 oz | 105 | 1.5 | 4 |
| **Kellogg's:** | | | |
| **To Go B'fast Shake,** Milk Choc., 10 fl.oz | 180 | 5 | 29 |
| **Knudsen:** | | | |
| **Recharge,** average, 8 fl.oz | 75 | 0 | 18 |
| **Simply Nutritious,** average, 8 fl.oz | 120 | 0 | 28 |
| **Kroger:** *Per 8 fl.oz Bottle* | | | |
| **Nutritional Shake,** all flavors | 190 | 7 | 23 |
| **Nutrition Shake,** Fortify Plus, av., | 350 | 11 | 50 |
| **La Brada:** | | | |
| **Lean Body,** Powder, av., 1.4 oz scoop | 155 | 3 | 8 |
| **RTD,** Lean Body, 17 fl.oz | 280 | 9 | 9 |
| **Lindora Protein Shakes:** | | | |
| Berry Cream Smoothie, 1 pkt | 100 | 1 | 7 |
| Prot. Choc. Shake, 1 sc., 1 oz | 110 | 1.5 | 10 |
| RTD: Chocolate, 8.5 fl.oz | 100 | 4 | 3 |
| Vanilla, 8.5 fl.oz | 110 | 4 | 3 |
| **Liquid Ice:** Black, 8.3 fl.oz | 110 | 0 | 26 |
| Other flavors, 8.3 fl.oz | 120 | 0 | 28 |
| **Liquid Lightning,** Reg., 12 fl.oz | 120 | 0 | 31 |
| **Met-Rx:** | | | |
| **51 Shakes,** average, 15 fl.oz | 250 | 2 | 6 |
| **Meal Repl. Powder,** av., 2.5 oz | 255 | 2.5 | 20 |
| **N.O.S. Pumped,** all flav., 16.9 fl.oz | 60 | 0 | 11 |

| Monster: | C | F | Cb |
|---|---|---|---|
| **Energy:** Regular, 16 fl.oz | 210 | 0 | 54 |
| Lo-Carb, 16 fl.oz | 25 | 0 | 7 |
| M-80, 16 fl.oz | 180 | 0 | 46 |
| Mixxd (with juice), 16 fl.oz | 220 | 0 | 54 |
| **Java Monster:** All flav., 15 fl.oz | 190 | 3 | 33 |
| Light, Vanilla, 15 fl.oz | 95 | 3 | 13 |
| **Shakes,** 16 fl.oz can | 220 | 4 | 20 |
| **MRM:** Whey, 1 scoop, 0.9 oz | 100 | 1.5 | 4 |
| Low Carb Protein, 1 scoop, 1.1 oz | 120 | 2.5 | 2 |
| Veggie Meal Replacement, 1.7 oz | 190 | 5 | 14 |
| **Mtn Dew AMP:** *Per 16 fl.oz* | | | |
| **Energy:** Orig.; Strawb. Limeade | 220 | 0 | 58 |
| Cherry Blast; Trop. Punch, av. | 110 | 0 | 28 |
| **Game Fuel Charged,** all flav. | 90 | 0 | 24 |
| **Muscle Milk** *(Cytosport)*: | | | |
| **Gainer,** powder, av. all flav., 2.85 oz | 315 | 4.5 | 55 |
| **Non Dairy RTD:** All flavors, 17 fl.oz | 320 | 15 | 13 |
| **100 Calorie Shakes,** av., 11 fl.oz | 100 | 1.5 | 6 |
| **Coffee House,** average, 11 fl.oz | 135 | 4 | 7 |
| **Collegiate,** average, 11 fl.oz | 235 | 6 | 28 |
| **Genuine,** average, 11 fl.oz | 160 | 4.5 | 6 |
| **Pro Series,** av. all flavors, 14 fl.oz | 200 | 2.5 | 9 |
| **Yogurt Protein Shakes,** 16 fl.oz | 260 | 4.5 | 28 |
| **Muscle Tech:** | | | |
| Mass-Tech Extremme 2000, | | | |
| Vanilla, 7 scoops, 20 oz | 2060 | 5 | 443 |
| Nitro Tech, Ripped, average, 1.5 oz | 170 | 4 | 4 |
| **Myoplex** *(EAS)*: | | | |
| **Ready To Drink Shakes:** | | | |
| Keto, German Choc., 11 fl.oz | 200 | 17 | 3 |
| Shred, Muscle Mocha, 16 fl.oz | 210 | 2 | 8 |
| **Powder:** Ketogenics, 2.32 oz pkt | 400 | 32 | 5 |
| Muscle Armor, 0.9 oz scp | 95 | 0 | 6 |
| Original, 0.9 oz scoop | 300 | 6 | 21 |
| Lite, 1.9 oz pkt | 180 | 2 | 24 |
| **Nature's Best:** | | | |
| **Isopure Powder:** | | | |
| Orig., all flav., 1.75 oz | 300 | 1 | 25 |
| Anytime Energy, all flav., 0.2 oz | 5 | 0 | 1 |
| Plant Based Prot., av., 1 sc. | 110 | 1.5 | 3 |
| **Isopue RTD:** Cocotein, all, 16 fl.oz | 100 | 0 | 6 |
| Mass, all flavors, 20 fl.oz | 50 | 0 | 53 |
| **Nestle Health Science,** | | | |
| **Diabetishield,** Mixed Berry, 8 fl.oz | 150 | 0 | 30 |
| **No-Fear:** Regular, 16 fl.oz | 260 | 0 | 72 |
| Sugar Free, 16 fl.oz | 20 | 0 | 2 |
| **NOS,** High Performance Energy: | | | |
| Orig.; Nitro Mango, 16 fl.oz | 210 | 0 | 54 |
| Sonic Sour; Power Punch, 16 fl.oz | 220 | 0 | 53 |
| **Nutrament** *(Nestle)*, all flav., 12 fl.oz | 360 | 10 | 52 |

## Energy/Protein Drinks (Cont)

| | C | F | Cb |
|---|---|---|---|
| **Nutrilite** *(Amway)*: | | | |
| **BodyKey Meal Replacement Shakes:** | | | |
| Powder, av. all flavors, 1.2 oz scoop | 110 | 3 | 8 |
| **Optifast:** *(Nestle)*: | | | |
| HP Shake Mix, 1 pkg | 200 | 6 | 10 |
| RTD Shakes & Shake Mix Pdr, 8 fl.oz | 160 | 3.5 | 18 |
| **Optimum Nutrition:** | | | |
| **Gold Standard:** | | | |
| 100% Whey, av. all flavors, 1 oz scp | 125 | 1.5 | 4 |
| Gainer, av. all flav., 7.9 oz scoop | 770 | 10 | 113 |
| **Hydro Whey,** average, 1.4 oz scoop | 145 | 1 | 3 |
| **Protein Water,** average, 16 fl.oz | 85 | 0 | 2 |
| **Optisource** *(Nestle)*, | | | |
| **Very High Prot. Drink,** all flav., 8 fl.oz | 200 | 6 | 12 |
| **Orgain:** | | | |
| **Nutritional Shake:** Organic, all, 11 fl.oz | 250 | 7 | 32 |
| Vegan, Smooth Chocolate, 11 fl.oz | 220 | 6 | 25 |
| **Protein Shake,** Vegan, Choc., 14 fl.oz | 150 | 5 | 15 |
| **Powerade,** average, 12 fl.oz | 80 | 0 | 21 |
| **Premier Protein** *(Premier Nutrition)*: | | | |
| **Clear,** 16.9 fl.oz | 90 | 0 | 1 |
| **Shakes,** average, 11 fl.oz bottle | 160 | 3 | 5 |
| **Propel,** Vitamin Boost, all flav., 20 fl.oz | 10 | 0 | 2 |
| **Protein2O:** *Per 16.89 fl.oz* | | | |
| **Protein Water:** 15g Protein + Energy, | | | |
| Blueb. Raspb.; Cherry Lemonade, av | 70 | 0 | 1 |
| 10g Protein, all flavors | 60 | 0 | 5 |
| **Pure Protein:** *Per 11 fl.oz Bottle or Can* | | | |
| **30 Gram Shakes,** average | 140 | 2 | 6 |
| **35 Gram Shakes:** Banana | 150 | 1 | 1 |
| Average other flavors | 165 | 1 | 3 |
| **Powder,** av., 1 scoop, 1.16 oz | 130 | 2 | 6 |
| **Red Bull:** | | | |
| **Energy Drink:** Average, 8.4 fl.oz | 110 | 0 | 28 |
| 12 fl.oz can | 160 | 0 | 40 |
| Sugar-Free, 8.4 fl.oz | 5 | 0 | 3 |
| Zero Calories, 8.4 fl.oz | 0 | 0 | 0 |
| **Revival:** | | | |
| **Protein Water,** all flavors, 1.2 oz pkt | 70 | 0 | 2 |
| **Soy Mix, unsweetened:** | | | |
| Plain, 2 scoops, 0.95 oz | 105 | 1 | 4 |
| Average all flavors, 1 pkt | 115 | 2.5 | 5 |
| **Soy Mix with Fructose:** Van., 1 pkt | 220 | 2 | 31 |
| Averae other flavors 1 pkt | 235 | 2.5 | 35 |
| **Rhino's:** Energy, av. all flav, 3.5 ml | 50 | 0 | 11 |
| Rush, all flavors, 8 fl.oz | 0 | 0 | 0 |
| **Rip It,** Energy Fuel, all flav., 16 fl.oz | 200 | 0 | 52 |
| **Rockstar:** *Per 16 fl.oz Can* | | | |
| **Energy Drink:** Punched, av. | 270 | 0 | 62 |
| Sugar Free | 20 | 0 | 0 |

| | C | F | Cb |
|---|---|---|---|
| **Rumble,** | | | |
| **Supershakes,** all flav. 12 fl.oz | 250 | 8 | 26 |
| **Rush:** *Per 8.4 fl.oz* | | | |
| **Energy Drink:** Regular | 120 | 0 | 32 |
| with Maca, 8 fl.oz | 130 | 0 | 30 |
| **Skratch Labs:** | | | |
| **Hydration Drink Mix:** *16 fl. oz Prepared* | | | |
| Anytime Mix, all flav., 1 scoop, 0.46 oz | 50 | 0 | 12 |
| Hyper Hydration, Passion Fruit, 0.8 oz | 80 | 0 | 17 |
| Sports, average, 0.76 oz | 80 | 0 | 20 |
| Wellness, average, 0.75 oz | 70 | 0 | 18 |
| **Recovery Mix,** av., 1.76 oz | 200 | 3.5 | 35 |
| **Slim-Fast:** Orig. Prot. Shakes, av., 11 fl.oz | 180 | 5 | 24 |
| **Advanced:** High Prot. Shakes, 11 fl.oz | 180 | 9 | 6 |
| Smoothie Mix, av., 1 scoop, 0.9 oz | 110 | 3.5 | 8 |
| **Diabetic Wt. Loss,** av., 1 sc., 0.9 oz | 100 | 7 | 11 |
| **Keto Meal Shake,** av., 2 sc., 1.34 oz | 190 | 15 | 9 |
| **SoBe:** *Per 20 fl.oz bottle* | | | |
| **Elixirs,** average | 250 | 1 | 63 |
| **Green Tea** | 200 | 0 | 52 |
| **Water:** Pacific Coconut | 8 | 0 | 21 |
| 0-Cal Water, all flavors | 0 | 0 | 0 |
| **Solixir,** Energy Drink, av. all, 12 fl.oz | 55 | 0 | 13 |
| **Special K,** Protein Shakes, av. all flav. | 185 | 5 | 23 |
| **Speed,** Vitamin Energy Drink, 16 fl.oz | 240 | 0 | 56 |
| **Spiru-Tein:** | | | |
| **Gold Shake,** Chocolate, 1 scoop, 1.2 oz | 90 | 0 | 21 |
| **High Protein Energy Meal Shakes:** | | | |
| Average all flavors, 1 scoop, 1.2 oz | 105 | 0.5 | 14 |
| **Plus,** Vanilla, 1 scoop, 1.2 oz | 120 | 0 | 18 |
| **Whey Protein Powder,** 1 sc., 1.2 oz | 125 | 2 | 15 |
| **Starbucks,** Refreshers, av.,12 fl.oz | 90 | 0 | 26 |
| **Doubleshot Energy** ~ *See page 37* | | | |
| **Steaz:** Energy, all flav., 12 fl.oz | 135 | 0 | 35 |
| Zero Calorie, Berry, 12 fl.oz | 0 | 0 | 0 |
| **Twin Lab,** Whey Fuel, 1 scoop, 1.4 oz | 150 | 3.5 | 5 |
| **Vega,** Protein Shake, av., 11 fl.oz | 170 | 4.5 | 14 |
| **Venom:** Mojave Rattler, 16 fl.oz | 45 | 0 | 8 |
| Av. other varieties, 16 fl.oz | 225 | 0 | 57 |
| Low Calorie, all flavors | 15 | 0 | 9 |
| *Note: Low Calorie options carbs contain 8g Erythritol* | | | |
| **Vital Whey** *(Well Wisdom)*, | | | |
| Natural, 1 scoop, 0.7 oz | 85 | 1 | 2 |
| **Weider:** 100% Whey, 1 sc., 1.4 oz | 160 | 3 | 12 |
| Dynamic Wt Gainer, av., 4.5 oz | 460 | 2 | 96 |
| Mega Mass: 2000, av., 3.5 oz | 400 | 7 | 61 |
| 4000, average, av., 3.5 oz | 400 | 7 | 60 |
| **XS** *(Amway)*, Energy Drink 8.4 oz | 10 | 0 | 0 |
| **Zola Acai:** | | | |
| **Original Acai,** 8 fl.oz | 140 | 3.5 | 26 |
| **Coconut Water,** Espresso, 8 fl.oz | 60 | 0 | 14 |
| **Hydrating Energy,** Dragon Fruit, 12 fl.oz | 110 | 0 | 26 |
| **Spark. Energy Water,** all flav., 12 fl.oz | 10 | 0 | 3 |

## Quick Guide    C  F  Cb

### Orange Juice
*Average ~ Fresh*

| | C | F | Cb |
|---|---|---|---|
| 1/2 Cup, 4 fl.oz | 55 | 0 | 13 |
| Small Glass, 6 fl.oz | 85 | 0 | 19 |
| Regular Cup 8 fl.oz | 110 | 0.5 | 26 |
| Regular Glass, 12 fl.oz | 160 | 0.5 | 39 |
| 10 fl.oz Bottle | 140 | 0.5 | 32 |
| 11.5 fl.oz Can | 160 | 0.5 | 37 |
| 16 fl.oz Bottle | 225 | 1 | 52 |
| 20 fl.oz Bottle | 280 | 1 | 64 |

### Juices ~ Generic

*Average All Brands:*

| | C | F | Cb |
|---|---|---|---|
| Aloe Vera Juice, unsweetened, 2 oz | 10 | 0 | 0 |
| Apple Juice: 8 fl.oz | 120 | 0 | 29 |
| 10 fl.oz Bottle | 145 | 0.5 | 36 |
| 16 fl.oz | 235 | 0.5 | 58 |
| Cactus Water, 1 Cup, 8 oz | 25 | 0 | 6 |
| Carrot Juice: Fresh, 6 fl.oz | 35 | 0 | 8 |
| Sweetened, 6 fl.oz | 75 | 0 | 17 |
| Coconut Water, 8 fl.oz | 50 | 0.5 | 9 |
| Cranberry Juice, Cocktail/Blend | 140 | 0 | 34 |
| Fruit Blends, average all, 8 fl.oz | 110 | 0 | 27 |
| Fruit Nectars, average all, 8 fl.oz | 140 | 0 | 36 |
| Grape Juice, 8 fl.oz | 155 | 0 | 38 |
| Grapefruit Juice, 8 fl.oz | 95 | 0 | 22 |
| Lemon/Lime Juice: 1 Tbsp | 5 | 0 | 1 |
| 1 cup, 8 fl.oz | 50 | 0.5 | 16 |
| Concentrate, 1 tsp | 0 | 0 | 0 |
| Noni Juice: | | | |
| Tahitian, 2 Tbsp, 1 fl.oz | 15 | 0 | 3 |
| Tahiti Traders, 1 fl.oz | 20 | 0 | 5 |
| Papaya/Peach Nectar, av., 8 fl.oz | 140 | 0 | 36 |
| Passion Fruit Juice, Fresh: | | | |
| Purple, 1 cup, 8 fl.oz | 125 | 0 | 34 |
| Yellow, 1 cup, 8 fl.oz | 80 | 1.5 | 14 |
| Pear Nectar, 8 fl.oz | 150 | 0 | 40 |
| Pineapple Juice, 8 fl.oz | 130 | 0 | 32 |
| Pomegranate Juice, 8 fl.oz | 160 | 0 | 40 |
| Prune Juice, 8 fl.oz | 180 | 0 | 45 |
| Strawberry/Raspberry Juice, 8 fl.oz | 100 | 0 | 23 |
| Tangerine Juice, 8 fl.oz | 105 | 0.5 | 25 |
| Tomato Juice, 8 fl.oz | 40 | 0 | 10 |
| Vegetable Juice, 8 fl.oz | 45 | 0 | 11 |
| Wheat Grass Juice: | | | |
| 1 fl.oz 'Shot' | 10 | 0 | 1.5 |
| 2 fl.oz 'Shot' | 20 | 0 | 3 |

## Quick Guide    C  F  Cb

### Fruit Smoothies (Jamba Juice; Smoothie King)
*Average All Brands*

| | C | F | Cb |
|---|---|---|---|
| Fruit Only: 8 fl.oz | 115 | 0.5 | 29 |
| 12 fl.oz | 175 | 1 | 43 |
| 16 fl.oz | 230 | 1 | 58 |
| 24 fl.oz | 350 | 1 | 78 |
| Fruit + Non-Fat Milk/Soy: | | | |
| 12 fl.oz | 135 | 0 | 29 |
| 16 fl.oz | 155 | 0 | 37 |
| 24 fl.oz | 265 | 1 | 59 |
| Fruit + Non-Fat Frozen Yogurt/Sherbet: | | | |
| 12 fl.oz | 200 | 0.5 | 47 |
| 16 fl.oz | 265 | 1 | 63 |
| 24 fl.oz | 395 | 1.5 | 95 |

### Juice ~ Brands

*Per 8 fl.oz Unless Indicated*

**Apple & Eve:**

**100% Juice, No Sugar Added:**

| | C | F | Cb |
|---|---|---|---|
| Cherries & Berries; Cranb. Raspb., av. | 120 | 0 | 29 |
| Cranberry Apple | 130 | 0 | 33 |
| Cranberry Pomegranate | 140 | 0 | 34 |
| Fruitables, av. all flav., 6.75 fl.oz | 60 | 0 | 14 |
| Organic Quenchers, all flav., 6.75 fl.oz | 40 | 0 | 10 |

**Bolthouse Farms:** *Per 8 fl.oz*

| | C | F | Cb |
|---|---|---|---|
| Juice: 100% Carrot | 70 | 0 | 15 |
| 100% Pomegranate | 150 | 0 | 38 |
| Acai + 10 Superblend | 120 | 0 | 31 |
| Mango Ginger + Carrot | 110 | 0.5 | 27 |
| Orange + Carrot | 100 | 0 | 22 |
| Fruit Smoothies: Amazing Mango | 130 | 0 | 31 |
| Berry Boost | 120 | 0 | 27 |
| Blue Goodness | 170 | 1.5 | 41 |
| C-Boost | 110 | 0 | 27 |
| Green Goodness | 130 | 0 | 30 |
| Strawberry Banana | 130 | 0 | 32 |

**Bright & Early** *(Minute Maid),*

| | C | F | Cb |
|---|---|---|---|
| Orange Flavored Drink, 8 fl.oz | 110 | 0 | 30 |

**Cactus Cooler,** Orange Pineapple Blast,

| | C | F | Cb |
|---|---|---|---|
| 12 fl oz can | 150 | 0 | 40 |

**Campbell's:**

| | C | F | Cb |
|---|---|---|---|
| Tomato Juice: 5.5 fl.oz can | 30 | 0 | 7 |
| 8 fl.oz | 50 | 0 | 10 |

## Juice Brands (Cont) | C | F | Cb

*Per 8 fl.oz Unless Indicated*

**Califia Farms:** *Per 8 fl.oz Unless Indicated*

**Agua Fresca:**

| | C | F | Cb |
|---|---|---|---|
| Strawberry Basil | 80 | 0 | 20 |
| Watermelon Ginger Lime | 60 | 0 | 14 |
| **Ginger Limeade** | 90 | 0 | 21 |
| **Meyer Lemonade** | 80 | 0 | 21 |
| **Orange Juice,** 10. 5 fl.oz | 140 | 0.5 | 32 |
| **Tangerine** | 100 | 0 | 24 |

**Capri Sun:** *Per 6 fl.oz*

| | C | F | Cb |
|---|---|---|---|
| *100% Juice,* average, | 85 | 0 | 21 |
| **Juice Drinks,** | | | |
| (25% Less Sugar), all flavors | 50 | 0 | 14 |
| *Roarin' Waters,* all flav., 6 fl.oz | 30 | 0 | 8 |

**Clamato:** *Per 8 fl.oz*

| | C | F | Cb |
|---|---|---|---|
| Original Tomato Cocktail | 60 | 0 | 12 |
| Picante | 60 | 0 | 13 |
| Coco Joy, Coconut Water, 8.4 fl.oz | 30 | 0 | 7 |
| Coco Libre, Coconut Water, 11 fl.oz pkg | 60 | 0 | 14 |

**CocoZia,** Coconut Water:

| | C | F | Cb |
|---|---|---|---|
| 100% Organic, 11.1 fl.oz pkg | 70 | 0 | 16 |
| Original, 8 fl.oz | 40 | 0 | 10 |
| Chocolate, 8 fl.oz | 60 | 0.5 | 13 |

**Dole:** *Per 8 fl.oz*

| | C | F | Cb |
|---|---|---|---|
| **100% Pure,** Chilled or Frozen, av. | 120 | 0 | 28 |
| *Blended Juices,* average all flavors | 120 | 0 | 30 |

**Florida's Natural:** *Per 8 fl.oz*

| | C | F | Cb |
|---|---|---|---|
| Apple Juice | 120 | 0 | 29 |
| Cranberry Ruby Red Cocktail | 130 | 0 | 32 |
| Orange, No Pulp | 110 | 0 | 26 |
| 100% Blends: Orange Mango | 110 | 0 | 27 |
| Orange Pineapple | 130 | 0 | 31 |
| Orange Strawberry | 110 | 0 | 26 |
| Ruby Red Grapefruit, Original | 90 | 0 | 22 |

**Goya:** *Per 12 fl.oz Can*

| | C | F | Cb |
|---|---|---|---|
| **Nectar:** Guava; Tamarind | 240 | 0 | 59 |
| Mango | 230 | 0 | 56 |
| Papaya; Peach, average | 220 | 0 | 55 |
| Average other varieties | 220 | 0 | 55 |

*Per 8 fl.oz Unless Indicated*

**Great Value** *(Walmart):*

**100% Juice:** *Per 8 fl.oz*

| | C | F | Cb |
|---|---|---|---|
| Apple | 110 | 0 | 28 |
| Cranberry Pomegranate | 140 | 0 | 35 |
| Grape | 160 | 0 | 40 |
| Orange, all varieties | 110 | 0 | 26 |
| White Grape | 150 | 0 | 38 |

**Hansen's:**

**Juice Box:** *Per 6.75 fl.oz Box*

| | C | F | Cb |
|---|---|---|---|
| Awesome Apple; Loud Lemonade, av. | 90 | 0 | 23 |
| Burstin Berry; Totally Tropical | 100 | 0 | 24 |
| Strawberry Banana | 110 | 0 | 27 |

**Junior Juice,**

| | C | F | Cb |
|---|---|---|---|
| 100% Juice, av. of flavors, 4.23 oz box | 60 | 0 | 16 |

**Natural,** (64 fl.oz Bottles): *Per 8 fl.oz*

| | C | F | Cb |
|---|---|---|---|
| Apple | 120 | 0 | 28 |
| Apple Strawberry | 110 | 0 | 27 |
| Cranberry Apple | 110 | 0 | 27 |
| Cranberry Grape | 140 | 0 | 35 |
| Grape | 120 | 0 | 33 |
| White Grape | 140 | 0 | 36 |

**Hawaii's Own,** Frozen Concentrate,

| | C | F | Cb |
|---|---|---|---|
| 10% Juice, average all flavors, 8 fl.oz prepared | 105 | 0 | 27 |

**Hi-C Juice Drinks:** *Per 6.75 fl.oz Box*

| | C | F | Cb |
|---|---|---|---|
| Flashin' Fruit Punch | 90 | 0 | 25 |
| Orange Lavaburst | 90 | 0 | 25 |
| Poppin' Lemonade | 100 | 0 | 27 |

**Hood:** *Per 8 fl.oz*

| | C | F | Cb |
|---|---|---|---|
| Apple | 120 | 0 | 31 |
| Lemonade | 110 | 0 | 29 |
| Orange | 120 | 0 | 30 |

**Jamba Juice** ~ *See Fast-Foods Section*

**Juicy Juice** *(Nestle):*

| | C | F | Cb |
|---|---|---|---|
| Average all flavors: | | | |
| 4.23 fl.oz box | 60 | 0 | 15 |
| 6.75 fl.oz box | 100 | 0 | 24 |

**Kerns:**

**Nectars:** *Per 11.5 fl.oz Can*

| | C | F | Cb |
|---|---|---|---|
| Guava; Strawberry | 210 | 0 | 53 |
| Pear; Strawb. Banana, av. | 220 | 0 | 53 |
| Pineapple Coconut | 280 | 8 | 53 |

**L & A:** *Per 8 fl.oz*

| | C | F | Cb |
|---|---|---|---|
| All Cherry | 180 | 0 | 45 |
| All Cranberry | 60 | 0 | 14 |
| Papaya Delight | 130 | 0 | 32 |
| Pineapple Coconut | 140 | 3 | 28 |

## Juice Brands (Cont) | C | F | Cb

*Per 8 fl.oz Unless Indicated*

**Lakewood Organic:** *Per 8 fl.oz*

| | C | F | Cb |
|---|---|---|---|
| **Blends:** Acai Amazon Berry | 130 | 1.5 | 29 |
| Blueberry Blend | 120 | 0 | 31 |
| Cranberry Lemonade | 100 | 0 | 24 |
| Lemonade | 100 | 0 | 25 |
| Pineapple Coconut | 190 | 8 | 29 |
| Pomegranate Lemonade | 100 | 0 | 26 |
| Super Kale | 100 | 0 | 24 |
| Super Tomato | 70 | 0 | 15 |
| Super Veggie | 60 | 0 | 13 |
| **Pure:** Apple | 120 | 0 | 30 |
| Beet | 100 | 0 | 23 |
| Blueberry | 110 | 0 | 26 |
| Carrot | 90 | 0 | 21 |
| Cranberry | 80 | 0 | 19 |
| Noni | 5 | 0 | 1 |
| Orange | 120 | 0 | 28 |
| Pineapple | 130 | 0 | 31 |
| Pink Grapefruit | 100 | 0 | 24 |
| Prune | 180 | 0 | 42 |

**Langers:** *Per 8 fl.oz*

| | C | F | Cb |
|---|---|---|---|
| **100% Juice:** Apple Cider | 120 | 0 | 28 |
| Apple Juice | 120 | 0 | 28 |
| Red/White Grape Juice | 160 | 0 | 40 |
| **Juice Cocktails (27% Juice):** | | | |
| Blueberry Cranberry | 135 | 0 | 34 |
| Cranberry | 140 | 0 | 35 |
| Cranberry Grape | 165 | 0 | 41 |
| Cranberry Raspberry | 140 | 0 | 35 |
| **20% Juice,** all flavors | 120 | 0 | 30 |

**Martinellli's:** *Per 8 fl.oz*

| | C | F | Cb |
|---|---|---|---|
| **Juice,** 100% Apple, all varieties | 140 | 0 | 35 |
| **Sparkling:** Apple Cider | 140 | 0 | 35 |
| Apple-Cranberry | 110 | 0 | 27 |
| Apple Grape | 120 | 0 | 31 |
| Apple-Mango/Pomegranate | 140 | 0 | 34 |
| Apple-Pear/Marionberry, av. | 125 | 0 | 31 |

**Minute Maid:**

**15.2 fl.oz Bottles:** *Per Bottle*

| | C | F | Cb |
|---|---|---|---|
| Apple Juice | 210 | 0 | 52 |
| Cranb. Apple Raspberry | 230 | 0 | 61 |
| Cranberry Grape | 270 | 0 | 74 |
| Pineapple Orange | 220 | 0 | 55 |

*Per 8 fl.oz Unless Indicated*

**Minute Maid (Cont):** | C | F | Cb

| | C | F | Cb |
|---|---|---|---|
| **Orange Juice,** | | | |
| Pure, No Pulp, 8 fl.oz | 110 | 0 | 26 |
| **Coolers,** average all flavors, 6.75 fl.oz | 100 | 0 | 26 |
| **Kid's Juice Boxes,** 100% Juice, | | | |
| Apple White Grape, 6.75 fl.oz | 90 | 0 | 22 |
| **Light Juices:** Orange, 8 fl.oz | 50 | 0 | 13 |
| With Tea; Light Lemonade, 8 fl.oz | 15 | 0 | 3 |
| **Soft Frozen Concentrate,** | | | |
| Limeade, 3 fl.oz tube | 70 | 0 | 19 |

**Mott's:**

| | C | F | Cb |
|---|---|---|---|
| **100% Juice:** | | | |
| Original Apple, 8 fl.oz | 120 | 0 | 29 |
| Apple White Grape, 6.75 fl.oz | 130 | 0 | 31 |
| Fruit Punch, 4.23 fl.oz | 60 | 0 | 15 |
| Light, Apple, 8 fl.oz | 50 | 0 | 12 |
| **Juice Drink:** | | | |
| Fruit Punch Rush, 8 fl.oz | 60 | 0 | 16 |
| Strawberry Boom, 8 fl.oz | 60 | 0 | 15 |
| Wild Grape Surge, 8 fl.oz | 60 | 0 | 16 |
| **Medleys:** | | | |
| Apple, 8 fl.oz | 110 | 0 | 25 |
| Grape, 8 fl.oz | 140 | 0 | 33 |
| **Mott's For Tots (47-54% Juice):** | | | |
| 40% Less Sugar: | | | |
| Apple Wh. Grape; Fruit Punch, 8 fl.oz | 70 | 0 | 17 |
| Average other flavors, 8 fl.oz | 60 | 0 | 16 |

**Naked Juice:** *Per 15.2 fl.oz*

| | C | F | Cb |
|---|---|---|---|
| **100% Juice,** No Sugar Added: | | | |
| O-J | 210 | 0 | 51 |
| Orange Mango | 250 | 0 | 59 |
| Pomegranate Blueberry | 290 | 0 | 68 |
| **100% Juice Smoothie,** No Sugar Added: | | | |
| Berry Blast; Strawb. Banana | 250 | 0 | 55 |
| Mighty Mango | 290 | 0 | 68 |
| **Boosted:** Acai Machine | 300 | 6 | 59 |
| Blue Machine | 170 | 0 | 40 |
| Green Machine | 270 | 0 | 63 |
| Power-C Machine | 230 | 0 | 55 |
| Red Machine | 320 | 9 | 59 |
| **Coconut Water:** Pure, 16.9 fl.oz | 80 | 0 | 21 |
| Kale Coconut, 16.9 fl.oz | 120 | 0 | 30 |
| Pineapple Coconut, 8 fl.oz | 50 | 0 | 13 |

| Juice Brands (Cont) | C | F | Cb |
|---|---|---|---|

*Per 8 fl.oz Unless Indicated*

**Nantucket Nectars:**

**100% Juice:** *Per 16 fl.oz*

| | | | |
|---|---|---|---|
| Peach Orange | 270 | 0 | 64 |
| Pineapple Orange Banana | 290 | 0 | 69 |
| Pomegranate Cherry | 230 | 0 | 57 |
| Premium Orange Juice | 220 | 0 | 51 |
| Pressed Apple | 240 | 0 | 59 |
| **Juice Cocktail,** Cranberry | 240 | 0 | 59 |

**Juice Drinks:** *Per 16 fl.oz*

| | | | |
|---|---|---|---|
| Orange Mango | 220 | 0 | 59 |
| Pineapple Orange Guava | 210 | 0 | 52 |
| Pomegranate Pear | 230 | 0 | 57 |
| Red Plum | 220 | 0 | 53 |
| Watermelon Strawberry | 220 | 0 | 55 |
| **Lemonade,** Squeezed | 180 | 0 | 47 |

**Newman's Own:** *Per 8 fl.oz*

| | | | |
|---|---|---|---|
| Lemonade, Regular; Pink | 110 | 0 | 27 |
| Limeade | 140 | 0 | 34 |

**Fruit Juice Cocktail:**

| | | | |
|---|---|---|---|
| Gorilla Grape | 110 | 0 | 29 |
| Orange Mango Tango | 130 | 0 | 33 |

**Northland:** *Per 8 fl.oz*

**100% Juice:**

| | | | |
|---|---|---|---|
| Blueberry Blackberry Acaí | 110 | 0 | 25 |
| Cranb. Blackberry/Raspberry, av. | 110 | 0 | 25 |
| Cranberry Cherry | 140 | 0 | 35 |
| Cranberry Grape | 100 | 0 | 25 |
| Cranberry Mango | 120 | 0 | 29 |
| **Superfruits,** Raspb. Pomegr. Goji | 130 | 0 | 32 |

**Ocean Spray:** *Per 8 fl.oz*

**Juice Cocktails:**

| | | | |
|---|---|---|---|
| Blueberry; Cranberry | 110 | 0 | 28 |

**100% Juice Blends:**

| | | | |
|---|---|---|---|
| Citrus Tangerine Orange | 110 | 0 | 28 |
| Cranberry Concord Grape | 130 | 0 | 33 |
| Cranberry Mango | 120 | 0 | 30 |
| Cranberry Raspberry | 120 | 0 | 30 |

**Juice Drinks:**

| | | | |
|---|---|---|---|
| Cran-Apple | 120 | 0 | 31 |
| Cran-Grape | 120 | 0 | 31 |
| Cran-Tangerine | 110 | 0 | 28 |
| **Diet Juice Drinks,** all flavors | 5 | 0 | 2 |
| **Light Juice Drinks,** av. all flavors | 50 | 0 | 13 |
| **Sparkling,** av. all flavors, 8.4 fl.oz | 85 | 0 | 22 |
| **Wave,** average all flavors, 8 fl.oz | 80 | 0 | 20 |

*Per 8 fl.oz Unless Indicated*

| | C | F | Cb |
|---|---|---|---|

**Odwalla:**

**100% Juice:** *Per 15.2 fl.oz Bottle*

| | | | |
|---|---|---|---|
| Berry Greens | 160 | 0 | 39 |
| Groovin' Greens | 150 | 0 | 37 |
| Orange | 210 | 0 | 47 |

**Smoothies:** *Per 15.2 fl.oz Bottle*

| | | | |
|---|---|---|---|
| Citrus C Monster | 240 | 0 | 58 |
| Mango Tango | 260 | 0 | 65 |
| Mo' Beta | 250 | 0 | 59 |
| Original Superfood | 240 | 0 | 58 |
| Red Rhapsody | 210 | 0 | 52 |
| Strawberry C Monster | 240 | 0 | 58 |

**Orange Julius:**

**Originals:** *Per Medium*

| | | | |
|---|---|---|---|
| Mango P'apple, 22.2 oz | 450 | 0 | 114 |
| Orange, 18.2 oz | 270 | 0 | 68 |
| Pina Colada, 21.6 oz | 470 | 7 | 99 |
| Strawberry Banana, 20.9 oz | 530 | 8 | 114 |

**Smoothies ~** *See Fast-Foods Section*

| | | | |
|---|---|---|---|
| **Orangina,** 10 fl.oz bottle | 130 | 0 | 32 |

**Pom Wonderful,**

**100% Juice (8 fl.oz Bottle),**

| | | | |
|---|---|---|---|
| Pom Blueberry/Cherry/Pomegranate | 150 | 0 | 37 |

**R.W. Knudsen:** *Per 8 fl.oz*

**Organic, 100% Juice:** Apple

| | | | |
|---|---|---|---|
| Apple | 110 | 0 | 28 |
| Concord Grape | 150 | 0 | 39 |
| Cranberry Blueberry | 120 | 0 | 31 |

**Natural, 100% Juice:**

| | | | |
|---|---|---|---|
| Mango Peach | 120 | 0 | 30 |
| Papaya Nectar | 130 | 0 | 32 |
| Razzleberry | 110 | 0 | 28 |
| Rio Red Grapefruit | 140 | 0 | 34 |

**Just Juice:**

| | | | |
|---|---|---|---|
| Just Blueberry | 100 | 0 | 24 |
| Just Black Cherry | 150 | 0 | 36 |
| Just Black Currant | 110 | 0 | 25 |
| **Simply Nutritious:** Mega C | 120 | 0 | 30 |
| Average other flavors | 125 | 0 | 31 |

**Sparkling:** Blueberry; Cranberry, av.

| | | | |
|---|---|---|---|
| Blueberry; Cranberry, av. | 110 | 0 | 28 |
| Cherry; Pomegranate | 130 | 0 | 32 |
| Organic Pear | 120 | 0 | 31 |

## Juice Brands (Cont) — C F Cb

*Per 8 fl.oz Unless Indicated*

**R.W. Knudsen (Cont):**

| | C | F | Cb |
|---|---|---|---|
| **Sensible Sippers:** *Per 4.23 fl.oz* | | | |
| Organic Apple; Fruit Punch | 30 | 0 | 7 |
| Organic Berry | 35 | 0 | 9 |
| **Very Veggie,** Original, 8 fl.oz | 60 | 0 | 12 |
| **ReaLemon – ReaLime:** | | | |
| Lemon/Lime Juice (from concentrate): | | | |
| 1 teaspoon | 0 | 0 | 0 |
| 2Tbsp, 1 fl.oz | 10 | 0 | 2.5 |
| **Santa Cruz:** *Per 8 fl.oz* | | | |
| **Organic, 100% Juice:** | | | |
| Apple; Red Tart Cherry | 120 | 0 | 30 |
| Concord/White Grape | 160 | 0 | 39 |
| Orange Mango | 120 | 0 | 29 |
| Pear Nectar | 130 | 0 | 33 |
| **Carbonated Beverages,** | | | |
| Lemonade, 10.5 fl.oz can | 130 | 0 | 32 |
| **Lemonade:** Regular; Peach; Mango | 90 | 0 | 22 |
| Cherry | 100 | 0 | 26 |
| Raspberry; Strawberry, average | 90 | 0 | 24 |
| **Simply Orange Juice Company:** | | | |
| **Lemonade; Limeade,** average | 120 | 0 | 31 |
| **Mixed Berry; Fruit Punch; Tropical** | 100 | 0 | 26 |
| **Orange Juice,** | | | |
| with or without pulp | 110 | 0 | 26 |
| **Snap·E· Tom,** | | | |
| **Tomato & Chili Cocktail,** | | | |
| 11.5 fl.oz can | 70 | 0 | 15 |
| **Snapple:** *Per 16 fl.oz Bottle* | | | |
| **Juice Drink Blends:** | | | |
| Go Bananas; Rasp. Peach, av. | 225 | 0 | 55 |
| Grapeade; Lemonade; Orangeade | 190 | 0 | 46 |
| Fruit Punch | 200 | 0 | 48 |
| **Diet,** Cranberry Raspberry | 20 | 0 | 5 |
| **Ssips,** Juice Boxes, | | | |
| av. all flavors, 6 fl.oz box | 80 | 0 | 21 |
| **Stonyfield Farm:** *Per 10 fl.oz Bottle* | | | |
| **Smoothies:** Strawb.; Wild Berry | 230 | 3 | 39 |
| Peach | 230 | 3 | 42 |
| **6 oz Bottle,** Strawb. Banana | 140 | 2 | 25 |

*Per 8 fl.oz Unless Indicated* — C F Cb

| | C | F | Cb |
|---|---|---|---|
| **SunnyD:** | | | |
| **Original:** *Per 64 fl.oz Ctn* | | | |
| Orange, all var., 8 fl.oz | 50 | 0 | 15 |
| **Blends,** 64 fl.oz Containers, | | | |
| average all flavors, 8 fl.oz | 60 | 0 | 15 |
| **Baja Juice:** *Per 12 fl.oz Bottles* | | | |
| Red Punch | 170 | 0 | 43 |
| Other flavors | 190 | 0 | 46 |
| **Chillers:** *Pe 16 fl.oz* | | | |
| Blue Raspberry | 110 | 0.5 | 28 |
| Grape | 120 | 0 | 30 |
| **Sunsweet:** *Per 8 fl.oz* | | | |
| **Plum Smart:** Original | 160 | 0 | 36 |
| Light | 60 | 0 | 15 |
| **Prune Juice:** Original | 180 | 0 | 42 |
| Light | 100 | 0 | 26 |
| **Trader Joe's:** | | | |
| **All Natural Pasteurized,** 32/64 fl.oz Bottle: *Per 8 fl.oz* | | | |
| 100% Cranberry | 70 | 0 | 16 |
| Blueberry Pomegranate | 140 | 0 | 34 |
| Just Blueberry | 100 | 0 | 24 |
| Just Pomegranate | 150 | 0 | 37 |
| Mango PassionFruit | 130 | 0 | 32 |
| Omega Orange Carrot | 110 | 0 | 26 |
| **Organic,** 32/64 fl.oz Bottle: *Per 8 fl.oz* | | | |
| 100% Pomegranate | 140 | 0 | 35 |
| Apple Juice | 120 | 0 | 30 |
| Concord Grape Juice | 160 | 0 | 39 |
| Cranberry | 70 | 0 | 18 |
| Grapefruit Sunset; Lemonade | 120 | 0 | 30 |
| Mango Nectar | 130 | 0 | 32 |
| Pink Lemonade | 130 | 0 | 32 |
| Strawberry Lemonade | 120 | 0 | 29 |
| White Grape Juice | 160 | 0 | 40 |
| **Joe's Kids:** *Per 6.75 oz Box* | | | |
| From Concentrate: Apple | 90 | 0 | 23 |
| Apple Grape | 100 | 0 | 24 |
| White Grape | 120 | 0 | 30 |
| 10% Juice, Lemonade | 90 | 0 | 22 |
| **Sparkling Juices,** 25.4 fl.oz Bottle: | | | |
| Blueberry, 8 fl.oz | 120 | 0 | 30 |
| Cranberry, 8 fl.oz | 140 | 0 | 35 |
| Pomegranate, 8 fl.oz | 130 | 0 | 31 |

## Juice Brands (Cont)   **C**  **F**  **Cb**

*Per 8 fl.oz Unless Indicated*

| | C | F | Cb |
|---|---|---|---|
| **Tree Top:** | | | |
| **100% Juice Concentrates:** | | | |
| **64 fl.oz Bottle:** *Per 8 fl.oz* | | | |
| Apple Berry/Grape, average | 125 | 0 | 32 |
| Apple Cranb.; Or. Passionfruit, av. | 115 | 0 | 28 |
| **11.5 fl.oz Can:** *Per Can* | | | |
| Apple Berry/Grape, av. | 180 | 0 | 46 |
| **6.75 fl.oz Box**, average | 105 | 0 | 26 |
| **Smoothie**, Ban. Strawb., 4.5 fl.oz | 100 | 0 | 23 |
| **Tropicana:** | | | |
| **20% Juice,** 15.2 fl.oz Bottle, | | | |
| Cranberry | 270 | 0 | 66 |
| **Farmstand,** 32 fl.oz bottle, | | | |
| average all flavors, 8 fl.oz | 120 | 0 | 27 |
| **100% Juice Pure Premium:** | | | |
| Grapefruit, 15.2 fl.oz | 170 | 0 | 42 |
| Ruby Red Grapefruit, 15.2 fl.oz | 250 | 0 | 59 |
| Strawberry Kiwi, 15.2 fl.oz | 230 | 0 | 58 |
| **Trop50,** 50% less sugar, 59 fl.oz bottle, | | | |
| average all flavors, 8 fl.oz | 50 | 0 | 13 |
| **Trop Twisters,** 20 fl.oz bottle: | | | |
| Or. Strawb. Banana Burst | 330 | 0 | 80 |
| Tropicana Twister , 20 fl.oz | 340 | 0 | 85 |
| **Tropics,** 59 fl.oz container, | | | |
| average all flavors, 8 fl.oz | 125 | 0 | 30 |
| **Tru Nopal:** | | | |
| **Cactus Water:** 1 Cup, 8 fl.oz | 25 | 0 | 6 |
| 16.9 fl.oz carton | 50 | 0 | 12 |
| **Turkey Hill:** *Per 8 fl.oz* | | | |
| **All Natural Lemonade:** Classic | 100 | 0 | 26 |
| Blackberry | 110 | 0 | 27 |
| Regular Lemonade flavors | 120 | 0 | 29 |
| Fruit Punch | 100 | 0 | 26 |
| Orangeade | 110 | 0 | 26 |
| **V8 Juices & Drinks** *(Campbell's)*: | | | |
| **Original/Spicy 100% Vegetable Juice:** | | | |
| 5.5 fl.oz can | 35 | 0 | 7 |
| 8 fl.oz cup | 50 | 0 | 10 |
| 11.5 fl.oz can | 70 | 0 | 14 |
| 12 fl.oz bottle | 75 | 0 | 15 |
| **Blends:** Pineapple Passion, 8 fl.oz | 70 | 0 | 17 |
| Red Radiance, 8 fl.oz | 70 | 0 | 17 |
| Healthy Greens; Carrot Mango, 8 fl.oz | 60 | 0 | 14 |
| **V-Fusion:** Average all flavors | 115 | 0 | 28 |
| Light Varieties, av. all flavors | 50 | 0 | 13 |
| **Veryfine:** | | | |
| **100%:** Apple, 8 fl.oz | 120 | 0 | 29 |
| Apple Strawb., Krazy Kiwi, 11.5 fl.oz | 170 | 0 | 43 |
| Orange, 8 fl.oz | 120 | 0 | 30 |

*Per 8 fl.oz Unless Indicated*

| | C | F | Cb |
|---|---|---|---|
| **Vita Coco:** | | | |
| **Coconut Water:** 8 fl.oz | 45 | 0 | 11 |
| with Pineapple, 8 fl.oz | 60 | 0 | 15 |
| Chocolate, 11 fl.oz | 90 | 3 | 16 |
| **Walnut Acres:** *Per 8 fl.oz* | | | |
| **Organic:** Apple; Cranberry, av. | 110 | 0 | 28 |
| Apricot; Raspberry | 130 | 0 | 32 |
| Cherry | 140 | 0 | 34 |
| Incredible Vegetable | 50 | 0 | 12 |
| Mango Nectar | 120 | 0 | 29 |
| **Welch's:** *Per 8 fl.oz Unless Indicated* | | | |
| **100% Juice:** Concord Grape | 140 | 0 | 36 |
| Red Grape juice | 160 | 0 | 41 |
| White Grape | 140 | 0 | 38 |
| White Grape Cherry/Peach | 140 | 0 | 34 |
| **Fruit Shots,** all flavors, 5.5 fl.oz can | 90 | 0 | 22 |
| **Frozen Concentrates,** | | | |
| 100% Juice, Grape; all var., 2 fl oz | 140 | 0 | 39 |
| **Light Juice,** 52 fl.oz Bottle | | | |
| Concord/White Grape, 8 fl.oz | 45 | 0 | 12 |
| **Sparkling Juice Cocktail:** | | | |
| Blueberry Grape, 8 fl.oz | 150 | 0 | 38 |
| Other flavors, 8 fl.oz | 160 | 0 | 40 |
| **Zola:** | | | |
| **Acai:** *Per 12 fl.oz Bottle* | | | |
| Original | 185 | 3 | 38 |
| with Blueberry/Pomegranate | 180 | 3 | 38 |
| **Coconut Water, 17.5 oz Can:** | | | |
| Original, | 50 | 0 | 13 |
| Chocolate, 8 fl.oz | 50 | 0 | 12 |
| Espresso, 8 fl.oz | 60 | 0 | 13 |

---

### CALORIEKING PORTION WATCH

| ORANGE JUICE | C | Cb |
|---|---|---|
| 8 fl.oz | 110 | 26 |
| 16 fl.oz | 220 | 52 |
| 24 fl.oz | 330 | 78 |
| 32 fl.oz | 440 | 104 |

## Quick Guide    **C** **F** **Cb**

### Cow's Milk ~ Average All Brands
**Whole (3.25% fat):**

| | C | F | Cb |
|---|---|---|---|
| 2 Tbsp, 1 fl.oz | 20 | 1 | 1.5 |
| 1 Cup, 8 fl.oz | 150 | 8 | 12 |
| 1 Large Glass, 12 fl.oz | 220 | 12 | 17 |
| 1 Pint, 16 fl.oz | 295 | 16 | 22 |
| 1 Quart, 946 ml | 590 | 32 | 44 |

**Reduced-Fat (2% fat):**

| | | | |
|---|---|---|---|
| 2 Tbsp, 1 fl.oz | 15 | 0.5 | 1.5 |
| 1 Cup, 8 fl.oz | 120 | 5 | 12 |
| 1 Large Glass, 12 fl.oz | 180 | 7.5 | 18 |
| 1 Pint, 16 fl.oz | 245 | 10 | 23 |
| 1 Quart, 946 ml | 490 | 20 | 46 |

**Light/Low-Fat (1% fat):**

| | | | |
|---|---|---|---|
| 2 Tbsp, 1 fl.oz | 13 | 0.3 | 1.5 |
| 1 Cup, 8 fl.oz | 100 | 2.5 | 12 |
| 1 Large Glass, 12 fl.oz | 150 | 4 | 18 |
| 1 Pint, 16 fl.oz | 205 | 5 | 25 |
| 1 Quart, 946 ml | 410 | 10 | 49 |

**Fat Free/Skim (0% fat):**

| | | | |
|---|---|---|---|
| 2 Tbsp, 1 fl.oz | 10 | 0 | 1.5 |
| 1 Cup, 8 fl.oz | 90 | 0.5 | 13 |
| 1 Large Glass, 12 fl.oz | 135 | 0.5 | 19 |
| 1 Pint, 16 fl.oz | 180 | 1 | 26 |

**Half & Half ~** *See Page* [89]

### SWITCH & SAVE

*Switch from whole milk to either 2%, 1% or 0% milk and save significant calories.*

*Per 8 oz Cup/Glass*

**WHOLE MILK** 3.3% Fat 150 Cals

| | SAVE |
|---|---|
| **2% MILK** 120 Cals | SAVE 30 Cals |
| **1% MILK** 100 Cals | SAVE 50 Cals |
| **0% FAT-FREE** 90 Cals | SAVE 60 Cals |

*Switching to low-fat or fat-free milk also greatly reduces saturated fat.*

## Other Milks    **C** **F** **Cb**

**Buttermilk:** *Average All Brands*

| | C | F | Cb |
|---|---|---|---|
| Reduced-Fat (2%), 1 cup, 8 fl.oz | 120 | 5 | 10 |
| Low-Fat (1%), 1 cup, 8 fl.oz | 100 | 2.5 | 12 |

**Lactose Free:**

| | | | |
|---|---|---|---|
| *Lactaid 100:* Whole | 160 | 8 | 13 |
| 2% Reduced-Fat | 130 | 5 | 12 |
| 1% Low-Fat | 110 | 2.5 | 13 |
| Fat Free; Calcium Enriched | 90 | 0 | 13 |
| *Smart Balance,* FF + Omega-3s & Vit. E | 100 | 0 | 14 |

**Lower Calorie/Carb Dairy Drinks:** *Per 8 fl.oz Cup*

| | | | |
|---|---|---|---|
| Calorie Countdown (*Hood*): | | | |
| 2% Reduced-Fat: Plain | 70 | 4.5 | 3 |
| Chocolate | 80 | 4.5 | 6 |
| Fat-Free | 35 | 0 | 4 |

### Goat/Sheep Milk, Kefir

**Goat's Milk** *(Meyenberg):*

| | | | |
|---|---|---|---|
| Whole, 1 cup, 8 fl.oz | 140 | 7 | 11 |
| Low-Fat (1%), 8 fl.oz | 100 | 2.5 | 11 |
| Evaporated, reconst., 8 fl.oz | 140 | 8 | 12 |

**Kefir:** *Per 8 fl.oz*

| | | | |
|---|---|---|---|
| *Lifeway:* Original, Plain | 150 | 8 | 12 |
| Greek, Plain, whole milk | 210 | 14 | 12 |
| Lowfat, average all flavors | 140 | 1.5 | 20 |
| *Nancy's:* Plain, low fat | 140 | 3 | 17 |
| Fruit flavors, average | 205 | 2.5 | 38 |
| *Trader Joe's:* Plain, 1% | 110 | 2.5 | 8 |
| Strawberry | 160 | 2 | 21 |
| **Sheep's Milk,** Whole, 1 cup | 265 | 17 | 13 |

### Canned & Dried Milk

**Condensed:** Sweetened, 2 T., 1 fl.oz

| | | | |
|---|---|---|---|
| | 130 | 3 | 22 |
| Low Fat, 2 Tbsp | 120 | 1.5 | 23 |
| Fat-Free, 2 Tbsp | 110 | 0 | 24 |

**Evaporated:** Whole, 2 Tbsp

| | | | |
|---|---|---|---|
| | 40 | 3 | 3 |
| Whole, 1/2 cup, 4 fl.oz | 170 | 10 | 13 |
| *Carnation:* Low Fat, 2 Tbsp, 1 oz | 25 | 0.5 | 3 |
| 1/2 cup, 4 fl.oz | 115 | 2.5 | 14 |
| Fat-Free, 2 Tbsp, 1 oz | 25 | 0 | 4 |

**Dried:** Whole, 1/4 cup, 1 oz

| | | | |
|---|---|---|---|
| | 160 | 9 | 12 |
| Skim/Non-Fat, 1/3 cup | 80 | 0 | 12 |
| Made-up, 1 cup, 8 fl.oz | 80 | 0 | 12 |
| Buttermilk (sweet cream): 1 oz | 110 | 2 | 14 |
| Non-Fat, 1 Tbsp | 25 | 0 | 3 |
| *Carnation,* Malted, dry, 3 Tbsp, 0.7 oz | 90 | 2 | 15 |
| *Horlick's,* Malt Powder, dry, 1 oz | 180 | 4 | 27 |

### Soy/Non-Dairy Drinks ~ See Page 49

### Quick Guide

| | C | F | Cb |
|---|---|---|---|

**Chocolate Milk:**
*Average All Brands:*

| | C | F | Cb |
|---|---|---|---|
| **Whole Milk,** (3.3%): | | | |
| 8 fl.oz cup | 220 | 8 | 29 |
| 1 Pint, 16 fl.oz | 440 | 16 | 58 |
| **Reduced-Fat,** (2%): | | | |
| 8 fl.oz cup | 190 | 5 | 30 |
| 1 Pint, 16 fl.oz | 380 | 10 | 60 |
| **Low-Fat,** (1%): | | | |
| 8 fl.oz cup | 160 | 3 | 26 |
| 1 Pint, 16 fl.oz | 315 | 5 | 52 |

### Flavored Milk ~ Brands

| | C | F | Cb |
|---|---|---|---|
| **Ready-To-Drink:** *Per 8 fl.oz Cup Unless Indicated* | | | |
| Albertson's, Choc Milk | 180 | 2.5 | 29 |
| **Great Value** *(Walmart)*, | | | |
| Low Fat Choc. Milk, 8 oz | 140 | 2.5 | 21 |
| **Hood:** Chocolate | 220 | 8 | 30 |
| Low-Fat (1%), Chocolate | 160 | 2.5 | 28 |
| **Horizon Organic:** | | | |
| Low-Fat: | | | |
| Chocolate with Omega 3 | 150 | 2.5 | 23 |
| Vanilla with Omega 3 | 150 | 2.5 | 22 |
| **Kellogg's:** | | | |
| To Go, Breakfast Shakes: *Per 10 fl.oz* | | | |
| Chocolate; Strawberry, av. | 190 | 5 | 30 |
| **Mixes,** average all flavors, | | | |
| 1 packet | 130 | 0.5 | 26 |
| **Kroger,** Simple Truth, | | | |
| Choc Milk, Low-Fat, 1% | 150 | 2.5 | 22 |
| **Land O Lakes:** *Per 8 fl.oz* | | | |
| **Grip 'n Go:** | | | |
| Swiss Chocolate (2% red-fat) | 190 | 5 | 26 |
| Strawberry (whole milk) | 190 | 8 | 22 |
| **Muscle Milk** ~ *See Energy Protein Drinks* | | | |
| **Nesquik:** *Per 8 fl.oz* | | | |
| **Low Fat,** average all flavors | 140 | 2.5 | 24 |
| **Chocolate:** Fat Free, 8 fl.oz | 95 | 0 | 24 |
| No Sugar Added | 100 | 2 | 13 |
| **Prairie Farms:** *Per 8 fl.oz* | | | |
| Chocolate, 2% Reduced Fat | 180 | 5 | 26 |
| Strawberry, 1% Low Fat | 160 | 2.5 | 28 |
| **Ralphs,** | | | |
| Choc., Low-Fat, 8 fl.oz | 210 | 2.5 | 36 |

**Bottled Coffee Drinks ~ See Page 37**

### Flavored Milk ~ Brands (Cont)

| | C | F | Cb |
|---|---|---|---|
| **Ready-To-Drink:** | | | |
| **TruMoo:** | | | |
| **Chocolate/Strawberry**: | | | |
| Whole, 8 fl.oz | 220 | 8 | 29 |
| 1% Low-Fat: 8 fl.oz | 140 | 2.5 | 20 |
| 14 fl.oz Bottle | 250 | 5 | 35 |
| Fat-free, 8 fl.oz | 120 | 0 | 20 |
| **High Protein 1% (25g),** | | | |
| average all flavors, 8 fl.oz | 205 | 2.5 | 31 |
| **Yoo-Hoo:** Chocolate,15.5 fl.oz bottle | 230 | 2 | 51 |
| Strawberry, 6.5 fl.oz | 100 | 0.5 | 22 |

**Bottled Coffee Drinks** ~ *See Page 37*

### Shakes

| | C | F | Cb |
|---|---|---|---|
| **Arby's:** *Per Small Size* | | | |
| Jamocha, Ultimate Choc., | 440 | 12 | 75 |
| **Burger King:** *Per Medium 16 oz* | | | |
| **Hand Spun Shakes:** Chocolate | 760 | 21 | 131 |
| Strawberry | 640 | 15 | 113 |
| Vanilla | 580 | 15 | 98 |
| **Other flavors** ~ *See Fast Food Section* | | | |
| **Denny's:** *Per 16 oz* | | | |
| Cake Batter | 1090 | 52 | 147 |
| Chocolate | 870 | 43 | 111 |
| Chocolate Peanut Butter | 1080 | 66 | 111 |
| Oreo | 1050 | 56 | 125 |
| Peanut Butter Banana | 1030 | 65 | 99 |
| Strawberry | 760 | 34 | 110 |
| Vanilla | 800 | 43 | 97 |
| **Hardees,** all flavors, av., 14 oz | 710 | 33 | 87 |
| **McDonalds,** McCafe Shakes: | | | |
| Chocolate/Strawberry, average: | | | |
| 12 fl.oz cup | 530 | 16 | 87 |
| 16 fl.oz cup | 635 | 18 | 104 |
| 22 fl.oz cup | 850 | 24 | 141 |
| **Other Restaurants** ~ *See Fast-Foods Section* | | | |

### Smoothies

| | C | F | Cb |
|---|---|---|---|
| *Made Up Ready-To-Drink:* | | | |
| **8 fl. oz Milk/Soy + Fruit:** *Per 12 fl.oz* | | | |
| *Average all flavors:* | | | |
| with Whole Milk | 300 | 8 | 50 |
| + Ice Cream, 1 scoop | 400 | 13 | 62 |
| with Non-Fat Milk | 240 | 0 | 50 |
| **Kroger/Ralph's Smoothies:** *Per 8 fl.oz* | | | |
| Mixed Berry | 210 | 2.5 | 40 |
| Strawberry Banana | 200 | 2.5 | 37 |

**Freshens; Jamba Juice; TCBY** ~ *See Fast-FoodsObis*

**Bottled Coffee Drinks ~ See Page 37**

## Nut, Rice & Cereal Drinks

*Per 8 fl.oz Cup Unless Indicated*

| | C | F | Cb |
|---|---|---|---|
| **Almond Breeze** (Blue Diamond): | | | |
| **Almond Milk:** Original | 60 | 2.5 | 8 |
| Chocolate; Vanilla, av. | 90 | 2.5 | 16 |
| **Red. Sugar,** Orig;Van., av. | | | |
| Original; Vanilla, av. | 45 | 2.5 | 6 |
| **Unsweetened:** | | | |
| Original; Vanilla; Choc. av. | 35 | 2.5 | 1 |
| **Blends:** | | | |
| Almond Cashew: Original | 60 | 2.5 | 8 |
| Vanilla | 80 | 2 | 15 |
| Almond Coconut: Original | 60 | 3 | 7 |
| Vanilla, unsweetened | 40 | 3.5 | 1 |
| **Hint of Honey,** Regular; Vanilla, av. | 55 | 2.5 | 8 |
| **Nog** | 70 | 1.5 | 14 |
| **Almond Dream** ~ *See Dream* | | | |
| **Amazake,** | | | |
| **Oh So Original,** Rice Shake | 150 | 0 | 31 |
| **Better Than Milk:** | | | |
| **Rice Vegan Powder Mix,** | | | |
| Orig.; Van., 2 Tbsp, 0.7 oz | 70 | 0 | 17 |
| **Cacique,** | | | |
| **Original Horchata,,** 12 fl.oz | 230 | 5 | 46 |
| **Califia Farms:** *Per 8 fl.oz Cup* | | | |
| **Almond Milk:** Original | 60 | 4 | 6 |
| Unsweetened | 35 | 3 | 1 |
| Chocolate | 90 | 4.5 | 11 |
| Vanilla | 50 | 3 | 4 |
| **Cashew,** Organic Homestyle | 120 | 10 | 6 |
| **Oatmilk,** unsweetened | 100 | 7 | 9 |
| **Don Jose:** *Per 8 fl.oz Cup* | | | |
| **Cereal Match** | 100 | 3 | 17 |
| **Horchata Rice Drink** | 140 | 4 | 25 |
| **Dream:** *Per 8 fl.oz Cup* | | | |
| **Almond Dream,** unsweetened | 30 | 3.5 | 3 |
| **Coconut Dream** ~ **See page 50** | | | |
| **Oat Dream:** Original; Vanilla, av. | 120 | 3.5 | 21 |
| Unsweetened | 70 | 3 | 8 |
| Chocolate | 170 | 3.5 | 32 |
| **Rice Dream:** Classic Orig./Enriched | 120 | 2.5 | 23 |
| Enriched: Unsweetened | 70 | 2.5 | 11 |
| Vanilla | 130 | 2.5 | 26 |
| Sprouted, unsweetened | 70 | 2.5 | 11 |
| **Soy Dream** ~ *See page 50* | | | |

Note: Rice/Oat/Nut Drinks are very low in protein. Unless enriched with prtein (and calcium), they are not suitable for infants as a substitute for milk or calcium-enriched soy drinks.

## Nut & Rice Drinks (Cont)

*Per 8 fl.oz Cup Unless Indicated*

| | C | F | Cb |
|---|---|---|---|
| **Milkadamia:** *Per 8 fl.oz Cup* | | | |
| **Macadamia Milk:** Original | 70 | 5 | 7 |
| Unsweetened, Orig./Vanilla | 50 | 5 | 1 |
| Latte da | 70 | 4.5 | 8 |
| **Pacific Foods:** *Per 8 fl.oz Cup* | | | |
| **Cashew,** Original | 70 | 4 | 8 |
| **Hazelnut,** Orig./Chocolate, av. | 120 | 4 | 18 |
| **Hemp:** Original | 140 | 6 | 19 |
| Unsweetened Orig./Vanilla | 60 | 4.5 | 0 |
| Chocolate | 200 | 6 | 32 |
| Vanilla | 170 | 6 | 23 |
| **Organic Almond:** Orig.; Vanilla, av. | 65 | 3 | 10 |
| Chocolate, single serve | 110 | 3 | 19 |
| **Silk:** *Per 8 fl.oz Cup* | | | |
| **Almond:** Original | 60 | 2.5 | 8 |
| Dark Chocolate | 100 | 2.5 | 19 |
| Unsweetened, Orig.; Vanilla | 30 | 2.5 | 1 |
| **Cashew:** Unsweetned Orig; Vanilla | 25 | 2 | 1 |
| Chocolate | 90 | 2 | 18 |
| **Protein:** | | | |
| Almond & Cashew: Original | 130 | 8 | 3 |
| Chocolate | 150 | 5 | 18 |
| Vanilla | 140 | 7 | 8 |
| **Trader Joe's:** | | | |
| **Rice Drinks:** *Per 8 fl.oz* | | | |
| Unsweetened: Original, Organic | 120 | 2.5 | 23 |
| Vanilla | 130 | 2.5 | 26 |

## Soy Milk ~ Ready-To-Drink

| | C | F | Cb |
|---|---|---|---|
| **365 Organic** (Whole Foods): *Per 8 fl.oz Cup* | | | |
| Original, unsweetened | 70 | 3.5 | 3 |
| Chocolate | 140 | 3.5 | 22 |
| Vanilla | 100 | 3.5 | 11 |
| **8th Continent:** *Per 8 fl.oz* | | | |
| Original/Complete Vanilla | 80 | 2.5 | 7 |
| Vanilla | 100 | 2.5 | 11 |
| Light: Original/Vanilla, av. | 55 | 2 | 4 |
| Chocolate | 90 | 1.5 | 12 |
| **Better Than Milk,** Original | 90 | 1.5 | 18 |
| **Edensoy:** *Per 8 fl.oz Cup* | | | |
| **Organic:** Original | 140 | 5 | 14 |
| Unsweetened | 120 | 6 | 5 |
| Carob; Cocoa, average | 185 | 4 | 30 |
| Vanilla | 150 | 3 | 24 |
| **Extra:** Original | 130 | 4 | 13 |
| Vanilla | 150 | 3 | 23 |
| **Great Value** (Walmart), Orig. Soy | 100 | 4 | 9 |

## Soy Milk ~ Ready-To-Drink (Cont)

*Per 8 fl.oz Unless Indicated*   **C**  **F**  **Cb**
**Odwalla:** *Per 15.2 fl.oz Bottle*

**Soy & Dairy Protein Shakes:**

| | C | F | Cb |
|---|---|---|---|
| Chocolate | 410 | 8 | 53 |
| Strawberry | 320 | 7 | 37 |
| Vanilla | 380 | 7 | 46 |

**Pacific:** *Per 8 fl.oz Cup*

| | C | F | Cb |
|---|---|---|---|
| **Soy,** Organic, Orig., unswtnd | 90 | 4 | 5 |
| **Select Soy,** Vanilla | 80 | 2.5 | 11 |
| **Ultra Soy,** Original | 140 | 5 | 13 |

**Pearl** *(Kikkoman): Per 8 fl.oz Cup*

| | C | F | Cb |
|---|---|---|---|
| **Organic:** Original; Crmy Van. | 110 | 3.5 | 12 |
| Unsweetened | 80 | 2.5 | 6 |
| Chocolate; Coffee, av. | 150 | 4 | 22 |
| Green Tea | 110 | 3.5 | 13 |

**Silk** *(Whitewave): Per 8 fl.oz Cup*

| | C | F | Cb |
|---|---|---|---|
| **Organic:** Original; Vanilla, av. | 105 | 4 | 10 |
| Chocolate | 150 | 5 | 19 |
| Very Vanilla | 130 | 3.5 | 18 |
| **Light,** Original | 60 | 2 | 5 |
| **Unsweetened:** Original | 80 | 4 | 3 |
| Vanilla | 80 | 4 | 4 |

**Slim-Fast** ~ *See Page 40*

**Soy Dream** *(Dream): Per 8 fl.oz Cup*

| | C | F | Cb |
|---|---|---|---|
| **Enriched:** Original | 100 | 4 | 8 |
| Vanilla | 120 | 4 | 14 |

**Soylent:**

**Ready To Drink Bottles:**

| | C | F | Cb |
|---|---|---|---|
| Bridge, Chocolate, 11 fl oz | 80 | 10 | 10 |
| Cacao,14 fl.oz | 400 | 21 | 37 |
| Cafe, av. all flavors, 14 fl. oz | 400 | 21 | 36 |
| Original; Strawberry, 14 fl. oz | 400 | 21 | 36 |
| Vanilla, 14 fl.oz | 400 | 21 | 33 |

**Soy Slender** *(Westsoy): Per 8 fl.oz Cup*

| | C | F | Cb |
|---|---|---|---|
| Cappuccino; Vanilla; Chocolate | 70 | 3 | 4 |

**Trader Joe's:** *Per 8 fl.oz*

| | C | F | Cb |
|---|---|---|---|
| **Soy Milk:** Original | 110 | 2 | 13 |
| Chocolate | 130 | 2.5 | 23 |
| Vanilla | 100 | 2 | 16 |
| **Organic:** Original | 130 | 3.5 | 18 |
| Chocolate | 120 | 3 | 17 |
| Vanilla | 130 | 3 | 19 |

## Soy Milk ~ Ready-To-Drink (Cont)

**WestSoy:** *Per 8 fl.oz Cup*   **C**  **F**  **Cb**

| | C | F | Cb |
|---|---|---|---|
| **Soy Milk:** Chocolate Peppermint Stick | 180 | 3.5 | 30 |
| Organic: Original | 130 | 3.5 | 18 |
| Unsweetened: Plain | 100 | 5 | 4 |
| Vanilla | 100 | 4.5 | 5 |
| Organic Plus, Plain/Vanilla | 110 | 4.5 | 11 |
| Low-Fat: Plain | 90 | 2 | 15 |
| Vanilla | 120 | 2 | 23 |
| Non-Fat: Plain | 70 | 0 | 10 |
| Vanilla | 80 | 0 | 12 |

## Soy Powder Mix

*1 oz (¼ cup) mix makes 8 fl.oz Cup*

| | C | F | Cb |
|---|---|---|---|
| **Soy Protein Isolate,** dry, 1 oz | 95 | 1 | 2 |

**Better Than Milk:**

| | C | F | Cb |
|---|---|---|---|
| Original, 2 Tbsp | 90 | 1.5 | 18 |
| Vanilla, 2 Tbsp | 90 | 1.5 | 18 |

**Now:**

**Soy Protein Isolate:**

| | C | F | Cb |
|---|---|---|---|
| Plain, ⅓ cup, 0.8 fl.oz | 90 | 0.5 | 0.5 |
| Chocolate, 1 scp, 1.6 oz | 160 | 1.5 | 9 |
| Vanilla, 1 scoop, 1.6 oz | 180 | 2.5 | 13 |

**Soylent:**

**Meal Replacement Powders:**

| | C | F | Cb |
|---|---|---|---|
| Original, ⅔ cup, 3.2 oz | 400 | 19 | 42 |
| Cacao, 2 rounded scoops, 3.2 oz | 400 | 20 | 41 |
| Cafe Mocha, ⅔cup, 3.2 oz | 400 | 20 | 41 |

**Whole Foods:**

| | C | F | Cb |
|---|---|---|---|
| Chocolate, with Spirulina, 1 oz | 100 | 1 | 10 |
| Vanilla, with Spirulina, 1 oz | 100 | 0 | 11 |

## Coconut Milk Drinks

**Califia Farms:** *Per 8 fl.oz Cup*

| | C | F | Cb |
|---|---|---|---|
| **Go Coconuts,** Coconut Milk/ Water | 45 | 4 | 2 |

**Coconut Dream** *(Dream): Per 8 fl.oz Cup*

| | C | F | Cb |
|---|---|---|---|
| Original | 80 | 5 | 7 |
| Unsweetened | 60 | 5 | 1 |
| Vanilla | 90 | 5 | 9 |

**Great Value,**

| | C | F | Cb |
|---|---|---|---|
| Original Unsweetened | 50 | 5 | 1 |
| **Pacific,** Original Unsweetened | 45 | 4 | 1 |

**Silk:** *Per 8 fl.oz Cup*

| | C | F | Cb |
|---|---|---|---|
| Original | 70 | 4.5 | 6 |
| Unsweetened | 40 | 4 | 1 |

**So Delicious:** *Per 8 fl.oz cup*

| | C | F | Cb |
|---|---|---|---|
| Unweeetened | 45 | 4.5 | 1 |

**Trader Joes:** *Per 8 fl.oz cup*

| | C | F | Cb |
|---|---|---|---|
| Unsweetened | 60 | 5 | 1 |
| Vanilla | 90 | 5 | 9 |

(Enriched with calcium + vitamins D & B12)

## Quick Guide  C  F  Cb

**Cola:**

**Drinks:** *Average all Brands*

| | C | F | Cb |
|---|---|---|---|
| 8 fl.oz Cup/Can | 100 | 0 | 26 |
| 12 fl.oz Can | 150 | 0 | 39 |
| 16 fl.oz Bottle | 200 | 0 | 52 |
| 20 fl.oz Bottle | 250 | 0 | 65 |
| 24 fl.oz (Pepsi) | 300 | 0 | 84 |
| 1-Liter Bottle (34 fl.oz) | 400 | 0 | 100 |
| 2-Liter Bottle (68 fl.oz) | 800 | 0 | 200 |

**Other Soda Drinks:** *Per 12 fl.oz, average all brands*

| | C | F | Cb |
|---|---|---|---|
| Club Soda | 0 | 0 | 0 |
| Cream Soda | 190 | 0 | 48 |
| Ginger Ale | 125 | 0 | 31 |
| Lemonade, Regular/Pink | 180 | 0 | 45 |
| Orange | 180 | 0 | 45 |
| Root Beer | 150 | 0 | 39 |
| Tonic Water | 125 | 0 | 32 |
| Mineral Water: Plain | 0 | 0 | 0 |
| Sweetened/flavored | 150 | 0 | 37 |
| with Fruit Juice | 120 | 0 | 30 |
| Soda Water/Seltzer: Plain/Diet | 0 | 0 | 0 |
| Sweetened/flavored | 155 | 0 | 39 |
| with Fruit Juice | 160 | 0 | 40 |

## Fountain, Movie Theater & Take-Out

*Average All Flavors*

| | C | F | Cb |
|---|---|---|---|
| **Small Cup,** 12 fl.oz: No Ice | 160 | 0 | 40 |
| with ⅓ Ice | 120 | 0 | 30 |
| **Regular,** 16 fl.oz: No Ice | 215 | 0 | 53 |
| with ⅓ Ice | 160 | 0 | 40 |
| **Medium,** 22 fl.oz: No Ice | 295 | 0 | 73 |
| with ⅓ Ice | 220 | 0 | 55 |
| **Large,** 32 fl.oz: No Ice | 430 | 0 | 105 |
| with ⅓ Ice | 320 | 0 | 80 |

*Note: ⅓ Cup of Ice = ¼ Cup Liquid*

## Soft Drink ~ Brands

*Per 12 fl.oz Unless Indicated*

| | C | F | Cb |
|---|---|---|---|
| A&W: Root Beer, 20 fl.oz | 290 | 0 | 78 |
| Ten, 20 fl.oz | 10 | 0 | 3 |
| **Albertson's:** | | | |
| **Super Chill:** Cola | 160 | 0 | 43 |
| Root Beer | 180 | 0 | 48 |
| Barq's: Root Beer | 170 | 0 | 47 |
| Diet | 0 | | |
| Big Red, Soda, 12fl.oz | 150 | 0 | 38 |
| Blue Sky, Natural Soda, Cola | 170 | 0 | 43 |

## Soft Drink Brands (Cont)

*Per 12 fl.oz Unless Indicated*  C  F  Cb

| | C | F | Cb |
|---|---|---|---|
| **Bubble Up,** Lemon-Lime Soda, 8 fl.oz | 110 | 0 | 28 |
| Cactus Cooler | 150 | 0 | 40 |
| **Canada Dry:** | | | |
| Club Soda; Diet Ginger Ale | 0 | 0 | 0 |
| Ginger Ale; Tonic Water, av. | 140 | 0 | 36 |
| Cheerwine | 150 | 0 | 42 |
| **Coca-Cola:** | | | |
| Classic; Orange Vanilla | 140 | 0 | 39 |
| Calif. Raspberry; Georgia Peach | 140 | 0 | 37 |
| Cherry; Vanilla | 150 | 0 | 42 |
| Diet Coke; Zero | 0 | 0 | 0 |
| Energy: Regular, 8.45 fl.oz | 105 | 0 | 26 |
| No Sugar Added, 8.45 fl.oz | 3 | 0 | 1.5 |
| Life | 90 | 0 | 24 |
| **Crush:** | | | |
| Grape; Orange | 160 | 0 | 43 |
| Peach; Pineapple, average | 190 | 0 | 51 |
| Strawberry | 170 | 0 | 46 |
| Dad's: Cream Soda | 200 | 0 | 51 |
| Root Beer | 165 | 0 | 42 |
| Diet Rite, Pure Zero | 0 | 0 | 0 |
| **Dr Pepper:** *Per 12 fl.oz Can* | | | |
| Regular | 150 | 0 | 40 |
| Cherry | 160 | 0 | 43 |
| Ten | 10 | 0 | 3 |
| Fanta: Orange | 160 | 0 | 44 |
| Zero, all flavors | 0 | 0 | 0 |
| Fresca, all flavors | 0 | 0 | 0 |
| GuS, average all flavors | 95 | 0 | 23 |
| Hansen's: *Per 12 fl.oz* | | | |
| **Natural Cane Sugar:** | | | |
| Creamy Root Beer | 170 | 0 | 45 |
| Original Cola | 160 | 0 | 41 |
| Pomegranate | 130 | 0 | 35 |
| Diet, all flavors | 0 | 0 | 0 |
| **Hawaiian Punch:** | | | |
| Aloha Morning, 40% less sugar, Orange/Strawb./Mixed Berry Citrus | 60 | 0 | 13 |
| Average other flavors | 60 | 0 | 14 |
| **Henry Weinhard's:** Root Beer | 170 | 0 | 43 |
| Orange/Vanilla Cream, av. | 180 | 0 | 44 |
| Hires, Root Beer | 170 | 0 | 45 |
| IBC: Cream Soda; Black Cherry | 175 | 0 | 44 |
| Root Beer | 160 | 0 | 40 |
| Icee: Cola; Orange; Lemon Lime, 6 fl.oz | 80 | 0 | 20 |
| Average other flavors | 80 | 0 | 21 |
| Jarritos, all flavors, 8 fl.oz | 110 | 0 | 28 |
| Jelly Belly, all flavors | 180 | 0 | 42 |
| Jolt, Cola | 150 | 0 | 41 |

## Soft Drink Brands (Cont)

*Per 12 fl.oz Unless Indicated*

| | C | F | Cb |
|---|---|---|---|
| **Jones Soda:** | | | |
| Regular, all flavors, 12 fl.oz | 170 | 0 | 42 |
| Stripped, all flavors, 12 fl.oz | 30 | 0 | 8 |
| Zilch, sugar free, 12 fl.oz | 0 | 0 | 0 |
| **Kool Aid,** Bursts, av., 6.75 fl.oz | 35 | 0 | 9 |
| **Mello Yello,** Regular | 170 | 0 | 47 |
| **Mountain Dew:** All flavors | 170 | 0 | 46 |
| Diet varieties | 0 | 0 | 0 |
| Dewshine | 160 | 0 | 42 |
| Black Label, 16 fl.oz | 210 | 0 | 54 |
| **Mug,** Root Beer | 160 | 0 | 43 |
| **Natural Brew:** Chai Cola | 170 | 0 | 41 |
| Draft Root Beer | 170 | 0 | 43 |
| Outrageous Ginger Ale | 180 | 0 | 44 |
| Vanilla Cream Soda | 160 | 0 | 39 |
| **Nehi,** Peach | 190 | 0 | 51 |
| **Pepsi:** *Per 12 fl.oz* | | | |
| Regular; Caffeine Free | 150 | 0 | 41 |
| Diet Pepsi; Jazz; Pepsi One | 0 | 0 | 0 |
| Pepsi Next | 60 | 0 | 16 |
| **Pepsi True:** 7.5 fl.oz can | 60 | 0 | 17 |
| 12 fl.oz can | 100 | 0 | 27 |
| **Perrier,** Carbonated Water | 0 | 0 | 0 |
| **Pibb:** Xtra | 140 | 0 | 39 |
| Zero, Original | 0 | 0 | 0 |
| **RC Cola:** Regular | 160 | 0 | 43 |
| Ten | 10 | 0 | 3 |
| **Reed's,** Ginger Brew, | | | |
| all varieties | 130 | 0 | 33 |
| **7·UP:** Lemon Lime; Cherry | 140 | 0 | 39 |
| Diet flavors | 0 | 0 | 0 |
| Ten, Lemon Lime | 10 | 0 | 3 |
| **Safeway:** *Per 8 fl.oz* | | | |
| **Refreshe:** Cola; Lem. Lime, av. | 110 | 0 | 28 |
| Grape | 140 | 0 | 36 |
| Mtn Breeze; Strawberry | 120 | 0 | 30 |
| Refreshe Ice, all flavors, 17 fl.oz | 0 | 0 | 0 |
| **Santa Cruz,** Lemonade, 12 fl.oz | 130 | 0 | 32 |
| **Schweppes:** Ginger Ale | 120 | 0 | 33 |
| Tonic Water | 130 | 0 | 33 |
| **Shasta:** Cream Soda | 190 | 0 | 47 |
| Cherry Cola | 180 | 0 | 45 |
| Club Soda; Diet, all flavors | 0 | 0 | 0 |
| Dr. Shasta | 150 | 0 | 38 |
| Ginger Ale | 130 | 0 | 33 |
| Tiki Punch; Pineapple; Orange | 200 | 0 | 50 |
| Average other flavors | 170 | 0 | 41 |
| **Sierra Mist,** Lemon Lime | 120 | 0 | 30 |
| **Sprite:** Original, 12 fl.oz | 140 | 0 | 38 |
| Zero, all flavors | 0 | 0 | 0 |

*Per 12 fl.oz Unless Indicated*

| | C | F | Cb |
|---|---|---|---|
| **Squirt,** Ruby Red | 170 | 0 | 45 |
| **Stewarts:** Root Beer | 150 | 0 | 38 |
| Grape; Orange 'n Cream | 180 | 0 | 45 |
| **Sun Drop:** Citrus Soda, 20 fl.oz | 290 | 0 | 76 |
| Diet Citrus Soda | 10 | 0 | 1 |
| **Sunkist:** Orange, with sugar, 20 fl.oz | 170 | 0 | 44 |
| Pineapple, 20 fl.oz | 320 | 0 | 85 |
| **Surge,** Original 16 fl.oz | 230 | 0 | 62 |
| **Tab, Original** | 0 | 0 | 0 |
| **Tampico:** *Per 12 fl.oz* | | | |
| **Punch:** Blue Raspberry | 90 | 0 | 21 |
| Pineapple Coconut | 105 | 0 | 26 |
| Average other flavors | 90 | 0 | 21 |
| **Soda,** all flavors, 12 fl.oz | 180 | 0 | 42 |
| **Thomas Kemper:** *Per 12 fl.oz* | | | |
| Black Cherry | 170 | 0 | 44 |
| Ginger Ale; Vanilla Cream | 150 | 0 | 36 |
| Root Beer | 160 | 0 | 41 |
| **Trader Joe's:** | | | |
| **Sparkling:** | | | |
| French Berry Lemonade: | | | |
| 1 cup, 8 fl.oz | 130 | 0 | 31 |
| 1 bottle, 33.8 fl.oz | 520 | 0 | 124 |
| Lime Ade: 1 cup, 8 fl.oz | 110 | 0 | 28 |
| 1 bottle, 33.8 fl.oz | 440 | 0 | 108 |
| Pink Lemonade: 1 cup, 8 fl.oz | 130 | 0 | 31 |
| 1 Bottle, 33.8 fl.oz | 520 | 0 | 124 |
| **Vernors,** Ginger Soda, 20 fl.oz | 240 | 0 | 65 |
| **Virgil's,** Root Beer | 160 | 0 | 42 |
| **Walgreens:** *Per 20 fl.oz* | | | |
| Orchard Grape Soda | 300 | 0 | 84 |
| Cola; Zesty Lemon Lime, av. | 225 | 0 | 65 |
| Root Beer | 225 | 0 | 75 |
| **Zevia,** all flavors | 0 | 0 | 4 |
| (Contains between 4-7g Erythritol) | | | |

## Powdered Soft Drink Mixes

*Per 8 fl.oz Prepared, Unless Indicated*

| | C | F | Cb |
|---|---|---|---|
| **Country Time:** | | | |
| Lemonade; Pink Lemonade | 60 | 0 | 16 |
| Strawberry Lemonade | 80 | 0 | 19 |
| **Crystal Light** *(Kraft):* | | | |
| Fruit Drinks, all flavors, 1/2 tsp | 5 | 0 | 0 |
| Pure Fitness, average all flavors, 1 pkt | 15 | 0 | 4 |
| **Flavor Aid,** 1/8 package | 0 | 0 | 0 |
| **Kool-Aid,** sweetened, 0.6 oz | 60 | 0 | 16 |
| **Tang,** Regular, 2 Tbsp, 1 oz | 90 | 0 | 24 |

## Quick Guide

| | **C** | **F** | **Cb** |
|---|---|---|---|
| **Teas** | | | |
| **Regular:** Bag, Loose or Instant | | | |
| Brewed, 1 cup, 8 fl.oz | 2 | 0 | 0.5 |
| (Add extra for sugar/milk) | | | |
| **Herbal,** av. all flav., 1 cup | 2 | 0 | 0.5 |
| **Bubble Milk Tea,** w/ Pearls, 8 fl.oz | 175 | 0 | 41 |
| **Chai Tea Latte Mix,** 1 oz | 110 | 1 | 24 |
| **Kombucha Tea,** *Average all Brands:* | | | |
| Low Sugar, 1 cup, 8 fl.oz | 30 | 0 | 7 |
| Higher Sugar, 1 cup, 8 fl.oz | 50 | 0 | 12 |
| **Iced Tea** | | | |
| *Average All Brands* | | | |
| **Sweetened:** 8 fl.oz cup | 90 | 0 | 22 |
| 12 fl.oz glass/can | 140 | 0 | 35 |
| 16 fl.oz bottle | 180 | 0 | 45 |
| 20 fl.oz bottle | 225 | 0 | 55 |
| **Unsweetened,** 8 fl.oz | 0 | 0 | 0 |

## Iced Tea Mixes

*Per 8 fl.oz Made-Up*

| | **C** | **F** | **Cb** |
|---|---|---|---|
| **4C Iced Tea:** | | | |
| **Average all flavors,** 0.67 oz | 70 | 0 | 18 |
| **Totally Light,** all flavors | 0 | 0 | 0 |
| **Crystal Light,** sugar free | 5 | 0 | 0 |
| **Lipton:** | | | |
| **Sweetened:** Lemon | 70 | 0 | 17 |
| Mango; Peach | 80 | 0 | 19 |
| Unsweetened | 0 | 0 | 0 |
| Diet, all varieties | 5 | 0 | 1 |

## Bottled & Canned Teas

| | **C** | **F** | **Cb** |
|---|---|---|---|
| **Arizona:** *Per 8 fl.oz* | | | |
| **Brewed Tea:** Extra Sweet | 100 | 0 | 25 |
| Southern Style: Sweet | 130 | 0 | 33 |
| **Green Tea,** with Ginseng & Honey | 60 | 0 | 17 |
| **Half & Half,** Lite | 50 | 0 | 14 |
| **Iced Tea:** with Cranberry Juice | 80 | 0 | 22 |
| with Lemon Flavor | 100 | 0 | 25 |
| **White Tea,** Blueberry | 70 | 0 | 21 |
| **Fuze:** *Per 16.9 fl.oz* | | | |
| **Black Tea:** Blueberry; Summer Peach | 120 | 0 | 32 |
| Meyer Lemon | 10 | 0 | 3 |
| **Green Tea,** Tropical Mango | 10 | 0 | 3 |
| **Gold Peak,** Lemon, 18.5 fl.oz | 180 | 0 | 45 |
| **Health-Ade:** *Per 8 fl.oz* | | | |
| Original Kombucha | 30 | 0 | 7 |
| Blood Orange Carrot Ginger | 35 | 0 | 7 |
| Ginger Lemonade | 35 | 0 | 7 |
| Pink Lady Apple; Bubbly Rose | 40 | 0 | 9 |

## Bottled & Canned Teas (Cont)

| | **C** | **F** | **Cb** |
|---|---|---|---|
| **Honest Tea:** *Per 16.9 fl.oz Bottle* | | | |
| **Honey Green Tea** | 70 | 0 | 19 |
| **Peach; Raspberry** | 100 | 0 | 25 |
| **Lipton:** *Per 16.9 fl.oz Unless Indicated* | | | |
| **Brewed Iced Tea,** Sweetened, 12 fl.oz | 100 | 0 | 27 |
| **Green Tea,** Citrus | 100 | 0 | 28 |
| **Half & Half** | 100 | 0 | 26 |
| **Iced Tea:** Berry; Tropical | 90 | 0 | 22 |
| Lemon | 100 | 0 | 27 |
| Mango | 100 | 0 | 25 |
| Peach | 100 | 0 | 26 |
| **Nestea:** | | | |
| **Black Flash Brewed,** | | | |
| all flavors, average, 17.6 fl.oz | 100 | 0 | 24 |
| **Black Classic Tea,** average, 8 fl.oz | 50 | 0 | 13 |
| **POM:** | | | |
| **Antioxidant Super Tea:** *Per 12 fl.oz* | | | |
| Pomegranate: | | | |
| Honey Green Tea | 130 | 0 | 35 |
| Lemonade Tea | 140 | 0 | 35 |
| Peach Passion White Tea | 130 | 0 | 32 |
| Sweet Tea | 120 | 0 | 30 |
| **Snapple:** *Per 16 fl.oz* | | | |
| **Green Tea** | 120 | 0 | 31 |
| Diet Green Tea | 0 | 0 | 0 |
| **Half & Half** | 210 | 0 | 51 |
| **Lemon/ Raspberry Tea** | 150 | 0 | 37 |
| Diet Lemon/Raspberry Tea | 5 | 0 | 0 |
| **Straight Up Tea:** *Per 18.5 fl.oz Bottle* | | | |
| **Sorta Sweet** | 90 | 0 | 22 |
| **Sweet** | 180 | 0 | 45 |
| **SoBe,** Elixir, Green Tea, 20 fl.oz | 200 | 0 | 52 |
| **Ssips,** Lemon Iced Tea, 6.75 fl.oz | 70 | 0 | 17 |
| **Steaz,** Iced Green Tea, | | | |
| lightly sweetened, av., 16 fl.oz | 80 | 0 | 20 |
| **Tampico,** Iced Tea, | | | |
| Peach, Lemon, 8 fl.oz | 40 | 0 | 10 |
| **Tazo,** Org. Iced Black Tea, 13.8 fl oz | 60 | 0 | 15 |
| **TeaZazz,** NaturalZ,all flav., 12.8 fl.oz | 70 | 0 | 20 |
| **Trader Joe's:** | | | |
| Organic Tea & Lemonade | 100 | 0 | 25 |
| Hibiscus & Lemonade, 16 fl.oz | 40 | 0 | 9 |
| **Turkey Hill:** Iced Tea, 12 fl.oz | 120 | 0 | 31 |
| Peach Tea, 12 fl.oz | 140 | 0 | 34 |
| Green Tea, Mango, 12 fl.oz | 120 | 0 | 30 |
| **365 Organic** *(Whole Foods):* | | | |
| Unsweetened: Black Tea | 0 | 0 | 0 |
| Green Tea | 0 | 0 | 0 |

Note: Most breads have similar calories on a weight basis. However, volume may vary.

For example, 1 oz of bread may equal 1 slice regular bread or 2 slices of a lighter bread. It is best to weigh bread used and calculate using: 1 oz bread = 70 calories, 14g carb.

## Quick Guide

**C  F  Cb**

### Bread

**White or Wheat:** *Average Per Slice*

| | C | F | Cb |
|---|---|---|---|
| **Thin or Light,** 0.75 oz | 50 | 0.5 | 9 |
| **Sandwich slice,** 1 oz | 70 | 1 | 14 |
| **Thick or Large,** 1.5 oz | 105 | 1.5 | 18 |
| **Thick,** 2 oz | 140 | 2 | 23 |
| **Extra Thick,** 3 oz | 210 | 3 | 35 |
| **Whole Loaf:** 16 oz | 1120 | 15 | 185 |
| 24 oz Loaf | 1680 | 24 | 280 |

**Multi Grain/Whole Grain:** *Per Slice*

| | C | F | Cb |
|---|---|---|---|
| **Sandwich Slice,** 1 oz | 75 | 1.5 | 12 |
| **Thick Slice,** 2 oz | 150 | 2.5 | 25 |

**Toast:** *Based on same counts as White/Wheat as above*

**1 Slice (1 oz fresh):**

| | C | F | Cb |
|---|---|---|---|
| with 1 tsp butter/margarine | 105 | 5 | 12 |
| with 1 tsp "light" butter/marg. | 90 | 3.5 | 12 |
| with 2 tsp butter/margarine | 140 | 9 | 12 |
| with 2 tsp "light" butter/marg. | 110 | 6 | 12 |

## Breads

*Per Slice Unless Indicated*

| | C | F | Cb |
|---|---|---|---|
| **12-Grain,** 1.5 oz | 110 | 1.5 | 22 |
| **Bran style/Dark,** 1 oz | 70 | 1 | 14 |
| **Buttermilk,** average, 1.5 oz | 110 | 1 | 22 |
| **Challah,** 0.75 oz | 85 | 1.5 | 17 |
| **Chapati,** 1 oz | 110 | 3 | 18 |
| **Ciabatta,** 2 oz | 130 | 1 | 26 |
| **Cornbread,** average, 3 oz | 220 | 6 | 37 |
| **Cracked Wheat Sourdough,** 1.5 oz | 130 | 0.5 | 27 |
| **Croissants** ~ *See Page 134* | | | |
| **Crustless Bread,** regular, slice, 0.75 oz | 40 | 0.5 | 8.5 |
| **Crusts Only,** regular slice, 0.25 oz | 30 | 0 | 7 |
| **English Toasting,** 2 oz | 140 | 1.5 | 27 |
| **Flax & Grain,** 1.5 oz | 120 | 3 | 19 |
| **Foccacia:** Plain, 2 oz serve | 150 | 2.5 | 28 |
| Cheese & Garlic; Pesto, 2 oz serve | 160 | 6 | 21 |
| Tomato & Olive, 2 oz serve | 150 | 5 | 21 |

## Breads (Cont)

**C  F  Cb**

*Per Slice Unless Indicated*

| | C | F | Cb |
|---|---|---|---|
| **French Stick/Baguette,** 1 oz | 70 | 1 | 15 |
| **French Toast:** Slice, 1.5oz | 140 | 2 | 26 |
| *Aunt Jemima,* Sticks, av., 2 oz | 110 | 2 | 18 |
| **Garlic Bread/Toast:** | | | |
| Small slice + 1 tsp spread, 0.75 oz | 80 | 5 | 7 |
| Medium slice + 2 tsp spread, 1.5 oz | 160 | 10 | 14 |
| Thick slice + 3 tsp spread, 1.8 oz | 220 | 14 | 20 |
| *Pepperidge Farm,* 1 slice, 1.4 oz | 160 | 10 | 15 |
| **Hawaiian Sweet Bread,** 1.5 oz | 110 | 2 | 19 |
| **Hemp Bread,** 1.2 oz | 95 | 2 | 12 |
| **Italian Bread,** 2 oz | 140 | 1 | 28 |
| **Lower Carb,** (higher protein/fiber), average all brands, 1 oz | 60 | 1.5 | 9 |
| **MultiGrain,** 1.5 oz | 100 | 2 | 21 |
| **Naan Flatbread,** 2 oz | 160 | 3.5 | 29 |
| **Nut/Health Nut,** 1.35 oz | 90 | 1.5 | 18 |
| **Oatmeal/Oatbran Bread,** 1.5 oz | 90 | 0.5 | 19 |
| **Pita,** average all types: | | | |
| Small (4" diam), 1 oz | 90 | 0 | 18 |
| Large (6½" diam), 2 oz | 140 | 1.5 | 27 |
| Extra Large (9" diam), 4 oz | 300 | 1.5 | 60 |
| **Popovers,** (1), without butter | 130 | 2 | 18 |
| **Pumpernickel:** | | | |
| Cocktail/Party size | 30 | 0.5 | 6 |
| Large slice, 1.35 oz | 80 | 0 | 15 |
| **Raisin Bread,** 1 oz | 80 | 1 | 15 |
| **Rye:** 1 thin slice, av., 1 oz | 80 | 1 | 14 |
| 1 thick slice, 2 oz | 150 | 2 | 25 |
| Cocktail size, 0.4 oz | 25 | 0.5 | 4 |
| **Sandwich Pockets,** 2 oz | 140 | 1.5 | 27 |
| **Sourdough:** Regular, 1.5oz | 120 | 1 | 25 |
| French Style, 1 oz | 75 | 0 | 14 |
| **Spelt,** 1.6 oz | 130 | 1 | 26 |
| **Sprouted 7-Grain,** 1.5 oz | 110 | 0.5 | 18 |
| **Squaw,** 1.1 oz | 85 | 0.5 | 13 |
| **Tacos/Tortillas** ~ *See Page 172* | | | |
| **Turkish/Middle Eastern,** 1 oz | 80 | 1.5 | 16 |
| **Wheat-Free Breads:** Spelt, 1.6 oz | 130 | 1 | 26 |
| Rice, with Fruit Juice, 1.5 oz | 110 | 2 | 21 |
| Healthseed Rye, 1.6 oz | 90 | 1 | 20 |
| Millet, 1.5 oz | 100 | 1 | 20 |

## Bread ~ Brands

**C** **F** **Cb**

*Per Slice Unless Indicated*

| Item | C | F | Cb |
|---|---|---|---|
| **Bimbo:** Doble Fibra, 1 slice, 1.1 oz | 60 | 1 | 13 |
| Pan Blanco Grande, 1 slice, 1 oz | 75 | 0.5 | 14 |
| Pan Integral Wheat, 1 slice, 1 oz | 75 | 1 | 14 |
| **Ener-G,** Gluten-Free: | | | |
| Brown Rice Loaf, regular, 1 sl., 1.3 oz | 100 | 3 | 16 |
| **Classic White:** Regular, 1 sl., 1.4 oz | 110 | 6 | 15 |
| Light, 1 slice, 0.8 oz | 60 | 3.5 | 9 |
| **Multigrain:** Regular, 1 slice, 1.4 oz | 100 | 5 | 15 |
| Light, 1 slice, 0.8 oz | 60 | 3 | 9 |
| **Home Pride:** | | | |
| **Butter Top:** Wheat, 1 slice, 0.9 oz | 70 | 1 | 13 |
| White, 1 slice, 0.9 oz | 70 | 1 | 14 |
| **Nature's Harvest:** *Per Slice* | | | |
| 100% Whole Wheat, 1 oz | 70 | 1 | 14 |
| Light Multigrain, 0.7 oz | 40 | 0.5 | 8 |
| Granola, 0.9 oz | 70 | 1 | 13 |
| **Nature's Own:** *Per Slice* | | | |
| 100% Whole Grain, 0.9 oz | 70 | 1.5 | 12 |
| 100% Whole Wheat, 0.9 oz | 60 | 0.5 | 11 |
| Honey Wheat, 0.9 oz | 70 | 1 | 13 |
| **Oroweat:** *Per Slice* | | | |
| **100% Whole Wheat,** 1.3 oz | 90 | 1 | 16 |
| **22 Grains & Seeds:** Regular, 1.7 oz | 130 | 2.5 | 23 |
| Organic, Thin Sliced, 1 oz | 80 | 1.5 | 13 |
| Honey Wheat, 1.9 oz | 140 | 1.5 | 27 |
| Oatnut, 1.3 oz | 110 | 2 | 19 |
| Pocket Thins, av., | | | |
| ½ flatbread | 100 | 1.5 | 20 |
| Premium Italian, 1.1 oz | 80 | 5 | 16 |
| Sandwich Thins, av., 2 oz roll | 150 | 2 | 28 |
| **Pepperidge Farm:** *Per Slice* | | | |
| 100% Whole Wheat, soft, 1.9 oz | 140 | 1.5 | 25 |
| 15 Grain, 1.7 oz | 130 | 2.5 | 22 |
| Family, White Sandwich, 1.9 oz | 150 | 3 | 26 |
| Italian, w/ Sesame Seeds, 1.1 oz | 90 | 1.5 | 17 |
| Light Style, average, 2 oz | 45 | 0 | 9 |
| Swirl, Brown Sugar Cinn., 1.3 oz | 110 | 2 | 21 |
| Very Thin, 0.5 oz | 40 | 0 | 8 |
| **Roman Meal:** 12 Grain, 1 sl., 1.7 oz | 120 | 2 | 21 |
| Honey Split Top, 1 slice, 2 oz | 130 | 1.5 | 25 |
| **Sara Lee:** *Per Slice* | | | |
| 100% Whole Wheat, 0.9 oz | 60 | 1 | 12 |
| Cracked Wheat, 1.1 oz | 80 | 0.5 | 15 |
| Delightful, av.,1 slices, 0.8 oz | 45 | 5 | 9 |
| Honey Wheat, 0.9 oz | 70 | 0.5 | 13 |
| Sweet Hawaiian, 1.3 oz | 100 | 1.5 | 18 |
| **Trader Joe's:** Gourmet White, 1.5 oz | 120 | 3.5 | 19 |
| Sprouted Wheat Cranberry, 1.2 oz | 90 | 1 | 16 |
| **Wonder:** Classic White, 1 slice, 1oz | 70 | 0.5 | 14 |
| Whole Grain White, 1 slice, 1 oz | 60 | 1 | 12 |
| Whole Wheat, 1 slice, 0.9 oz | 60 | 0.5 | 11 |

## Biscuits, Bread Rolls & Buns

**C** **F** **Cb**

| Item | C | F | Cb |
|---|---|---|---|
| **Biscuits:** *Average, 2½" diameter* | | | |
| Plain/Butter Milk: | | | |
| Prepared from Recipe | 210 | 10 | 27 |
| Refrig. Dough, Baked | 95 | 4 | 13 |
| Brown 'n Serve, av., 1 oz | 70 | 1 | 13 |
| Refrigerated Dough: | | | |
| *Pillsbury,* Buttermilk Biscuit, | | | |
| (3), 2.25 oz | 150 | 2 | 30 |
| **Buns:** | | | |
| Frankfurter/Hot Dog: 1.25 oz | 110 | 1.5 | 21 |
| 1.5 oz | 130 | 2 | 25 |
| Hamburger: Regular, 1.5 oz | 110 | 1.5 | 22 |
| Large, 3 oz | 210 | 3 | 40 |
| Hoagie/Submarine, Plain, 2.3 oz | 200 | 1 | 38 |
| **Rolls:** | | | |
| Ciabatta Roll, 3.5 oz | 230 | 4 | 41 |
| Crescent Roll, Original, 1 oz | 100 | 6 | 11 |
| Dinner: | | | |
| 1 small, 1 oz | 90 | 1.5 | 17 |
| 1 medium (3" diam),1.5 oz | 110 | 1 | 23 |
| French: 1 medium 1.3 oz | 110 | 1.5 | 22 |
| 1 large, 3 oz | 230 | 2.5 | 42 |
| Kaiser: | | | |
| Small, 2 oz | 200 | 2.5 | 35 |
| Large, 3.5 oz | 350 | 4 | 61 |
| Plain, 6", average all, 2.5 oz | 200 | 1 | 38 |
| Sourdough, 1.3 oz | 110 | 1 | 21 |
| Wheat Rolls: Small, 1.2 oz | 100 | 1 | 17 |
| Medium, 1.8 oz | 130 | 1.5 | 23 |
| Large, 3.5 oz | 260 | 3 | 46 |

## Breadsticks, Croutons

| Item | C | F | Cb |
|---|---|---|---|
| **Breadsticks:** | | | |
| Salt Sticks, plain, 1 oz | 110 | 1 | 20 |
| Fresh baked (1), 2 oz | 180 | 2.5 | 34 |
| *Stella D'oro:* Original (1) | 45 | 1 | 7 |
| Sesame (1) | 50 | 2 | 7 |
| **Croutons:** Seasoned, 2 Tbsp, 0.3 oz | 35 | 1.5 | 4 |
| *Pepp. Farm,* Zesty Italian, 6 croutons | 30 | 1 | 5 |

## Bread Products

| Item | C | F | Cb |
|---|---|---|---|
| **Bread Crumbs,** dry: | | | |
| Plain or seasoned: 1 oz | 110 | 1.5 | 20 |
| 1 cup, 3.5 oz | 385 | 5 | 70 |
| **Corn Flake Crumbs,** 1 oz | 120 | 0 | 29 |
| **Graham Cracker Crumbs** *(Keebler)*,1 oz | 110 | 2.5 | 20 |
| **Bread Dough,** average: | | | |
| Frozen, 1 slice, 2 oz | 140 | 2 | 26 |
| Refrigerated: French, 1" sl. | 60 | 1 | 13 |
| Wheat; White, 1" slice | 80 | 2 | 14 |
| **Coating Mixes,** av., 2 Tbsp., 1 oz | 100 | 0.5 | 20 |
| **Stuffing:** Dry mix, average all,1 oz | 110 | 1 | 10 |
| Prepared, ½ cup, 4 oz | 180 | 9 | 22 |

| Quick Guide | C | F | Cb |
|---|---|---|---|

### Bagels
*Average All Brands*
**Plain/Onion:**

| | C | F | Cb |
|---|---|---|---|
| 1 mini/bagelette, 1 oz | 65 | 0.5 | 13 |
| 1 small bagel, 2 oz | 145 | 1 | 29 |
| 1 medium bagel, 3 oz | 220 | 1.5 | 43 |
| 1 large bagel, 4 oz | 290 | 2 | 57 |
| **Bagel Chips,** 1 oz | 130 | 4.5 | 19 |
| **Pizza Bagel Bites (Bagel Bites),** average all varieties., 4 pieces, 3 oz | 190 | 5.5 | 27 |
| **Bagel Crisps** (New York Style), average all varieties, 6 crisps, 1 oz | 130 | 5 | 17 |
| **Bagel Thins** (Thomas'), 1, 1.5 oz | 110 | 1 | 25 |

### Bagel ~ Brands

*Per Bagel*

| | C | F | Cb |
|---|---|---|---|
| **Bubba's:** Plain | 220 | 1.5 | 45 |
| Blueberry | 230 | 2 | 49 |
| Cinnamon Raisin | 230 | 1.5 | 48 |
| **Costco Bakery:** Plain | 330 | 1.5 | 70 |
| Cinnamon Raisin | 340 | 1.5 | 73 |
| Whole Grain | 300 | 5 | 56 |
| **Lender's,** Fresh, NY Style: | | | |
| Plain, 3.3 oz | 240 | 2 | 46 |
| Blueberry, 3.3 oz | 240 | 2 | 46 |
| Cinnamon, 3.3 oz | 240 | 2 | 46 |
| Whole Wheat, 3.3 oz | 240 | 2 | 46 |
| **Panera Bread:** Plain | 290 | 1.5 | 58 |
| Cinnamon Swirl & Raisin, 3.8 fl.oz | 320 | 2 | 66 |
| Everything, 4 oz | 300 | 2 | 58 |
| Whole Grain, 4.3 oz | 330 | 2.5 | 67 |
| **Sara Lee:** Plain, 3.4 oz | 260 | 1 | 52 |
| Blueberry, 3.4 oz | 260 | 1 | 54 |
| Cinnamon Raisin, 3.7 oz | 260 | 0.5 | 54 |
| Everything, 3.4 oz | 270 | 3 | 50 |
| Onion, 3.4 oz | 260 | 1 | 53 |
| **Western,** The Alternatives, av., 2 oz | 120 | 0.5 | 29 |

### Bagel Spreads

**Cream Cheese:**

| | C | F | Cb |
|---|---|---|---|
| Plain: 2 Tbsp, 1 oz | 100 | 9 | 1 |
| 2 oz mini-tub | 200 | 18 | 2 |
| Reduced Fat: 2 Tbsp, 1 oz | 60 | 5 | 2 |
| 2 oz mini-tub | 120 | 10 | 4 |
| **Flavors:** Lox, 1 oz | 90 | 8 | 2 |
| Honey Nut, 1 oz | 80 | 7 | 4 |
| Strawberry, 1 oz | 90 | 7 | 5 |
| Sundried Tomato, 1 oz | 80 | 7 | 2 |
| Vegetable, 1 oz | 90 | 8 | 2 |

### English Muffins

*Average All Brands*

| | C | F | Cb |
|---|---|---|---|
| **Plain/Whole Wheat:** Regular, 2 oz | 135 | 1.5 | 26 |
| Heavier, 2.5 oz | 155 | 2 | 31 |
| Super Size, 3.2 oz | 190 | 2 | 38 |
| **Raisin-Cinnamon,** 2.2 oz | 150 | 1 | 30 |

Note: Actual weight of packaged muffins can be 10-15% heavier than stated net weight.

### Rice Cakes

| | C | F | Cb |
|---|---|---|---|
| Regular size (1), average, 0.3 oz | 35 | 0.5 | 7.5 |
| **Hain,** Mini, White Cheddar (10), 1.2 oz | 70 | 2.5 | 11 |
| **Lundberg:** Brown Rice (1), 0.7 oz | 60 | 0.5 | 14 |
| Caramel Corn (1) | 80 | 0.5 | 17 |
| Cinnamon Toast (1), 0.8 oz | 80 | 0 | 20 |
| **Quaker:** Apple Cinn., 0.5 oz | 50 | 0 | 11 |
| Butter Popcorn, 0.3 oz | 35 | 0 | 8 |
| Tomato & Basil, 0.42 oz | 50 | 2 | 8 |
| White Cheddar, 0.4 oz | 45 | 0.5 | 8 |

### Tortillas & Shells

**Tortillas:** *Per Tortilla*

| | C | F | Cb |
|---|---|---|---|
| Corn Flour, White/Yellow: 6", 1 oz | 55 | 1 | 11 |
| 7", 1.2 oz | 75 | 1 | 14 |
| Wheat Flour: | | | |
| 6", 1.2 oz | 100 | 3 | 16 |
| 8", 1.4 oz | 130 | 4 | 20 |
| 10", 2.3 oz | 200 | 6 | 31 |

**Shells:** *Per Shell, without Fillings*

| | C | F | Cb |
|---|---|---|---|
| Corn Taco Shells: Mini, 3", 0.2 oz | 25 | 1 | 3 |
| Medium, 5", 0.5 oz | 60 | 2.5 | 8 |
| Large, 6½", 0.7 oz | 100 | 4.5 | 13 |
| Salad Shell, 10" | 310 | 17 | 34 |
| Tostada Shells, fried: | | | |
| White Corn, 5½" diam., 0.4 oz | 55 | 2.5 | 8 |
| Yellow Corn, 5½" diam., 0.5 oz | 80 | 3.5 | 11 |
| **Sopes,** 1 shell, 4" 2 oz | 110 | 1.5 | 23 |

**La Tortilla Factory:**

**Non GMO:** Hand Made Style,

| | C | F | Cb |
|---|---|---|---|
| White Corn & Wheat, 1.45 oz | 90 | 1 | 15 |
| Gluten Free, Casava Flour, 1.4 oz | 120 | 4.5 | 20 |
| Low Carb Flour, Burrito Size, 2.2 oz | 110 | 3.5 | 23 |
| Whole Wheat, Burrito Size, 2 oz | 170 | 4.5 | 31 |
| Traditional, Flour, Burrito Size, 2.2 oz | 180 | 4.5 | 31 |

**Mission Foods:**

**Corn,** Yellow/White, Super Soft:

| | C | F | Cb |
|---|---|---|---|
| Regular size, 2 Tortillas, 1.7 oz | 100 | 1.5 | 20 |
| **Flour,** Burrito Size (1), 2.47 oz | 200 | 4.5 | 34 |

## Quick Guide  C  F  Cb

### Cooked Cereals

| | C | F | Cb |
|---|---|---|---|
| **Barley,** pearled, cooked, 1 cup | 195 | 0.5 | 44 |
| **Buckwheat Groats,** roasted: | | | |
| Dry, 1/2 cup, 3 oz | 285 | 2 | 61 |
| Cooked, 1 cup, 6 oz | 155 | 1 | 34 |
| **Bulgur:** Dry, 1/2 cup, 2.5 oz | 240 | 1 | 53 |
| Cooked, 1 cup, 6.5 oz | 150 | 0.5 | 34 |
| **Corn/Hominy Grits:** | | | |
| Dry: Regular, 1/4 cup, 1.4 oz | 140 | 0.5 | 32 |
| Instant: 0.8 fl.oz packet | 75 | 0 | 18 |
| w/ Imitation Bacon Bits, 1 oz | 100 | 0.5 | 22 |
| Cooked, 3/4 cup, 6.5 oz | 110 | 0.5 | 23 |
| **Cream of Rice,** cooked, 3/4 cup, 6.5 oz | 95 | 0 | 21 |
| **Cream of Wheat:** | | | |
| Cooked: Regular, 3/4 cup, 6.5 oz | 95 | 0.5 | 20 |
| Instant, 3/4 cup, 6.5 oz | 105 | 0.5 | 21 |
| Quick, 3/4 cup, 6.5 oz | 100 | 0.5 | 22 |
| **Farina,** cooked, 3/4 cup, 6 oz | 95 | 0.5 | 19 |
| **Millet,** dry, 1/2 cup, 1.8 oz | 190 | 2 | 36 |
| **Oat Bran:** Raw, 1/3 cup, 1 oz | 70 | 2 | 19 |
| Cooked, 1/2 cup, 3.8 fl.oz | 45 | 1 | 13 |
| **Oatmeal:** | | | |
| Dry: Regular, 1/3 cup, 1 oz | 100 | 1.5 | 18 |
| Instant: Regular, average, 1 oz | 105 | 1.5 | 18 |
| Flavored, average, 1.5 oz | 165 | 2 | 34 |
| Cooked: Regular, 3/4 cup, 6 oz | 125 | 2.5 | 21 |
| 1 cup, 8 fl.oz | 165 | 3.5 | 28 |
| **Whole Wheat,** cooked, 3/4 cup, 6.5 oz | 115 | 0.5 | 25 |

### Brans, Wheat Germ, Add-Ons

| | C | F | Cb |
|---|---|---|---|
| **Bee Pollen Granules,** 1 Tbsp, 0.3 oz | 25 | 1 | 2 |
| **Bran:** | | | |
| **Oat Bran:** Raw, 1 Tbsp, 0.2 oz | 20 | 0.5 | 3 |
| 1/3 cup, 1 oz | 100 | 2 | 17 |
| **Rice Bran:** Raw, 1 Tbsp, 0.2 oz | 15 | 1 | 2.5 |
| 1/4 cup, 1 oz | 95 | 6 | 15 |
| **Fruit:** Dried, average, 1 oz | 70 | 0 | 18 |
| Banana, 1/2 medium | 55 | 0 | 14 |
| Prunes in Syrup (5), 3 oz | 90 | 0 | 23 |
| **Honey,** 1 Tbsp, 0.75 oz | 65 | 0 | 17 |
| **Lecithin Granules,** 1 Tbsp, 0.4 oz | 55 | 4 | 0.5 |
| **Nuts,** Almonds (6), 0.3 oz | 40 | 4 | 1.5 |
| **Psyllium Husks,** 1 Tbsp, 0.2 oz | 10 | 0 | 4 |
| **Wheat,** unprocessed, 1 Tbsp | 5 | 0 | 2 |
| **Wheat Germ:** Raw, 1 Tbsp, 0.3 oz | 25 | 0.5 | 4 |
| 1/4 cup, 1 oz | 105 | 3 | 15 |

## Hot/Cooked Cereals ~ Brands

*Per Serving, Dry Mix only*  C  F  Cb

| | C | F | Cb |
|---|---|---|---|
| **Albers,** | | | |
| Quick Grits, 1/4 cup, 1.4 oz | 140 | 0.5 | 31 |
| **B&G:** | | | |
| **Cream of Wheat Instant:** | | | |
| Original, 1 oz | 100 | 0 | 20 |
| Cinnabon; Maple Br. Sugar, 1.3 oz | 130 | 0 | 29 |
| **Bob's Red Mill:** | | | |
| **Brown Rice Farina,** 1/4 cup | 150 | 1 | 32 |
| **Thick Rolled Oats,** 1/2 cup, 2 oz | 220 | 3.5 | 40 |
| **Dr. McDougall's:** | | | |
| **Lower Sugar:** | | | |
| Apple Cinn. Oatmeal, 1 oz pkt | 120 | 2 | 22 |
| Maple Brown Sugar, 1.34 oz pkt | 140 | 2 | 27 |
| **Superfood Chia Crunch,** 1.3 oz pkt | 140 | 3 | 24 |
| **Great Value** *(Walmart):* | | | |
| **Instant Oatmeal:** | | | |
| Cinnamon Swirl, 1.6 oz | 160 | 2 | 34 |
| Original, 1 oz packet | 100 | 2 | 19 |
| **McCann's:** | | | |
| **Instant Irish Oatmeal:** | | | |
| Regular, 1 oz package | 100 | 2 | 19 |
| Apples & Cinn., 1.3 oz | 130 | 0 | 28 |
| Maple & Brown Sugar, 1.5 oz | 160 | 2 | 32 |
| **Malt-O-Meal:** Original; Choc., 1.2 oz | 130 | 0 | 27 |
| Maple Brown Sugar, 1/4 cup | 170 | 0 | 37 |
| **Natures Path:** | | | |
| **Oatmeal:** Flax Plus, 1.76 oz | 210 | 0 | 38 |
| Apple Cinnamon, 1.76 oz | 210 | 2.5 | 40 |
| Maple Nut, 1.7 oz | 210 | 4 | 38 |
| **NutriSystem,** | | | |
| Oatmeal, Maple Brown Sugar, 1 pkg | 150 | 1.5 | 29 |
| **Quaker:** | | | |
| **Gluten Free,** Instant, Orig., 1.23 oz pkt | 130 | 2.5 | 24 |
| **Instant Grits,** av. all flavors, 1 oz | 100 | 1 | 22 |
| **Quick Grits,** Original, 1/4 cup, 1.3 oz | 130 | 0.5 | 29 |
| **Instant Organic Oatmeal:** | | | |
| Original, 1 oz | 100 | 2 | 19 |
| Maple & Brn Sugar, 1.5 oz | 150 | 2 | 31 |
| **Old Fash'nd/Quick Oats,** 1/2 c., 1.4 oz | 150 | 3 | 27 |
| **Real Medleys:** | | | |
| Apple Walnut, 2.65 oz | 300 | 8 | 53 |
| Blueb. Hazelnut, 2.47 oz | 270 | 7 | 49 |
| Summer Berry, 2.47 oz | 250 | 3 | 51 |
| Super Grains: Ban. Walnut, 2.47 oz | 280 | 8 | 49 |
| Maple Pecan Raisin, 2.47 oz | 270 | 7 | 48 |
| **Wegmans:** | | | |
| **Instant Oatmeal:** Orig., 1 oz pkt | 100 | 2 | 19 |
| Raisin & Spice, 1.5 oz pkt | 150 | 1.5 | 33 |

# B Breakfast Cereals

## Quick Guide    **C**   **F**   **Cb**

### Cold Cereals
*Average All Brands*

| | C | F | Cb |
|---|---|---|---|
| Bran Flakes, 3/4 cup, 1 oz | **95** | 0.5 | 24 |
| Corn Flakes, 1 cup, 1 oz | **100** | 0 | 22 |
| Frosted Flakes, 3/4 cup, 1 oz | **110** | 0 | 27 |
| Granola, 100% Nat., 1/2 cup, 1.7 oz | **205** | 6 | 35 |
| Oat Bran Cereal, 1/2 cup, 1.5 oz | **145** | 3 | 25 |
| Puffed Rice, 1 cup. 0.5 oz | **55** | 0 | 13 |
| Puffed Wheat, 1 cup, 0.5 oz | **45** | 0 | 10 |
| Raisin Bran, 1/2 cup, 1 oz | **90** | 0.5 | 22 |
| Rice Crisps, 1 cup, 1 oz | **105** | 0.5 | 24 |
| Shredded Wheat, 1 biscuit, 1 oz | **85** | 0.5 | 20 |
| Wheat Flakes, 3/4 cup, 1 oz | **105** | 1 | 24 |

**Breakfast/Cereal Bars ~** *See Page 31*

## Ready-To-Eat Cereal ~ Brands

**Arrowhead Mills:**

| | C | F | Cb |
|---|---|---|---|
| **Flakes:** Amaranth, 1.2 oz | **140** | 2 | 26 |
| Kamut, 1 oz | **120** | 1 | 25 |
| Maple Buckwheat, 1.5 oz | **170** | 1 | 35 |
| Oat Bran, 1.2 oz | **140** | 2.5 | 24 |
| Spelt, 1 oz | **120** | 1 | 24 |
| Sweetened Rice, 1.65 oz | **180** | 1 | 40 |
| **Puffed:** Corn, 0.5 oz | **60** | 1 | 12 |
| Kamut, 0.5 oz | **50** | 0 | 11 |
| Millet, 0.5 oz | **60** | 0.5 | 11 |
| Rice, 0.5 oz | **60** | 0 | 14 |
| Wheat, 0.5 oz | **60** | 0 | 12 |
| **Shredded Wheat,** | | | |
| Bite Size, 1.7 oz | **190** | 1 | 38 |
| **Sprouted,** Corn Flakes, 1.3 oz | **110** | 1 | 25 |

**Back to Nature:** *Per 1/2 Cup*

| | C | F | Cb |
|---|---|---|---|
| **Granola:** Apple Blueberry, 1.76 oz | **190** | 2.5 | 37 |
| Chocolate Delight, 1.76 oz | **200** | 5 | 36 |
| Classic, 1.76 oz | **200** | 2.5 | 38 |
| Cranberry Pecan, 1.65 oz | **180** | 5 | 34 |
| Dark Chocolate Coconut, 1.76 oz | **230** | 11 | 31 |
| Honey Nut, 1.76 oz | **220** | 6 | 36 |
| Sunflower & Pumpkin Seed, 1.65 oz | **210** | 7 | 31 |
| Vanilla Almond Agave, 1.76 oz | **200** | 6 | 34 |
| **Granola Clusters:** | | | |
| Peanut Butter, 1.8 oz | **220** | 9 | 27 |
| Av. other varieties, 1.8 oz | **200** | 4.5 | 36 |

**Barbara's Bakery:**    **C**   **F**   **Cb**

**Classics, Organic & Sweetened:**

| | C | F | Cb |
|---|---|---|---|
| Brown Rice Crisps, 1.4 oz | **150** | 1 | 33 |
| Corn Flakes, 1.4 oz | **150** | 0 | 35 |
| Honest O's, Orig., 1.4 oz | **150** | 2 | 30 |
| **Morning Oat Crunch:** | | | |
| Original, 2 oz | **210** | 2.5 | 45 |
| Cinnamon, 2 oz | **220** | 2.5 | 46 |
| Vanilla Almond, 1.94 oz | **220** | 2.5 | 46 |
| **Puffins:** | | | |
| Original; Cinnamon, 1 oz | **90** | 1 | 24 |
| Honey Rice, 1 oz | **110** | 0.5 | 25 |
| Multigrain; Pumpkin, 1 oz | **110** | 0 | 25 |
| PB/PB & Choc., av., 1 oz | **115** | 1.5 | 24 |
| **Snackanimals,** all varieties, 1 oz | **110** | 0.5 | 26 |
| **Shredded Wheat,** 2 biscuits, 1.4 oz | **140** | 1 | 32 |
| **Spoonfuls,** Multigrain, 1.1 oz | **120** | 1.5 | 24 |
| **Squarefuls,** Multigrain, 1.95 oz | **200** | 1 | 47 |

**Bear Naked, Granola:**

| | C | F | Cb |
|---|---|---|---|
| **Fruit & Nut,** 1 oz | **140** | 6 | 20 |
| **Original Cinnamon,** 1 oz | **130** | 6 | 15 |
| **Peanut Butter,** 1.16 oz | **150** | 7 | 21 |
| **V'nilla Almond,** 1 oz | **120** | 2.5 | 22 |

**Bob's Red Mill,**

| | C | F | Cb |
|---|---|---|---|
| **Muesli,** Old Country Style, 1.23 oz | **140** | 3 | 23 |

**Cascadian Farm:**

| | C | F | Cb |
|---|---|---|---|
| **Buzz Crunch,** 2.1 oz | **230** | 3 | 47 |
| **Cinnamon Crunch,** 1 oz | **110** | 2.5 | 22 |
| **Graham Crunch,** 1 oz | **110** | 2 | 23 |
| **Granola:** Ancient Grains, 2 oz | **240** | 6 | 41 |
| French Vanilla Almond, 2 oz | **250** | 7 | 42 |
| Oats & Honey, 2.2 oz | **260** | 7 | 46 |
| **Honey Nut O's,** 1 oz | **110** | 1 | 25 |
| **Multi Grain Squares,** | | | |
| 1 cup, 1.9 oz | **210** | 1 | 44 |
| **Raisin Bran,** 1.8 oz | **180** | 1 | 41 |

**EnviroKidz:** *Per 1 oz*

| | C | F | Cb |
|---|---|---|---|
| **Amazon Frosted Flakes,** 1 oz | **120** | 0 | 27 |
| **Gorilla Munch,** 1 oz | **120** | 1 | 26 |
| **Leapin' Lemurs,** 1 oz | **120** | 1.5 | 25 |
| **Panda Puffs,** 1 oz | **130** | 3.5 | 23 |

**Erewhon:**

| | C | F | Cb |
|---|---|---|---|
| **Corn Flakes,** 1.2 oz | **130** | 0 | 30 |
| **Crispy Brown Rice,** 1 oz | **110** | 0.5 | 24 |
| **Cinn. Crispy Brown Rice,** | **110** | 0.5 | 23 |
| **Honey Rice Twice,** 1 oz | **120** | 0.5 | 25 |
| **Simply Vanilla Granola,** 1.94 oz | **240** | 6 | 41 |

### Ready-To-Eat Cereal (Cont)

**Ezekiel 4.9:**

| | C | F | Cb |
|---|---|---|---|
| **Sprouted Whole Grain Cereal:** | | | |
| Original, ½ cup, 2 oz | 190 | 1 | 40 |
| Almond, ½ cup, 2 oz | 200 | 3 | 38 |
| Golden Flax, ½ cup, 2 oz | 180 | 2.5 | 37 |
| **Sprouted Flakes:** Almond, ¾ c., 1.94 oz | 210 | 2.5 | 40 |
| Flax & Chia, ¾ cup, 1.94 oz | 210 | 3 | 42 |
| Original, ¾ cup, 1.94 oz | 210 | 2 | 41 |

**General Mills:**

| | C | F | Cb |
|---|---|---|---|
| **Apple/Blueberry/Strawberry,** | | | |
| **Cinn. Toast Crunch,** 1 oz | 120 | 3 | 22 |
| **Blueberry Toast Crunch,** 1 oz | 120 | 3 | 22 |
| **Cheerios:** *Per ¾ Cup Unless Indicated* | | | |
| Original, 1 cup, 1 oz | 100 | 2 | 20 |
| Apple Cinn., ¾ cup, 1 oz | 110 | 1.5 | 22 |
| Chocolate, ¾ cup, 1 oz | 100 | 1.5 | 21 |
| Frosted, ¾ cup, 1 oz | 100 | 1.5 | 22 |
| Fruity, ¾ cup, 1 oz | 100 | 1.5 | 21 |
| Honey Nut, ¾ cup, 1 oz | 110 | 1.5 | 22 |
| Multi Grain, 1 cup, 1oz | 110 | 1.5 | 24 |
| Protein: Oats & Honey, 1¼ c., 2 oz | 210 | 2.5 | 41 |
| Cinnamon Almond, 11/4 c., 2 oz | 220 | 4.5 | 40 |
| Very Berry, ¾ cup, 1 oz | 110 | 1.5 | 22 |
| **Chex:** Choc., ¾ cup, 1 oz | 130 | 2.5 | 26 |
| Cinnamon, ¾ cup, 1 oz | 120 | 2 | 25 |
| Corn, 1 cup, 1 oz | 120 | 0.5 | 26 |
| Honey Nut, ¾ cup, 1 oz | 120 | 0.5 | 28 |
| Rice, 1 cup, 1 oz | 100 | 0.5 | 23 |
| Vanilla, ¾ cup, 1 oz | 120 | 2 | 25 |
| Wheat, ¾ cup, 1.7 oz | 160 | 1 | 39 |
| **Cinn. Toast Crunch,** ¾ cup, 1 oz | 130 | 3 | 25 |
| **Fiber One:** Original, ½ cup, 1 oz | 60 | 1 | 25 |
| Honey Clusters, 1 cup, 1.8 oz | 170 | 1.5 | 44 |
| **French Toast Crunch,** ¾ cup, 1 oz | 110 | 1 | 24 |
| **Kix:** Original, 1¼ cups, 1 oz | 110 | 1 | 25 |
| Berry Berry; Honey, | | | |
| 1¼ cups, 1.2 oz | 120 | 1.5 | 28 |
| **Lucky Charms,** | | | |
| Original; Chocolate, ¾ cup, 1 oz | 110 | 1.5 | 23 |
| **Monster:** Berry varieties, 1 cup 1.2 oz | 130 | 1.5 | 28 |
| Count Chocula, ¾ cup, 1 oz | 100 | 1.5 | 23 |
| **Total,** Whole Grain, 1 oz | 110 | 0.5 | 25 |
| **Trix,** 1 cup, 1.1 oz | 120 | 1.5 | 27 |
| **Wheaties,** 1 oz | 100 | 0.5 | 23 |

**Great Value** *(Walmart):*

| | C | F | Cb |
|---|---|---|---|
| Apple Blasts, 1.2 oz | 120 | 0 | 29 |
| Cinnamon Crunch, ¾ cup, 1.1.oz | 120 | 1 | 25 |
| Cocoa Crunch, ¾ cup, 1 oz | 120 | 1.5 | 26 |
| Corn Flakes, 1 cup | 110 | 0 | 26 |
| Crunchy Raisin Bran, 1.87 oz | 190 | 1 | 20 |
| Extra Raisin Raisin Bran, 1 cup | 200 | 1 | 43 |
| Frosted Shredded Wheat, 1.9 oz | 180 | 1 | 42 |
| Fruit Spins, 1 cup, 1 oz | 110 | 1 | 25 |
| O's Oat, 1 oz | 120 | 1 | 23 |
| Toasted Multi-Grain Spins, | | | |
| 1 cup | 110 | 1.5 | 24 |

**Heartland:**

| | C | F | Cb |
|---|---|---|---|
| **Granola:** Original, ½ cup, 2 oz | 240 | 6 | 41 |
| Fruit & Nut Harvest, ½ c., 1.8 oz | 210 | 6 | 34 |
| Harvest Spice, ½ cup, 1.8 oz | 210 | 5 | 37 |
| Low-Fat varieties, ½ cup, 1.8 oz | 200 | 3 | 40 |
| Oat Bran, ½ cup, 1.4 oz | 160 | 3 | 23 |
| Raisin, ½ cup, 2 oz | 240 | 6 | 41 |

**Kashi:**

| | C | F | Cb |
|---|---|---|---|
| **7 Whole Grain:** Flakes, 1 cup, 1.8 oz | 170 | 0.5 | 41 |
| Honey Puffs, | | | |
| 1⅓ cups, 1.4 oz | 150 | 1 | 34 |
| Whole Grain Puffs, | | | |
| 1½ cups, 1.4 oz | 150 | 1.5 | 32 |
| **Go:** Original, 1¼ cups, 2 oz | 180 | 2 | 40 |
| Crunch: Original, ¾ cup, 2 oz | 190 | 3 | 38 |
| Chocolate, ¾ cup, 1.83 oz | 210 | 7 | 32 |
| Cinnamon Crisp, ¾ cup, 1.8 oz | 180 | 4 | 32 |
| Peanut Butter Crunch, ¾ c., 2 oz | 230 | 9 | 31 |

**Heart to Heart:**

| | C | F | Cb |
|---|---|---|---|
| Organic Honey Toasted Oat, 1 c., 1.5 oz | 150 | 5 | 34 |
| Organic Warm Cinnamon, 1 cup, 1.5 oz | 150 | 2.5 | 33 |

**Organic:**

| | C | F | Cb |
|---|---|---|---|
| Indigo Morning, 1 oz | 100 | 1 | 22 |
| Sprouted Grains, 1¼ cups, 2 oz | 190 | 1 | 45 |
| Sweet Potato Sunshine, 1 c., 1.8 oz | 190 | 1 | 43 |

**Whole Wheat Biscuit,**

| | C | F | Cb |
|---|---|---|---|
| Island Vanilla, 29 biscuits | 200 | 1 | 47 |

**Kellogg's:**

| | C | F | Cb |
|---|---|---|---|
| **All-Bran:** Original, ½ cup, 1 oz | 80 | 1 | 23 |
| Bran Buds, ⅓ cup, 1 oz | 80 | 1 | 24 |
| Compl. Wheat Flakes, 1.3 oz | 120 | 1 | 30 |
| **Apple Jacks,** 1 cup, 1 oz | 110 | 1 | 25 |
| **Cinnabon,** 1 cup, 1 oz | 120 | 2 | 25 |

*continued next page...*

# Breakfast Cereals

## Ready-To-Eat Cereal (Cont)

### Kellogg's (Cont):

| | C | F | Cb |
|---|---|---|---|
| **Corn Flakes,** Orig., 1 cup, 1 oz | 100 | 0 | 24 |
| **Cracklin' Oat Bran,** ³/₄ cup, 1.8 oz | 200 | 7 | 34 |
| **Crispix,** Original, 1 cup, 1 oz | 110 | 0 | 25 |
| **Despicable Me 3 Minion,** 1 c., 1.2 oz | 120 | 1 | 27 |
| **Froot Loops:** Original, 1 cup, 1 oz | 110 | 1 | 25 |
| Marshmallow, 1 cup, 1 oz | 110 | 1 | 26 |
| **Frosted Flakes:** *Per 1 oz* | | | |
| Chocolate, ³/₄ cup, 1 oz | 120 | 1 | 26 |
| w/ Marshmallows, 1.1 oz | 120 | 1 | 26 |
| Cinnamon, ³/₄ cup, 1 oz | 110 | 0 | 26 |
| Honey Nut, ³/₄ cup, 1 oz | 110 | 0 | 26 |
| Original Flakes, ³/₄ cup, 1 oz | 110 | 0 | 26 |
| w/ Marshmallows, 1 oz | 110 | 0 | 26 |
| **Happy Inside,** all flavors, 1.94 oz | 210 | 4 | 44 |
| **Honey Smacks,** 1.5 oz | 160 | 0.5 | 37 |
| **Krave,** Double Choc., 1.45 oz | 170 | 4.5 | 31 |
| **Mini-Wheats, Frosted:** | | | |
| Bite Size, Orig. (21), 1.8 oz | 190 | 1 | 46 |
| Little Bites: Orig., 1 c., 2 oz | 200 | 1 | 47 |
| Chocolate, 1 cup, 2 oz | 200 | 2 | 45 |
| Touch of Fruit In Middle, Raspberry (24), 2 oz | 190 | 1 | 45 |
| **Mini Wheats,** unfrosted: | | | |
| Bite Size (30), 1.8 oz | 190 | 1 | 45 |
| Little Bites, 1 cup, 2 oz | 200 | 1 | 47 |
| **Mueslix,** 1 cup, 2.36 oz | 250 | 3.5 | 50 |
| **Raisin Bran:** Reg., 1 c., 2 oz | 190 | 1 | 47 |
| Crunch, 1 cup, 1.94 oz | 190 | 1 | 46 |
| **Rice Krispies:** Orig., 1.2 oz | 130 | 0 | 29 |
| Treats, ³/₄ cup, 1 oz | 120 | 1 | 26 |
| **Smart Start,** Strong Heart, Antioxidants, 1¼ cups, 2.25 oz | 240 | 1 | 56 |
| **Special K:** Orig., 1¼ cups, 1.4 oz | 150 | 0.5 | 29 |
| Apple Cinnamon Crunch, 1.5 oz | 160 | 1.5 | 35 |
| Chocolate Almond, 1.5 oz | 160 | 2 | 34 |
| Chocolatey Delight, 1 cup, 1.48 oz | 170 | 3 | 34 |
| Cinn. Brown Sugar Crunch, 1.5 oz | 160 | 1 | 29 |
| Fruit & Yogurt, 1 cup, 1.48 oz | 160 | 1 | 36 |
| Nourish, C'nut Cranb. Alm., 1.94 oz | 210 | 4 | 43 |
| Red Berries, 1¼ cups, 1.4 oz | 140 | 0.5 | 34 |
| Vanilla Almond, 1.4 oz | 150 | 1.5 | 33 |
| **Strawberry Krispies,** 1.2 oz | 120 | 0 | 28 |

### Kind:
#### Clusters:
| | C | F | Cb |
|---|---|---|---|
| Cinn. Oat, with Flax, 1.76 oz | 190 | 5 | 34 |
| Dark Choc. Whole Grain, 2,3 oz | 240 | 6 | 38 |
| Maple Quinoa, with Chia, 1.76 oz | 200 | 4.5 | 34 |
| Peanut Butter Whole Grain, 2.3 oz | 260 | 8 | 37 |

### Malt-O-Meal:
| | C | F | Cb |
|---|---|---|---|
| **Apple Zings,** 1 cup, 1 oz | 110 | 0.5 | 25 |
| **Cocoa Dyno-Bites,** 1 oz | 110 | 1 | 26 |
| **Coco Roos,** 0.9 oz | 100 | 1 | 23 |
| **Frosted Flakes,** 1.2 oz | 130 | 0 | 30 |
| **Fruity Dyno-Bites,** 1 oz | 110 | 1 | 24 |
| **Frosted Mini Spooners,** 1.94 oz | 190 | 1 | 45 |
| **Golden Puffs,** ³/₄ cup, 1 oz | 110 | 0 | 26 |
| **Honey Nut Scooters,** 1 oz | 120 | 1.5 | 24 |
| **Marshmallow Mateys,** 1 oz | 120 | 1 | 25 |
| **Peanut Butter Cups,** 1 oz | 130 | 4 | 23 |
| **Raisin Bran,** 1 cup, 2 oz | 200 | 1 | 47 |

### Nature's Path:
#### Flax Plus:
| | C | F | Cb |
|---|---|---|---|
| Maple Pecan Crunch, 2.1 oz | 240 | 8 | 41 |
| Multibran Flakes, 1.4 oz | 150 | 2 | 31 |
| **Heritage Flakes,** 1.4 oz | 160 | 1.5 | 31 |
| **Sunrise:** Crunchy Honey, 1 oz | 120 | 1 | 26 |
| Crunchy Maple, 1 oz | 110 | 1 | 25 |
| **Superflakes,** Qi'a Cocoa Coconut, 1.94 oz | 240 | 7 | 39 |
| **Whole Os,** 1.4 oz | 160 | 2 | 33 |
| **Granola:** Coconut Chia, 1.94 oz | 270 | 11 | 36 |
| Coconut & Cashew Butter, 1 oz | 150 | 7 | 19 |
| Grain Free: Maple Almond, 1 oz | 180 | 15 | 5 |
| Vanilla Poppyseed, 1 oz | 180 | 15 | 6 |
| Honey Almond, 1 oz | 140 | 4.5 | 21 |
| Pumpkin Seed & Flax, 1.94 oz | 260 | 10 | 37 |
| Summer Berries, 1 oz | 140 | 4 | 22 |

### New England Natural Bakers:
#### Organic Granola:
| | C | F | Cb |
|---|---|---|---|
| Berry Coconut, unswtnd,1.5 oz | 250 | 12 | 31 |
| Blueberry Harvest, ½ cup, 2 oz | 220 | 6 | 34 |
| Cranberry Almond, ²/₃ cup, 2 oz | 240 | 9 | 36 |
| Granny Smith Apple ½ cup, 2 oz | 250 | 7 | 38 |

### NutriSystem:
| | C | F | Cb |
|---|---|---|---|
| **Granola Cereal,** 1 pkg | 160 | 2.5 | 30 |

### Peace:
#### Clusters & Flakes:
| | C | F | Cb |
|---|---|---|---|
| Mango Peach Passion, 1.94 oz | 230 | 2.5 | 46 |
| Maple Pecan, 1.94 oz | 240 | 6 | 42 |
| Vanilla Almond, 1.94 oz | 240 | 6 | 42 |
| Wild Berry, 1.94 oz | 220 | 3 | 44 |
| **Granola:** Coconut Craze, 1.94 | 270 | 12 | 37 |
| French Vanilla, 1.94 oz | 240 | 6 | 41 |
| Maple Pecan, 1.94 oz | 250 | 8 | 40 |
| **Purple Corn Flakes,** 1 oz | 90 | 1 | 23 |
| **Raisin Bran,** 1.94 oz | 170 | 0.5 | 42 |

## Ready-To-Eat Cereal ~ Brands (Cont)

| | C | F | Cb |
|---|---|---|---|

**Post:**

| | C | F | Cb |
|---|---|---|---|
| **Alpha Bits,** 1 cup, 1 oz | 100 | 1 | 22 |
| **Bran Flakes,** 1 cup, 1.3 oz | 110 | 1 | 29 |
| **CoCo Wheats,** 1.1 oz | 110 | 0 | 24 |
| **Golden Crisp,** 1 cup, 1.34 oz | 150 | 0.5 | 34 |
| **Grape-Nuts:** Original, 2 oz | 210 | 1 | 47 |
| Flakes, ³/₄ cup, 1 oz | 110 | 1 | 24 |
| **Great Grains:** | | | |
| Banana Nut Crunch, 1 cup, 1 oz | 230 | 4.5 | 45 |
| Cranb. Alm. Crunch, 1 cup, 2 oz | 210 | 3 | 44 |
| Crunchy Pecan, ³/₄ cup, 1.8 oz | 210 | 6 | 38 |
| **Honey Bunches of Oats:** | | | |
| Chocolate, 1.1 oz | 130 | 1.5 | 27 |
| Honey Roasted, 1 oz | 120 | 1.5 | 23 |
| Pecan & Maple Brown Sugar, 1 oz | 120 | 2.5 | 23 |
| With Almonds, 1.1 oz | 130 | 2.5 | 26 |
| W/ Cinnamon Bunches, 1 oz | 120 | 1.5 | 25 |
| **Honey-Comb,** 1.1 oz | 130 | 1 | 28 |
| **Malt O Meal ~ see Page 60** | | | |
| **Nutter Butter,** 1¹/₄ cups, 1.4 oz | 180 | 5 | 31 |
| **Oreo O's,** 1⅓ cups, 1.4 oz | 160 | 2 | 34 |
| **Pebbles,** av. all varieties, 1 oz | 115 | 1 | 24 |
| **Raisin Bran,** 1 cup, 2 oz | 190 | 1 | 47 |
| **Shredded Wheat,** Spoon Size: | | | |
| Original, 19 biscuits, 1.94 oz | 200 | 2.5 | 44 |
| Wheat & Bran, 2 oz | 210 | 1.5 | 47 |
| **Shredded Wheat,** Frosted, | | | |
| Choc. Strawb., 19 bisc., 1.94 oz | 200 | 2.5 | 44 |

**Quaker:**

| | C | F | Cb |
|---|---|---|---|
| **King Vitaman,** 1¹/₂ cups, 1 oz | 120 | 1 | 26 |
| **Life,** all types, ³/₄ cup, 1 oz | 120 | 1.5 | 25 |
| **Oatmeal Squares,** | | | |
| all varieties, 2 oz | 210 | 2.5 | 44 |
| **Quisps,** 1 cup 1 oz | 100 | 1.5 | 23 |
| **Simply Granola:** | | | |
| Apple Cranberry Almond, 1.7 oz | 200 | 5 | 37 |
| Oats, Honey, Raisins & Alm., 1.8 oz | 210 | 5 | 38 |

**Stop & Shop:**

| | C | F | Cb |
|---|---|---|---|
| **Fiber Select,** ¹/₂ cup, 1 oz | 50 | 0.5 | 23 |
| **Granola:** | | | |
| Oats & Honey, ¹/₂ c., 1.8 oz | 230 | 9 | 31 |
| **Oats & O's,** 1 cup, 1.1 oz | 110 | 1.5 | 22 |
| **Raisin Bran,** 1 cup, 2 oz | 190 | 1 | 46 |
| **Shredded Wheat,** Bite Size, 1 c., 1.5 oz | 140 | 1 | 33 |

**Sweet Home Farm:**

| | C | F | Cb |
|---|---|---|---|
| **Granola:** Blueberry, w/ Flax, 1.94 oz | 250 | 8 | 40 |
| Cinnamon, with Raisins, 1.94 oz | 200 | 3 | 43 |
| French Vanilla, with Alm., 1.94 oz | 250 | 8 | 40 |
| Honey Nut, with Alm., 1.94 oz | 260 | 10 | 37 |
| Maple Pecan, with Syrup, 1.94 oz | 250 | 8 | 40 |
| Pumpkin Flax, 1.94 oz | 240 | 9 | 37 |

**Trader Joe's:**

| | C | F | Cb |
|---|---|---|---|
| **Bran Flakes,** ³/₄ cup, 1 oz | 100 | 0.5 | 24 |
| **Cinnamon Squares,** 1 cup, 1.5 oz | 170 | 3 | 31 |
| **Clusters:** Raisin Bran, 1 cup, 2 oz | 190 | 3 | 41 |
| Super Nutty Toffee, ³/₄ cup, 2 oz | 250 | 9 | 38 |
| Vanilla Almond, ²/₃ cup, 2 oz | 220 | 8 | 34 |
| Av. other Flavors, 1 c., 2 oz | 230 | 8 | 40 |
| **Cornflakes,** 1 cup, 1 oz | 110 | 0 | 26 |
| **Frosted Flakes,** ³/₄ c., 1 oz | 110 | 0 | 24 |
| **High Fiber Cereal:** Reg., ²/₃ cup, 1 oz | 80 | 0.5 | 23 |
| Fruit & Nut, Multigrain, 1 oz | 90 | 1.5 | 25 |
| **Granola:** Gluten Free, ³/₄ cup, 2 oz | 60 | 12 | 35 |
| Low Fat, av., ³/₄ cup, 2 oz | 210 | 3 | 44 |
| Org., Apple/Mango, av., ²/₃ cup, 2 oz | 240 | 8 | 37 |
| **Joe's O's,** 1 cup, 1 oz | 110 | 2 | 20 |
| **Just The Clusters,** av., ²/₃ cup, 2 oz | 240 | 9 | 36 |
| **O's,** av. all flavours, ³/₄ - 1 cup, 1 oz | 120 | 2 | 24 |
| **Oatmeal (Instant):** *Per 1.4 oz Pkt* | | | |
| Ancient Grains | 160 | 6 | 24 |
| Mango;  Maple & Brown Sugar, av. | 160 | 2 | 32 |
| Unsweetened | 160 | 3.5 | 27 |
| **Oatmeal Complete:** Plain, 1.4 oz pkt | 170 | 3 | 29 |
| Maple Brown Sugar, 1.4 oz pkt | 210 | 3 | 38 |
| **Raisin Bran:** Regular, 1 cup, 2 oz | 170 | 1 | 44 |
| Clusters, 1 cup, 2 oz | 190 | 3 | 41 |
| w/ Pomegr. Blue. Flakes/Clusters, 1 c. | 210 | 2 | 44 |
| **Shredded Wheat,** 1 cup, 1.7 oz | 180 | 1 | 38 |
| **Toasted Oatmeal Flakes,** ³/₄ c., 1 oz | 110 | 1 | 23 |

**Udi's:**

| | C | F | Cb |
|---|---|---|---|
| **Granola:** Orig.; Cranberry, 2 oz | 270 | 10 | 41 |
| Au Naturel; Vanilla, av., 2 oz | 275 | 10 | 39 |

**Uncle Sam:**

| | C | F | Cb |
|---|---|---|---|
| **Original,** Wheat Berry, | | | |
| ³/₄ cup, 1.94 oz | 210 | 6 | 37 |
| **Skinner's Raisin Bran,** 1.94 oz | 200 | 1 | 45 |
| **Weetabix,** 2 bisc., 1.3 oz | 130 | 1 | 29 |

**Wegmans:**

| | C | F | Cb |
|---|---|---|---|
| **Chocolaty Rice Crisps,** 1.5 oz | 170 | 1.5 | 37 |
| **Crunchy Raisin Bran,** 1.8 oz | 190 | 1 | 44 |
| **Granola:** | | | |
| Oats & Honey, with Alm., 1.1 oz | 130 | 2 | 26 |
| Vanilla & Almonds,  1 oz | 140 | 4 | 22 |
| **Shredded Wheat,** | | | |
| Frosted Bite Size, 2 oz | 210 | 1 | 50 |

**Whole Foods 365:**

| | C | F | Cb |
|---|---|---|---|
| **Corn Flakes,** 1 cup, 1 oz | 110 | 0 | 26 |
| **Frosted Flakes,** 1 oz | 110 | 0 | 27 |
| **Honey Flakes & Oat Clusters,** 1 oz | 120 | 1 | 25 |
| **Protein & Fiber Crunch,** 1.8 oz | 190 | 1 | 33 |
| **Raisin Bran,** 1 cup, 2 oz | 180 | 1 | 44 |
| **Wheat Squares:** | | | |
| Bite Sized, 1.7 oz | 180 | 1 | 38 |
| Frosted, 1 cup, 1.9 oz | 210 | 1 | 45 |

## Ready-to-Eat | **C** | **F** | **Cb**

*Per Piece/Slice*

| | C | F | Cb |
|---|---|---|---|
| **Angel Food,** Plain: without oil, 2 oz | 145 | 0 | 33 |
| with oil, 2 oz | 145 | 1 | 27 |
| with Cream Frosting | 255 | 7 | 45 |
| **Almond Croissant,** 5 oz | 620 | 35 | 67 |
| **Apple Danish,** 5 oz | 450 | 18 | 67 |
| **Apple Pie ~** *See Pies/Tarts Page 134* | | | |
| **Baklava,** 1½" square, 1.75 oz | 200 | 10 | 27 |
| **Banana Cake,** with Butter Cream, 2 oz | 230 | 9 | 37 |
| **Banana Walnut Cake,** 3 oz | 270 | 11 | 40 |
| **Bear Claw,** 4.5 oz | 540 | 24 | 71 |
| **Black Forest,** 3 oz | 345 | 11 | 59 |
| **Brownie:** Small, 2" Square, 1 oz | 130 | 8 | 14 |
| Large, 3 oz | 390 | 24 | 42 |
| **Bundt Cakes,** average all types: | | | |
| 3 oz slice | 300 | 13 | 42 |
| Mini-Bundt, 5 oz | 500 | 22 | 70 |
| **Cannoli's:** Mini, 1 oz | 85 | 3 | 11 |
| Regular, 2.5 oz | 215 | 8 | 28 |
| **Carrot Cake:** Plain, 3 oz | 300 | 16 | 37 |
| with Cream Cheese Frosting | 400 | 22 | 48 |
| **Cheesecake:** | | | |
| Small serving, 3 oz | 240 | 13 | 26 |
| Large serving, 5 oz | 400 | 21 | 44 |
| with Low-Fat Cheese/Fruit, 3 oz | 170 | 4 | 28 |
| *Denny's,* NY Style, 5oz | 510 | 34 | 43 |
| **Chocolate Cake:** | | | |
| with Chocolate Frosting, 4 oz | 415 | 18 | 62 |
| without Frosting, ¹⁄₁₂ of 9", 3.5 oz | 340 | 14 | 51 |
| **Chocolate Croissant,** 4.25 oz | 470 | 26 | 54 |
| **Chocolate Eclair,** w/ custard, 3.5 oz | 260 | 16 | 24 |
| **Chocolate Fudge Cake,** 3 oz | 270 | 12 | 40 |
| **Chocolate Meringue,** 2.5 oz | 320 | 13 | 48 |
| **Churros,** 1 stick, 1.5 oz | 165 | 8 | 21 |
| **Cinnamon Crumb Cake,** 2.5 oz | 260 | 9 | 40 |
| **Cinnamon Rolls:** Small, 2 oz | 220 | 8 | 34 |
| Regular, 4 oz | 440 | 16 | 68 |
| Large, 6 oz | 660 | 24 | 102 |
| **Brands ~** *See Page 67* | | | |
| **Coffee Cake,** 2 oz | 180 | 6 | 30 |
| **Concha:** Small, 2 oz | 240 | 9 | 33 |
| Large (5" diameter), 5.5 oz | 615 | 23 | 85 |
| **Cream Puff,** custard filled, 4.6 oz | 335 | 20 | 30 |
| **Cream Horn,** 3 oz | 210 | 5 | 36 |
| **Crumble Coffee Cake,** 4.5 oz | 500 | 25 | 65 |
| **Danish Pastries:** | | | |
| Small, 2.5 oz | 250 | 14 | 25 |
| Large, 5 oz | 500 | 28 | 50 |
| **Donuts ~** *See Page 66* | | | |
| **Eclair,** Chocolate, custard filled, 3.5 oz | 260 | 16 | 24 |
| **Fig Bars,** average | 160 | 3 | 31 |

## Ready-to-Eat (Cont) | **C** | **F** | **Cb**

*Per Piece/Slice*

| | C | F | Cb |
|---|---|---|---|
| **Fruit Cake,** Dark/Light, 2 oz | 185 | 5 | 34 |
| **Fudge Nut Brownie,** 3.5 oz | 380 | 18 | 54 |
| **Gingerbread,** from mix, 3" square | 210 | 4 | 41 |
| **Honey Bun,** 2.7 oz | 310 | 15 | 39 |
| **Jelly Roll,** ¹⁄₁₂ roll, 1.8 oz | 150 | 2 | 32 |
| **Key Lime Pie,** 4.3 oz | 400 | 25 | 41 |
| **Kringles:** Almond; Pecan, average | 205 | 12 | 24 |
| Blueberry: Cherry; Raspberry, av. | 165 | 8 | 24 |
| **Lady Finger,** 3 oz | 310 | 4.5 | 59 |
| **Lemon Cake,** 4 oz | 440 | 24 | 49 |
| **Lemon Poppy Seed Creme,** 1.6 oz | 180 | 9 | 23 |
| **Marble Cake,** 4 oz | 430 | 23 | 50 |
| **Mississippi Mud Pie,** 4 oz | 480 | 22 | 67 |
| **Mud Cake,** 4.5 oz | 380 | 20 | 44 |
| **Muffins ~** *See Page 67* | | | |
| **Palmier Cookie,** large, 4.5 oz | 490 | 25 | 62 |
| **Pineapple Upside Down Cake,** | | | |
| 2.5 oz | 230 | 9 | 36 |
| **Peach Melba,** 3.5 oz | 300 | 8 | 52 |
| **Pecan Sticky Roll,** 6.5 oz | 690 | 22 | 91 |
| **Pecan Twirls,** 1.3 oz | 170 | 7 | 26 |
| **Pies & Tarts ~** *See Page 134* | | | |
| **Pound Cakes:** Iced Lemon, 3.5 oz | 360 | 17 | 50 |
| Marble, 3.75 oz | 350 | 13 | 53 |
| **Raspberry Rugulah,** | | | |
| 1.2 oz | 110 | 9 | 7 |
| **Scone,** fruit, 2 oz | 200 | 9 | 30 |
| **Sponge Cake:** Plain, 2.5 oz | 220 | 10 | 33 |
| with Chocolate Frosting | 290 | 12 | 45 |
| with Cream & Strawberry Jam | 390 | 12 | 69 |
| **Starbucks Cakes ~** *Page 244* | | | |
| **Strawberry Cream Cake,** 4.7 oz | 400 | 27 | 33 |
| **Strudel Bites,** 0.75 oz | 60 | 2.5 | 9 |
| **Strudel,** fruit, av., 4.5 oz | 300 | 17 | 32 |
| **Swiss Rolls,** 1 oz | 135 | 6 | 19 |
| **Tiramisu,** 4.5 oz | 440 | 22 | 34 |
| **Turnovers,** fruit, average, 3 oz | 290 | 15 | 35 |

## Cupcakes

*Average all Varieties*

| | C | F | Cb |
|---|---|---|---|
| **Regular:** | | | |
| Cake only, 1.5 oz | 140 | 5.5 | 20 |
| Cake + Icing, 2.5 oz | 260 | 13 | 34 |
| **Large,** (Muffin Size): | | | |
| Cake only, 2.5 oz | 235 | 9 | 34 |
| Cake + Icing, 5 oz | 520 | 27 | 67 |
| **Mini,** (2-Bite): | | | |
| Cake only, 0.4 oz | 40 | 1.5 | 5.5 |
| Cake + Icing, 1 oz | 110 | 5.5 | 13 |
| **Icing Only:** Per 1 oz | 115 | 7 | 13 |
| Thick/Tall amount, 2.5 oz | 290 | 17 | 32 |

## Cakes ~ Brands   ⒸⒻⒸⒷ

**Albertson's Bakery:**
**Ring Cakes:** *Per 1/10 Cake*

| | C | F | Cb |
|---|---|---|---|
| Angel Food | 135 | 0 | 27 |

**Cake Slices:** *Per Slice Unless Indicated*

| | C | F | Cb |
|---|---|---|---|
| Banana Nut Loaf | 330 | 17 | 39 |
| Creme Cake (2), 3.2 oz | 300 | 12 | 43 |
| Cinn. Streusel (2), 3.2 oz | 350 | 18 | 43 |

**Bimbo Bakery:**

| | C | F | Cb |
|---|---|---|---|
| **Concha,** Vanilla, 2 oz | 260 | 6 | 35 |

**Pound Cakes:** *Per Slice*

| | C | F | Cb |
|---|---|---|---|
| Panquecitos, 1.8 oz | 170 | 4.5 | 29 |
| Pecan, 2.3 oz | 260 | 11 | 36 |
| Raisin, 2.3 oz | 240 | 9 | 38 |

**Bon Appetit Bakery:**

| | C | F | Cb |
|---|---|---|---|
| **Banana Bread,** 4 oz | 440 | 25 | 49 |
| **Cream Cheese Cake,** 4 oz slice | 430 | 24 | 49 |

**Danish:**

| | C | F | Cb |
|---|---|---|---|
| Apple (1), 5 oz | 210 | 11 | 25 |
| Bear Claw (1), 5 oz | 240 | 13 | 27 |
| Cheese & Berries (1), 5 oz | 250 | 14 | 26 |
| Vienna Cream (1), 5 oz | 240 | 14 | 27 |

**Slices:**

| | C | F | Cb |
|---|---|---|---|
| Cheesecake, 4 oz | 430 | 24 | 49 |
| Lemon Cake, 4 oz | 430 | 24 | 49 |
| Marble Cake, 4 oz | 430 | 24 | 50 |
| **Walnut Brownie,** 3.5 oz | 380 | 18 | 54 |

**Cheesecake Factory** ~ *See Fast-Foods Section*
**Entenmann's:** *Per Slice*

**Crumb Cakes:**

| | C | F | Cb |
|---|---|---|---|
| Butter French, 1.76 oz | 210 | 10 | 29 |
| Cheese-Filled Coffee, 1.9 oz | 200 | 10 | 25 |
| NY Style, 1/9 cake | 250 | 12 | 34 |

**Danish:**

| | C | F | Cb |
|---|---|---|---|
| Cherry Cheese, 1/8 cake | 180 | 6 | 28 |
| Pecan Twist, 1/6 cake | 260 | 16 | 27 |
| Raspberry Twist, 1.87 oz | 220 | 11 | 29 |

**Iced Cakes:**

| | C | F | Cb |
|---|---|---|---|
| Banana, 2.25 oz | 270 | 14 | 36 |
| Chocolate Fundge, 2.25 | 240 | 10 | 37 |
| Marshmallow Devil's Food, 2.25 oz | 260 | 13 | 36 |

**Loaf Cakes:** Banana Bread

| | C | F | Cb |
|---|---|---|---|
| Chocolate, 2 oz | 190 | 8 | 29 |
| Lemon, 1.9 oz | 210 | 10 | 28 |
| Marble, 2.75 oz | 280 | 11 | 39 |
| Vanilla Bean Iced Cake, 1/6 cake | 380 | 20 | 47 |
| Cinnamon Crunch, 1/6 loaf | 270 | 14 | 33 |

**Glenny's:**
**100 Calorie:**

| | C | F | Cb |
|---|---|---|---|
| Blondie, Choc. Chip, 1.5 oz | 100 | 4 | 15 |
| Brownies: Chocolate Chip, 1.5 oz | 100 | 4 | 12 |
| Peanut Butter, 1.5 oz | 100 | 4 | 15 |

**Muffins/Sweet Rolls ~ See Page 67**

**Great American Cookies:**
**Original Cookie Cakes:** *Per Slice*   ⒸⒻⒸⒷ

| | C | F | Cb |
|---|---|---|---|
| By the Slice, 4.4 oz | 530 | 25 | 75 |
| 14" Heart Shaped, 3 oz | 350 | 16 | 51 |
| with M&M, 3 oz | 360 | 17 | 52 |

**Great Value** *(Walmart):* *Per Slice*

| | C | F | Cb |
|---|---|---|---|
| **Chocolate Cup Cake,** (1), 2 oz | 200 | 6 | 35 |
| **Chocolate 3 Layer Cake,** 2.36 oz | 260 | 13 | 35 |
| **Lemon Flav. Shadow,** Cake, 2.6 oz | 360 | 18 | 49 |
| **Ultimate Vanilla,** 2.8 oz | 380 | 20 | 47 |

**Hostess:**
**Cup Cakes:**

| | C | F | Cb |
|---|---|---|---|
| 100 Calorie Packs, av., 3 minicakes | 100 | 2.5 | 21 |
| 8 Pack, Chocolate, 1 cake, 1.5 oz | 160 | 6 | 26 |
| **Ding Dongs,** (1) | 165 | 9 | 22 |
| **Ho Hos,** (1) | 120 | 5 | 18 |

**Twinkies:**

| | C | F | Cb |
|---|---|---|---|
| Original; Banana, av., (1) | 140 | 5 | 24 |
| Deep Fried: Original (1) | 220 | 9 | 32 |
| Chocolate (1) | 220 | 8 | 36 |
| **Zingers,** (2) | 250 | 9 | 41 |

**Donettes** ~ *Page 66*
**Little Debbie:**

**Boxed:**

| | C | F | Cb |
|---|---|---|---|
| Butterfly Cake (1), 2.1 oz | 270 | 2 | 39 |
| Cinn. Streusel Cake (1),1.6 oz | 180 | 7 | 26 |
| Cocoa Cremes (1), 1.4 oz | 170 | 8 | 24 |
| Cookies & Creme Cake (2) | 320 | 15 | 43 |
| Orange Creme Cake (1), 1.5 oz | 190 | 9 | 26 |
| Pumpkin Spice Cake Roll (1) | 260 | 11 | 39 |
| Red Velvet Creme Filled Cake, 2.57 oz | 330 | 16 | 45 |
| Zebra Cake, (1), 2.6 oz | 320 | 14 | 48 |

**Ne-Mo's:**

| | C | F | Cb |
|---|---|---|---|
| **Brookie,** (1), 1.5 oz | 160 | 7 | 26 |

**Bundt:**

| | C | F | Cb |
|---|---|---|---|
| Chocolate, 4 oz | 380 | 14 | 62 |
| Coconut Pineapple, 4 oz | 410 | 18 | 60 |
| Key Lime, 4 oz | 440 | 18 | 67 |
| Orange Dreamswirl | 440 | 18 | 67 |

**Cake Breads:**

| | C | F | Cb |
|---|---|---|---|
| Banana, 4 oz | 460 | 23 | 57 |
| Carrot, 4 oz | 450 | 22 | 56 |
| Cheese Coffee Cake, 4 oz | 460 | 21 | 62 |
| Wild Blueberry Bread, 4 oz | 430 | 20 | 58 |

**Cake Squares:**

| | C | F | Cb |
|---|---|---|---|
| Carrot, 3.6 oz | 390 | 21 | 47 |
| Banana; Chocolate, av, 3 oz | 300 | 12 | 45 |

**Crumble Cake:**

| | C | F | Cb |
|---|---|---|---|
| Blueberry (1), 4 oz | 390 | 17 | 54 |
| Cinnamon Streusel (1), 4 oz | 420 | 18 | 59 |
| Lemon Rasp. (1), 4 oz | 400 | 19 | 55 |

## Cakes ~ Brands (Cont)

| | C | F | Cb |
|---|---|---|---|
| **Pepperidge Farm:** | | | |
| **3-Layer Cakes:** *Per ⅛ Cake* | | | |
| Chocolate Fudge, 2.4 oz | 240 | 13 | 32 |
| Coconut, 2.4 oz | 250 | 12 | 34 |
| Creamy Red Velvet, 2.4 oz | 240 | 13 | 30 |
| German Chocolate, 2.4 oz | 240 | 12 | 31 |
| Key Lime; Vanilla, 2.4 oz | 240 | 12 | 34 |
| Lemon, 2.4 oz | 240 | 12 | 34 |
| **Turnovers (Frozen):** | | | |
| Apple; Blueb.; Cherry (1) | 260 | 13 | 31 |
| Chocolate (1) | 350 | 22 | 35 |
| Peach; Raspberry (1) | 270 | 13 | 34 |
| **Pop Tarts** *(Kellogg's): Each* | | | |
| Brown Sugar Cinnamon | 210 | 7 | 35 |
| Chocolate Chip | 210 | 6 | 36 |
| Cookies & Cream | 190 | 5 | 35 |
| Fruit/Frosted/Unfrosted, av. | 205 | 5 | 37 |
| **Prairie City:** | | | |
| **Ooey Gooey Butter Cake:** *Per 2 oz Package* | | | |
| Key Lime | 220 | 10 | 31 |
| Lemon | 210 | 9 | 32 |
| Original | 220 | 9 | 33 |
| Sea Salt Caramel | 230 | 10 | 33 |
| **Brownie,** Big n' Fudgy, 3.5 oz pkg | 440 | 23 | 58 |
| **Cinnamon Roll,** Bigger Big, 6 oz | 620 | 34 | 74 |
| **Safeway Select,** | | | |
| Molten Chocolate Lava Cake, 4.5 oz | 440 | 26 | 50 |
| **Sara Lee:** | | | |
| **Banana Cake,** 2.75 oz | 270 | 10 | 42 |
| **Carrot Cake,**[3.2] oz | 340 | 17 | 44 |
| **Cheesecakes:** | | | |
| Classic: Cheesecake, 4.27 oz | 330 | 17 | 37 |
| Cherry, 4.77 oz | 360 | 12 | 55 |
| Strawberry, 4.76 oz | 330 | 12 | 50 |
| French Style: Classic | 410 | 26 | 38 |
| Strawberry, 4.33 oz | 310 | 18 | 35 |
| NY Style: Original, 5 oz | 510 | 30 | 52 |
| Chocolate, 5 oz | 500 | 29 | 55 |
| Pumpkin, 5 oz | 480 | 30 | 46 |
| **Pound Cakes:** | | | |
| All Butter, 2.68 oz | 290 | 15 | 36 |
| Blueberry,, 2.57 oz | 230 | 8 | 38 |
| Lemon, 2.68 oz | 240 | 8 | 38 |
| Slices: Original, 1.4 oz | 150 | 5 | 24 |
| Double Chocolate, 1.5 oz | 150 | 5 | 24 |
| **Special K,** Pastry Crisps, | | | |
| all varieties, 1 pouch, 0.9 oz | 100 | 2 | 20 |

| | C | F | Cb |
|---|---|---|---|
| **Tastykake:** | | | |
| **Creme Filled Cupcakes:** | | | |
| Chocolate (2), 2.4 oz | 270 | 10 | 42 |
| Koffee Cake (2), 2.1 oz | 240 | 9 | 38 |
| Swirly Choc. (1), 2 oz | 200 | 6 | 35 |
| **Kandy Kake:** | | | |
| Chocolate (2), 1.3 oz | 180 | 9 | 24 |
| Peanut Butter (2), 1.3 oz | 190 | 10 | 20 |
| **Krimpets,** Butterscotch (2), 2 oz | 220 | 9 | 39 |
| **Krimpies,** Vanilla (2), 2.3 oz | 270 | 11 | 41 |
| **Kupid Kakes,** 5 oz | 150 | 5 | 24 |
| **Toaster Strudel** *(Pillsbury): Per 2 oz* | | | |
| **Boston Cream Pie** | 180 | 7 | 25 |
| **Cream Cheese,** | | | |
| average all varieties | 190 | 9 | 25 |
| **Fruit flavors,** all var. | 180 | 7 | 27 |
| **Trader Joe's:** | | | |
| **Bakery Fresh:** | | | |
| Apricot Almond Tart, | | | |
| 4 oz slice | 450 | 24 | 56 |
| Cheesecake Brownie Bites (1) | 110 | 7 | 9 |
| Chocolate Ganache Cake, 3 oz slice | 390 | 22 | 44 |
| Flourless Chocolate Cake, | | | |
| 1 slice, 2 oz | 260 | 17 | 23 |
| Lemon Cake, 3.3oz slice | 350 | 19 | 43 |
| Mini Carrot Cake, 5 oz | 450 | 19 | 68 |
| Whoopie Pie (1), 2.5 oz | 350 | 14 | 54 |
| Bread Cake: | | | |
| Banana Bonanza, 2.6 oz slice | 250 | 9 | 39 |
| Pumpkin Nut, 2.6 oz slice | 270 | 10 | 43 |
| Walnut Streusel Coffee, 2 oz slice | 180 | 8 | 25 |
| Zucchini Carrot, 2 oz slice | 200 | 7 | 32 |
| Loaf Cake: | | | |
| Cranberry Pumpkin, 2 oz slice | 140 | 2 | 30 |
| Pumpkin Nut, 2.6 oz slice | 270 | 10 | 43 |
| **Frozen:** | | | |
| Apple Raspberry Turnover, 3.2 oz | 280 | 14 | 34 |
| Chocolate Dilemma Cheesecake: | | | |
| Plain, 3.5 oz | 320 | 19 | 30 |
| Choc. Chip; Triple Choc., av., 3.5 oz | 345 | 20 | 35 |
| Tuxedo, 3.5 oz | 320 | 17 | 34 |
| Choc Lava Cake, 4 oz | 360 | 23 | 40 |
| Karat Cake, 3 oz slice | 320 | 19 | 37 |
| N.Y. Style Cheesecake, 4.5 oz slice | 400 | 28 | 32 |
| Tiramisu Torte, 3.2 oz slice | 230 | 12 | 24 |
| Tarts: | | | |
| Pear, 3.5 oz slice | 250 | 9 | 39 |
| Raspberry, 5 oz slice | 290 | 10 | 51 |
| Wild Blueberry, 3.5 oz slice | 260 | 6 | 52 |

## Cakes ~ Mixes

| | C | F | Cb |
|---|---|---|---|
| **Arrowhead Mills:** *Dry Mix Only* | | | |
| **Brownie Mix** *(Gluten Free):* | | | |
| All Purpose Mix, 1.4 oz | 130 | 1 | 28 |
| Fudge Brownie, 1 oz | 110 | 2 | 21 |
| **Cake Mix:** | | | |
| Chocolate, organic, 1.75 oz | 160 | 1 | 37 |
| Vanilla, 1/12 package, 1.7 oz | 160 | 0 | 37 |
| **Betty Crocker:** *Dry MixOnly* | | | |
| **Brownie Mix:** | | | |
| Dark Chocolate, 1 oz | 110 | 1 | 24 |
| Fudge, 0.9 oz | 100 | 1 | 23 |
| Mint Chip, 1.1 oz | 120 | 2 | 26 |
| Salted Caramel, 1.15 oz | 120 | 1.5 | 26 |
| Supreme: | | | |
| Chocolate Chunk, 1.2 oz | 130 | 2 | 26 |
| Fudge, 1.2 oz | 120 | 1.5 | 26 |
| Original, 1.2 oz | 120 | 1 | 27 |
| Triple Chunk, 1 oz | 120 | 2 | 25 |
| **Gluten Free Cake Mix:** | | | |
| Devils Food, 1.65 oz | 260 | 12 | 36 |
| Yellow, 1/10 Pkg | 260 | 11 | 37 |
| **Super Moiste Cake Mixes:** | | | |
| Butter Recipe Yellow, 1.5 oz | 160 | 1.5 | 36 |
| Butter Pecan, 1.5 oz | 160 | 1.5 | 36 |
| Carrot, 1.5 oz | 160 | 1.5 | 35 |
| Cherry Chip, 1.5 oz | 160 | 1.5 | 36 |
| Devil's Food; French Vanilla,1.5 oz | 160 | 1.5 | 35 |
| Lemon, 1.5 oz | 160 | 1.5 | 36 |
| Milk Chocolate, 1.5 oz | 160 | 1.5 | 35 |
| Triple Choc. Fudge, 1.5 oz | 160 | 2 | 34 |
| **Dessert Bars:** | | | |
| Coconut White Chip Oat Bar, 1.1 oz | 150 | 6 | 22 |
| Supreme: Cookie Brownie, 1.25 oz | 140 | 2.5 | 29 |
| Lemon, 1 oz | 130 | 3.5 | 24 |
| **Duncan Hines:** *Prepared as Directed* | | | |
| **Brownie Mix:** | | | |
| Chewy Fudge Brownie, 0.9 oz | 160 | 7 | 22 |
| Decadent: Caramel Turtle, 1.1 oz | 170 | 7 | 24 |
| Red Velvet, 1.1 oz | 170 | 7 | 25 |
| Triple Choc., 1.1 oz | 180 | 8 | 25 |
| **Cake Mix,** | | | |
| Classic, Dark Choc. Fudge, 1.5 oz | 260 | 13 | 33 |
| **Decadent:** | | | |
| Classic Carrot, 1.75 oz | 260 | 10 | 39 |
| German Chocolate, 1.75 oz | 300 | 15 | 37 |

| **Duncan Hines (Cont):** *Prep. As Directed* | C | F | Cb |
|---|---|---|---|
| **Signature:** | | | |
| Banana Supreme, 1.5 oz | 260 | 12 | 34 |
| Coconut Supreme, 1.5 oz | 260 | 12 | 34 |
| French Vanilla, 1.5 oz | 260 | 12 | 34 |
| Orange Supreme, 1.5 oz | 260 | 12 | 34 |
| Red Velvet, 1.5 oz | 260 | 13 | 33 |
| **Jell-O:** *Prepared As Directed* | | | |
| **No Bake:** | | | |
| Lemon Meringue Pie, 1.75 oz | 200 | 3 | 43 |
| **Krusteaz:** *Prepared As Directed* | | | |
| **Bars:** Meyer Lemon, 2" Bar | 140 | 5 | 26 |
| Pumpkin Pie, 1/18 pkg | 150 | 6 | 24 |
| Raspberry, 2" Bar | 150 | 6 | 22 |
| **Pillsbury:** *Dry Mix Only* | | | |
| **Brownies, Premium Mix:** | | | |
| Cheesecake Swirl, 1 oz | 110 | 1.5 | 25 |
| **Chocolate:** | | | |
| Extreme, 1 oz | 120 | 2 | 24 |
| Chunk, 1 oz | 120 | 2.5 | 24 |
| Walnut, 1.1 oz | 130 | 3 | 25 |
| Raspberry Cheesecake Swirl, 1 oz | 110 | 1.5 | 25 |
| **Cakes:** | | | |
| **Coffee Cakes,** Cinnamon Struesel | 310 | 12 | 49 |
| **Funfetti:** Bold Purple, 1.4 oz | 140 | 1.5 | 32 |
| Neon Yellow, 1.4 oz | 140 | 1.5 | 31 |
| **Moist Supreme:** | | | |
| Devils Food, 1.5 oz | 160 | 2 | 35 |
| White/Yellow, 1.5 oz | 160 | 1.5 | 35 |

## Cake Frostings

| **Betty Crocker:** | C | F | Cb |
|---|---|---|---|
| **Rich & Creamy,** | | | |
| average all flavors, 2 Tbsp, 1.2 oz | 135 | 5 | 22 |
| **Whipped,** av. all flavors.,2 T., 0.9 oz | 100 | 4.5 | 15 |
| **Cool Whip,** Original, 2 Tbsp, 0.3 oz | 25 | 1.5 | 2 |
| **Duncan Hines:** | | | |
| **Creamy Homestyle,** av. all flav., 2T. | 140 | 6 | 23 |
| **Whipped,** av. all flavors, 3 Tbsp | 150 | 7 | 21 |
| **Pillsbury:** *Per 2 Tbsp* | | | |
| **Creamy Supreme:** | | | |
| Choc Fudge; Milk Choc., 1.2 oz | 130 | 6 | 21 |
| Classic White; Vanilla, 1.2 oz | 140 | 5 | 22 |
| **Fluffy,** av. all flavors, 2 Tbsp, 0.8 oz | 100 | 5 | 14 |
| **Funfetti,** av. all flavors, 2 Tbsp,1.2 oz | 140 | 5 | 23 |
| **Sugar Free,** average, 2 Tbsp, 1.1 oz | 100 | 6 | 16 |

## Quick Guide | C | F | Cb

### Donuts
*Average All Brands*

| | C | F | Cb |
|---|---|---|---|
| **Cake:** Plain, 1.8 oz | 205 | 12 | 23 |
| Chocolate Iced, 2 oz | 255 | 14 | 29 |
| Sugared, 0.8 oz | 205 | 10 | 29 |
| **Non-Cake,** Glazed, 2 oz | 225 | 11 | 29 |

### Croissant-Donuts
(Includes Cronuts/Frissants)
*Average all Brands*

| | C | F | Cb |
|---|---|---|---|
| Cream-filled, 3.5 oz | 430 | 26 | 45 |
| Custard-filled, 3.5 oz | 360 | 19 | 45 |

**Extra Listings** ~ *See CalorieKing.com*
*(Cronut is a trademark of Dominique Ansel Bakery, New York)*

## Donuts ~ Brands

**Albertson's:**
**Donut Holes:**

| | C | F | Cb |
|---|---|---|---|
| Glazed Old Fashioned (4) | 240 | 12 | 31 |
| Powdered Sugar (4) | 210 | 12 | 24 |
| **Gem Donuts:** Plain Cake (3) | 190 | 12 | 20 |
| Cinnamon Sugar (3) | 240 | 15 | 23 |
| Glazed (1) | 140 | 6 | 21 |

**Bon Appetit:**
**Mini Donuts:**

| | C | F | Cb |
|---|---|---|---|
| Chocolate (4) | 270 | 16 | 29 |
| Crumb (4) | 240 | 12 | 32 |
| Powdered (4) | 250 | 12 | 34 |

**Dunkin':**

| | C | F | Cb |
|---|---|---|---|
| **Apple Crumb** | 320 | 15 | 42 |
| **Apple N' Spice** | 260 | 14 | 29 |
| **Barvarian Kreme** | 270 | 15 | 31 |
| **Blueberry Butternut** | 420 | 17 | 60 |
| **Blueberry Crumb Cake** | 380 | 18 | 50 |
| **Boston Kreme** | 300 | 16 | 37 |
| **Chocolate Frosted Cake** | 350 | 19 | 40 |
| **Chocolate Headlight** | 330 | 18 | 39 |
| **Choc. Peanut Butter Flav. Cream** | 360 | 19 | 44 |
| **Glazed Chocolate** | 340 | 19 | 38 |
| **Jelly Filled** | 270 | 14 | 32 |
| **Powdered** | 320 | 19 | 33 |
| **Vanilla Creme** | 330 | 20 | 35 |

**Extra Listings** ~ *See Fast Food Section*

## Donuts ~ Brands (Cont) | C | F | Cb

**Entenmann's:**
**8 Pack:** *Per Donut*

| | C | F | Cb |
|---|---|---|---|
| Plain | 220 | 13 | 24 |
| Crumb Topped | 250 | 12 | 36 |
| Glazed | 260 | 13 | 34 |
| Rich Frosted | 290 | 19 | 30 |

**Pop'ems:**

| | C | F | Cb |
|---|---|---|---|
| Pumpkin (4) | 230 | 13 | 29 |
| Rich Frosted (4) | 320 | 23 | 28 |

**Hostess:**

| | C | F | Cb |
|---|---|---|---|
| **Mini Donettes:** Crumb, 6-pack, 4 oz | 430 | 18 | 63 |
| Frosted, 6-pack, 3 oz | 360 | 22 | 38 |
| Powdered, 6-pack, 3 oz | 340 | 17 | 43 |

**Krispy Kreme:**

| | C | F | Cb |
|---|---|---|---|
| **Apple Fritter,** 3.5 oz | 350 | 19 | 42 |
| **Chocolate:** Iced Cake, 2.5 oz | 280 | 13 | 37 |
| Iced Custard Filled, 3 oz | 300 | 15 | 37 |
| Iced Glazed Cruller, 2.5 oz | 260 | 10 | 40 |
| Iced Glazed, 2.2 | 240 | 11 | 33 |
| Iced Kreme Filled, 3 oz | 350 | 19 | 41 |
| Iced Glazed w/ Sprinkles, 2.3 oz | 250 | 11 | 36 |
| **Cinnamon Twist,** 1.9oz | 210 | 11 | 26 |
| **Glazed Cruller,** 1.9 oz | 210 | 10 | 29 |

**Glazed Doughnut Holes:**

| | C | F | Cb |
|---|---|---|---|
| Original (5) | 220 | 11 | 25 |
| Blueberry (4) | 190 | 7 | 28 |
| Cake (4) | 190 | 8 | 28 |
| Chocolate Cake (4) | 180 | 7 | 27 |
| **Glazed Kreme Filled,** 3 oz | 340 | 19 | 40 |
| **Maple Iced Glazed,** 2.2 oz | 240 | 11 | 34 |
| **New York Cheesecake,** 3.3 oz | 310 | 17 | 35 |
| **Original Glazed,** 1.7 oz | 190 | 11 | 22 |
| **Powdered Cake,** 2.3 oz | 240 | 11 | 29 |
| **Traditional Cake,** 2 oz | 230 | 12 | 26 |

**Little Debbie,**

| | C | F | Cb |
|---|---|---|---|
| Donut Sticks, 1.9 oz | 270 | 16 | 29 |

**Tastykake:**

| | C | F | Cb |
|---|---|---|---|
| **Cinnamon,** (3), 2 oz | 230 | 11 | 31 |
| **Mini:** Crunch, 3 oz pkg | 330 | 13 | 50 |
| Powdered Sugar, 2.5 oz pkg | 300 | 14 | 41 |

## Quick Guide | C | F | Cb

### Muffins: Ready-To-Eat
*Average All Brands*

| | C | F | Cb |
|---|---|---|---|
| Small, 1 oz | 90 | 3.5 | 14 |
| Medium, 2 oz | 185 | 6.5 | 28 |
| Large, 3 oz | 275 | 10 | 42 |
| Extra Large, 4 oz | 365 | 13 | 57 |
| Giant, 6 oz | 550 | 20 | 84 |
| Super Size, 8 oz | 730 | 27 | 112 |

### Muffins Ready-To-Eat ~ Brands

| | C | F | Cb |
|---|---|---|---|
| **Albertsons:** | | | |
| **Minis:** Banana Nut (2) | 200 | 12 | 20 |
| Blueberry (2) | 180 | 10 | 21 |
| Honey Raisin Bran (2) | 170 | 7 | 24 |
| **Entenmann's,** | | | |
| Blueberry; Choc. Chip; Corn (1), av. | 190 | 9 | 25 |
| **Garden Lites:** Chocolate (1), 2 oz | 120 | 4 | 21 |
| Banana Choc. Chip (1), 2 oz | 120 | 3 | 23 |
| Blueberry Oat (1), 2 oz | 120 | 2 | 25 |
| Av. other flavors (1), 1 oz | 70 | 2 | 13 |
| **Great Value** *(Walmart):* | | | |
| **Double Banana Filled,** (1), 4 oz | 360 | 16 | 52 |
| **Double Blueberry Filled,** (1), 4 oz | 430 | 16 | 65 |
| **Triple Chocolate Filled,** (1), 4 oz | 420 | 18 | 61 |
| **Little Debbie:** Banana Nut (1), 1.9 oz | 210 | 9 | 30 |
| Blueberry (1), 1.9 oz | 190 | 8 | 27 |
| Chocolate Chip (1), 1.9 oz | 210 | 9 | 28 |
| **My Favorite Muffin:** *Per Large* | | | |
| **Banana Nut** | 650 | 38 | 71 |
| **Blueberry** | 590 | 28 | 78 |
| **Boston Cream Pie** | 740 | 33 | 105 |
| **Chocolate Chip** | 790 | 39 | 100 |
| **Lemon Poppyseed** | 670 | 32 | 90 |
| **Otis Spunkmeyer:** | | | |
| **Banana,** 2 oz | 220 | 10 | 30 |
| **Blueberry,** 2 oz | 210 | 9 | 29 |
| **Choc. Chip Minis (3),** 2.25 oz | 270 | 14 | 32 |
| **Starbucks** ~ *See Fast-Foods Section* | | | |
| **Trader Joe's:** *Per Muffin* | | | |
| **Apple Cranberry,** 4.8 oz | 220 | 5 | 38 |
| **Banana Chocolate Chip,** 4 oz | 400 | 18 | 57 |
| **Carrot,** 4 oz | 320 | 11 | 52 |
| **Triple Berry,** 4 oz | 310 | 11 | 49 |
| **Vitalicious:** | | | |
| **VitaTops:** Deep Choc./Choc Mint, 2 oz | 100 | 1.5 | 26 |
| Wild Blueberry, 2 oz | 120 | 2 | 25 |
| Protein, hoc. P'nut Butter, 2 oz | 150 | 4 | 23 |
| Sugar free, Velvety Choc., 2 oz | 90 | 2 | 24 |
| **Weight Watchers,** | | | |
| Blueb.; Double Choc, av., 2.5 oz | 185 | 2.5 | 42 |

## Muffin Mixes | C | F | Cb

*Per Muffin, Prepared*

| | C | F | Cb |
|---|---|---|---|
| **Betty Crocker:** Banana Nut | 170 | 8 | 22 |
| Cinnamon Streusel | 190 | 8 | 27 |
| Wild Blueberry | 160 | 6.5 | 24 |
| Pouch Mix, with Milk: | | | |
| Banana Nut | 130 | 4 | 24 |
| Blueberry | 130 | 3 | 23 |
| Chocolate Chip | 130 | 3 | 23 |
| **Krusteaz:** | | | |
| **Choc Chunk** | 260 | 12 | 33 |
| **Lemon Poppyseed** | 170 | 4 | 31 |
| **Oat Bran** | 180 | 4.5 | 32 |
| **Trader Joe's,** Triple Berry | 150 | 2 | 28 |

## Sweet Rolls & Buns

Note: It is best to weigh for accuracy as actual weight can be 10-50% higher than label weight·

*Per Sweet Roll or Bun Unless Indicated*

| | C | F | Cb |
|---|---|---|---|
| **Bimbo,** Bimbolete, 2.2 oz | 250 | 10 | 36 |
| **Bon Appetit,** | | | |
| Cinnamon Roll, 2.5 oz | 230 | 8 | 34 |
| **Cinnabon:** Classic | 880 | 37 | 127 |
| Caramel Pecanbon | 1080 | 51 | 146 |
| **Cloverhill Bakery,** | | | |
| Jumbo Glazed Honey Bun, 4.75 oz | 600 | 35 | 64 |
| **Entenmann's,** Cinn. Swirl Bun, 3 oz | 320 | 14 | 44 |
| **Little Debbie:** | | | |
| **Honey Bun:** 2.3 oz | 280 | 16 | 32 |
| Individual: 3 oz Bun | 360 | 20 | 41 |
| 4 oz Bun | 480 | 26 | 56 |
| with White Icing, 4 oz | 490 | 25 | 60 |
| **Pecan Spinwheels:** Single, 1 oz | 100 | 3.5 | 17 |
| 2 Pack, 2.1 oz | 210 | 7 | 32 |
| **O&H Danish:** *Per 1.95 oz* | | | |
| **Kringles:** Apple | 180 | 7 | 26 |
| Almond; Turtle, average | 215 | 10 | 30 |
| Cinn. Roll; Cream Cheese, average | 205 | 11 | 26 |
| Wisconsin, | 170 | 5.5 | 28 |
| **Pillsbury:** | | | |
| **Sweet Rolls,** Refrigerated: *Per Roll Unless Indicated* | | | |
| Cinnamon, w/ Crm Cheese Icing | 140 | 4.5 | 23 |
| Cinn., Flaky w/ Butter Cream Icing | 160 | 7 | 23 |
| Twists, Flaky Cinnamon, with Icing | 160 | 7 | 23 |
| **Grands,** Refrigerated: *Per Roll* | | | |
| Cinnabon: Cinnamon Roll, | | | |
| with Cream Cheese Icing | 300 | 7 | 54 |
| Caramel Rolls, with Icing, 3.5 oz | 300 | 8 | 53 |
| Flaky Supreme Cinnamon Roll, | | | |
| with Icing, 3.5 oz | 360 | 17 | 47 |
| **7-Eleven:** Iced Honey Bun, 6 oz | 820 | 58 | 68 |
| Glazed Honey Bun, 5 oz | 620 | 35 | 70 |
| **Sara Lee,** Cinnamon Roll, 2.4 oz | 260 | 12 | 33 |

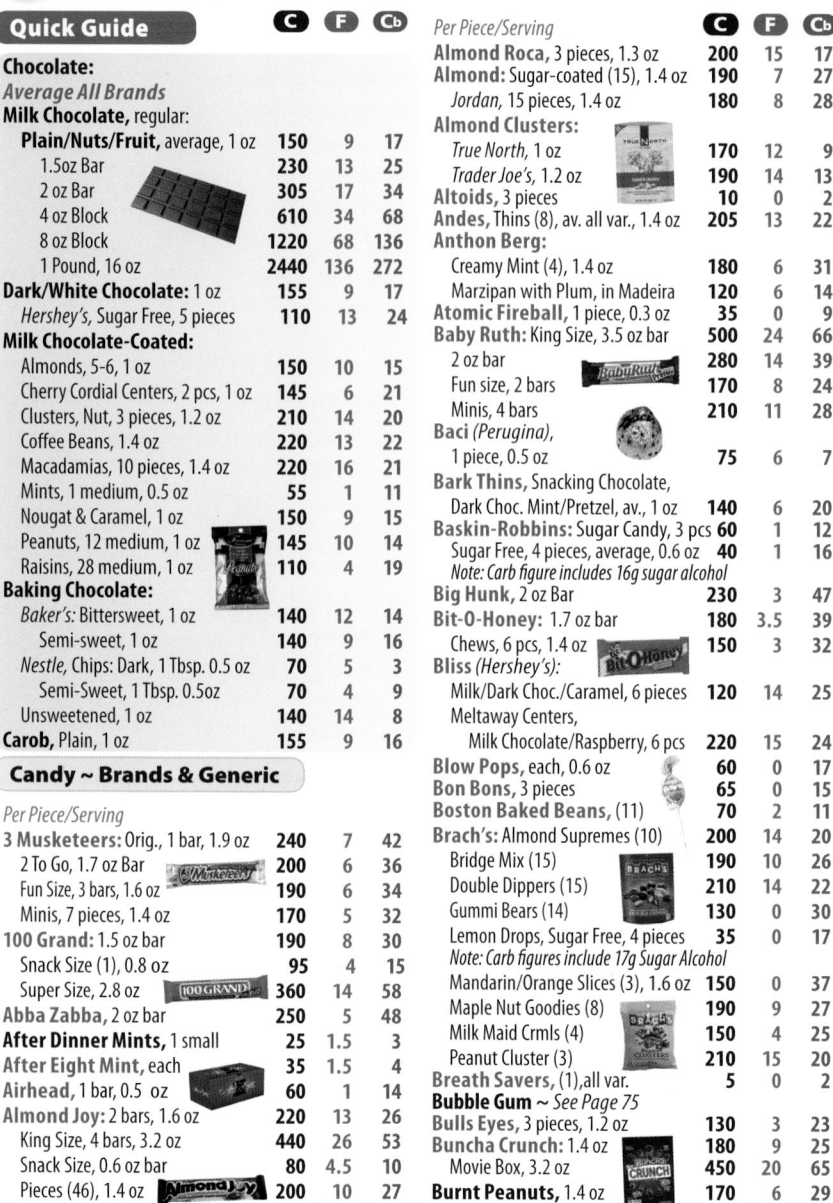

## Quick Guide

**C** **F** **Cb**

**Chocolate:**
*Average All Brands*
**Milk Chocolate,** regular:

| | C | F | Cb |
|---|---|---|---|
| **Plain/Nuts/Fruit,** average, 1 oz | 150 | 9 | 17 |
| 1.5oz Bar | 230 | 13 | 25 |
| 2 oz Bar | 305 | 17 | 34 |
| 4 oz Block | 610 | 34 | 68 |
| 8 oz Block | 1220 | 68 | 136 |
| 1 Pound, 16 oz | 2440 | 136 | 272 |
| **Dark/White Chocolate:** 1 oz | 155 | 9 | 17 |
| *Hershey's,* Sugar Free, 5 pieces | 110 | 13 | 24 |

**Milk Chocolate-Coated:**

| | C | F | Cb |
|---|---|---|---|
| Almonds, 5-6, 1 oz | 150 | 10 | 15 |
| Cherry Cordial Centers, 2 pcs, 1 oz | 145 | 6 | 21 |
| Clusters, Nut, 3 pieces, 1.2 oz | 210 | 14 | 20 |
| Coffee Beans, 1.4 oz | 220 | 13 | 22 |
| Macadamias, 10 pieces, 1.4 oz | 220 | 16 | 21 |
| Mints, 1 medium, 0.5 oz | 55 | 1 | 11 |
| Nougat & Caramel, 1 oz | 150 | 9 | 15 |
| Peanuts, 12 medium, 1 oz | 145 | 10 | 14 |
| Raisins, 28 medium, 1 oz | 110 | 4 | 19 |

**Baking Chocolate:**

| | C | F | Cb |
|---|---|---|---|
| *Baker's:* Bittersweet, 1 oz | 140 | 12 | 14 |
| Semi-sweet, 1 oz | 140 | 9 | 16 |
| *Nestle,* Chips: Dark, 1 Tbsp. 0.5 oz | 70 | 5 | 3 |
| Semi-Sweet, 1 Tbsp. 0.5oz | 70 | 4 | 9 |
| Unsweetened, 1 oz | 140 | 14 | 8 |
| **Carob,** Plain, 1 oz | 155 | 9 | 16 |

## Candy ~ Brands & Generic

*Per Piece/Serving*

| | C | F | Cb |
|---|---|---|---|
| **3 Musketeers:** Orig., 1 bar, 1.9 oz | 240 | 7 | 42 |
| 2 To Go, 1.7 oz Bar | 200 | 6 | 36 |
| Fun Size, 3 bars, 1.6 oz | 190 | 6 | 34 |
| Minis, 7 pieces, 1.4 oz | 170 | 5 | 32 |
| **100 Grand:** 1.5 oz bar | 190 | 8 | 30 |
| Snack Size (1), 0.8 oz | 95 | 4 | 15 |
| Super Size, 2.8 oz | 360 | 14 | 58 |
| **Abba Zabba,** 2 oz bar | 250 | 5 | 48 |
| **After Dinner Mints,** 1 small | 25 | 1.5 | 3 |
| **After Eight Mint,** each | 35 | 1.5 | 4 |
| **Airhead,** 1 bar, 0.5 oz | 60 | 1 | 14 |
| **Almond Joy:** 2 bars, 1.6 oz | 220 | 13 | 26 |
| King Size, 4 bars, 3.2 oz | 440 | 26 | 53 |
| Snack Size, 0.6 oz bar | 80 | 4.5 | 10 |
| Pieces (46), 1.4 oz | 200 | 10 | 27 |

*Per Piece/Serving*

**C** **F** **Cb**

| | C | F | Cb |
|---|---|---|---|
| **Almond Roca,** 3 pieces, 1.3 oz | 200 | 15 | 17 |
| **Almond:** Sugar-coated (15), 1.4 oz | 190 | 7 | 27 |
| *Jordan,* 15 pieces, 1.4 oz | 180 | 8 | 28 |
| **Almond Clusters:** | | | |
| *True North,* 1 oz | 170 | 12 | 9 |
| *Trader Joe's,* 1.2 oz | 190 | 14 | 13 |
| **Altoids,** 3 pieces | 10 | 0 | 2 |
| **Andes,** Thins (8), av. all var., 1.4 oz | 205 | 13 | 22 |
| **Anthon Berg:** | | | |
| Creamy Mint (4), 1.4 oz | 180 | 6 | 31 |
| Marzipan with Plum, in Madeira | 120 | 6 | 14 |
| **Atomic Fireball,** 1 piece, 0.3 oz | 35 | 0 | 9 |
| **Baby Ruth:** King Size, 3.5 oz bar | 500 | 24 | 66 |
| 2 oz bar | 280 | 14 | 39 |
| Fun size, 2 bars | 170 | 8 | 24 |
| Minis, 4 bars | 210 | 11 | 28 |
| **Baci** *(Perugina),* | | | |
| 1 piece, 0.5 oz | 75 | 6 | 7 |
| **Bark Thins,** Snacking Chocolate, | | | |
| Dark Choc. Mint/Pretzel, av., 1 oz | 140 | 6 | 20 |
| **Baskin-Robbins:** Sugar Candy, 3 pcs | 60 | 1 | 12 |
| Sugar Free, 4 pieces, average, 0.6 oz | 40 | 1 | 16 |
| *Note: Carb figure includes 16g sugar alcohol* | | | |
| **Big Hunk,** 2 oz Bar | 230 | 3 | 47 |
| **Bit-O-Honey:** 1.7 oz bar | 180 | 3.5 | 39 |
| Chews, 6 pcs, 1.4 oz | 150 | 3 | 32 |
| **Bliss** *(Hershey's):* | | | |
| Milk/Dark Choc./Caramel, 6 pieces | 120 | 14 | 25 |
| Meltaway Centers, | | | |
| Milk Chocolate/Raspberry, 6 pcs | 220 | 15 | 24 |
| **Blow Pops,** each, 0.6 oz | 60 | 0 | 17 |
| **Bon Bons,** 3 pieces | 65 | 0 | 15 |
| **Boston Baked Beans,** (11) | 70 | 2 | 11 |
| **Brach's:** Almond Supremes (10) | 200 | 14 | 20 |
| Bridge Mix (15) | 190 | 10 | 26 |
| Double Dippers (15) | 210 | 14 | 22 |
| Gummi Bears (14) | 130 | 0 | 30 |
| Lemon Drops, Sugar Free, 4 pieces | 35 | 0 | 17 |
| *Note: Carb figures include 17g Sugar Alcohol* | | | |
| Mandarin/Orange Slices (3), 1.6 oz | 150 | 0 | 37 |
| Maple Nut Goodies (8) | 190 | 9 | 27 |
| Milk Maid Crmls (4) | 150 | 4 | 25 |
| Peanut Cluster (3) | 210 | 15 | 20 |
| **Breath Savers,** (1),all var. | 5 | 0 | 2 |
| **Bubble Gum** ~ *See Page 75* | | | |
| **Bulls Eyes,** 3 pieces, 1.2 oz | 130 | 3 | 23 |
| **Buncha Crunch:** 1.4 oz | 180 | 9 | 25 |
| Movie Box, 3.2 oz | 450 | 20 | 65 |
| **Burnt Peanuts,** 1.4 oz | 170 | 6 | 29 |

## Candy ~ Brands & Generic (Cont)

*Per Piece/Serving*

| | C | F | Cb |
|---|---|---|---|
| **Butterfinger:** 2 oz bar | 270 | 11 | 43 |
| King Size (3 bars), 3.5 oz | 480 | 18 | 75 |
| Fun Size, (1), 0.8 oz | 100 | 4 | 15 |
| Giant, (Pieces in Choc.), | | | |
| ¼ bar, 1 oz | 150 | 8 | 21 |
| Miniatures: | | | |
| 1 piece, 0.4 oz | 45 | 2 | 8 |
| 4 pieces, 1.4 oz | 180 | 8 | 32 |
| Crisp Bar: Original, 2 oz bar | 270 | 11 | 43 |
| King Size, 3 pieces, 2 oz | 310 | 17 | 38 |
| Minis, 2 bars, 1.4 oz | 210 | 11 | 25 |
| Snackerz: | | | |
| Single, 1.3 oz | 170 | 8 | 23 |
| Fun Size, 2 pcs, 1.2 oz | 150 | 7 | 21 |
| King Size, 10 pcs, 1.4 oz | 190 | 8 | 25 |
| **Butter Mints,** 7 pieces, 0.5 oz | 50 | 0 | 12 |
| **Butterscotch:** 3 pieces | 60 | 0 | 15 |
| Discs (*Walgreens*), 3 pieces, 0.6 oz | 70 | 0 | 17 |
| **Cadbury:** Caramello Bar, 1.6 oz | 220 | 10 | 29 |
| Caramel Egg, 1.2 oz | 170 | 8 | 22 |
| Dairy Milk Bar, 7 pcs, 1.4 oz | 200 | 11 | 23 |
| Mini Eggs (Candy), 12 pcs, 1.4 oz | 190 | 8 | 28 |
| **Candy Apple,** medium, 6.5 oz | 280 | 0 | 60 |
| **Candy Cane,** medium, 5", 0.5 oz | 40 | 0 | 14 |
| **Candy Corn,** 20 pieces, 1.4 oz | 150 | 0 | 38 |
| **Candy Jar Mix** (*Jewel*), 3 pcs, 0.6 oz | 60 | 0 | 14 |
| **Candy Necklace** (*Smarties*), (1), 0.8 oz | 90 | 0.5 | 20 |
| **Caramels:** Each, 0.4 oz | 40 | 1 | 8 |
| Chocolate, each, 0.3 oz | 25 | 0.3 | 6 |
| Creams (3), 1.3 oz | 130 | 3 | 23 |
| **Caramel Popcorn,** ⅔ cup | 150 | 6 | 23 |
| Cella's, | | | |
| Milk Choc. Cherries, 3 pieces, 1.5 oz | 160 | 6 | 27 |
| **Certs,** Breath Mints, 1 piece | 5 | 0 | 2 |
| **Charleston Chew:** | | | |
| Chocolate Bar (1), 1.4 oz | 160 | 4.5 | 30 |
| Mini Bars, 13 pieces | 190 | 6 | 34 |
| **Charms:** Blow Pop | 60 | 0 | 17 |
| Flat Pop, 0.5 oz | 50 | 0 | 14 |
| **Chew-ets,** Peanut Chews, | | | |
| Original (4), 1.6 oz | 230 | 12 | 29 |
| **Chewz,** 1 roll, 1 oz | 120 | 1 | 28 |
| **Chick O Stick,** 2 oz | 240 | 9 | 42 |

*Per Piece/Serving*

| | C | F | Cb |
|---|---|---|---|
| **Chunky Bar** (*Nestlé*), | | | |
| King Size, 2.5 oz | 340 | 19 | 44 |
| **Chupa Chups,** 1 Pop | 50 | 0 | 12 |
| **Cinn. Buttons** (*Walgreens*), 3 pieces | 60 | 0 | 16 |
| **Cinnamon Disks** (*Walmart*), 3 pieces | 70 | 0 | 18 |
| **Circus Peanuts** (*Spangler*), | | | |
| 6 pieces, 1.3 oz | 165 | 0 | 41 |
| **CocoaVia,** Orig., 0.8 oz | 100 | 6 | 12 |
| **Coconut Stacks,** (8) | 320 | 16 | 46 |
| **Coffee Go,** Candy, (4) | 60 | 1 | 12 |
| **Conversation Hearts** (*Necco*): | | | |
| Small (40), 1.4 oz | 160 | 0 | 39 |
| 1 large | 10 | 0 | 3 |
| **Cookie Dough Bites,** 1.4 oz | 200 | 10 | 27 |
| **Cote d'Or:** Dark 86% Coca, 4 pcs | 270 | 22 | 14 |
| Dark, 70%, Orange, 3.5 oz | 575 | 46 | 34 |
| Dark, Raspberry, 3.5 oz | 580 | 46 | 34 |
| Milk, Intense, 3.5 oz | 575 | 40 | 45 |
| **Cotton Candy,** 1 oz | 110 | 0 | 28 |
| **Cough Drops ~** *See Page 75* | | | |
| **Cracker Jack,** ½ cup, 1 oz | 120 | 2 | 23 |
| **Creme Savers:** | | | |
| 3 pieces, 0.5 oz | 60 | 1 | 11 |
| Sugar-Free, 3 pieces | 30 | 1 | 8 |
| **Crisped Rice,** Choc Chip, 1 bar, 1 oz | 115 | 4 | 20 |
| **Crows,** 11 pieces, 1.4 oz | 130 | 0 | 33 |
| **Crunch Bar ~** *See Nestle* | | | |
| **Dots,** 11 dots, 1.4 oz | 130 | 0 | 33 |
| **Double Dip Stick,** 1 stick | 15 | 0.5 | 3 |
| Dove: | | | |
| **Milk Choc:** Singles Bar, 1.4 oz | 220 | 13 | 24 |
| Large Tablet Bar, 9 pcs, 1.5 oz | 230 | 13 | 25 |
| Choc. Cov. Almonds, 13 pcs, 1.4 oz | 220 | 15 | 19 |
| Promises: Milk Choc., 1 pce, 0.3 oz | 45 | 2.5 | 5 |
| w/ Caramel, 1 piece, 0.3 oz | 40 | 2 | 5 |
| w/ Peanut Butter, 1 pce, 0.3 oz | 45 | 3 | 4 |
| Swirls, all var., 9 pieces 1.5 oz | 230 | 14 | 25 |
| **Dark Choc:** Singles Bar, 1.3 oz | 220 | 13 | 24 |
| Large Tablet Bar, 9 pcs, 1.5 oz | 220 | 14 | 25 |
| Choc. Cov. Almds, 13 pcs, 1.4 oz | 210 | 15 | 19 |
| Promises, Almond, 1 piece, 0.3 oz | 40 | 3 | 4 |
| Swirls, Raspberry, 9 pcs, 1.4 oz | 220 | 14 | 24 |
| **Sugar Free,** all flav., 5 pcs, 1.4 oz | 195 | 15 | 21 |
| **Dum Dum Pops** (*Spangler*), 1 pop | 25 | 0 | 7 |
| **Drops** (*Hershey's*): | | | |
| Cookies 'n' Creme, 14 pieces, 1.5 oz | 210 | 11 | 26 |
| Milk Chocolate, 15 pieces, 1.4 oz | 200 | 12 | 25 |

## Candy ~ Brands & Generic (Cont)

| Per Piece/Serving | C | F | Cb |
|---|---|---|---|
| **English Toffee,** 1 piece, 0.4 oz | 70 | 4 | 6 |
| **5th Avenue:** 2 oz bar | 260 | 12 | 38 |
| King Size, 3.5 oz | 440 | 20 | 64 |
| **Fannie May:** | | | |
| Mint Meltaway (1) | 230 | 15 | 24 |
| Pixie (1), 1.5 oz | 210 | 12 | 24 |
| Trinidad (1), 1.5 oz | 200 | 12 | 23 |
| **Fast Break (Reese's):** 2 oz bar | 260 | 12 | 35 |
| 3.5 oz bar | 460 | 22 | 62 |
| **Ferrero Rocher:** 1 piece | 75 | 5 | 5 |
| 3 pieces, 1.3 oz | 220 | 16 | 16 |
| Rondnoir, 3 pieces, 1 oz | 180 | 13 | 14 |
| **Fifty 50 Snack Bars:** | | | |
| **Milk Chocolate:** | | | |
| 5 pieces, 1 oz | 135 | 11 | 14 |
| Almond, 5 pieces, 1 oz | 135 | 12 | 14 |
| Crunch Bar, 7 pcs, 1 oz | 140 | 12 | 16 |
| **Dark Chocolate,** 5 pieces, 1 oz | 120 | 11 | 15 |
| *Note: Carb figures include 9-12g Sugar Alcohol* | | | |
| **Fluffy Stuff** *(Charms),* | | | |
| Cotton Candy, 1.4 oz | 150 | 0 | 40 |
| **Fondant:** Choc-coated, 1.2 oz | 125 | 3 | 27 |
| Mint, 1 oz | 105 | 0 | 25 |
| **Fran's:** Gold Bar, Macadamia (1) | 250 | 14 | 27 |
| GoldBite, Almond (1) | 120 | 7 | 13 |
| **Fruit Drops,** (1), ¹⁄₄ oz | 20 | 0 | 4 |
| **Fruit Gems** *(Sunkist),* (4), 1.4 oz | 130 | 0 | 33 |
| **Fruit Leathers,** average, 0.5 oz | 50 | 0.5 | 12 |
| **Fruit Pastilles** *(Rowntree),* 1 roll | 185 | 0 | 45 |
| **Fruit Roll-Ups** *(Betty Crocker/Sunkist),* | | | |
| 1 roll, 0.5 oz | 50 | 1 | 12 |
| **Fruit Runts** *(Walgreens),* | | | |
| 12 pieces | 60 | 0 | 14 |
| **Fruit Flavored Shapes** *(Betty Crocker),* | | | |
| all varieties, 0.8 oz | 80 | 0 | 19 |
| **Fudge:** | | | |
| Chocolate; Mint, 1 oz | 130 | 8 | 14 |
| P'nut Butter & Choc., 1 oz | 130 | 8 | 13 |
| *Brevin's:* Cashew, 1 oz | 195 | 9 | 28 |
| Triple Decker, 1 oz | 165 | 7 | 25 |
| **Ghirardelli:** | | | |
| **3 oz Bars:** Dark Choc., 4 squares | 220 | 17 | 23 |
| Filled, P'nut Butter, 4 squares | 250 | 17 | 22 |
| Intense Dark Bars, | | | |
| Ev'ng Dream, 3 pcs | 190 | 15 | 20 |
| **Squares:** | | | |
| Dark Choc., (4), 1.5 oz | 210 | 16 | 23 |
| Milk & Caramel (3), 1.5 oz | 220 | 12 | 27 |
| Sea Salt Escape (4), 1.5 oz | 210 | 15 | 24 |

| Per Piece/Serving | C | F | Cb |
|---|---|---|---|
| **Godiva:** | | | |
| **Bars:** Milk/Dark, av., 1.5 oz | 230 | 14 | 26 |
| Extra Dark: 75%, 1.5 oz | 230 | 17 | 18 |
| 85%, 1.4 oz | 260 | 21 | 14 |
| **Chocoiste:** Dk Choc. Cherries (12) | 190 | 7 | 30 |
| Milk Chocolate Cashews (14) | 230 | 15 | 19 |
| **Hearts:** Dark Ganache (4) | 200 | 12 | 23 |
| Milk Praline (4) | 220 | 13 | 23 |
| **Go Lightly:** | | | |
| Assorted Toffee, 5 pieces, 1 oz | 85 | 2 | 24 |
| Fruit Chews, 5 pieces, 1 oz | 95 | 2 | 26 |
| Hard Candy, Assorted (4), 0.5 oz | 45 | 0 | 15 |
| *Note: Carb figures include 15-25g sugar alcohol* | | | |
| **Goobers Peanuts,** 1 package, 1.4 oz | 200 | 13 | 21 |
| **Good & Plenty** *(Hershey's),* (33), 1.4 oz | 140 | 0 | 35 |
| **GooGoo Clusters,** 1 piece, 1.8 oz | 240 | 12 | 30 |
| **Gum** ~ *See Page 75* | | | |
| **Gum Drops:** 1 small, 0.1 oz | 15 | 0 | 3 |
| 5 pieces, 0.5 oz | 75 | 0 | 15 |
| **Gummi** *(Shur Fine):* | | | |
| Bears (15), 1.4 oz | 130 | 0 | 29 |
| Chewy Sweet Tarts (4) | 160 | 0 | 36 |
| Worms (9), 1.5 oz | 140 | 0 | 31 |
| **Guylian:** | | | |
| **Bars:** Dark Chocolate (3), 1 oz | 150 | 12 | 11 |
| Milk Choc. w/ Hazelnuts (3),1 oz | 170 | 11 | 15 |
| **No Sugar Added Bars:** | | | |
| Milk Chocolate, 3 squares | 150 | 11 | 16 |
| 54% Cocoa, Dark Choc., 3 sqrs. | 140 | 11 | 16 |
| **Seashells:** | | | |
| Bar, 1.4 oz | 210 | 13 | 21 |
| Boxed, Originals (1), 0.4 oz | 60 | 4 | 6 |
| Truffles, (1), 0.4 oz | 70 | 5.5 | 5 |
| **Heath:** Original (1), 1.4 oz | 210 | 13 | 24 |
| King Size, 2.8 oz | 410 | 22 | 49 |
| Snack Size, 3 pieces, 1.5 oz | 230 | 14 | 27 |
| **Hershey's:** | | | |
| **Cookie Layer Crunch,** av., 1.4 oz | 300 | 17 | 36 |
| **Cookies 'n' Creme,** 1.55 oz Bar | 230 | 12 | 26 |
| **Milk Chocolate:** | | | |
| Bars: 1.55 oz | 220 | 13 | 26 |
| with Almonds, 1 bar, 1.4 oz | 210 | 14 | 21 |
| King Size, 1 Bar, 2.5 oz | 370 | 22 | 44 |
| Kisses, 9 pieces, av., 1.4 oz | 200 | 12 | 25 |
| Nuggets: 4 pieces, 1.4 oz | 200 | 13 | 20 |
| w/ Toffee & Alm., 4 pcs, 1.3 oz | 200 | 13 | 21 |
| **Extra Dark Choc.,** 4 pcs, 1.4 oz | 180 | 14 | 21 |
| **Simple Pleasures,** 6 pcs, av. | 180 | 8 | 29 |
| **Special Dark Choc.,** 1.5 oz bar | 190 | 12 | 25 |
| **Sugar Free Choc.,** 5 pieces, 1.4 oz | 160 | 13 | 24 |

## Candy ~ Brands & Generic (Cont)

*Per Piece/Serving*

| | C | F | Cb |
|---|---|---|---|
| **Hershey's, (Cont):** | | | |
| **Pot of Gold Chocolate Asstd:** | | | |
| Carmel, 4 pieces, 1.4 oz | 190 | 10 | 26 |
| Av. other var., 4 pieces, 1.4 oz | 210 | 12 | 24 |
| **Candy-Coated Eggs:** | | | |
| Milk Chocolate: (8) 1.2 oz | 170 | 8 | 27 |
| w/ Almonds (8) 1.2 oz | 200 | 12 | 18 |
| **Honeycomb:** Plain, 1 oz | 115 | 0 | 27 |
| Choc-coated, 2 pieces | 180 | 7 | 31 |
| **Hot Tamales,** | | | |
| 20 pieces, 1.4 oz | 150 | 0 | 36 |
| **Hugs ~ See Kisses** | | | |
| **Jawbreakers** *(Sathers)*, (15), 0.6 oz | 60 | 0 | 16 |
| **Jells** *(Joyva)*, Raspb., 3 pieces, 1.6 oz | 160 | 0 | 38 |
| **Jelly Beans,** average all brands: | | | |
| Small Size (Jelly Belly): 1 bean | 5 | 0 | 1 |
| 12 beans, 0.5 oz | 50 | 0 | 13 |
| Regular Size: 1 bean | 10 | 0 | 2 |
| 10 beans, 1 oz | 105 | 0 | 26 |
| Large Size: 1 bean | 15 | 0 | 38 |
| 10 beans, 1.5 oz | 150 | 0 | 38 |
| Sugar Free, | | | |
| average all brands, 25 beans, 1 oz | 60 | 0 | 26 |
| *Note: Carb figure include 26g sugar alcohol* | | | |
| **Jelly Belly:** 25 beans, 1 oz | 105 | 0 | 26 |
| 3.5 oz package | 360 | 0 | 90 |
| Sugar Free, | | | |
| 25 beans, 1 oz | 60 | 0 | 26 |
| *Note: Carb figure include 26g sugar alcohol* | | | |
| Chocolate Dips: | | | |
| All flavors: 1 bean | 4 | 0 | 1 |
| 10 beans | 40 | 1 | 8 |
| 2.8 oz bag | 300 | 8 | 62 |
| **Jelly Rings** *(Jewel)*, 5 pieces, 1.4 oz | 110 | 0 | 26 |
| **Jolly Rancher:** | | | |
| Bites: Soft, 15 pieces | 150 | 1.5 | 32 |
| Sours, 16 pieces | 130 | 0 | 34 |
| Crunch 'N Chew, 1 oz pkg | 160 | 0.5 | 40 |
| Filled Fruity Bites, 22 pieces | 140 | 1 | 31 |
| Gummies, 9 pieces | 120 | 0 | 28 |
| Hard Candy, 3 pieces | 70 | 0 | 17 |
| Jelly Beans/Sours, 1.4 oz | 140 | 0 | 36 |
| Lollipops (1), 0.55 oz | 60 | 0 | 15 |
| **Jujubes,** all varieties (52), 1.4 oz | 110 | 0 | 28 |
| **Juju Bears,** 5 pieces | 130 | 0 | 34 |
| **Juju Mix (Sathers),** 11 pieces, 1.5 oz | 150 | 0 | 36 |
| **Jujyfruits,** 16 pieces, 1.4 oz | 120 | 0 | 32 |
| **Junior Caramels:** 13 pieces, 1.5 oz | 190 | 6 | 33 |
| Mini, 2 boxes, 1 oz | 130 | 4 | 23 |

*Per Piece/Serving*

| | C | F | Cb |
|---|---|---|---|
| **Junior Mints:** 1.8 oz | 220 | 4 | 45 |
| 16 pieces, 1.4 oz | 170 | 3 | 35 |
| **Justin's,** Peanut Butter Cups, | | | |
| Milk Choc, 2 cups, 1.4 oz pkg | 200 | 14 | 18 |
| **Kinder Joy,** 1 egg, 0.7 oz | 110 | 6 | 12 |
| **Kisses** *(Hershey's)*: | | | |
| **Milk Chocolate:** (1), 0.16 oz | 25 | 1.5 | 3 |
| (9), 1.4oz | 200 | 12 | 25 |
| with Almonds (9), 1.4 oz | 200 | 13 | 22 |
| Caramel Filled (9), 1.5 oz | 190 | 9 | 27 |
| Air Delights (11), 1.4 oz | 200 | 12 | 24 |
| Cookies 'n' Creme (9), 1.5 oz | 220 | 12 | 26 |
| Hugs (9), 1.4 oz | 210 | 12 | 24 |
| **Special Dark,** (9), 1.4 oz | 180 | 12 | 25 |
| **Kit Kat** *(Nestle)*: | | | |
| **Halloween:** | | | |
| Miniatures, 1.34 oz bar | 190 | 12 | 22 |
| Snack Size: Triple Choc. 1.48 oz | 200 | 11 | 27 |
| White Choc., 1.48 oz | 220 | 11 | 27 |
| **Milk Chocolate:** 4 pce bar, 1.5 oz | 210 | 11 | 28 |
| Extra Crispy, 1.6 oz bar | 220 | 12 | 29 |
| King Size, 8 pcs, 3 oz bar | 420 | 22 | 56 |
| Minis, 5 pieces | 210 | 11 | 28 |
| Snack Size, 6 pcs, 1.5 oz | 210 | 11 | 27 |
| **White Chocolate,** 4 pcs, 1.5 oz | 220 | 12 | 28 |
| **Lemon Drops:** (4), 0.6 oz | 60 | 0 | 16 |
| *Walgreens,* Sugar Free (3), 0.6 oz | 50 | 0 | 17 |
| **Lemonhead,** (26), 1.4 oz | 140 | 0 | 36 |
| **Lance,** Peanut Bar, 2.2 oz | 340 | 19 | 29 |
| **Licorice:** | | | |
| Average all varieties, 1oz | 100 | 0 | 25 |
| Chews *(Panda)*, (1) | 10 | 0 | 3 |
| Tid Bits (1) | 10 | 0 | 2 |
| Twists: Black/Red, av., 1 pc | 35 | 0 | 8 |
| Sugar Free, 1 piece | 15 | 0 | 2.5 |
| **American Licorice Co.:** | | | |
| Natural Vines: Black (9), 1.4 oz | 140 | 1 | 33 |
| Strawberry (9), 1.4 oz | 150 | 1 | 34 |
| Red Vines (4), 1.4 oz | 140 | 0 | 34 |
| Sip-n-Chew, 1 oz package | 100 | 1 | 23 |
| Snaps (31), 1.4 oz | 140 | 0.5 | 33 |
| Sour Punch (6), 1.4 oz | 150 | 0.5 | 34 |
| Super Ropes (1), 2 oz | 200 | 0 | 46 |
| **Lifesavers:** Large size, 1 candy | 15 | 0 | 3 |
| Regular: All flavors, 1 candy | 10 | 0 | 3 |
| 1 Roll (14 candies), 1.2 oz | 140 | 0 | 35 |
| Creme Savers, 3 pcs, 0.5 oz | 60 | 1 | 11 |
| Pep-o-mint (3), 0.2 oz | 20 | 0 | 5 |
| Fruit Splosion (10), 1.4 oz | 130 | 0 | 31 |
| Sugar-Free, Pep-O-Mint (4), 0.5 oz | 35 | 0 | 14 |
| *Note: Carb figure includes 14g sugar alcohol* | | | |

## Candy ~ Brands & Generic (Cont)

| Per Piece/Serving | C | F | Cb |
|---|---|---|---|
| **Lik-m-aid** *(Nestle)*, Fun Dip, 1 package | 50 | 0 | 13 |
| **Lindt:** Lindor Truffles (1), average | 75 | 6 | 5 |
| **Swiss Milk Chocolate Bars:** | | | |
| 70% Cocoa, 4 pieces | 220 | 17 | 13 |
| Classic, with Hazelnuts, 10 pieces | 230 | 16 | 20 |
| Raspberry filled, 7 pieces | 200 | 10 | 25 |
| **Dark Choc. Truffles,** | | | |
| with filling, 7 pieces | 240 | 18 | 18 |
| **Lollipops:** Mini, 0.3 oz | 25 | 0 | 6 |
| Small, 0.5 oz | 50 | 0 | 12 |
| Medium, 1 oz | 100 | 0 | 25 |
| Giant (4" diam), 7 oz | 790 | 0 | 198 |
| **M & M's:** | | | |
| **Dark Chocolate:** 1.5 oz package | 210 | 10 | 29 |
| Peanuts, 1.5 oz | 220 | 12 | 25 |
| **Halloween:** | 210 | 10 | 29 |
| Mini, Whitet Candy Corn Choc., 1.5 oz | 220 | 11 | 29 |
| White Pumpkin Pie Candy, 1.5 oz | 210 | 11 | 29 |
| **Milk Chocolate:** 28 piece, 1 oz | 145 | 6.5 | 21 |
| 1.5 oz package | 210 | 9 | 30 |
| 1.7 oz package | 240 | 10 | 34 |
| Almond Choc., 1.5 oz | 220 | 12 | 25 |
| Minis, 1 tube, 1 oz | 150 | 7 | 21 |
| **Peanut:** 28 pieces, 1 oz | 155 | 8 | 17 |
| 1.75 oz pkg | 250 | 13 | 30 |
| **Peanut Butter,** 1.6 oz pkg | 240 | 14 | 26 |
| **Premiums:** Chocolate Trio, 1.5 oz | 230 | 14 | 25 |
| Mint Thrills, 1.5 oz | 240 | 14 | 25 |
| **Pretzels,** 1/2 pkg, 1.4 oz | 180 | 6 | 29 |
| **Snack Mix,** av. 1/3 cup, 1.5 oz | 200 | 9 | 25 |
| **Mamba Sours,** Fruit Chews, | | | |
| 6 pieces, 1 oz | 100 | 1 | 22 |
| **Marshmallow Egg,** 1 egg, 1 oz | 120 | 3 | 22 |
| **Mary Jane** *(Necco)*, 5 pieces, 1.4 oz | 160 | 3.5 | 32 |
| **Marshmallows:** Firm/Soft, 1 oz | 90 | 0 | 23 |
| Regular size, 4 pieces, 1 oz | 100 | 0 | 24 |
| Mini-Marshmallow, 2/3 cup, 1 oz | 95 | 0 | 24 |
| *Joyva,* Choc-coated Twists | 95 | 2 | 10 |
| *Fluff,* 2 Tbsp, 0.6 oz | 60 | 0 | 15 |
| *Kraft:* Creme, 0.5 oz | 45 | 0 | 11 |
| Funmallows, 2/3 cup, 1 oz | 100 | 0 | 24 |
| Jet-Puffed, 5 pieces, 1 oz | 100 | 0 | 24 |
| Mini, 1 oz | 90 | 0 | 23 |
| **Marzipan,** 2 Tbsp, 1.4 oz | 160 | 4 | 29 |
| **Mauna Loa,** Mountains, 4 pcs | 230 | 17 | 21 |
| **Mexican Hats,** (7), 1.4 oz | 120 | 0 | 30 |
| **Mentos:** Regular | 10 | 0 | 3 |
| Sugar Free | 5 | 0 | 2 |
| **Mike & Ike:** | | | |
| Original: 2.1 oz package | 220 | 0 | 55 |
| 23 pieces, 1.4 oz | 140 | 0 | 36 |
| **Milk Duds,** 1 box, 1.8 oz | 230 | 8 | 38 |

| Per Piece/Serving | C | F | Cb |
|---|---|---|---|
| **Milky Way** *(Mars):* | | | |
| **Bars:** Single, 2 oz | 240 | 9 | 37 |
| Fun Size, 2 bars, 1.2 oz | 160 | 6 | 24 |
| To Go, 1.8 oz | 230 | 9 | 36 |
| Minis, 5 pieces, 1.5 oz | 190 | 7 | 30 |
| Midnight Bars: 1.8 oz | 230 | 8 | 36 |
| Minis, 5 pieces, 1.4 oz | 190 | 7 | 30 |
| Simply Caramel, 1.9 oz | 250 | 11 | 37 |
| **Mints:** Uncoated, 3 pieces | 70 | 0 | 17 |
| 1 mint , medium | 7 | 0 | 1 |
| 1 large mint | 15 | 0 | 3 |
| **Mon Cheri** *(Ferrero)*, 4 pieces, 2 oz | 260 | 18 | 20 |
| **Mounds:** 1.75 oz bar | 240 | 13 | 28 |
| King Size, 4 pieces, 3.5 oz | 480 | 26 | 56 |
| Snack Size, 1 piece, 0.6 oz | 80 | 4.5 | 10 |
| **Mr Goodbar:** 1.8 oz bar | 250 | 17 | 26 |
| King Size, 2.6 oz bar | 380 | 26 | 38 |
| **Munch Bar,** 1.4 oz | 220 | 15 | 18 |
| **Necco,** Candy Wafers (40), 2 oz | 220 | 0 | 56 |
| **Nestle:** Original, 1.6 oz bar | 220 | 11 | 30 |
| Fun Size, 3 bars, 1.4 oz | 180 | 9 | 26 |
| Miniatures, 4 bars, 1.4 oz | 200 | 10 | 27 |
| Buncha Crunch, 1/3 cup, 1.2 oz | 180 | 9 | 25 |
| Crunch Crisp, 1.8 oz | 240 | 13 | 32 |
| **Newman's Own:** | | | |
| **Milk Choc.:** Caramel Cups (3) | 160 | 8 | 21 |
| Peanut Butter Cups (3) | 180 | 12 | 17 |
| **Dark Choc.:** Caramel Cups (3) | 160 | 9 | 20 |
| Peanut Butter Cups (3) | 180 | 13 | 16 |
| **Nips,** all varieties, 2 pieces, 0.5 oz | 60 | 2 | 11 |
| **Nougat:** 3 pieces, 1.5 oz | 170 | 1 | 39 |
| Chocolate Covered, 1 oz | 125 | 4 | 22 |
| **Nuggets** ~ *See Hershey's* | | | |
| **Nutrageous Bar** *(Reese's)*, 1.8 oz | 260 | 16 | 28 |
| **Oh Henry!:** Fun Size, 0.9 oz | 120 | 5 | 16 |
| 1.8 oz bar | 230 | 11 | 33 |
| **Orange Slices:** | | | |
| *Jewel,* 3 pieces, 1.5 oz | 140 | 0 | 35 |
| *Walgreens,* 4 pieces, 1.6 oz | 160 | 0 | 39 |
| **Pastel Mints** *(Walgreens)*, 20 pieces | 60 | 0 | 14 |
| **PayDay Bar:** 1.8 oz bar | 240 | 13 | 27 |
| King Size, 3.5 oz bar | 440 | 24 | 50 |
| Snack Size, 0.7 oz | 90 | 5 | 10 |
| Avalanche, 1.8 oz bar | 250 | 13 | 29 |
| **Peanut Bar** *(Planter's)*, 1.6 oz | 240 | 14 | 21 |
| **Peanut Butter Cups** ~ *See Reese's; Newman's Own* | | | |
| **Peanut Brittle:** 1 piece, 1.5 oz | 190 | 5 | 32 |
| Sugar Free *(Russell Stover)*, | | | |
| 4 pieces, 1.3 oz | 140 | 10 | 24 |

## Candy ~ Brands & Generic (Cont)

*Per Piece/Serving* **© 🄕 🄒ᵇ**

| | C | F | Cb |
|---|---|---|---|
| **Peanuts,** choc-covered, 14 pieces | 230 | 14 | 23 |
| **Pearson's,** Mint Patties, (5), 1.3 oz | 150 | 2.5 | 31 |
| **Peppermints:** 7 small, 0.5 oz | 60 | 0 | 15 |
| *Brach's,* Star Brites (3) | 60 | 0 | 16 |
| **Pez,** 1 roll | 35 | 0 | 9 |
| **Planters,** | | | |
| Double Peanut Bar, 1.6 oz | 240 | 14 | 21 |
| **Pop Rocks,** 0.4 oz package | 35 | 0 | 9 |
| **Pot of Gold** *(Hershey's):* | | | |
| Assortment: Caramel, 4 pieces | 190 | 10 | 25 |
| Nut, 4 pieces | 210 | 13 | 23 |
| **Pretzels:** Choc-covered, Mini (6) | 200 | 9 | 25 |
| White Chocolate Bites (23), 1.4 oz | 200 | 9 | 25 |
| **Pretzel Flipz** *(Nestlé),* 8 pcs, 1 oz | 130 | 5 | 20 |
| **Raisinets:** | | | |
| Milk Choc: 1.58 oz pkg | 190 | 8 | 32 |
| Movie Pack, 3.5 oz | 380 | 16 | 64 |
| Dark Chocolate, ¼ cup, 1.6 oz | 180 | 8 | 32 |
| **Reese's:** | | | |
| **Clusters,** 3 pieces, 1.5 oz | 220 | 12 | 24 |
| **Crispy Crunchy Bar:** 1.7 oz | 260 | 18 | 22 |
| 2 pieces, 1.2 oz | 170 | 10 | 19 |
| King Size, 3 oz | 480 | 32 | 40 |
| **Fast Break,** 2 oz bar | 260 | 12 | 35 |
| **Halloween:** PB Pumpkins, 1.2 oz | 180 | 10 | 18 |
| Snack Size (2), 1.2 oz | 180 | 10 | 19 |
| **P'nut Butter Chips,** 0.5 oz | 80 | 4 | 8 |
| **P'nut Butter Cups:** | | | |
| Milk Choc: (2), 1.5 oz | 210 | 13 | 24 |
| Miniatures (5), 1.5 oz | 220 | 13 | 26 |
| Minis (11) | 200 | 12 | 23 |
| Big Cup (1), 1.4 oz | 200 | 12 | 22 |
| Sugar Free, Minis (5), 1.4 oz | 180 | 13 | 27 |
| **Dark Chocolate (2),** 1.5 oz | 210 | 14 | 23 |
| **Pieces,** Peanut Butter (51) | 200 | 9 | 25 |
| **Sticks:** 1.5 oz pkg | 220 | 13 | 23 |
| King Size, 3 oz pkg | 440 | 26 | 46 |
| Snack Size (1), 0.6 oz | 90 | 5 | 9 |
| **Snacksters,** 1 package, 0.8 oz | 100 | 4 | 14 |
| **Whipps,** 1.5 oz | 230 | 9 | 37 |
| **Rice Krispies Treats** *(Kellogg's),* | | | |
| 1 bar, average all varieties, 0.8 oz | 95 | 2.5 | 17 |
| **Riesen,** Choc. Chew, 4 pcs, 1.3 oz | 170 | 6 | 28 |
| **Rocky Road,** Milk/Dark, 1.8 oz bar | 240 | 11 | 34 |
| **Roca Thins,** 3 pieces, av. all var. | 210 | 14 | 24 |
| **Rolo:** Regular, all var., 1.7 oz roll | 220 | 10 | 33 |
| Mini Chews, Caramel in milk choc. (11) | 190 | 9 | 26 |
| **Root Beer Barrels,** (3), 0.6 oz | 60 | 0 | 17 |

*Per Piece/Serving* **© 🄕 🄒ᵇ**

| | C | F | Cb |
|---|---|---|---|
| **Russell Stover Candy:** | | | |
| **Boxed Chocolates Choc. Coated:** | | | |
| Assorted (2), 1.2 oz | 150 | 7 | 22 |
| Cherry Cordials (3), 0.4 oz | 150 | 5 | 25 |
| Dairy Crm Caramels (2), 1.2 oz | 160 | 7 | 22 |
| Elegant Collection (3), 1.6 oz | 210 | 10 | 25 |
| French Choc. Mints (4), 1.4 oz | 220 | 13 | 22 |
| Nut, Chewy & Crisp Centers (2) | 160 | 8 | 21 |
| **Sugar Free:** | | | |
| Ass'td Hard Candies (3), 1.6 oz | 210 | 16 | 24 |
| Bags: Caramel (3), 1.3 oz | 180 | 8 | 25 |
| Coconut (3), 1.5 oz | 160 | 10 | 28 |
| Mint Patty (3), 1.5 oz | 180 | 12 | 26 |
| Peanut Butter Cups (2), 1.2 oz | 160 | 12 | 17 |
| Pecan Delight (2), 1.2 oz | 160 | 12 | 19 |
| *Note: Carbohydrate figures include sugar alcohol* | | | |
| **Salt Water Taffy** *(Brach's),* (5) | 170 | 2.5 | 36 |
| **Seashells** *(Guylian),* (4), 1.6 oz | 260 | 17 | 24 |
| **See's Candies:** | | | |
| Almond Royal (5) | 190 | 13 | 18 |
| Butterscotch Chews (5) | 210 | 12 | 27 |
| Krispy's: Caffe Latte (5) | 180 | 8 | 27 |
| Mint (5) | 170 | 8 | 27 |
| Little Pops: | | | |
| Butterscotch (4), 0.5 oz | 60 | 2 | 12 |
| Av. other flavors (4) | 55 | 3 | 10 |
| Lollypops, average, 0.7 oz | 90 | 3 | 17 |
| Milk Molasses Chips ( 6), 1.4 oz | 180 | 8 | 27 |
| Milk Peppermints, 2 pieces, 1.3 oz | 150 | 4 | 28 |
| Peanut Brittle Bar, 1 oz | 150 | 10 | 15 |
| Peanut Butter Patties (2), 1.2 oz | 170 | 10 | 16 |
| Peppermint Twists (3) | 60 | 0 | 15 |
| Toffee-ettes, 3 pieces | 270 | 21 | 18 |
| **Sugar Free:** | | | |
| Dark Bar, 1.5 oz | 180 | 16 | 24 |
| Dark Walnut Clusters (4), 1.5 oz | 230 | 21 | 17 |
| Peanut Brittle, 1.5 oz | 170 | 14 | 17 |
| *Note: Carbohydrate figures include 12-18 g sugar alcohol* | | | |
| **Skinny Cow:** | | | |
| Dreamy Clusters, all var., 1 pouch | 120 | 6 | 20 |
| Heavenly Crips, all varieties, 1 bar | 110 | 6 | 14 |
| **Skittles:** Original, 2 oz | 230 | 2.5 | 52 |
| Sour, 1.8 oz | 200 | 2 | 44 |
| Tropical; Wild Berry, 2.2 oz | 250 | 2.5 | 56 |
| Fun Size, 1 bag, 0.5 oz | 60 | 1 | 14 |
| Tear & Share, 4 oz bag | 420 | 4.5 | 93 |
| **Skor,** Toffee Bar (1), 1.4 oz | 200 | 12 | 25 |
| **Smarties:** Candy Rolls (1), 0.3 oz | 25 | 0 | 6 |
| Giant, 1 roll, 1 oz | 100 | 0 | 25 |

## Candy ~ Brands & Generic (Cont)

*Per Piece/Serving*

| Snickers: | C | F | Cb |
|---|---|---|---|
| **Milk Chocolate:** 1.9 oz bar | 250 | 12 | 33 |
| Fun Size, 2 bars, 1.2 oz | 160 | 8 | 21 |
| To Go Bar, 1.6 oz | 220 | 10 | 29 |
| Almond Bar, 1.8 oz | 230 | 11 | 32 |
| Protein Bar, 2 oz | 200 | 7 | 18 |
| P'nut Butter Squared, 2 bars, 1.8 oz | 250 | 13 | 30 |
| Miniatures: (4) | 170 | 8 | 22 |
| Sugar Free, 5 pcs | 180 | 13 | 27 |
| **Dark Chocolate Bar,** 1.8 oz | 250 | 12 | 31 |
| **Sno Caps,** $^1/_4$ cup, 1.4 oz | 180 | 8 | 30 |
| **Soft 'N Chewy,** Butter Toffee, 1 piece | 30 | 0.5 | 5 |
| **Sorbee,** Crystal Light Hard Candy (4) | 25 | 0 | 13 |

*Note: Carb figure includes Isomalt which has fewer calories than sugar.*

| | C | F | Cb |
|---|---|---|---|
| **Sour Patch:** Kids, average, 2 oz | 210 | 0 | 52 |
| Extreme, 1.8 oz | 190 | 0 | 47 |
| **Spearmint Leaves:** | | | |
| *Jewel,* 5 pieces, 1.4 oz | 140 | 0 | 35 |
| *Walgreens,* 4 pieces, 1.6 oz | 160 | 0 | 39 |
| **Spree Candies:** Original, 15 pieces | 50 | 0 | 13 |
| Chewy, 8 pieces | 60 | 0 | 13 |
| **Starburst:** | | | |
| Candy Canes, 0.5 oz | 70 | 0 | 18 |
| Fruit Chews: Original (1) | 20 | 0.5 | 4 |
| 8 pieces, 1.4 oz | 160 | 3.5 | 33 |
| Gummibursts, 9 pieces, 1.4 oz | 130 | 0 | 31 |
| Jellybeans, 1.5 oz | 150 | 0 | 37 |
| **Starlight Mints,** 3 pieces, 0.5 oz | 60 | 0 | 15 |
| **Suckers** *(Walgreens),* 1 piece, 0.4 oz | 45 | 0 | 11 |
| **Sugar Babies,** Original, 1.4 oz | 160 | 1.5 | 37 |
| **Sugar Coated Peanuts,** 1 oz | 120 | 8 | 10 |
| **Sunbursts Sunflowers** *(Kimmie):* | | | |
| ChocoRocks Milk, 3.5 oz | 525 | 25 | 67 |
| Habanero Corn, 3.5 oz | 500 | 23 | 70 |
| Sunburst Mix, Milk, 3.5 oz | 500 | 28 | 55 |
| **Swedish Fish,** 7 pieces, 1.5 oz | 150 | 0 | 38 |
| **SweeTARTS:** | | | |
| Orig., 8 pieces, 0.5 oz | 50 | 0 | 13 |
| Mini Chewy, 23 pieces, 0.5 oz | 50 | 0.5 | 12 |
| **Symphony** *(Hershey's):* | | | |
| **Milk Choc:** 1.5 oz bar | 220 | 14 | 23 |
| Large Block: 5 pieces, 1.4 oz | 200 | 12 | 22 |
| w/ Alm. & Toffee, 5 pcs, 1.3 oz | 200 | 13 | 21 |

*Per Piece/Serving*

| Taffy, | C | F | Cb |
|---|---|---|---|
| Fruit Chews, 1 piece | 20 | 0.5 | 4 |
| **Take 5** *(Hershey's):* Orig., 1.5oz | 200 | 11 | 25 |
| King Size, 2.3 oz | 300 | 16 | 37 |
| Snack Size, 2 pcs, 1 oz | 150 | 8 | 19 |
| **3 Musketeers:** | | | |
| Original, 1.9 oz | 240 | 7 | 42 |
| 2 To Go, 1 bar, 1.6 oz | 200 | 6 | 35 |
| Fun Size, 3 bars, 1.6 oz | 190 | 6 | 34 |
| Minis, 7 pieces, 1.4 oz | 170 | 5 | 32 |
| **Tang-a-Roos,** 1 roll | 25 | 0 | 6 |
| **Terry's:** Chocolate Orange (5), 1.5 oz | 230 | 12 | 27 |
| Dark Chocolate Orange (5), 1.5 oz | 240 | 13 | 28 |
| **Tic Tac,** all flavors, 1 piece | 2 | 0 | 0 |
| **Toblerone:** 1.3 oz bar | 190 | 10 | 22 |
| 1.8 oz bar | 270 | 15 | 31 |
| 3.5 oz bar | 540 | 30 | 63 |
| 5.3 oz Package, 5 pieces, 1.5 oz | 230 | 13 | 27 |
| **Toffees,** Regular, 1 oz | 160 | 9 | 18 |
| **Tootsie Pops,** (1), 0.6 oz | 60 | 0 | 15 |
| **Tootsie Roll:** 2.3 oz roll | 245 | 2 | 55 |
| Midgees, 1.4 oz | 140 | 3 | 28 |
| **Truffles:** Reg., 1 piece, 0.4 oz | 60 | 4 | 6 |
| Large *(Godiva),* 0.8 oz | 110 | 6.5 | 12 |
| Extra Large *(J.Schmidt),* 1.5 oz | 220 | 13 | 24 |
| **Turtles:** Original, 1 piece, 0.6 oz | 85 | 5 | 10 |
| Sugar Free, 1 piece, 0.4 oz | 50 | 3.5 | 7 |
| **Twists,** Licorice; Strawb., sugar free, | | | |
| 7 pieces, 1.4 oz | 90 | 0 | 25 |
| **Twix:** | | | |
| **Caramel:** 2 cookies, 1.8 oz | 250 | 12 | 34 |
| Fun Size, 2 cookies, 1.7 oz | 250 | 14 | 27 |
| 4 To Go, 1 cookie, 0.8 oz | 110 | 5 | 15 |
| 6 To Go, 1 cookie, 0.5 oz | 80 | 4 | 11 |
| Minis, 3 pieces, 1 oz | 150 | 7 | 20 |
| **Peanut Butter:** | | | |
| Single, 2 cookies, 1.7 oz | 250 | 14 | 27 |
| 4 to Go, 1 cookie, 0.8 oz | 250 | 12 | 34 |
| **Twizzlers:** Cherry Bites (17), 1.4 oz | 140 | 0.5 | 32 |
| Cherry Nibs, 29 pieces, 1.4 oz | 140 | 1 | 32 |
| Pull 'n' Peel, Cherry, 1 piece, 1.2 oz | 110 | 0.5 | 26 |
| Twists, Strawb., 1.3 oz | 120 | 0.5 | 29 |
| **U-No Bar,** 1.5 oz | 250 | 17 | 22 |
| **Weight Watchers** *(Whitman's):* | | | |
| Caramel Medallions (3) | 160 | 9 | 24 |
| Coconut (3) | 150 | 9 | 23 |
| English Toffee Squares (3) | 150 | 9 | 21 |
| Mint Patties (3) | 150 | 9 | 23 |
| Peanut Butter Cups (4) | 180 | 8 | 31 |
| Pecan Crowns (3) | 160 | 10 | 24 |

## Candy ~ Brands & Generic (Cont)

*Per Piece/Serving* | **C** | **F** | **Cb**
|---|---|---|---|
| **Werther's:** | | | |
| Hard Candy: Original (3), 0.5 oz | 70 | 1.5 | 14 |
| Sugar-Free Original (5) | 40 | 1.5 | 15 |
| *Note: Carb figure includes 14g sugar alcohol* | | | |
| Soft, Chocolate Caramel (4), 1.4 oz | 190 | 8 | 28 |
| **Whatchamacallit:** 1.5 oz Bar | 230 | 12 | 28 |
| King Size Bar, 2.5 oz | 370 | 20 | 45 |
| **Whitman's, Boxed Chocolates:** | | | |
| Sampler (4), 1.6 oz | 220 | 12 | 27 |
| 12 oz Box, 3 pieces, 1.2 oz | 170 | 9 | 21 |
| Reserve, 7 oz Box, 2 pieces, 1.2 oz | 160 | 9 | 21 |
| Sugar Free, 10 oz Box, 3 pcs, 1.5 oz | 190 | 13 | 25 |
| **Whoppers,** av. all varieties, 18 pcs | 190 | 7 | 31 |
| **Wonka:** | | | |
| Bar (1), 2.5 oz | 360 | 19 | 49 |
| Exceptional Bars, average, 4 pieces | 200 | 13 | 23 |
| Gobstopper, 9 pieces, 0.5 oz | 60 | 0 | 14 |
| **Laffy Taffy:** Ropes, all var., 0.8 oz | 80 | 1.5 | 18 |
| Stretchy & Tangy, all var., 1.5 oz | 150 | 3.5 | 29 |
| Nerds, Giant, Chewy, 1.8 oz package | 180 | 0 | 42 |
| **Yogurt Candy,** | | | |
| Coated Raisins, 27 pieces, 1.4 oz | 180 | 8 | 28 |
| **York:** Mints, (3) | 10 | 0 | 3 |
| Peppermint Pattie, reg, 1.4 oz | 140 | 2.5 | 31 |
| Pieces (50) | 170 | 8 | 28 |
| **Zagnut,** 1.75 oz bar | 220 | 9 | 35 |
| **Zero Bar:** 1.8 oz bar | 230 | 8 | 37 |
| King Size, 3.5 oz | 400 | 14 | 68 |

## Gum

*Per Piece* | **C** | **F** | **Cb**
|---|---|---|---|
| **Bazooka** | 15 | 0 | 4 |
| **Beechies** | 6 | 0 | 2 |
| **Big League Chews** | 10 | 0 | 2 |
| **Bubble Yum:** Original | 25 | 0 | 6 |
| Sugarless | 10 | 0 | 3 |
| Candilicious | 30 | 0 | 2 |
| **Carefree,** Sugarless/Regular | 5 | 0 | 2 |
| **Chiclet** | 5 | 0 | 1 |
| **Dentyne** | 5 | 0 | 0.5 |
| **Double Bubble Ball** | 20 | 0 | 5 |
| **Estee,** Bubble/Regular | 5 | 0 | 2 |
| **Extra** (Wrigley's), Sugar-Free | 5 | 0 | 2 |
| **Freshen-Up** | 10 | 0 | 3 |
| **Hubba Bubba:** Regular | 25 | 0 | 6 |
| Sugar-free, average | 14 | 0 | 0.5 |
| **Ice Breakers** | 5 | 0 | 2 |
| **Jolt Gum** | 5 | 0 | 2 |
| **Super Bubble** | 15 | 0 | 4 |
| **Trident,** Orig.; White | 5 | 0 | 1 |
| **Wrigley's,** all flavors | 10 | 0 | 2 |

## Carob Candy

| | **C** | **F** | **Cb** |
|---|---|---|---|
| *Per Piece/Serving* | | | |
| **Carob,** Plain/Natural, 1 oz | 155 | 9 | 15 |
| **Carob Coated:** Raisins, 1 oz | 130 | 8 | 15 |
| Almonds/Peanuts, 1 oz | 150 | 10 | 14 |
| Caramels, 1 oz | 110 | 4 | 18 |
| Dates, 1 oz | 125 | 5 | 20 |
| Malt Balls, 1 oz | 135 | 8 | 15 |
| Soybeans | 145 | 9 | 16 |
| Trail/Party Mix, 1 oz | 150 | 9 | 15 |

## Cough Drops

| | **C** | **F** | **Cb** |
|---|---|---|---|
| *Per Drop/Piece* | | | |
| **Beech Nut,** 1 drop | 10 | 0 | 2 |
| **CVS,** Honey Lemon Cough Drops | 15 | 0 | 4 |
| **Diabetic Tussin** | 0 | 0 | 0 |
| **Halls, Defense Vitamin C:** Regular | 15 | 0 | 4 |
| Sugar Free | 5 | 0 | 3 |
| Fruit Breezers | 15 | 0 | 4 |
| Menthol Drops: Regular | 15 | 0 | 4 |
| Sugar Free | 5 | 0 | 4 |
| Plus | 20 | 0 | 5 |
| **Listerine** (Amer. Chicle), Lozenge | 10 | 0 | 2 |
| **Luden's,** Throat Drops: Reg., all var. | 10 | 0 | 2 |
| Sugar Free | 0 | 0 | 0 |
| **Pine Bros,** Cough Drops | 10 | 0 | 2 |
| **Ricola,** Cough Drops: | | | |
| Natural Herbs | 10 | 0 | 3 |
| Sugar-Free Lemon Mint | 0 | 0 | 1 |
| **Rolaids,** Sodium Free | 5 | 0 | 1 |
| **Sathers,** Peppermint Lozenges | 15 | 0 | 3 |
| **Sucrets** (Beecham), Lozenges | 10 | 0 | 2.5 |
| **Wintergreen,** Lozenges | 15 | 0 | 3 |

*Eat at least 5 servings of fruit and vegetables every day . . . and Enjoy Better Health!*

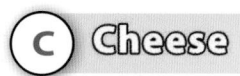

# C — Cheese

## Quick Guide

**C** **F** **Cb**

### Firm/Hard Cheeses
**American, Cheddar, Jack, Swiss:**
**Average All Brands**
**Regular Cheese:**

| | C | F | Cb |
|---|---|---|---|
| Thin Deli slice, 0.8 oz | 80 | 6 | 0.5 |
| 1 oz slice/piece | 110 | 9 | 0.5 |
| 8 oz package | 880 | 72 | 3 |
| **Cubes:** 1" cube, 0.6 oz | 70 | 5.5 | 0.5 |
| 1¼" cube, 1 oz | 115 | 9 | 0.5 |
| **Diced,** 1 cup, 4.5 oz | 510 | 41 | 3 |
| **Melted,** ¼ cup, 2 oz | 245 | 20 | 1 |
| **Shredded:** ¼ cup, 1 oz | 110 | 9 | 0.5 |
| 1 cup, 4 oz | 440 | 36 | 2 |

## Cheese & Cheese Products

*Per 1 oz Unless Indicated*

| | C | F | Cb |
|---|---|---|---|
| **Almond** (Lisanatti), Chunks, average | 50 | 1 | 3 |
| **American:** | | | |
| Regular: 1 slice, 1 oz | 105 | 9 | 0.5 |
| *Kraft,* Regular, 0.67 oz slice | 60 | 4 | 1 |
| *Land O'Lakes,* 0.67 oz slice | 70 | 4 | 2 |
| Reduced Fat: | | | |
| *Alpine Lace,* Yellow/White, 1 oz | 90 | 6 | 2 |
| *Borden* 2%, 1 slice, 0.8 oz | 50 | 3 | 2 |
| *Kraft,* 2% Milk, 0.67 oz | 45 | 2.5 | 1 |
| *Land O Lakes,* | | | |
| 2% Milk, 1 oz | 90 | 6 | 2 |
| **Babybel** (Laughing Cow), Mini: | | | |
| Original (1), 0.75 oz | 70 | 6 | 0 |
| Light (1), 0.75 oz | 50 | 3 | 0 |
| Light Original (1), 0.75 oz | 50 | 3 | 0 |
| Gouda (1), 0.75 oz | 70 | 6 | 0 |
| Mozzarella (1), 0.75 oz | 50 | 3.5 | 0 |
| **Blue/Bleu:** *Average all Brands* | | | |
| Crumbled, ¼ cup, 1 oz | 100 | 8 | 0 |
| Light, 0.8 oz | 35 | 1.5 | 2 |
| **Brie:** Average, 1 oz | 95 | 8 | 0 |
| *Alouette,* 1 oz | 100 | 9 | 1 |
| **Camembert,** 1 oz | 85 | 7 | 0 |
| **Caraway,** 1 oz | 105 | 8 | 1 |
| **Castello,** 1 oz | 120 | 12 | 0 |
| **Cheddar:** | | | |
| Regular: Medium/Sharp, av., 1 oz | 110 | 9 | 1 |
| Shredded, ¼ cup, 1 oz | 110 | 9 | 1 |
| *Cracker Barrel:* Extra Sharp, 1 oz | 110 | 10 | 0 |
| Vermont Sharp White, 1 oz | 110 | 10 | 0 |

## Cheese & Cheese Products (Cont)

*Per 1 oz Unless Indicated*

**C** **F** **Cb**

| | C | F | Cb |
|---|---|---|---|
| **Cheddar (Cont):** | | | |
| Reduced Fat, 2% Milk, | | | |
| *Kraft,* Shredded, 1 oz | 90 | 6 | 1 |
| Curds, Cheddar Cheese, | | | |
| **Cheese Curds** ~ *See Cottage Cheese* | | | |
| **Cheese Logs** (Kaukauna), average | 100 | 7 | 4 |
| **Cheez Whiz** ~ *See Dips* | | | |
| **Cheshire,** 1 oz | 110 | 9 | 1.5 |
| **Colby,** Regular, 1 oz | 110 | 8 | 0 |
| **Colby-Jack:** | | | |
| Big Slice, 0.8 oz | 90 | 7 | 0 |
| **Cottage Cheese (Curds):** *Average All Brands* | | | |
| Creamed (4% milk fat): | | | |
| 2 Tbsp, 1 oz | 30 | 1 | 1.5 |
| ½ cup, 4 oz | 110 | 5 | 4 |
| with fruit, ½ cup, 4 oz | 115 | 4 | 5 |
| Reduced-Fat (2%): 2 Tbsp, 1 oz | 25 | 0.5 | 1 |
| ½ cup, 4 oz | 100 | 3 | 4 |
| Low-Fat (1%): 2 Tbsp, 1 oz | 20 | 0.5 | 1 |
| ½ cup, 4 oz | 80 | 1 | 3 |
| Fat-Free/Non-Fat: 2 T., 1 oz | 20 | 0 | 1 |
| ½ cup, 4 oz | 80 | 0 | 5 |
| **Cottage Cheese (Curds):** *Brands* | | | |
| *Fiber One,* 1% Fat, ½ c., 4 oz | 80 | 2 | 8 |
| *Friendship:* | | | |
| 1% Low-Fat with Pineapple, 5 oz | 150 | 1.5 | 22 |
| Nonfat with Pineapple, ½ cup, 4 oz | 110 | 0 | 18 |
| Pot Style, 2%, ½ cup, 4 oz | 100 | 2.5 | 4 |
| *Hood,* Low Fat, 4 oz | 90 | 1.5 | 5 |
| *Knudsen/Breakstone's:* | | | |
| Free, Non-Fat, ½ cup, 4.25 oz | 80 | 0 | 7 |
| 2% Milk Fat, ½ cup, 4 oz | 90 | 2.5 | 6 |
| On the Go!, | | | |
| Low-Fat, 4 oz carton | 90 | 2.5 | 7 |
| *Lactaid,* 1% Low-Fat, 1½ cup, 4 oz | 80 | 1 | 7 |
| *Light n' Lively:* | | | |
| Fat-Free, ½ cup, 4.4 oz | 80 | 0 | 8 |
| Low-Fat, ½ cup, 4.4 oz | 80 | 1.5 | 6 |
| Breaded & Fried: | | | |
| *A&W,* 5 oz | 570 | 40 | 27 |
| *Culver's,* Wisconsin, 5.3 oz | 510 | 25 | 51 |

## Cheese & Cheese Products (Cont)

*Per 1 oz Unless Indicated*  **C** **F** **Cb**

| | C | F | Cb |
|---|---|---|---|
| **Cream Cheese:** *Average All Brands* | | | |
| Regular/Soft: | | | |
| 2 Tbsp, 1 oz | 95 | 10 | 1 |
| 3 oz package | 290 | 29 | 3.5 |
| 8 oz package | 780 | 78 | 9 |
| Light, Plain, 1 oz | 60 | 4.5 | 2.5 |
| Fat-Free, Plain, 1 oz | 30 | 0 | 2 |
| *Better Than Cream Cheese (Tofutti),* | | | |
| all varieties, 1 oz | 85 | 5 | 9 |
| *Easy Cheese* (Kraft), | | | |
| American, 2 Tbsp, 1.2 oz | 80 | 6 | 1 |
| **Edam,** 1 oz | 100 | 8 | 0.5 |
| **Farmer,** Low-Fat, 1 oz | 40 | 2.5 | 0 |
| **Feta:** Regular, 1 oz | 75 | 6 | 1 |
| Crumbled, ½ cup, 2.5 oz | 190 | 15 | 3 |
| *Athenos,* Reduced-Fat, | | | |
| 1 oz | 50 | 3 | 1 |
| **Fontina,** 2 Tbsp, 1 oz | 110 | 9 | 0.5 |
| *Galaxy,* Cheese Substitute: | | | |
| Grated Parmesan Flavor, 2 tsp, 0.2 oz | 15 | 0.5 | 0 |
| Slices: Mozzarella, 1 slice, 0.6 oz | 40 | 3 | 0.5 |
| Cheddar, 1 slice, 0.67 oz | 35 | 2 | 5 |
| **Goat's Milk Cheese:** | | | |
| Chevre: Original, 2 Tbsp | 75 | 6 | 0.5 |
| Semi-Soft, 1 oz | 100 | 8.5 | 1 |
| Hard, 1 oz | 130 | 10 | 0.5 |
| *Chavrie,* Logs: | | | |
| Original, 2 Tbsp, 1 oz | 80 | 7 | 1 |
| Sundried Tomato & Garlic, 1 oz | 80 | 6 | 2 |
| Pyramid, Original, 1 oz | 50 | 3.5 | 1 |
| Gjetost, fresh, 1 oz | 130 | 8 | 12 |
| Myzithra, grated, 1 oz | 80 | 4 | 2 |
| Gorgonzola, 1 oz | 100 | 8 | 0.5 |
| *Galbani,* Dolcelatte, 1 oz | 95 | 8 | 1 |
| **Gouda,** 1 oz slice | 100 | 8 | 0.5 |
| **Gruyere,** 1 oz | 115 | 9 | 1 |
| **Handi-Snacks** (Kraft): | | | |
| Breadsticks 'n Cheez Single, 1 oz | 110 | 4.5 | 14 |
| Ritz Crackers 'n Cheez Dip, 1 oz | 100 | 6 | 11 |
| **Havarti** (Land O'Lakes), 0.7 oz | 80 | 6 | 1 |
| **Jarlsberg:** Average, 1 oz | 100 | 8 | 0 |
| Reduced Fat, shredded, 1 oz | 70 | 3.5 | 0 |
| **Labneh,** (Lebanese Cream Chse), 1.8 oz | 70 | 4 | 4 |

## Cheese & Cheese Products (Cont)

*Per 1 oz Unless Indicated*  **C** **F** **Cb**

| | C | F | Cb |
|---|---|---|---|
| *Laughing Cow,* Wedges: | | | |
| Creamy Asiago (1) | 35 | 1.5 | 1 |
| Swiss: Original Creamy (1) | 50 | 4 | 1 |
| Light Swiss (1) | 35 | 1.5 | 1 |
| *Lifetime,* Cholesterol Reducing, | | | |
| Low Fat, all varieties, 1 Slice, 1 oz | 45 | 1.5 | 1 |
| **Limburger,** 1 oz | 95 | 8 | 0 |
| **Mascarpone,** av., 1 oz | 125 | 13 | 0.5 |
| **Mexican:** | | | |
| *Cacique:* Asadero, sliced | 70 | 5 | 1 |
| Cotija | 100 | 8 | 0 |
| Enchilado; Manchego | 90 | 7 | 0 |
| Panela | 80 | 7 | 0 |
| Queso Fresco | 80 | 6 | 0 |
| Queso Quesadilla | 90 | 7 | 0 |
| Ranchero | 80 | 6 | 0 |
| *Chi-Chi's,* Salsa Con Quéso, Mild | 45 | 3 | 4 |
| *El Mexicano:* Asadero, Regular | 90 | 7 | 0 |
| Cotija, grated, 2 Tbsp | 40 | 3 | 0 |
| *Kraft,* Mexican Four Cheese; Taco, | | | |
| Shredded, | 100 | 8 | 0 |
| *Sargento,* 4 Cheese Mexican | 110 | 9 | 2 |
| *Supremo,* Quéso Chihuahua, 1 oz | 100 | 8 | 0 |
| *Verole,* Quéso Oaxaca, 1 oz | 70 | 8 | 0 |
| **Monterey Jack:** | | | |
| Regular, shredded, 1 oz | 100 | 8 | 1 |
| *Land O Lakes,* Co-Jack, 1 oz | 110 | 9 | 1 |
| *Kraft,* 1" cube, 1 oz | 100 | 9 | 0 |
| **Mozzarella:** | | | |
| Whole Milk: Average 1 oz | 85 | 6.5 | 0.5 |
| *Land O'Lakes/Polly-O:* | | | |
| Slice, average, 1 oz | 80 | 6 | 1 |
| String, 1 oz | 90 | 6 | 1 |
| Fat-Free, | | | |
| *Kraft,* Shredded, 1 oz | 45 | 0 | 2 |
| Reduced Fat, | | | |
| *Kraft,* 2% Milk Fat | 70 | 5 | 1 |
| Part Skim: | | | |
| *Borden/Kraft,* Shredded | 80 | 5 | 2 |
| *Kraft,* String | 80 | 6 | 0 |
| *Polly-O,* Shredded, 1 oz | 80 | 5 | 0 |
| **Muenster:** | | | |
| Regular, 1 oz | 105 | 9 | 0.5 |
| Low-Fat, 1 oz | 85 | 5 | 1 |

## Cheese & Cheese Products (Cont)

| Per 1 oz Unless Indicated | C | F | Cb |
|---|---|---|---|
| **Parmesan:** | | | |
| Fresh/Block, Dry, 1 oz | 110 | 7.5 | 1 |
| Grated (Packaged): 2 tsp | 20 | 1.5 | 0 |
| 1 oz | 120 | 8 | 1 |
| ½ cup, 1.8 oz | 215 | 14 | 2 |
| *Kraft,* Reduced-Fat Topping, 1 Tbsp | 20 | 1 | 2 |
| ***Philadelphia:*** | | | |
| **Cream Cheese:** Original, 2 T. 1 oz | 80 | 7 | 2 |
| 3 oz package | 240 | 21 | 6 |
| **Flavored:** | | | |
| Blueberry, 1.16 oz | 80 | 4.5 | 7 |
| Chive & Onion, 1.1 oz | 80 | 7 | 2 |
| Pinapple, 1 oz | 70 | 4.5 | 5 |
| Salmon, 1.1 oz | 70 | 5 | 2 |
| Strawberry, 1.1 oz | 80 | 6 | 5 |
| **⅓ Less Fat:** Plain, 2 T., 1 oz | 70 | 5 | 3 |
| Neufchatel, 2 T., 1 oz | 70 | 6 | 1 |
| **Fat-Free,** Plain, 1 oz | 30 | 0 | 3 |
| **Cheesecake Filling,** 3 oz | 240 | 17 | 6 |
| **Milk/White Chocolate:** | | | |
| 2 Tbsp, 1.27 oz | 110 | 6 | 12 |
| **Dark Chocolate,** 2 T., 1.23 oz | 100 | 5 | 12 |
| **Whipped:** | | | |
| Original, 0.8 oz | 50 | 4.5 | 2 |
| Mixed Berry, 0.7 oz | 50 | 3.5 | 5 |
| **Pizza Four Cheese,** shredded, | | | |
| *Kraft/Sargento,* Regular, av., 1 oz | 90 | 7 | 1 |
| **Port de Salut,** 1 oz | 100 | 8 | 0 |
| **Port Wine** *(Kaukauna/WisPride):* | | | |
| 10 oz Ball, 1 oz | 100 | 6 | 4 |
| 10 oz Log, 2 Tbsp, 1 oz | 100 | 7 | 4 |
| 11.3 oz Tub, 0.85 oz | 80 | 6 | 3 |
| **Provolone:** Regular, 1 oz | 100 | 7.5 | 0.5 |
| *Alpine Lace,* Reduced-Fat, 1 oz | 80 | 6 | 1 |
| *Sargento,* 1 slice, 0.67 oz | 70 | 5 | 0 |
| **Pub** *(President),* average all varieties | 75 | 7 | 1 |
| **Quark:** 40% fat | 45 | 3 | 2 |
| 20% fat | 30 | 1.5 | 1 |
| Skim/Non-Fat | 20 | 0 | 1.5 |
| **Rice Cheese Chunks** *(Lisanatti),* | | | |
| average, 1 oz | 60 | 3 | 2 |

## Cheese & Cheese Products (Cont)

| Per 1 oz Unless Indicated | C | F | Cb |
|---|---|---|---|
| **Ricotta Cheese:** | | | |
| Whole Milk: 1 oz | 50 | 3.5 | 1 |
| ½ cup, 4.5 oz | 215 | 16 | 4 |
| Part Skim: 1 oz | 40 | 2 | 1.5 |
| ½ cup, 4.5 oz | 170 | 10 | 6 |
| Light/Low-Fat: 1 oz | 25 | 1 | 1.5 |
| ½ cup, 4.5 oz | 125 | 5 | 6 |
| Fat-Free, ½ cup, 4.5 oz | 100 | 0 | 10 |
| Baked Ricotta, 2 oz | 130 | 9 | 3 |
| **Romano:** Block/Loaf | 110 | 8 | 1 |
| Grated: 1 oz | 120 | 9 | 1 |
| 1 Tbsp, 0.2 oz | 20 | 1.5 | 0 |
| **Roquefort,** 1 oz | 105 | 9 | 0.5 |
| **Sheep's Milk,** (Manchego), | | | |
| *Trader Joes/Wegman's,* 1 oz | 120 | 10 | 0 |
| **Soy Cheese:** | | | |
| *Trader Joe's,* Cheddar flavor, 0.7 oz | 45 | 2 | 3 |
| *Soy Kaas:* Cheddar, 1 oz | 50 | 2 | 8 |
| Monterey Jack, 1 oz | 60 | 4 | 0 |
| *Soy Sation,* Chunks, | | | |
| all varieties, 1 oz | 60 | 3 | 2 |
| **Smoked Cheddar,** average, 1 oz | 110 | 10 | 0 |
| **Stilton,** average, 1 oz | 110 | 10 | 0 |
| **String:** | | | |
| Regular, average all brands | 80 | 6 | 0.5 |
| *Kraft,* Twist-Ums & String-ums, | | | |
| Super Long, 1 stick, 1.1 oz | 90 | 6 | 1 |
| Light/Lite: | | | |
| *Frigo,* String (1), 0.85 oz | 50 | 2.5 | 0.5 |
| *Polly-O,* String, | | | |
| 2% Red-Fat, 1 oz | 70 | 4.5 | 0 |
| *Sargento:* 1 piece, 1 oz | 80 | 6 | 1 |
| Light, , 0.75 oz | 50 | 2.5 | 1 |
| **Swiss:** Regular, 1 oz | 110 | 8 | 1.5 |
| *Alpine Lace,* Reduced-Fat, 1 oz | 90 | 6 | 1 |
| *Kraft Singles,* 2% Milk, 0.75 oz | 60 | 4.5 | 1 |
| **Tilsit,** 1 oz | 100 | 7.5 | 0.5 |
| ***Tofutti,*** Better Than Cream Cheese, | | | |
| all flavors, 2 Tbsp | 60 | 5 | 2 |
| **Tybo,** 1 oz | 100 | 7 | 0.5 |
| ***Velveeta*** *(Kraft):* | | | |
| Original, 1 oz | 80 | 5 | 3 |
| Reduced Fat, 2% Milk, 1 oz | 60 | 3 | 4 |
| Mexican, 1 oz | 60 | 4 | 3 |
| Queso Blanco, Mild, 1 oz | 70 | 4 | 3 |

## Dips/Spreads  **C** **F** **Cb**

*Per 2 Tbsp, 1 oz, Unless Indicated*

### Average All Brands

| | C | F | Cb |
|---|---|---|---|
| Avocado/Guacamole | 45 | 4 | 2 |
| Baba Ghanoush (Eggplant/Sesame) | 70 | 6 | 2 |
| Cheese Fondue, ½ cup, 4 oz | 260 | 15 | 4 |
| French Onion Dip | 60 | 4.5 | 3 |
| Hummus: 2 Tbsp | 50 | 1 | 5 |
| ½ cup, 4.5 oz | 220 | 4.5 | 23 |
| Tzatziki (Cucumber/Yogurt) | 30 | 2.5 | 2 |
| **Clearman's,** Original Spread | 150 | 16 | 0 |
| **De La Casa,** 5 Layer Party Dip | 45 | 2.5 | 4 |
| **Fritolay,** French Onion Dip, 2 Tbsp | 60 | 5 | 3 |

**Fritos:** *Per 2 Tbsp*

**Dips:**

| | C | F | Cb |
|---|---|---|---|
| Bean; Hot Bean w/ Jalapeno | 35 | 1 | 5 |
| Jalapeno Cheddar Cheese | 40 | 2.5 | 3 |
| Mild Cheddar | 40 | 3 | 3 |
| **Guiltless Gourmet,** | | | |
| Black Bean/Spicy Black Bean Dip | 40 | 0 | 7 |
| **Heluva Good Cheese,** | | | |
| French Onion Dip, 2 Tbsp | 50 | 4.5 | 2 |
| **Kaukauna** *(Wisconsin):* | | | |
| Spreadable Cheddar, | | | |
| Sharp/Smokey Cheddar | 80 | 6 | 3 |

**Kemps:** *Per 2 Tbsp*

| | C | F | Cb |
|---|---|---|---|
| **Dips:** French Onion | 60 | 5 | 2 |
| Ranch Style | 60 | 5 | 2 |
| Top The Tater, | | | |
| Taco Fiesta; Veggie Ranch, av. | 60 | 5 | 3 |
| **Kroger,** Dips, all varieties | 60 | 5 | 2 |

**Kraft:** *Per 2 Tbsp*

| | C | F | Cb |
|---|---|---|---|
| **Dips:** Average all varieties | 60 | 5 | 3 |
| Cheez Whiz: Orig., 1.2 oz | 90 | 7 | 4 |
| Light | 80 | 3.5 | 6 |

*Salsa Con Queso ~ See Velveeeta*

| | C | F | Cb |
|---|---|---|---|
| **Spreads:** Olive & Pimento, 1.1 oz | 80 | 6 | 3 |
| Old English Sharp; Roka Blue, av | 88 | 7 | 3 |

**Marzetti:** *Per 2 Tbsp*

| | C | F | Cb |
|---|---|---|---|
| **Dips:** Chocolate Fruit, 2 Tbsp | 110 | 1 | 25 |
| Old Fashioned Caramel, 1.25 oz | 130 | 4 | 22 |
| Veggie: Dill, Light, 1.1 oz | 60 | 5 | 4 |
| Ranch, 1 oz | 110 | 12 | 2 |
| Light Ranch, 1.1 oz | 60 | 5 | 4 |

## Dips/Spreads (Cont)  **C** **F** **Cb**

*Per 2 Tbsp, 1 oz, Unless Indicated*

**Marie's:**

| | C | F | Cb |
|---|---|---|---|
| **Dips:** Buttermilk Ranch; Crmy Dill. av. | 100 | 10 | 2 |
| Guacamole | 40 | 3 | 3 |

**Naturally Fresh:** *Per 2 Tbsp*

| | C | F | Cb |
|---|---|---|---|
| **Dips:** Chocolate, 1.3 oz | 90 | 0 | 23 |
| Crm Cheese Strawb., 1 oz | 90 | 3 | 15 |
| Caramel, 1 oz | 100 | 4 | 16 |

**Old Dutch:**

| | C | F | Cb |
|---|---|---|---|
| **Dips:** French Onion, 1 oz | 50 | 5 | 5 |
| Mild Cheddar, 1 oz | 40 | 3 | 2 |
| Nacho Cheese, 1 oz | 35 | 2.5 | 2 |

**Old El Paso:** *Per 2 Tbsp*

| | C | F | Cb |
|---|---|---|---|
| **Dips:** Cheese & Salsa, 1.2 oz | 40 | 3 | 3 |
| Thick N' Chunky Salsa | 10 | 0 | 2 |

**Price's:** *Per 2 Tbsp*

| | C | F | Cb |
|---|---|---|---|
| **Dips:** Pimiento Cheese | 90 | 7 | 4 |
| Light Pimiento | 50 | 3 | 3 |

**Stop & Shop:** *Per 2 Tbsp*

| | C | F | Cb |
|---|---|---|---|
| **Dips:** Veggie | 100 | 10 | 3 |
| Sour Cream French Onion | 60 | 4.5 | 2 |

**TGI Fridays,**

| | C | F | Cb |
|---|---|---|---|
| Spinach, Cheese & Artichoke Dip, 1 oz | 30 | 2 | 2 |
| **Toby's,** Original Tofu Spread, 2 Tbsp | 80 | 8 | 2 |

**Tostitos:**

| | C | F | Cb |
|---|---|---|---|
| **Dips:** Chunky Salsa, 2 Tbsp | 10 | 0 | 2 |
| Creamy Spinach, 2 Tbsp | 50 | 4 | 2 |
| Salsa Con Queso, 2 Tbsp | 40 | 2.5 | 5 |

**Wise:** *Per 2 Tbsp*

| | C | F | Cb |
|---|---|---|---|
| **Dips:** French Onion | 60 | 5 | 3 |
| Salsa con Queso | 45 | 3 | 3 |

***New Diet Aid
- The Refrigerator Air Bag!***

**POOF!**

| Condiments, Sauces | C | F | Cb |
|---|---|---|---|

*Average of Brands & Homemade*

**Apple Sauce:**
| | | | |
|---|---|---|---|
| Sweetened, ¼ cup, 2.5 oz | 55 | 0 | 13 |
| Unsweetened, ¼ cup, 2 oz | 25 | 0 | 7 |

**Barbecue Sauce:**
| | | | |
|---|---|---|---|
| Regular, av. all flavors, 2 Tbsp, 1 oz | 40 | 0 | 10 |
| *Bull's Eye*, Original, 1 oz | 60 | 0 | 14 |
| **Bearnaise Sauce,** ¼ cup, 2.5 oz | 190 | 19 | 5 |
| **Buffalo Wing Sce:** Hon. Mustard, 1 T. | 40 | 3 | 3 |
| Average other varieties, 1 Tbsp | 25 | 2 | 2 |
| **Cheese,** h/made, ¼ cup, 2.5 oz | 150 | 10 | 12 |
| **Chef-Mate,** Hot Dog, ¼ cup | 70 | 2.5 | 9 |
| **Chili Sauce** *(Heinz)*, 1 Tbsp | 20 | 0 | 5 |
| **Cocktail Sauce:** ¼ cup | 110 | 0 | 15 |
| *Walden Farms*, Fat-Free, 1 Tbsp | 0 | 0 | 0 |
| **Cranberry Sauce,** av. all varieties: 2 T. | 45 | 0 | 11 |
| ¼ cup, 2.5 oz | 110 | 0 | 27 |
| **Demi Glaze Gold,** 2 tsp | 30 | 0.5 | 3 |
| **Honey Mustard** *(French's)*, 2 Tbsp | 60 | 0.5 | 12 |
| **Horseradish:** 1 tsp | 2 | 0 | 0 |
| *Kraft*, 1 tsp | 15 | 1.5 | 1 |
| **Ketchup:** Regular, 1 Tbsp | 15 | 0 | 4 |
| *Heinz:* Reduced Sugar, 1 Tbsp | 5 | 0 | 1 |
| Simply Heinz, 1 Tbsp | 15 | 0 | 4 |

**Mole:**
| | | | |
|---|---|---|---|
| *Dona Maria*, av. all varieties. 2 T. | 150 | 10 | 10 |
| *Rogelio Bueno*, 2 Tbsp, 1 oz | 160 | 11 | 12 |
| **Mushroom Sce,** ½ cup, 2 oz | 50 | 2 | 5 |
| **Mustard,** average, 1 tsp | 5 | 0 | 0.5 |
| **Pesto Sauce,** ¼ cup, 2 oz | 270 | 28 | 2 |
| **Pizza Sauce,** ¼ cup, 2 oz | 30 | 0 | 6 |
| **Seafood Cocktail Sce,** ¼ cup | 60 | 0 | 15 |
| **Soy Sauce:** Average all, 1 Tbsp | 10 | 0 | 1 |
| *Kikkoman*, Lite Soy, 1 Tbsp | 10 | 0 | 1 |
| **Spaghetti Sce,** ½ cup, 4.5 oz | 135 | 6 | 19 |

**Steak Sauce:**
| | | | |
|---|---|---|---|
| *Kraft*, A1, 1 Tbsp, 0.5 oz | 15 | 0 | 3 |
| *Lea & Perrins*, 1 Tbsp, 0.5 oz | 20 | 0 | 5 |
| **Strawb. Puree Sauce,** Unsweet., 2 T. | 10 | 0 | 2 |

**Sweet & Sour Sauce:**
| | | | |
|---|---|---|---|
| *Contadina*, 1.2 oz | 40 | 1 | 8 |
| *Kraft*, 1 Tbsp | 60 | 0 | 13 |
| **Tabasco Sauce,** 1 tsp | 2 | 0 | 0 |
| **Taco Sauce,** average all, 2 Tbsp, 1 oz | 10 | 0 | 1 |
| **Tartar Sauce:** *(Heinz)*, 2 Tbsp, 1 oz | 120 | 11 | 4 |
| *Hellmann's*, Regular, 2 Tbsp, 1 oz | 80 | 7 | 4 |
| *McCormick*, Fat-Free, 2 Tbsp, 1 oz | 30 | 0 | 7 |
| **Teriyaki Sauce** *(Kikkoman)*, 1 T., 0.5 oz | 15 | 0 | 2 |
| **Vinegar,** White or Wine, 2 T. | 4 | 0 | 1 |
| **White Sauce,** ½ cup, 5 oz | 130 | 7 | 10 |
| **Worcestershire Sauce,** 1 tsp | 5 | 0 | 1 |

| Pickles & Relish | C | F | Cb |
|---|---|---|---|

*Average All Brands*

| | | | |
|---|---|---|---|
| **Bread & Butter Pickles,** 4 sl.,1 oz | 25 | 0 | 6 |
| **Chutney,** 2 Tbsp, 1.25 oz | 50 | 0.5 | 11 |

**Dill Pickles:**
| | | | |
|---|---|---|---|
| Slices, 4 slices, 1 oz | 4 | 0 | 1 |
| 1 large, (3¾"x 1¼" diam.), 2.25 oz | 12 | 0 | 3 |
| Extra large (4"x 1¾" diam.), 5 oz | 30 | 0 | 6 |
| Halves: Small, 1 oz | 3 | 0 | 0.5 |
| Large, 2.5 oz | 8 | 0 | 2 |
| **Gherkins,** sweet, 1 medium, 1 oz | 30 | 0 | 7 |
| **Green Chiles,** chopped, 2 Tbsp | 5 | 0 | 1 |
| **Horseradish,** 1 Tbsp | 10 | 0 | 2 |
| **Jalapenos,** pickled (2), 2 oz | 10 | 0.5 | 2 |
| **Jalapeno Relish,** 1 Tbsp, 0.5 oz | 5 | 0 | 1 |
| **Mustard,** av. all brands, 1 tsp | 5 | 0 | 0.5 |
| **Peppers,** Hot/Mild (1), 1.5 oz | 20 | 0 | 4 |
| **Pickled:** Beets, ½ cup, 4 oz | 75 | 0 | 19 |
| Cocktail Onion, 1 onion | 2 | 0 | 0 |
| Red Cabbage, ½ cup, 3 oz | 65 | 0 | 15 |
| **Pickles:** Sweet, 2 Tbsp, 1 oz | 35 | 0 | 8 |
| Large (3" x ¾ diam.),1.25 oz | 40 | 0 | 10 |
| Pickle in a Pouch, 1 large | 12 | 0 | 3 |

**Relishes:**
| | | | |
|---|---|---|---|
| Cranberry-Orange, 1 Tbsp | 30 | 0 | 7 |
| Hot Dog *(Heinz)*, 1 T., 0.5 oz | 17 | 0 | 3 |
| S'wich Spread, 1 tsp | 20 | 1 | 5 |
| Sweet Pickle, 1 Tbsp, 0.5 oz | 20 | 0 | 5 |
| Sweet Cauliflower, 1 oz | 35 | 0 | 8 |
| Sugar Free Relish, 1 tsp | 5 | 0 | 1 |
| Sweet Gherkins (2), 1 oz | 5 | 0 | 1 |

**Sauerkraut,**
| | | | |
|---|---|---|---|
| Drained, 1 cup, 5 oz | 25 | 0 | 6 |

| Salsa | | | |
|---|---|---|---|

*Average all Types:*

| | | | |
|---|---|---|---|
| Regular, w/out oil, 2 T., 1 oz | 15 | 0 | 3.5 |
| Made with oil, 2 Tbsp, 1 oz | 40 | 3 | 8 |
| **La Victoria,** 2 Tbsp, 1 oz | 10 | 0 | 2 |
| **Old El Paso,** 1 Tbsp, 1 oz | 10 | 0 | 3 |
| **TGI Friday's,** 1.2 oz | 15 | 0 | 4 |

## Quick Guide
**C F Cb**

### Cookies:
**Average All Brands:** *Per Cookie*

| | C | F | Cb |
|---|---|---|---|
| **Biscotti:** Small, 0.5 oz | 70 | 3 | 10 |
| Regular, 1 oz | 140 | 6.5 | 18 |
| **Chocolate Chip:** | | | |
| Small/Thin, 0.5 oz | 70 | 3.5 | 9 |
| Regular, 1 oz | 140 | 7 | 18 |
| Large (*Mrs Fields*), 3 oz | 350 | 17 | 45 |
| Extra Large, 4 oz | 555 | 28 | 73 |
| **Oatmeal/Oatmeal Raisin:** | | | |
| Small/Thin, 0.5 oz | 65 | 2.5 | 10 |
| Regular, 1 oz | 130 | 5 | 20 |
| Large (*Mrs Fields*), 2.5 oz | 330 | 14 | 44 |
| Extra Large, 4 oz | 510 | 20 | 78 |
| **Peanut Butter:** | | | |
| Small/Thin, 0.5 oz | 70 | 3.5 | 9 |
| Regular, 1 oz | 135 | 7 | 17 |
| Large (*Mrs Fields*), 2.5 oz | 330 | 17 | 41 |
| Extra Large, 4 oz | 540 | 27 | 67 |
| **Low-Fat Cookies:** | | | |
| Choc Chip (Low-Fat), (1), 0.5 oz | 65 | 2 | 10 |
| Oatmeal Raisin (Fat-Free), (1), 1 oz | 95 | 0.5 | 22 |
| Peanut Butter (Low-Fat), (1), 1 oz | 105 | 5 | 15 |

## Quick Guide

### Crackers
**Average All Brands:** *Per Cracker Unless Indicated*

| | C | F | Cb |
|---|---|---|---|
| **Cheese Crackers:** | | | |
| Plain: 1" square | 5 | 0 | 0.5 |
| Bag, single serving, 1 oz | 140 | 7 | 16 |
| Cheese/P'nut Butter filled | 30 | 1.5 | 4 |
| **Crispbread,** Rye | 35 | 0 | 8 |
| **Grahams,** 2½" square | 30 | 0.5 | 5 |
| **Melba Toast,** Plain, 1 piece | 20 | 0 | 4 |
| **Matzo,** Plain, 1 oz | 110 | 0.5 | 23 |
| **Oyster/Soup,** ½ cup | 95 | 2 | 17 |
| **Rice:** 1 crackers | 70 | 1.5 | 11 |
| Oriental Style, 1 oz | 130 | 3.5 | 23 |
| **Saltines,** 5 crackers | 65 | 2 | 11 |
| **Snack-type,** 1 round cracker | 15 | 1 | 2 |
| **Soda Crackers** (*Saltine*), 2 | 25 | 1 | 4.5 |
| **Water Cracker** (*Carr's*), Original | 15 | 0.5 | 2.5 |
| **Wheat:** | | | |
| Wheat Thins | 10 | 0.5 | 1.5 |
| Cheese/Peanut Butter filled | 35 | 2 | 4 |

### Cookies & Crackers ~ Brands

*Per Cookie/Cracker, Unless indicated* **C F Cb**

| | C | F | Cb |
|---|---|---|---|
| **Albertsons:** | | | |
| Animal Crackers (6), 1 oz | 130 | 3.5 | 22 |
| **Chocolate Chip:** | | | |
| Original (3), 1 oz | 150 | 7 | 20 |
| Chewy (2), 1 oz | 130 | 6 | 18 |
| Chunky (1), 0.5 oz | 80 | 3.5 | 10 |
| **Chocolate S'wich Cremes:** (3) 1 oz | 150 | 6 | 25 |
| Double Filled (2), 1 oz | 140 | 6 | 22 |
| Fudge Graham (3), 1 oz | 140 | 7 | 18 |
| Fudge Wafer (3), 1 oz | 140 | 8 | 18 |
| Fudge Marshmallow Ring | 120 | 5 | 19 |
| Pinwheels, Chocolate Marshmallow | 120 | 5 | 20 |
| Vanilla Wafers (9), 1 oz | 140 | 4 | 25 |
| **Graham:** Cinnamon (2) | 150 | 3 | 28 |
| Honey (2), 1 oz | 140 | 2 | 28 |
| **Annie's:** | | | |
| **Bunny Grahams:** | | | |
| Honey, 1 oz | 130 | 4 | 20 |
| Other varieties, 1 oz | 130 | 4.5 | 22 |
| Gluten Free: Cocoa & Vanilla, 1 oz | 120 | 3.5 | 22 |
| SnickerDoodle, Cinn. Sugar, 1 oz | 140 | 4.5 | 22 |
| **Crackers:** | | | |
| **Cheddar Bunnies:** | | | |
| Regular, 1 oz Snack Pack | 140 | 6 | 19 |
| Extra Cheesy, 1 oz | 150 | 7 | 18 |
| White Cheddar; Whole Wheat, 1 oz | 145 | 7 | 19 |
| **Arnott's:** | | | |
| **Tim Tams:** Original; Chewy C'rml (2) | 190 | 9 | 26 |
| Classic Dark; Dark Mint (2) | 190 | 10 | 25 |
| **Austin:** | | | |
| **Sandwich Crackers:** *Per Package* | | | |
| Cheese: with Cheddar Cheese | 190 | 10 | 23 |
| with Peanut Butter | 190 | 10 | 23 |
| with PB & Jelly | 190 | 9 | 25 |
| Toasty | | | |
| **Barbara's Bakery:** | | | |
| **Snackimals:** | | | |
| Choc Chip; Vanilla, 1 oz | 140 | 4.5 | 23 |
| Oatmeal, 1 oz | 130 | 4 | 20 |

## Cookies & Crackers ~ Brands (Cont)

*Per Cookie/Cracker, Unless Indicated* **C** **F** **Cb**

**BelVita** *(Nabisco)*:

**Breakfast Biscuits:**

| | C | F | Cb |
|---|---|---|---|
| Crunchy, 1 pack (4 biscuits), average | 230 | 8 | 36 |
| Soft Baked, 1 biscuit, average | 190 | 7 | 32 |
| **Bites,** (46), av., 1.8 oz | 230 | 8 | 37 |

**Blue Diamond:**

| | | | |
|---|---|---|---|
| **Nut Thins:** Almond,(19),1 oz | 130 | 2 | 24 |
| Cheddar Cheese, 2 oz bag | 250 | 7 | 41 |
| Country Ranch (17); Pecan (16), 1 oz | 130 | 3.5 | 23 |

**Brent & Sam's:**

**Natural:** *Per 2 Cookies*

| | | | |
|---|---|---|---|
| Key Lime White Choc. | 120 | 6 | 16 |
| White Choc. Macadamia | 130 | 7 | 14 |

**Soft Baked:** *Per 1 Cookie*

| | | | |
|---|---|---|---|
| Choc. Chunk; Snickerdoodle | 130 | 4.5 | 20 |
| Oatmeal Raisin | 140 | 6 | 20 |

**Carr's:**

| | | | |
|---|---|---|---|
| **Crackers:** Orig.; Cracked Pepper (4) | 60 | 1 | 10 |
| Roasted Garlic & Herbs (4) | 50 | 1 | 10 |
| Rosemary (4) | 70 | 2.5 | 11 |
| Toasted Sesame (4) | 60 | 1.5 | 10 |

**Cheez•It** ~ *See Sunshine, Page 87*

**Chips Ahoy!** ~ *See Nabisco, Page 85*

**Country Choice:**

**Sandwich Cremes,**

| | | | |
|---|---|---|---|
| all varieties, 2 pieces | 130 | 5 | 19 |

**Snacking:**

| | | | |
|---|---|---|---|
| Ginger Snaps (5); Vanilla Wafers (7) | 140 | 5 | 22 |
| Iced Oatmeal (4) | 120 | 4 | 21 |

**Dr. Kracker:**

| | | | |
|---|---|---|---|
| **Crispbread:** Klassic 3 Seed (1) | 100 | 4 | 15 |
| Pumpkin Seed Cheddar (1) | 100 | 4.5 | 13 |
| **Snackers,** Pumpkin Seed Cheddar (8) | 125 | 5 | 13 |

**Ener-G Cookies** (Gluten Free):

| | | | |
|---|---|---|---|
| Cinnamon (1) | 80 | 4.5 | 11 |
| Ginger (1), ½ oz | 50 | 1.5 | 10 |
| Sunflowr (1), 1.2 oz | 120 | 10 | 13 |

**Erin Baker's:**

**Original Breakfast:** *Per 3 oz*

| | | | |
|---|---|---|---|
| Banana Walnut | 310 | 8 | 55 |
| Peanut Butter | 330 | 11 | 50 |

**Minis:** *Per 1 oz Cookie*

| | | | |
|---|---|---|---|
| Peanut Butter | 100 | 3.5 | 16 |
| Dble Chocolate; Oatmeal Raisin, av. | 100 | 2.5 | 18 |

**Famous Amos:**

**Bite Size:** Choc. Chip,

| | | | |
|---|---|---|---|
| 4 Cookies, 1 oz | 140 | 7 | 20 |
| Choc. Chip & Pecans (4) | 150 | 8 | 18 |

*Per Cookie/Cracker, Unless Indicated* **C** **F** **Cb**

**Fig Newtons** ~ *See Nabisco, Page 85*

**Fifty50:**

| | | | |
|---|---|---|---|
| **Chocolate Chip (4)** | 170 | 9 | 22 |
| **Hearty Oatmeal (4)** | 160 | 7 | 24 |
| **Wafers,** average all varieties, (4) | 150 | 9 | 17 |

**Gamesa:**

| | | | |
|---|---|---|---|
| **Animalitos,** 14 cookies, 1 oz | 110 | 1 | 25 |
| **Arcoiris Marshmallow,** | | | |
| 2 oz pkg, 6 cookies | 220 | 5 | 38 |
| **Chocolatines Marshmallow,** | | | |
| 2 cookies, 1 oz | 130 | 5 | 18 |
| **Chokis,** Chocolate Chip, 1.4 oz pkg | 190 | 9 | 27 |
| **Emperador:** Cream Cookie Sandwich | | | |
| Lemon Creme, 1 pkg, 6 cookies | 270 | 8 | 45 |
| Av. other flavors, 1 pkg, 6 cookies | 360 | 12 | 57 |
| **Fruitbars,** average, 1 cookie, 1 oz | 110 | 4.5 | 18 |
| **Giro,** 3 cookies, 1 oz | 140 | 6 | 20 |
| **Mamut,** Choc Marshmallow, | | | |
| 1 cookie, 1 oz | 130 | 5 | 19 |
| **Marias,** 8 cookies, 1 oz | 120 | 2 | 24 |
| **Sugar Wafers,** (3), average, 1.2 oz | 160 | 7 | 25 |

**Girl Scouts Cookies:**

| | | | |
|---|---|---|---|
| **Caramel DeLites/Samoas,** (2), av. | 145 | 8 | 18 |
| **Girl Scout S'Mores (2)** | 180 | 9 | 25 |
| **Peanut Butter S'wich,** (3) | 170 | 9 | 19 |
| **Shortbread (4)** | 120 | 4.5 | 19 |
| **Thin Mints (4)** | 160 | 7 | 22 |

**Goldfish Crackers** ~ *See Pepperidge Farm, Page 86*

**Goya:**

| | | | |
|---|---|---|---|
| **Lady Fingers ,** 1 oz | 130 | 1 | 25 |
| **Maria,** 5 cookies, 1 oz | 130 | 3 | 24 |
| **Wafers,** average all flavors, | | | |
| 4 wafers, 1 oz | 150 | 7 | 20 |

**Grandma's:**

**Homestyle:** *Per Cookie*

| | | | |
|---|---|---|---|
| Chocolate Brownie | 190 | 8 | 27 |
| Chocolate Chip | 200 | 10 | 25 |
| Minis, 1 pkg | 210 | 8 | 31 |
| Oatmeal Raisin | 180 | 7 | 26 |
| Peanut Butter | 190 | 10 | 22 |

**Sandwich Cremes:**

| | | | |
|---|---|---|---|
| Peanut Butter (5) | 200 | 9 | 25 |
| Vanilla (5) | 190 | 9 | 27 |
| Minis, 1 pkg | 240 | 1 | 34 |

## Cookies & Crackers ~ Brands (Cont)

*Per Cookie/Cracker, Unless Indicated* **C** **F** **Cb**

**Great American Cookies:**

| | C | F | Cb |
|---|---|---|---|
| Chewy Choc. Supreme | 200 | 9 | 29 |
| Chewy Pecan Supreme | 230 | 12 | 31 |
| Double Fudge with Reese's | 230 | 11 | 33 |
| Original, w/ Reese's or M&M's | 240 | 12 | 31 |
| Peanut Butter w/ M&M's | 250 | 14 | 29 |
| White Chunk Macadamia | 250 | 14 | 30 |

**Double Doozies:**

| | C | F | Cb |
|---|---|---|---|
| Original, 5.3 oz | 690 | 34 | 94 |
| M&M Big Bite, 2.5 oz | 340 | 17 | 46 |

**Cookie Cakes:**

| | C | F | Cb |
|---|---|---|---|
| 16", 3.5 oz | 460 | 22 | 67 |
| 16" M&M, 4 oz | 500 | 24 | 73 |
| Heart Shaped, 3.5 oz | 440 | 21 | 64 |

**Great Value** *(Walmart):*

**Chocolate Chip Chippers:**

| | C | F | Cb |
|---|---|---|---|
| Chewy (2), 1 oz | 150 | 6 | 21 |
| Chunky (2), 1.3 oz | 160 | 8 | 21 |
| Classic (3), 1.3 | 170 | 8 | 22 |
| Fig Bars, (1) | 120 | 2 | 24 |
| Fudge Marshmallow, (1) | 130 | 5 | 20 |
| Ginger Snaps, (4) | 130 | 4 | 22 |
| Pecan Shortbread, (2) | 160 | 9 | 19 |
| Twist & Shout, (2) | 140 | 7 | 20 |

**Crackers:**

| | C | F | Cb |
|---|---|---|---|
| Buttery Rounds, (4), 0.5 oz | 70 | 4 | 8 |
| Buttery Smooth, (4), 0.5 oz | 70 | 2.5 | 11 |
| Cheddar Cheese, (28), 1 oz | 150 | 8 | 18 |

**Joseph's:**

**Sugar Free:**

| | C | F | Cb |
|---|---|---|---|
| Almond; Chocolate Chip (4) | 95 | 5 | 13 |
| Coconut (4) | 95 | 4.5 | 14 |
| Average other varieties (4) | 95 | 4 | 15 |

*Note: Carb figures include 6 grams Maltitol*

**Kashi:** *Per Cookie*

| | C | F | Cb |
|---|---|---|---|
| Chocolate Almond Butter | 130 | 5 | 19 |

**Oatmeal:**

| | C | F | Cb |
|---|---|---|---|
| Dark Chocolate | 130 | 5 | 20 |
| Raisin Flax | 120 | 4.5 | 20 |

**Crackers:**

| | C | F | Cb |
|---|---|---|---|
| Original 7 Grain, (15) | 120 | 3.5 | 20 |
| Fire Roasted Veggie, (15) | 120 | 3.5 | 20 |

**Pita Crisps:**

| | C | F | Cb |
|---|---|---|---|
| 7 Grain Sea Salt (11), 1 oz | 120 | 3 | 23 |
| Garlic Pesto (11), 1 oz | 120 | 3 | 23 |

*Per Cookie/Cracker, Unless Indicated* **C** **F** **Cb**

**Keebler:**

**Animals:**

| | C | F | Cb |
|---|---|---|---|
| Crackers, Pouch, 1 oz | 120 | 3.5 | 22 |
| Frosted Cookies (8) | 160 | 8 | 22 |

**Chips Deluxe:** Original (2)

| | C | F | Cb |
|---|---|---|---|
| Chips Deluxe: Original (2) | 160 | 8 | 19 |
| Chocolate Lovers (2) | 170 | 9 | 20 |
| Coconut (2) | 160 | 9 | 18 |
| Deluxe Triple Choc (2) | 150 | 8 | 20 |
| Soft 'n Chewy (2) | 140 | 6 | 21 |

Rainbow:

| | C | F | Cb |
|---|---|---|---|
| Choc. Chip wih M&M's (2) | 160 | 8 | 20 |
| Choc. Chip Minis, with M&M's, 5 cookies, 1 oz | 140 | 7 | 19 |
| Danish Wedding, (5) | 160 | 8 | 22 |

**E.L. Fudge:** Original (2)

| | C | F | Cb |
|---|---|---|---|
| E.L. Fudge: Original (2) | 170 | 7 | 25 |
| Chocolate (2) | 170 | 7 | 26 |
| Double Stuffed (2) | 180 | 9 | 24 |
| Vanilla (2) | 180 | 7 | 26 |

**Fudge Shoppe:**

| | C | F | Cb |
|---|---|---|---|
| Coconut Dreams (2) | 140 | 8 | 17 |
| Deluxe Grahams (3) | 140 | 7 | 18 |

Fudge Sticks:

| | C | F | Cb |
|---|---|---|---|
| Original (3) | 150 | 8 | 20 |

Fudge Stripes:

| | C | F | Cb |
|---|---|---|---|
| Birthday (2) | 140 | 6 | 19 |
| Original (2) | 140 | 6 | 19 |
| Mini, Original, 2 oz pkg | 280 | 13 | 38 |
| Grasshopper (4) | 150 | 7 | 20 |
| Gripz, Chips Deluxe, 0.9 oz pouch | 120 | 5 | 18 |
| Oatmeal: With Raisins (2) | 130 | 6 | 19 |
| Country Style (2) | 130 | 6 | 19 |
| Pitter Patter, P'nt Butter Creme (2) | 140 | 6 | 19 |

**Sandies Shortbread Cookies:**

| | C | F | Cb |
|---|---|---|---|
| Cashew (2) | 170 | 9 | 19 |
| Classic (2) | 160 | 9 | 19 |
| Pecan (2) | 170 | 10 | 18 |
| Toffee (2) | 160 | 9 | 20 |

**Simply Made Cookies:**

| | C | F | Cb |
|---|---|---|---|
| Butter (2) | 140 | 7 | 18 |
| Chocolate Chip (2) | 140 | 7 | 17 |
| Chocolate S'wich (2) | 140 | 6 | 20 |
| PB Chocolate Chip (2) | 140 | 8 | 15 |
| Soft Batch, Chocolate Chip (2) | 150 | 7 | 21 |

**Vienna Fingers:**

| | C | F | Cb |
|---|---|---|---|
| Creme Filled (2) | 150 | 6 | 23 |
| Reduced Fat (2) | 140 | 4.5 | 24 |
| Wafers, Vanilla (8) | 140 | 5 | 23 |

*continued next page...*

## Cookies & Crackers ~ Brands (Cont)

*Per Cookie/Cracker, Unless Indicated*  **C** **F** **Cb**

**Keebler (Cont):**

**Crackers:**

| | C | F | Cb |
|---|---|---|---|
| **Club:** Original (4) | 70 | 3 | 9 |
| Reduced Fat (5) | 70 | 2 | 12 |
| **Grahams:** Original (8) | 130 | 3.5 | 22 |
| Honey (8) | 140 | 4.5 | 24 |
| **Town House:** Original (5) | 80 | 5 | 9 |
| Reduced Fat (6) | 60 | 1.5 | 12 |
| Flatbread Crisps, all flavors (8) | 70 | 2 | 11 |
| Pita: Mediterranean Herb (6) | 70 | 2.5 | 12 |
| Parmesan Cheese Basil (6) | 70 | 2.5 | 11 |

**Kroger:**

| | C | F | Cb |
|---|---|---|---|
| **Chip Mates:** Orig. (3), 1.5 oz | 150 | 7 | 22 |
| Chunky (2), 1 oz | 120 | 6 | 17 |
| Peanut Butter (2), 1 oz | 120 | 7 | 15 |
| White Chip (2), 1 oz | 120 | 6 | 16 |
| **Chocolate Sandwich:** | | | |
| Original (3), 1.2 oz | 150 | 6 | 24 |
| Double Filled (2), 1 oz | 140 | 6 | 22 |
| Olde Southern Pecan Shortbread (2) | 150 | 9 | 16 |
| Vanilla Wafers (7) | 130 | 3.5 | 23 |

**Crackers:**

| | C | F | Cb |
|---|---|---|---|
| **Grahams,** Orig.; Honey, (4) | 120 | 3 | 20 |
| **Saltines,** Original (5), 0.5oz | 60 | 1.5 | 10 |

**Lance:** *Per Pack of 6 Cookies/Crackers*

| | C | F | Cb |
|---|---|---|---|
| **Choc-O-Lunch/Van-O-Lunch,** av. | 220 | 8 | 34 |

**Crackers:**

**Captain's Wafers:**

| | C | F | Cb |
|---|---|---|---|
| Grilled Cheese | 190 | 9 | 25 |
| PB & Honey | 200 | 9 | 23 |

**Cracker Sandwiches:**

| | C | F | Cb |
|---|---|---|---|
| Malt, with Peanut Butter Filling | 180 | 8 | 20 |
| Nekot, Peanut Butter | 240 | 11 | 33 |
| Nip Chee, Cheddar Cheese | 200 | 9 | 24 |
| Toastchee, Peanut Butter | 220 | 11 | 25 |
| Toasty, Peanut Butter | 190 | 9 | 21 |
| Wholegrain, Cheddar Cheese | 200 | 10 | 26 |

**Little Debbie:**

| | C | F | Cb |
|---|---|---|---|
| Crml Apple Oatmeal Pies (1), 1.23 oz | 140 | 4.5 | 24 |
| Chocolate Chip Cream Pie (1), 3 oz | 380 | 16 | 58 |

**Little Debbie (Cont):**  **C** **F** **Cb**

| | C | F | Cb |
|---|---|---|---|
| Cookies & Cream (1) | 160 | 7.5 | 22 |
| Happy Campers, Strawberry (1) | 140 | 4 | 25 |
| Marshmallow Puffs (1) | 160 | 5 | 25 |
| Oatmeal Creme Pie (1) | 170 | 7 | 26 |
| Star Crunch (1) | 150 | 6 | 22 |

**Lu:**

| | C | F | Cb |
|---|---|---|---|
| Petit Ecolier Dark Chocolate (2) | 130 | 6 | 17 |
| Petit Ecolier, Milk Chocolate (2) | 130 | 6 | 17 |
| Pim's, Orange (2), 0.9 oz | 100 | 3 | 17 |

**Manischewitz:**

**Crackers:**

| | C | F | Cb |
|---|---|---|---|
| **Tam Tams:** Original (10) | 110 | 4 | 16 |
| Everything; Garlic (10) | 140 | 5 | 19 |

**Mary's Gone Crackers:**

| | C | F | Cb |
|---|---|---|---|
| **Chocolate Chip Cookies,** (2) | 130 | 6 | 19 |

**Crackers:**

| | C | F | Cb |
|---|---|---|---|
| **All Flavors,** (13) | 140 | 5 | 21 |
| **Super Seed,** Classic (12) | 160 | 8 | 9 |

**Miss Meringue:**

**Meringue Classiques:**

| | C | F | Cb |
|---|---|---|---|
| Cappuccino (4), 1 oz | 110 | 0 | 26 |
| Mint Choc. Chip (4), 1 oz | 120 | 1.5 | 25 |
| Triple Chocolate (4), 1 oz | 120 | 1.5 | 25 |
| Vanilla Rainbow/Van. (4), 1 oz | 110 | 0 | 27 |

**Meringue Minis,** Low Fat:

| | C | F | Cb |
|---|---|---|---|
| Mini: Chocolate Chip (12), 1 oz | 130 | 1.5 | 27 |
| Mint Chocolate Chip (12), 1 oz | 120 | 1.5 | 26 |

**Meringue Minis,** Fat Free:

| | C | F | Cb |
|---|---|---|---|
| Peppermint Crush (9), 1 oz | 110 | 0 | 25 |
| Rainbw Vanilla; Vanilla (13), 1 oz | 110 | 0 | 27 |
| **Meringue Petites:** Cafe au Lait (7) | 100 | 0 | 25 |
| Toasted Coconut (6) | 120 | 2.5 | 23 |

**Mother's:**

| | C | F | Cb |
|---|---|---|---|
| **Circus Animal,** (7), 1 oz | 150 | 7 | 20 |
| **Chocolate Chips,** (4) | 150 | 7 | 20 |
| **Coconut Cocadas,** (4), 1 oz | 140 | 7 | 17 |
| **Double Fudge,** (2), 1.3 oz | 190 | 8 | 27 |
| **English Tea,** (2), 1.4 oz | 190 | 8 | 28 |
| **Iced Oatmeal,** (4), 1.2 oz | 150 | 6 | 23 |
| **Taffy,** (2), 1.3 oz | 190 | 9 | 28 |

**Mrs Fields Cookies** ~ *See Page 219*

## Cookies & Crackers ~ Brands (Cont)

*Per Cookie/Cracker, Unless Indicated* **C** **F** **Cb**

### Nabisco Cookies:

**Chips Ahoy!, Chocolate Chip:**

| | C | F | Cb |
|---|---|---|---|
| Original: | | | |
| 3 cookies, 1.2 oz | 160 | 8 | 22 |
| Single Serve, 2 oz | 280 | 14 | 38 |
| Reduced Fat (2), 1.2 oz | 150 | 6 | 24 |
| Mini Choc. Chips: | | | |
| Big Bag, 5 cookies, 1oz | 150 | 7 | 19 |
| Go Pak, 14 cookies, 1 oz | 150 | 7 | 20 |
| Snak Sak, 5 cookies, 1.1 oz | 160 | 7 | 21 |
| Chewy: Regular (2), 1.1 oz | 140 | 6 | 21 |
| Brownie Filled (1), 0.65 oz | 80 | 3.5 | 12 |
| Chunky: Choc. Chunk (2), 1.2 oz | 160 | 8 | 20 |
| White Fudge Chocolate (1) | 80 | 4 | 11 |
| Hot Cocoa (2), 1.1 oz | 150 | 7 | 22 |
| Oreo Creme, (2), 1.1 oz | 150 | 7 | 21 |
| Peanut Butter, (1), 0.7 oz | 90 | 4 | 13 |

**Lorna Doone:**

| | C | F | Cb |
|---|---|---|---|
| 100 Calorie Pack, | | | |
| Shortbread Cookie Crisps (6), 0.7 oz | 100 | 3 | 16 |
| Shorbreads: 1 oz cookie | 140 | 7 | 20 |
| 1.5 oz cookie | 210 | 10 | 28 |
| **Mallomars** (1), 1 oz | 120 | 5 | 18 |

**Newtons:**

| | C | F | Cb |
|---|---|---|---|
| 100% Whole Grain: | | | |
| Blueberry (2), 1 oz | 100 | 1.5 | 22 |
| Fig (2), 1 oz | 110 | 0 | 22 |
| Strawberry 92), 1 o | 100 | 2 | 21 |
| Original Fig: 2 cookies, 1.1 oz | 110 | 2 | 22 |
| Fat-Free, 2 cookies, 1 oz | 90 | 0 | 23 |

**Nilla Wafers:**

| | C | F | Cb |
|---|---|---|---|
| 8 wafers, 1 oz | 140 | 6 | 21 |
| Reduced-Fat (8), 1 oz | 120 | 1.5 | 24 |
| Vanilla, 1 oz pkg | 120 | 3 | 22 |

**Nutter Butter:**

| | C | F | Cb |
|---|---|---|---|
| Peanut Butter Sandwich: | | | |
| 16 oz package, 2 cookies, 1 oz | 140 | 6 | 19 |
| 4.8 oz package, 2 cookies, 0.9 oz | 120 | 5 | 16 |
| 1.9 oz package | 270 | 11 | 39 |
| **Bites**, 1 package, 1.73 oz | 240 | 10 | 34 |
| **Wafer**, 5 patties, 1.2 oz | 160 | 9 | 19 |
| **Oreo Berry,** (2) 1 oz | 140 | 6 | 20 |
| **Oreo Cool Mint,** (2), 1 oz | 140 | 7 | 21 |

**Oreo Chocolate/Golden:** *Average All fillings*

| | C | F | Cb |
|---|---|---|---|
| 100 Calorie Pack, Thin Crisps (6) | 100 | 2 | 19 |
| Original: 1 cookie | 55 | 2.5 | 8 |
| 3 cookies, 1.2 oz | 165 | 7 | 25 |

---

*Per Cookie/Cracker, Unless Indicated* **C** **F** **Cb**

### Nabisco (Cont):

**Oreo, Choc./Golden (Cont):** *Average All Fillings*

| | C | F | Cb |
|---|---|---|---|
| Original Continued: | | | |
| Reduced Fat (3), 1.2 oz | 150 | 5 | 27 |
| Mini Bite: Bite Size (9), 1 oz | 130 | 6 | 21 |
| 15 oz Pack | 200 | 8 | 30 |
| Go-Paks, average, 3.5 oz | 490 | 22 | 70 |
| Chewy, 1.2 oz | 150 | 7 | 21 |
| Double Stuf: | | | |
| 2 cookies, 1 oz | 145 | 7 | 21 |
| Single Serve, 1.5 oz | 210 | 10 | 30 |
| Fudge Cremes: 1 cookie | 60 | 3 | 8 |
| 3 cookies | 190 | 9 | 24 |
| Thins, all flavors, 1 oz | 140 | 6 | 21 |
| Triple Double Chocolate (1), 0.75 oz | 100 | 5 | 15 |
| **Oreo Peanut Butter Creme,**(2) 1 oz | 140 | 6 | 20 |

**Teddy Grahams:**

| | C | F | Cb |
|---|---|---|---|
| Single Serve: Honey (24), 1 oz | 120 | 4 | 21 |
| Cinnamon (24), 1 oz | 120 | 4 | 21 |

### Nabisco Crackers:

**Barnum's Animals:**

| | C | F | Cb |
|---|---|---|---|
| 8 crackers, 1 oz Pack | 120 | 3.5 | 22 |
| Snack Saks, 1.2 oz Pack | 140 | 4 | 24 |

**Cheese Nips:**

| | C | F | Cb |
|---|---|---|---|
| Cheddar: 29 pieces, 1 oz | 150 | 6 | 19 |
| Mini, Despicable Me, 1 oz Pack | 130 | 4 | 19 |

**Honey Maid:**

| | C | F | Cb |
|---|---|---|---|
| Grahams (8) average all varieties, | 130 | 3 | 24 |
| Honey, low fat (8), 1.24 oz | 140 | 2 | 29 |

**Premium:**

| | C | F | Cb |
|---|---|---|---|
| Original: 5 crackers, 0.5 oz | 70 | 1.5 | 12 |
| Minis (17), 0.5 oz | 70 | 2 | 11 |
| Unsalted Tops(5), 0.5 oz | 70 | 1.5 | 13 |
| Rounds: Original (6), 0.5 oz | 60 | 1.5 | 12 |
| Wholegrain (6), 0.5 oz | 60 | 1.5 | 11 |
| Soup & Oyster (22), 0.5 oz | 60 | 1.5 | 11 |
| **Teddy Graham Crackers,** 1 oz pkt | 120 | 4 | 21 |
| **Triscuit:** Original (6 ), 1 oz | 120 | 3.5 | 20 |
| Reduced Fat (6), 1 oz | 110 | 2.5 | 21 |
| Brown Rice & Wheat (6), | | | |
| average all varieties | 130 | 3 | 22 |
| Thin Crisps, Original (7) | 130 | 4.5 | 21 |

**Wheat Thins:** *Per 9 oz Box*

| | C | F | Cb |
|---|---|---|---|
| Original (16), 1.1 oz | 140 | 5 | 22 |
| Reduced Fat (16), 1 oz | 130 | 3 | 22 |
| Av. other flav. (14), 1.1 oz | 140 | 5 | 21 |
| Multigrain (14), 1.1 oz | 130 | 4 | 22 |
| Popped, av. all flavors, 24 pcs | 125 | 3 | 23 |

---

*Per Cookie/Cracker, Unless Indicated* **C** **F** **Cb**

**Nana's:** *Per Cookie*

| | C | F | Cb |
|---|---|---|---|
| **Choc. Chip; Oatmeal Raisin, av.** | 410 | 17 | 59 |
| **Coconut Chip; Peanut Butter, av.** | 370 | 18 | 50 |
| **Double Chocolate** | 420 | 20 | 58 |
| **Gluten Free:** Choc. Crunch | 360 | 12 | 62 |
| Ginger | 360 | 10 | 64 |
| Lemon | 360 | 14 | 60 |
| **Cookie Bars,** average | 150 | 6 | 23 |
| **Bites,** P'Nut Butter (1), 1 oz | 130 | 6 | 17 |

**Newman's Own Organics:**

| | C | F | Cb |
|---|---|---|---|
| **Alphabet:** Chocolate (10) | 110 | 3 | 21 |
| Other varieties (10) | 120 | 3 | 21 |
| **Double Choc Chip,** (5) | 150 | 8 | 22 |
| **Fig Newman's:** | | | |
| Fat-Free (2) | 100 | 0 | 24 |
| Low Fat & Wheat/Dairy-Free (2) | 110 | 1.5 | 23 |
| Strawberry (2) | 110 | 1.5 | 22 |
| **Newman-O's:** Original (2) | 130 | 5 | 20 |
| Choc.; Hint O Mint Creme, (2), av. | 130 | 5 | 20 |
| Peanut Butter (2) | 120 | 5 | 18 |
| **Oatmeal Chocolate Chip,** (2) | 140 | 6 | 23 |
| **Orange Chocolate Chip,** (2) | 160 | 7 | 22 |

**Nonni's:**

**Biscotti:**

| | C | F | Cb |
|---|---|---|---|
| Original, 1 piece, 0.8 oz | 90 | 3 | 14 |
| Av. other varieties, 1 piece, 0.8 oz | 110 | 4 | 17 |
| **THINAddictives:** Cranb. Alm., 1 oz | 130 | 4.5 | 20 |
| Chocolate varieties, average, 1 oz | 140 | 5 | 21 |
| Pistachio/Mango Coconut Alm., 1 oz | 145 | 6 | 18 |

**Oreo Cookies** ~ *See Nabisco, Page 85*

**Payaso:**

| | C | F | Cb |
|---|---|---|---|
| **Animalitos,** 19 pieces | 120 | 1.5 | 23 |
| **Marias,** (8) | 120 | 2.5 | 22 |
| **Orejitas Finas,** (4) | 100 | 5 | 13 |

**Pepperidge Farm:**

**Cookies:**

**Chunk:** *Per Cookie*

| | C | F | Cb |
|---|---|---|---|
| Chesapeake, Dark Chocolate Pecan | 140 | 8 | 20 |
| Lexington, Milk Chocolate, Toffee Almond | 130 | 7 | 16 |
| Monauk, Milk Chocolate | 140 | 6 | 22 |
| Nantucket, Dble Dark Chocolate | 140 | 7 | 19 |
| Sausalito, Milk Choc. Macadamia | 130 | 7 | 17 |
| Tahoe, White Chocolate Macadamia | 130 | 7 | 17 |

*Per Cookie/Cracker, Unless Indicated* **C** **F** **Cb**

**Pepperidge Farm (Cont):**

| | C | F | Cb |
|---|---|---|---|
| **Brown Butter Rum,** (3) | 130 | 6 | 20 |
| **Brussels** (3) | 150 | 7 | 20 |
| **Lemon** (4) | 160 | 8 | 21 |
| **Geneva** (3) | 160 | 9 | 19 |
| **Milano:** Crunchy Almond Slices (3) | 150 | 8 | 17 |
| Dark Chocolate (2) | 180 | 9 | 22 |
| Double Milk Chocolate (2) | 130 | 7 | 17 |
| Dulce De Leche (2) | 130 | 7 | 16 |
| **Pirouettes,** (2), av. all var. | 120 | 5 | 19 |
| **Tahiti,** Coconut (2) | 170 | 10 | 17 |

**Crackers:**

| | C | F | Cb |
|---|---|---|---|
| **Cracker Trio,** (3) | 60 | 2 | 9 |
| **Golden Butter,** (4) | 70 | 2.5 | 11 |
| **Harvest Wheat,** (2) | 50 | 2 | 7 |
| **Goldfish Crackers:** | | | |
| **Cheddar:** ½cup, 1.1 oz | 140 | 5 | 20 |
| Carton, small, 2 oz | 280 | 10 | 40 |
| Lunch Pack, 0.9 oz pouch | 120 | 4.5 | 17 |
| **Flavor Blasted,** av., (56) | 140 | 4 | 20 |
| **Grahams,** av., (35) | 140 | 5 | 22 |
| **Parmesan,** (60) | 140 | 5 | 20 |
| **Pizza,** (55) | 140 | 5 | 20 |
| **Pretzel,** (43) | 130 | 2.5 | 24 |
| **Wholegrain Cheddar,** (55) | 140 | 5 | 19 |

**Ritz:**

| | C | F | Cb |
|---|---|---|---|
| **Originals:** Original (5) | 80 | 4.5 | 10 |
| Roasted Veg. (5) | 80 | 3.5 | 10 |
| Whole Wheat (5) | 70 | 2.5 | 10 |
| **Bits,** Peanut Butter (12) | 150 | 8 | 18 |
| **Crisp & Thins,** all varieties (21) | 130 | 4.5 | 21 |
| **Toasted Chips:** | | | |
| Original (13) | 130 | 4 | 20 |
| Cheddar (12) | 30 | 6 | 19 |
| Sour Cream & Onion (12) | 130 | 6 | 19 |

**Safeway Select:**

| | C | F | Cb |
|---|---|---|---|
| **Homestyle,** Oatmeal Raisin, 1 oz | 130 | 6 | 18 |
| **Indulgent:** Double Choc Chunk, 1 oz | 130 | 7 | 18 |
| Milk Chocolate Macadamia Nut, 1 oz | 140 | 8 | 17 |
| **Gourmet Sandwich Cremes:** | | | |
| Maple Creme (2) | 170 | 7 | 25 |
| Raspberry Swirl (2) | 130 | 5 | 20 |
| Strawberry Swirl (2) | 130 | 6 | 19 |

**Sedano's:**

| | C | F | Cb |
|---|---|---|---|
| **Cinnamon,** (5) | 160 | 6 | 24 |
| **Maria,** (5) | 120 | 3 | 22 |

**Shar Gluten Free** ~ *See CalorieKing.com*

## Cookies & Crackers ~ Brands (Cont)

*Per Cookie/Cracker, Unless Indicated*  **C**  **F**  **Cb**

**Special K:** *Per 1 oz Serving*

| | C | F | Cb |
|---|---|---|---|
| **Crackers,** all varieties (14) | 130 | 4.5 | 21 |
| **Cracker Chips,** 0.9 oz pouch | 100 | 3.5 | 18 |

**Stella D'Oro:**

| | | | |
|---|---|---|---|
| Breakfast Treats (1), av. all var. | 90 | 2.5 | 15 |
| Margherite: Chocolate (2) | 130 | 6 | 19 |
| Vanilla (2) | 120 | 4 | 20 |
| Roman Egg Biscuits, 1 oz | 130 | 4.5 | 19 |
| Swiss Fudge (3) | 180 | 9 | 22 |

**Toast & Sponge:**

| | | | |
|---|---|---|---|
| Almond Toast (2) | 100 | 1.5 | 20 |
| Anisette Sponge (3) | 90 | 1 | 18 |

**Streit's:**

**Flavored Wafers:**

| | | | |
|---|---|---|---|
| Chocolate (3) | 160 | 9 | 19 |
| Vanilla (3) | 170 | 11 | 18 |

**Sunshine:**

**Cheez-It:**

| | | | |
|---|---|---|---|
| **Crackers:** Original, 1 oz | 150 | 8 | 17 |
| Grab & Go, 2 oz pouch | 290 | 15 | 32 |
| White Cheddar, 1 oz | 140 | 7 | 17 |
| Whole Grain, 0.75 oz pouch | 100 | 3.5 | 14 |
| **Big,** 1 oz | 150 | 8 | 17 |
| **Snack Mix:** Classic, 1 oz | 140 | 5 | 20 |
| Double Cheese, 0.9 oz | 120 | 5 | 17 |

**Trader Joe's:**

| | | | |
|---|---|---|---|
| 100 Calorie Packs, average | 100 | 2.5 | 18 |
| Almond Windmill (2) | 140 | 6 | 18 |
| Charmingly Chewy Choc Chip (2) | 130 | 5 | 20 |
| Cherry Granola (2) | 110 | 4 | 18 |
| **Chocolate Chip:** Small (4) | 140 | 7 | 18 |
| Large, singles, 1.7 oz | 280 | 14 | 35 |
| Deep Dish: ⅒ cookie, 1.6 oz | 200 | 9 | 28 |
| ¼ Cookie, 4 oz | 500 | 23 | 70 |
| Vegan (1) | 130 | 6 | 18 |
| Caramel Cashew (3) | 140 | 7 | 16 |
| Crispy Crunchy Choc. Chip (12) | 150 | 9 | 19 |
| Crispy Oatmeal Choc. Chip (12) | 150 | 7 | 19 |
| Dark Choc Chunks with almonds (3) | 140 | 7 | 17 |
| **Dunkers:** Chocolate Chip (2) | 160 | 7 | 21 |
| Choc. Coated Choc. Chip (2) | 190 | 9 | 25 |

*Per Cookie/Cracker, Unless Indicated*  **C**  **F**  **Cb**

**Trader Joe's (Cont):**

| | C | F | Cb |
|---|---|---|---|
| Ginger Snaps, Gluten Free (5) | 140 | 6 | 21 |
| Highbrow Chocolate (2) | 140 | 7 | 17 |
| Joe Joe's Sandwich Cremes, Chocolate/ Vanilla (2) | 130 | 6 | 19 |
| Macarons A La Parisienne (2) | 90 | 3 | 10 |
| Meringues, Vanilla (4) | 110 | 0 | 27 |
| Oatmeal Raisin, 1.8 oz | 270 | 12 | 35 |
| Pecan Southern Style (4) | 150 | 9 | 15 |
| **Thins:** Meyer Lemon (9) | 130 | 4.5 | 22 |
| Toasted Coconut (8) | 130 | 4.5 | 22 |
| Triple Choc Chunk, 1 oz | 140 | 7 | 20 |
| Ultimate Vanilla Wafers (5) | 120 | 6 | 15 |
| Way More Chocolate Chip (3) | 160 | 11 | 14 |

**Crackers:**

| | | | |
|---|---|---|---|
| Multigrain (14) | 150 | 6 | 22 |
| Savory Thin Edaname (38) | 120 | 2 | 21 |
| Water (4) | 60 | 1 | 12 |

**Triscuits** ~ *See Page 85*

**Voortman:** *Per Cookie Unless Indicated*

| | | | |
|---|---|---|---|
| Almond Delight | 120 | 6 | 16 |
| Chocolate Chip | 90 | 4 | 13 |
| Coconut | 100 | 5 | 9 |
| Coconut Dark Chocolate | 90 | 5 | 10 |
| Fudge Striped Almonette | 110 | 6 | 13 |
| Iced Almonettes | 100 | 4.5 | 11 |
| Oatmeal Choc Chip | 90 | 4 | 12 |
| **Sugar Free:** Choc Chip | 90 | 4.5 | 14 |
| Fudge Striped Shortbread | 130 | 8 | 17 |
| Oatmeal | 90 | 4.5 | 14 |
| Wafers (3), average all flavors | 140 | 8 | 18 |

**Whole Foods (365 Organic):**

| | | | |
|---|---|---|---|
| Chocolate Chip (2) | 150 | 7 | 21 |
| Classic Fig Bars (2) | 140 | 2.5 | 27 |
| Lemon Wafers (7) | 110 | 3 | 19 |
| Oatmeal (2) | 130 | 4.5 | 20 |
| Sandwich Cremes; Sugar, (2), average | 130 | 5 | 20 |

## Cookie ~ Mixes

*As Packaged*

**Betty Crocker:**

**Cookie Mix:** *Per 3 Tbsp Mix*

| | | | |
|---|---|---|---|
| Double Chocolate Chunk | 110 | 2.5 | 21 |
| Reeses PB & Choc. Chunk | 130 | 5 | 20 |
| Snickerdoodle | 110 | 1.5 | 24 |
| Walnut Chocolate Chip | 120 | 3.5 | 20 |

**Limited Edition,**

| | | | |
|---|---|---|---|
| Snowball, 2 Tbsp Mix, 1 cookie | 100 | 3 | 18 |

# C Cookies ~ Refrigerated ◇ Crispbread

| Thaw, Bake & Serve | **C** | **F** | **Cb** |

*Per Cookie/Cracker Unless Indicated*

**Pillsbury Cookies:**

**Refrigerated Cookie Dough:** *Per Cookie*

| | C | F | Cb |
|---|---|---|---|
| Chocolate Chip Cookie, 1 oz | **130** | 6 | 17 |
| P'nut Butter, 1.1 oz | **130** | 6 | 19 |
| Sugar, 1 oz | **160** | 7 | 23 |

**Ready To Bake:**

| | | | |
|---|---|---|---|
| Choc. Chunk?Chip Cookies, 1.34 oz | **170** | 7 | 24 |
| Choc. Chunk & Chip Cookies, | **170** | 7 | 24 |
| Sugar Cookies, 1 oz | **120** | 5 | 18 |
| **Melts:** Caramel Brownie (1) | **140** | 5 | 22 |
| S'mores Sensation (1) | **150** | 6 | 23 |
| **Sugar Shapes,** (2), av. all var.,1 oz | **120** | 6 | 15 |

**Refrigerated Sweet Buns/Rolls~** *See Page 67*

**Toll House (Nestle):**

**Refrigerated Doughs:** *Per Cookie*

| | | | |
|---|---|---|---|
| **Bars:** Chocolate Chip | **90** | 4 | 11 |
| P'B Chocolate Chip | **80** | 4.5 | 10 |
| Sugar Bar | **80** | 3.5 | 11 |
| Walnut Chocolate Chip | **90** | 4.5 | 11 |
| Blueberry Lemon (1) | **80** | 3 | 4 |
| Peanut Butter (1) | **130** | 7 | 15 |
| Pecan Turtle Delight (1) | **160** | 7 | 24 |
| Triple Chip (1) | **90** | 4.5 | 4 |

**Ultimates Refrigerated Dough:** *Per Cookie*

| | | | |
|---|---|---|---|
| Chocolate Chip Lovers | **180** | 9 | 23 |
| Chocolate Pecan Deluxe | **190** | 10 | 22 |
| Choc. P'nut Butter Deluxe | **180** | 9 | 23 |
| Dark Chocolate Delight | **160** | 8 | 21 |
| Pecan Turtle Delight | **160** | 7 | 23 |

| Crispbreads | **C** | **F** | **Cb** |

*Per Crispbread Unless Indicated*

**Finn Crisp:**

| | C | F | Cb |
|---|---|---|---|
| **Classic:** Caraway | **20** | 0 | 4 |
| High Fibre | **40** | 0.5 | 7 |
| Sourdough | **20** | 0.5 | 4 |
| Traditional | **40** | 0.5 | 7 |
| **Round:** Multigrain | **50** | 0 | 7.5 |
| Original | **45** | 0.5 | 8 |

**New York Flatbread Crisps,**

| | | | |
|---|---|---|---|
| Sesame, 0.4 oz | **50** | 1.5 | 8 |
| **Ry-Krisp:** Natural (2) | **50** | 0 | 11 |
| Seasoned (2) | **50** | 0 | 11 |
| Sesame (2) | **50** | 0 | 9 |

**Ryvita:**

| | | | |
|---|---|---|---|
| **Crackerbreads,** Original; Ched. Chse | **20** | 0 | 4 |
| **Crispbreads,** Original; Dark | **35** | 0 | 6.5 |

**WASA:**

**Crisp'n Light Thins:**

| | | | |
|---|---|---|---|
| Fiber (2), 0.7 oz | **60** | 1 | 14 |
| Hearty (1), 0.5 oz | **50** | 0 | 12 |
| Light Rye (2), 0.5 oz | **60** | 0 | 15 |
| Whole Grain (1), 0.5 oz | **40** | 0 | 10 |

| Matzos | | | |

**Manischewitz:**

| | C | F | Cb |
|---|---|---|---|
| **Matzo:** Egg & Onion, 1 oz | **80** | 0.5 | 17 |
| Thin Salted/Tea, average, 0.9 oz | **95** | 0 | 20 |
| Whole Wheat, 1 oz | **110** | 1 | 21 |
| Yolk Free, 1.2 oz | **100** | 0 | 20 |

**Crackers:**

| | | | |
|---|---|---|---|
| **Tam Tam Snack::** Original (10), 1 oz | **110** | 4 | 16 |
| Everything; Onion (10), 1 oz | **140** | 5 | 19 |
| Rye (10), 1 oz | **110** | 4 | 16 |

**Streit's:**

| | | | |
|---|---|---|---|
| **Lightly Salted,** (1) | **110** | 0.5 | 23 |
| **Unsalted Matzos,** (1) | **100** | 0 | 23 |

## Quick Guide

**C** **F** **Cb**

### Cream
*Average All Brands*

**Half & Half Cream:**

| | C | F | Cb |
|---|---|---|---|
| 1 Tbsp, 0.5 oz | 20 | 1.5 | 0.5 |
| 2 Tbsp, 1 oz | 40 | 3 | 1 |
| ¼ cup, 2 oz | 80 | 6 | 2 |
| **Light:** Coffee/table (20% fat): 1 Tbsp | 30 | 3 | 0.5 |
| 2 Tbsp, 1 oz | 60 | 6 | 0.5 |

**Sour Cream:**

| | C | F | Cb |
|---|---|---|---|
| **Regular:** 1 Tbsp, 0.5 oz | 25 | 2.5 | 1 |
| 1 cup, 8 oz | 445 | 45 | 7 |
| **Low-Fat/Light:** 1 Tbsp, 0.5 oz | 20 | 1.5 | 1 |
| 2 Tbsp, 1 oz | 40 | 3 | 2 |
| **Fat-Free:** Av., 2 Tbsp, 1 oz | 20 | 0 | 3 |
| *Knudsen*, 2 Tbsp, 1 oz | 30 | 0 | 2 |
| *Kroger*, 2 Tbsp, 1 oz | 20 | 0 | 3 |

**Sour Cream Substitute:**

| | C | F | Cb |
|---|---|---|---|
| *Albertson's*, 2 Tbsp, 1 oz | 60 | 5 | 2 |
| *Tofutti*, Sour Supreme, 2 Tbsp, 1 oz | 85 | 5 | 9 |

**Whipping Cream:**
**Heavy,** (37% fat):

| | C | F | Cb |
|---|---|---|---|
| 1 Tbsp fluid/2 Tbsp whipped | 50 | 5.5 | 0.5 |
| ½ cup whipped | 105 | 11 | 1 |
| 1 cup whipped | 410 | 44 | 3.5 |

**Light,** (30% fat):

| | C | F | Cb |
|---|---|---|---|
| 1 Tbsp fluid/2 Tbsp whipped | 45 | 4.5 | 0.5 |
| ½ cup fluid/1 cup whipped | 350 | 37 | 3.5 |

## Coconut Cream/Milk

**Coconut Cream,** (Canned):
**Plain/unsweetened:** 2 Tbsp, 1 oz

| | C | F | Cb |
|---|---|---|---|
| Plain/unsweetened: 2 Tbsp, 1 oz | 75 | 6.5 | 3 |
| ½ cup, 4 oz | 285 | 26 | 12 |

**Sweetened:**

| | C | F | Cb |
|---|---|---|---|
| *Coco Lopez:* 1 oz | 130 | 5 | 21 |
| ½ cup, 4 oz | 520 | 20 | 84 |

**Coconut Milk:** (Canned):

| | C | F | Cb |
|---|---|---|---|
| *Thai Kitchen:* Lite, ⅓ cup, 2 fl.oz | 50 | 4.5 | 1 |
| Premium/Organic, 2 fl.oz | 115 | 10 | 4 |
| Unsweetened, ⅓ cup | 140 | 14 | 3 |
| **Coconut Water,** (Center), 1 cup | 45 | 0.5 | 9 |

## Whipped Toppings

*Average All Brands*

| | C | F | Cb |
|---|---|---|---|
| **Cream (Pressurized):** 2 Tbsp | 20 | 1.5 | 1 |
| ¼ cup | 40 | 3.5 | 2 |
| **Cream Topping,** Lite, 2 Tbsp | 20 | 1 | 3 |

## Whipped Toppings (Cont)

**Kraft:**
**Cool Whip:** Regular, Original, ⅓ oz

| | C | F | Cb |
|---|---|---|---|
| Cool Whip: Regular, Original, ⅓ oz | 25 | 1.5 | 2 |
| Extra Creamy, 2 Tbsp | 25 | 2 | 2 |
| Lite, Sugar Free, ¼ oz | 20 | 1 | 3 |
| Free, 2 Tbsp, 0.3 oz | 20 | 0 | 3 |
| Seasons Delight, Fr. Vanilla, 0.3 oz | 25 | 1.5 | 2 |
| **Dream Whip Mix,** ⅟₁₆ envelope | 10 | 0 | 1 |

**Reddi-wip:**

| | C | F | Cb |
|---|---|---|---|
| **Original,** 2 Tbsp, 0.3 oz | 15 | 1 | 1 |
| **Extra Creamy,** 2 Tbsp, 0.3 oz | 15 | 1 | 1 |
| **Fat-Free,** 2 Tbsp, 0.3 oz | 5 | 0 | 1 |
| **Chocolate,** 2 Tbsp, 0.3 oz | 15 | 1 | 1 |

## Creamers (Non-Dairy)

**Powder:**
**Coffee-Mate/Cremora/N-Rich:**

| | C | F | Cb |
|---|---|---|---|
| **Original:** 1 tsp | 10 | 0.5 | 1 |
| **Lite,** 1 tsp | 10 | 0 | 2 |
| **Flavors:** Av., 0.4 oz | 60 | 3 | 9 |
| Fat-Free, average, 4 tsp | 50 | 0 | 11 |
| Sugar Free, Chocolate, 0.2 oz | 30 | 0.5 | 2 |

**Liquid/Refrigerated:**
*Per Tablespoon*

**Baileys,** Coffee Creamer,

| | C | F | Cb |
|---|---|---|---|
| all flavors, 1 Tbsp, 15ml | 25 | 0.5 | 5 |
| **Califia Farms,** all flavors, 1 Tbsp | 15 | 0 | 4 |

**Coffee-Mate:** *Per Tbsp, 15 ml Unless Indicated*

| | C | F | Cb |
|---|---|---|---|
| **Flavors:** Average all flavors | 35 | 1.5 | 5 |
| Fat-Free, all flavors | 25 | 0 | 5 |
| Sugar free, all flavors | 15 | 1 | 2 |
| **Shelf Stable,** Ital. Swt Creme | 35 | 1.5 | 5 |
| **Unflavored:** Original | 20 | 1 | 2 |
| Fat-Free | 10 | 0 | 1 |
| **2Go,** all flavors, 5 ml | 25 | 1.5 | 3 |
| **Natural Bliss,** all flavors | 35 | 1.5 | 5 |
| **Hood,** Country Creamer, 1 Tbsp | 20 | 1.5 | 2 |

**International Delight:** *Per Tbsp*
**American/Classic/Coffee House:**

| | C | F | Cb |
|---|---|---|---|
| Regular, all flavors | 35 | 1.5 | 6 |
| Fat-Free, all flavors | 30 | 0 | 7 |
| Sugar-Free, all flav. | 20 | 2 | 1 |
| **Simply Pure,** all flavors | 30 | 1 | 5 |

**Kroger:** *Per Tbsp*

| | C | F | Cb |
|---|---|---|---|
| **Coffee Creamers:** Original | 20 | 1 | 3 |
| Caramel Vanilla; Hazelnut | 35 | 1.5 | 6 |
| Fat-free, Hazelnut | 30 | 0 | 6 |
| **Silk:** Almond, Vanilla | 20 | 1 | 3 |
| Soy: Original | 20 | 1.5 | 2 |
| Hazelnut | 30 | 1.5 | 4 |

# D Desserts ~ Puddings ◆ Gelatin

## Ready-To-Serve | C | F | Cb

**Hunt's:**
**Snack Pack Puddings:**
**5.5 oz Container:**

| | C | F | Cb |
|---|---|---|---|
| Chocolate | 180 | 3.5 | 34 |
| Butterscotch | 170 | 4 | 33 |
| Vanilla | 170 | 4.5 | 32 |

**3.3 oz Container:**

| | C | F | Cb |
|---|---|---|---|
| Butterscotch | 100 | 2.5 | 20 |
| Choc./Fudge; Tapioca, av. | 110 | 2 | 20 |
| Vanilla | 100 | 2.5 | 19 |
| Sugar Free: Chocolate | 70 | 3.5 | 14 |
| Vanilla | 60 | 3 | 11 |
| **Juicy Gels:** All flav., 5.5 oz | 160 | 0 | 39 |
| All flavors, 3.25 | 90 | 0 | 23 |
| Sugar Free, Cherry, 3.25 oz | 5 | 0 | 1 |
| **Naturals:** Choc., 3.8 oz | 130 | 2.5 | 24 |
| Vanilla, 3.8 oz | 130 | 3.5 | 22 |

**Jell-O** *(Kraft):*

| | C | F | Cb |
|---|---|---|---|
| **Gelatin:** Orig., av. all flav., 3.4 oz | 70 | 0 | 17 |
| Sugar Free, 3.2 oz | 10 | 0 | 0 |
| **Puddings:** *4 Packs* | | | |
| Choc. Vanilla Swirls, 3.5 oz | 110 | 1.5 | 24 |
| Strawberry Cheesecake, 3.5 oz | 130 | 2 | 25 |
| **Sugar Free Puddings:** *4 Packs* | | | |
| Chocolate Vanilla, 3.6 oz | 60 | 1.5 | 10 |
| Creme Brule Rice Pudding, 3.6 oz | 70 | 2 | 12 |
| **Temptations:** Lem. Meringue Pie, 3.4 oz | 80 | 1.5 | 17 |
| Strawberry Cheesecake, 3.5 oz | 130 | 2.5 | 25 |

**Kozy Shack:**

| | C | F | Cb |
|---|---|---|---|
| **Flan,** Creme Caramel, 1 cup, 4 oz | 150 | 3 | 27 |
| **Original Puddings:** | | | |
| Chocolate, 4.6 oz | 140 | 2.5 | 27 |
| Cinn. Raisin Rice, 4.6 oz | 140 | 2.5 | 26 |
| French Vanilla Rice, 4.6 oz | 140 | 2.5 | 24 |
| Original Rice, 4.6 oz | 130 | 2.5 | 24 |
| Tapioca, 4.6 oz | 130 | 2 | 25 |
| **Simply Well Puddings,** | | | |
| average all flavors | 90 | 2 | 13 |

**Kroger:** *Per Container*
**4 Pack Puddings:** *Per 3.25 oz*

| | C | F | Cb |
|---|---|---|---|
| Butterscotch | 100 | 2.5 | 20 |
| Chocolate | 100 | 2.5 | 19 |

**Swiss Miss:**
**Puddings:** *Per 4 oz Cup*

| | C | F | Cb |
|---|---|---|---|
| Classic Butterscotch | 130 | 3.5 | 22 |
| Creamy : Milk Choc. | 150 | 3.5 | 27 |
| Vanilla | 140 | 3.5 | 24 |
| Old Fashioned Tapioca | 140 | 3.5 | 24 |
| Triple Chocolate Dream | 160 | 4 | 27 |

## Homemade Puddings | C | F | Cb

| | C | F | Cb |
|---|---|---|---|
| Apple Tapioca, ½ cup | 150 | 0 | 32 |
| Bread Pudding, ½ cup | 250 | 8 | 40 |
| Blancmange, ½ cup | 140 | 5 | 19 |
| Chocolate, ½ cup | 190 | 6 | 30 |
| Crème Brulée, ½ cup | 400 | 35 | 16 |
| Plum Pudding, 2 oz | 170 | 3 | 32 |
| Rice, with Raisins, ½ cup | 200 | 4 | 38 |
| Sponge Pudding, 3.5 oz | 340 | 16 | 45 |
| Tapioca Cream, ½ cup | 110 | 4 | 15 |
| Trifle, ½ cup | 180 | 7 | 26 |

## Custards

**Custard Mix** *(Jello/Royal Flan),* average:

| | C | F | Cb |
|---|---|---|---|
| Dry, ¼ of 2.9 oz package, 0.7 oz | 80 | 0 | 19 |
| Prepared: whole milk, ½ cup | 155 | 4 | 25 |
| 2% milk, ½ cup | 140 | 2.5 | 25 |
| Non-Fat milk, ½ cup | 125 | 0 | 25 |
| **Home Made Egg Custard:** | | | |
| With Whole Milk, ½ cup | 170 | 8 | 18 |
| With 2% Milk, ½ cup | 155 | 6.5 | 18 |

## Gelatin • Parfait • Jell-O

**Jell-O:**
**Gelatin Dessert Mix:** *Dry Mix Only*

| | C | F | Cb |
|---|---|---|---|
| All flavors, 0.8 oz | 80 | 0 | 19 |
| Sugar free, all flavors, 0.3 oz | 10 | 0 | 0 |

**Instant Pudding & Pie Filling:** *Dry Mix Only*

| | C | F | Cb |
|---|---|---|---|
| Butterscotch, 0.9 oz | 90 | 0 | 23 |
| Choc.,; Choc Fudge, av., 1 oz | 105 | 0 | 25 |
| White Chocolate, 0.8 oz | 100 | 0 | 23 |
| Sugar free, Fat-Free: | | | |
| Chocolate var., 0.3 oz | 40 | 0 | 8 |
| Other flavors, 0.3 oz | 25 | 0 | 6 |

**No Bake Dessert Mix:** *Dry Mix Only*

| | C | F | Cb |
|---|---|---|---|
| Cheesecake: Real, 1.8 oz | 210 | 5 | 41 |
| Cherry, 2.2 oz | 210 | 4 | 42 |
| Strawberry, 2.4 oz | 200 | 4 | 43 |
| Oreo, 2 oz | 260 | 8 | 47 |
| Pumpkin Style Pie, 1.2 oz | 130 | 1.5 | 29 |
| **Ida Mae,** Strawberry Parfait | 90 | 2 | 18 |
| **Reser's,** Parfaits, av. all flavors, 3.9 oz | 105 | 2 | 19 |

## Meringues

| | C | F | Cb |
|---|---|---|---|
| Meringue Swirl, ½ oz | 50 | 0 | 8 |
| Meringue Shell, 1 oz | 100 | 0 | 16 |

## Egg ~ Egg Dishes (E)

### Chicken Eggs — C | F | Cb

| Item | C | F | Cb |
|---|---|---|---|
| **Fresh Eggs:** | | | |
| **Raw:** | | | |
| Small | 55 | 4 | 0 |
| Medium | 65 | 4 | 0 |
| Large | 70 | 5 | 0 |
| Extra Large | 80 | 5.5 | 0 |
| Jumbo | 90 | 6 | 0 |
| **Egg Yolk,** 1 extra large | 55 | 4.5 | 0 |
| **Egg White,** 1 extra large | 17 | 0 | 0 |
| **Dried Egg Powder:** | | | |
| **Whole Egg:** ¼ cup, 1 oz | 170 | 12 | 0 |
| 1 Tbsp | 30 | 2 | 0 |
| **Egg White,** ¼ cup, 1 oz | 105 | 0 | 0 |
| **Egg Yolk,** ¼ cup, 1 oz | 195 | 18 | 0 |

### Egg Substitutes

¼ Cup (Equivalent to 1 Egg) ~ Zero Cholesterol

| Item | C | F | Cb |
|---|---|---|---|
| **All Whites** (Crystal Farms), 1.6 oz | 25 | 0 | 0 |
| **Better 'n Eggs** (Crystal Farms): | | | |
| Regular, ¼ cup, 2 oz | 30 | 0 | 1 |
| **Egg Beaters** (ConAgra): | | | |
| 100% Egg White 3 Tbsp | 25 | 0 | 0 |
| Original, 3 Tbsp, 1.6 oz | 25 | 0 | 0.5 |
| Southwestern Style, 3 Tbsp, 1.6 oz | 20 | 0 | 0.5 |
| **Egg Replacer** (Ener-g), 1.5 tsp | 15 | 0 | 4 |
| **Egg Substitute** (Albertson's), ¼ cup | 30 | 0 | 1 |
| **Naturegg** (Burnbrae Farms), | | | |
| Simply Egg White, ¼ cup, 2 oz | 30 | 0 | 0 |
| **Vegan Egg Substitute:** | | | |
| **Aquafaba,** ¼ cup, 2 oz | 10 | 0 | 2 |

Liquid from cooked/canned beans or chickpeas. Replaces eggs and egg whites in recipes.
Extra Info: www.aquafaba.com

### Other Eggs

| Item | C | F | Cb |
|---|---|---|---|
| Duck, 1 large, 2.5 oz | 130 | 9.5 | 0 |
| Goose, 1 large, 5 oz | 280 | 19 | 0 |
| Quail, 3 eggs, 1 oz | 42 | 3 | 0 |
| Turkey, 1 large, 3 oz | 135 | 9.5 | 0 |
| Turtle, 1 egg, 1.75 oz | 75 | 5 | 0 |

### Omega-3 Fat Enriched

| Item | C | F | Cb |
|---|---|---|---|
| **Egg·Land's Best,** 1 large | 60 | 4 | 0 |
| **Horizon Organic,** 1 large | 70 | 4.5 | 1 |

Note: Cholesterol content is the same as regular eggs.

### Cooked Eggs — C | F | Cb

| Item | C | F | Cb |
|---|---|---|---|
| **Boiled Egg:** Same as Raw Egg | | | |
| **Hard-Cooked,** Small, peeled | 65 | 4 | 0 |
| **Fried Egg:** | | | |
| With fat: 1 large egg | 105 | 9 | 0.5 |
| 2 small eggs | 175 | 13 | 1 |
| No fat/nonstick pan, 1 large | 75 | 5 | 0.5 |
| **Deviled Egg,** 2 halves | 145 | 13 | 0.5 |
| **Eggs Benedict,** (2), on Toast or English Muffin | 860 | 56 | 25 |
| **Eggs Florentine,** (2), on Toast or English Muffin | 890 | 59 | 25 |
| **Pickled Egg,** 1 large | 80 | 5.5 | 0 |
| **Poached Egg,** 1 large | 65 | 4 | 0 |
| **Quiche** (Homemade): | | | |
| Egg & Bacon, 1 slice, 5.3 oz | 580 | 43 | 27 |
| Ham & Cheese, 1 slice, 5.3 oz | 475 | 33 | 29 |
| **Scotch Egg,** 1 egg | 300 | 21 | 16 |
| **Scrambled Eggs:** | | | |
| 1 large egg: | | | |
| With 1 Tbsp milk + 1 tsp fat | 120 | 9 | 1 |
| With 1 Tbsp skim milk/no fat | 85 | 5.5 | 1 |
| 2 large eggs: | | | |
| With 2 Tbsp milk + 2 tsp fat | 260 | 20 | 2 |
| With 2 Tbsp skim milk, w/o fat | 180 | 11 | 2 |

### Omelets

| Item | C | F | Cb |
|---|---|---|---|
| **1 Egg:** | | | |
| Plain (with 1 tsp fat) | 125 | 10 | 0.5 |
| With: ½ oz cheese | 175 | 15 | 0.5 |
| ½ oz cheese + ½ oz ham | 200 | 16 | 0.5 |
| **2 Eggs:** | | | |
| Plain (with 2 tsp fat) | 250 | 20 | 1 |
| With: 1 oz cheese | 360 | 29 | 2 |
| 1 oz cheese +1 oz ham | 410 | 32 | 2 |
| **3 Eggs:** | | | |
| Plain (with 1 Tbsp fat) | 360 | 29 | 1.5 |
| With: 2 oz cheese | 580 | 47 | 2.5 |
| 2 oz cheese+2 oz ham | 680 | 53 | 2.5 |
| **Extras,** Tomato/Onion/Veggies, 2 oz | 20 | 0 | 4.5 |
| **Egg Substitute** (EggBeaters): | | | |
| 2 eggs (½ cup) + 1 tsp fat | 100 | 4 | 2 |
| 3 eggs (¾ cup) + 2 tsp fat | 160 | 8 | 3 |
| Extras: 1 oz Cheese | 110 | 9 | 1 |
| 1 oz Ham | 50 | 3 | 1 |

### Egg Nog

| Item | C | F | Cb |
|---|---|---|---|
| **Average all Brands,** ½ cup, 4 oz | 170 | 9.5 | 17 |
| **Borden,** Regular, 4 fl.oz | 160 | 8 | 18 |
| **Hood,** Golden, ½ cup, 4 fl.oz | 180 | 9 | 22 |
| **Horizon,** Light/Low-Fat, | 130 | 3 | 23 |

## Breakfast Sides | C | F | Cb

**Toast:**

| | C | F | Cb |
|---|---|---|---|
| Plain, 1 thick slice | 85 | 1 | 13 |
| With: 2 tsp butter/marg. | 155 | 9 | 13 |
| 3 tsp/1 Tbsp fat | 190 | 13 | 13 |
| **English Muffin:** | | | |
| Plain, 2 oz | 130 | 1 | 26 |
| With 3 tsp fat | 230 | 12 | 26 |
| **Bacon,** 2 strips | 70 | 5 | 0 |
| **Ham,** lean, 2 oz | 100 | 3 | 0 |
| **Hash Brown:** | | | |
| ½ cup, 3 oz | 125 | 6.5 | 14 |
| 1 cup serving, 6 oz | 250 | 13 | 28 |
| **Sausages,** 2 oz link | 180 | 16 | 1.5 |

## Frozen Egg Breakfasts

**Jimmy Dean:**
**Breakfast Sandwich:** *Per Sandwich*

| | C | F | Cb |
|---|---|---|---|
| Biscuit, Sausage, Egg & Cheese | 410 | 29 | 26 |
| Croissant, Egg, Red Peppers, Onions | | | |
| & Jack Cheese | 290 | 16 | 27 |
| Muffin, Meat Lovers | 480 | 34 | 26 |
| **Omelets:** *Per Omelet* | | | |
| Three Cheese | 290 | 23 | 4 |
| Ham & Cheese | 250 | 19 | 4 |

**MorningStar Farms,**
**Breakfast Muffin Sandwich,**

| | C | F | Cb |
|---|---|---|---|
| Veggie Sausage, Egg & Chse | 210 | 8 | 20 |

**Pillsbury:**
**Toaster Scrambles:**

| | C | F | Cb |
|---|---|---|---|
| Bacon | 190 | 10 | 18 |
| Bacon & Sausage | 190 | 11 | 18 |
| Ham | 180 | 10 | 17 |

**Red Baron:**
**Biscuit Scrambles:**

| | C | F | Cb |
|---|---|---|---|
| Bacon (1), 5.85 oz | 440 | 21 | 47 |
| Sausage (1), 5.85 oz | 430 | 20 | 47 |

**Frozen Pancake/Waffles** ~ *See Page 132*
**Toaster Pastries** ~ *See Page 64*

## Frozen Egg Rolls

**Kahiki:** *Each, without sauce*

| | C | F | Cb |
|---|---|---|---|
| **Chicken; Vegetable,** av., 2.3 oz | 150 | 3.5 | 26 |
| **Pork,** 2.8 oz | 190 | 5 | 31 |
| **Lotus Restaurant:** | | | |
| **Imperial,** Chicken/Pork (1) | 160 | 6.5 | 24 |
| **Vegetarian,** (1) | 120 | 5 | 20 |

**Pagoda Express:** *Each, with Sauce*

| | C | F | Cb |
|---|---|---|---|
| **Chicken** | 160 | 4 | 24 |
| **Pork** | 180 | 7 | 23 |
| **Pork & Shrimp** | 180 | 7 | 23 |
| **Vegetable** | 140 | 4 | 24 |

## Fast-Foods/Restaurants | C | F | Cb

**Arby's,**

| | C | F | Cb |
|---|---|---|---|
| Bacon, Egg & Cheese Croissant | 440 | 27 | 29 |
| **Au Bon Pain,** 2 Egg on Plain Bagel | 390 | 11 | 51 |

**Bob Evans:**
**Omelets, Low Calorie:**

| | C | F | Cb |
|---|---|---|---|
| Border Scramble | 840 | 53 | 55 |
| Western | 740 | 43 | 52 |

**Bojangles:** Cheddar 'Bo'

| | C | F | Cb |
|---|---|---|---|
| Cheddar 'Bo' | 510 | 31 | 42 |
| Bacon, Egg & Cheese Biscuit | 480 | 28 | 42 |

**Bruegger's:**
**Bagel:** Egg & Cheese, 6.8 oz

| | C | F | Cb |
|---|---|---|---|
| Egg & Cheese, 6.8 oz | 450 | 14 | 62 |
| Western, 9.2 oz | 560 | 25 | 64 |

**Burger King:**

| | C | F | Cb |
|---|---|---|---|
| **Burrito,** Egg-Normous | 910 | 55 | 73 |
| **Croissan'wich:** | | | |
| Bacon, Egg & Cheese | 340 | 18 | 30 |
| Ham, Egg & Cheese | 330 | 16 | 31 |
| King, with Double Sausage | 700 | 51 | 31 |

**Carl's Jr:**

| | C | F | Cb |
|---|---|---|---|
| **Burrito:** Bacon & Egg | 570 | 35 | 32 |
| Big Country | 740 | 45 | 55 |
| Loaded Breakfast | 760 | 48 | 46 |
| Steak & Egg | 630 | 36 | 37 |

**Chick-fil-A,** Chicken, Egg & Cheese,

| | C | F | Cb |
|---|---|---|---|
| on Sunflower Multigrain Bagel | 480 | 18 | 51 |
| **Del Taco,** Bacon Breakfast Burrito | 640 | 36 | 38 |

**Denny's:** *With Hashbrowns, Without Bread*
**Omelette:**

| | C | F | Cb |
|---|---|---|---|
| Loaded Veggie | 600 | 43 | 25 |
| Ultimate | 820 | 66 | 25 |

**Dunkin Donuts:**

| | C | F | Cb |
|---|---|---|---|
| **Bagel,** Bacon, Egg & Cheese | 520 | 18 | 67 |
| **Croissant,** Saus., Egg & Cheese | 700 | 50 | 41 |

**Eat 'N Park:**
**Omelette:**

| | C | F | Cb |
|---|---|---|---|
| Ham & Cheese | 535 | 35 | 5 |
| Meat Lovers | 725 | 55 | 3 |

**Hardee's:**

| | C | F | Cb |
|---|---|---|---|
| **Biscuit:** Loaded Omelet | 490 | 28 | 40 |
| Sausage & Egg | 560 | 39 | 39 |
| **IHOP:** 2 Eggs, Scrambled | 220 | 17 | 2 |
| Omelette, Spinach & Mushroom | 890 | 70 | 20 |

**Jack in the Box:**

| | C | F | Cb |
|---|---|---|---|
| **Biscuit:** Bacon, Egg & Cheese | 410 | 25 | 26 |
| Saus., Egg & Cheese | 535 | 38 | 27 |

**McDonald's:**

| | C | F | Cb |
|---|---|---|---|
| **Biscuit:** Bacon, Egg & Cheese, reg. | 450 | 24 | 40 |
| **McMuffin,** Egg | 300 | 12 | 30 |

**Whataburger,** Breakfast Platter,

| | C | F | Cb |
|---|---|---|---|
| with Bacon | 740 | 52 | 36 |

## Quick Guide  🅒 🅕 🅒ᵇ

### Butter
*Average All Brands*

| | | C | F | Cb |
|---|---|---|---|---|
| **Regular:** 1 tsp, 0.2 oz | | 35 | 4 | 0 |
| 1 Tbsp, 0.5 oz | | 100 | 11 | 0 |
| 2 Tbsp, 1 oz | | 205 | 23 | 0 |
| 1 Stick, ½ cup, 4 oz | | 810 | 92 | 0 |
| 1 Pound, 2 cups, 16 oz | | 3255 | 368 | 0 |
| **Light:** Regular, 40% Fat | | | | |
| 1 tsp, 0.2 oz | | 30 | 3 | 0 |
| 1 Tbsp, 0.5 oz | | 70 | 7.5 | 0 |
| 2 Tbsp, 1 oz | | 140 | 15 | 0 |
| **Whipped Butter:** Regular | | | | |
| 1 tsp, 0.1 oz | | 20 | 2.5 | 0 |
| 1 Tbsp, 0.3 oz | | 65 | 7.5 | 0 |
| 1 Stick, 2.7 oz | | 545 | 62 | 0 |
| **Whipped Light Butter** *(Land O Lakes)*: | | | | |
| 1 tsp, 0.15 oz | | 15 | 1.5 | 0 |
| 1 Tbsp, 0.4 oz | | 45 | 5 | 0 |
| 2 Tbsp, 0.8 oz | | 90 | 10 | 0 |

**Unsalted ~** *Same as Salted*

### Flavored Butter/Spreads

*Average All Brands*

| | C | F | Cb |
|---|---|---|---|
| **Honey Butter,** (60% Fat): | | | |
| 1 Tbsp, 0.5 oz | 90 | 8 | 4 |
| *Downey's,* 2% Fat, | | | |
| 1 Tbsp, 0.5 oz | 60 | 1 | 11 |
| **Garlic Butter,** (80% Fat): | | | |
| 1 Tbsp, 0.5 oz | 100 | 11 | 0 |
| **Sweet Cream Butter:** | | | |
| *Land O Lakes:* Reguar, 1 Tbsp | 100 | 11 | 0 |
| Honey Butter Spread, 1 Tbsp | 70 | 6 | 4 |

### Butter & Butter Blends

*Per 1 Tablespoon*

| | C | F | Cb |
|---|---|---|---|
| **Challenge:** Stick, 0.5 oz | 100 | 11 | 0 |
| Tub, Whipped, 0.3 oz | 70 | 7 | 0 |
| **Brummel & Brown,** | | | |
| Spread Made with Yogurt, 0.5oz | 45 | 5 | 0 |
| **Land O'Lakes:** | | | |
| **Sticks,** Original, 0.5oz | 100 | 11 | 0 |
| **Tubs,** Butter With Olive Oil, 0.5 oz | 90 | 10 | 0 |

### Ghee (Clarified Butter)  🅒 🅕 🅒ᵇ

(Example ~ *Purity Farms*)
Note: Ghee is 100% fat compared to
regular butter (80% fat + 20% water)

| | C | F | Cb |
|---|---|---|---|
| 1 tsp, 0.2 oz | 45 | 5 | 0 |
| 1 Tbsp, 0.5 oz | 120 | 14 | 0 |

### Light & Reduced Fat Spreads

*Per Tablespoon*

| | C | F | Cb |
|---|---|---|---|
| **bestlife,** | | | |
| Buttery Spread, 0.5 oz | 60 | 6 | 0 |
| **Benecol:** Regular, 0.5 oz | 70 | 8 | 0 |
| Light, 0.5 oz | 50 | 5 | 0 |
| **Blue Bonnet:** | | | |
| Stick, Light Spread, 0.5 oz | 50 | 5 | 0.5 |
| Tub, Orig. Soft Spread, 0.5 oz | 60 | 6 | 0.5 |
| **Country Crock** *(Shedd's)*: Stick, 0.5 oz | 80 | 8 | 0 |
| **Tubs:** Original Spread, 0.5 oz | 50 | 6 | 0 |
| Light Spread, 0.5 oz | 35 | 4 | 0 |
| Churn Style, 0.5 oz | 50 | 6 | 0 |
| **Fleischmann's:** | | | |
| Orig., Soft Spread, 0.4 oz | 60 | 7 | 0 |
| Olive Oil Spread, 0.4 oz | 60 | 7 | 1 |
| Unsalted Spread, 0.4 oz | 60 | 7 | 0 |
| **I Can't Believe It's Not Butter!:** | | | |
| **Tubs:** Original Spread, 0.5 oz | 60 | 6 | 0 |
| Light, 0.5 oz | 40 | 4 | 0 |
| Olive Oil Spread, 1 Tbsp | 60 | 6 | 0 |
| **Parkay:** | | | |
| Original Spread, 0.4 oz | 70 | 7 | 0.5 |
| Spray, 5 sprays | 0 | 0 | 0 |
| Squeeze Bottle, 0.5 oz | 70 | 8 | 0 |
| **Promise:** Activ, Spread, 0.5 oz | 45 | 5 | 0 |
| Buttery Spread, 0.5 oz | 80 | 8 | 0 |
| Light Spread, 0.5 oz | 45 | 5 | 0 |
| **Smart Balance:** | | | |
| **Tubs,** Buttery Spread: | | | |
| Original, 0.4 oz | 80 | 9 | 0 |
| EVOO, 0.4 oz | 60 | 7 | 0 |
| Light EVOO, 0.4 oz | 50 | 5 | 0 |
| Light with Flaxseed Oil. 0.5 oz | 50 | 5 | 0 |
| Omega 3: Reg., 0.5 oz | 80 | 9 | 0 |
| Light, 0.5 oz | 50 | 5 | 0 |

### Butter Substitutes

| | C | F | Cb |
|---|---|---|---|
| **Butter Buds:** | | | |
| **Butter Flavored:** Mix, 1 tsp | 5 | 0 | 2 |
| Sprinkles, 1 tsp | 10 | 0 | 2 |
| **Earth Balance,** | | | |
| Original, 1 Tbsp | 100 | 11 | 0 |
| **Molly McButter,** 1 tsp | 5 | 0 | 1 |
| **Sunsweet,** (Butter/Oil Replacement), | | | |
| Lighter Bake, 1 Tbsp, 0.7 oz | 35 | 0 | 9 |

# F Fats ~ Spreads & Oils ◇ Mayo

## Animal Fats/Lards    C   F   Cb

*Average All Types*
**Beef Tallow/Drippings, Lard (Pork),**
**Chicken, Duck, Goose, Turkey:**

| | C | F | Cb |
|---|---|---|---|
| 1 Tbsp, 0.5 oz | 115 | 13 | 0 |
| 2¼ Tbsp, 1 oz | 255 | 28 | 0 |
| 1 cup, 7.3 oz | 1850 | 205 | 0 |
| ½ pound, 8 oz | 2040 | 227 | 0 |

**Ghee/Butter/ Oil** ~ *See Page 93*

## Vegetable Shortening

*Average All Types*

| | | | |
|---|---|---|---|
| 1 Tbsp, 0.5 oz | 115 | 13 | 0 |
| 2¼ Tbsp, 1 oz | 250 | 28 | 0 |
| 1 cup, 7.3 oz | 1810 | 205 | 0 |

## Vegetable Oils

Includes almond, avocado, canola, corn, coconut, flaxseed, grapeseed, linseed, mustard, olive, palm, peanut, rice bran, safflower, sesame, sunflower, soybean, wheat germ. Note: Oil is 100% fat.

| | | | |
|---|---|---|---|
| 1 tsp, 0.2 oz | 45 | 5 | 0 |
| 1 Tbsp, 0.5 oz | 120 | 14 | 0 |
| 2 Tbsp, 1 oz | 240 | 28 | 0 |
| 1 cup, 7.3 oz | 1930 | 205 | 0 |

## Fish Oils

*Average All Types*
(Includes Cod Liver, Herring,
Salmon, Sardines): 1 Tbsp, 0.5 oz    **125**   **14**   **0**

## Cooking Sprays/Squeezes

Cooking Sprays: (PAM, Mazola, I Can't Believe It's Not Butter, Weight Watchers, Wesson):

| | | | |
|---|---|---|---|
| *Pam:* ¼ second spray | 2 | 0 | 0 |
| 1-3 second spray | 6 | 1 | 0 |
| *I Can't Believe It's Not Butter,* | | | |
| Original Spray | 0 | 0 | 0 |
| *Parkay,* Buttery Spray | 0 | 0 | 0 |

## Olestra (Olean)    C   F   Cb

**Olestra** *(Olean)*    **0**   **0**   **0**
Note: Olean is Procter & Gamble's brand name for Olestra – a no-calorie cooking oil that gives snacks (like potato chips, tortilla chips and crackers) taste and texture without adding fat or calories.
**Examples:**
• **Frito-Lay,** Light Products
  *(Lays, Ruffles, Tostitos, Doritos)*
• **Pringles,** Fat-Free Potato Crisps

## Quick Guide

### Mayonnaise:    C   F   Cb
**Regular:** *Per 1 Tbsp, 0.5 oz Unless Indicated*

| | C | F | Cb |
|---|---|---|---|
| Average All Brands | 90 | 10 | 0 |
| **Best Foods, Hellman's; Kraft:** | | | |
| Original/Real | 90 | 10 | 0 |
| ½ cup, 4 oz | 720 | 80 | 0 |
| **Hain,** Safflower Mayonnaise | 100 | 11 | 0 |
| **Spectrum,** Canola Mayo | 100 | 11 | 0 |
| **Light/Reduced Fat:** *Per 1 Tbsp, 0.5 oz* | | | |
| **Best Foods/Hellman's** | 35 | 3.5 | 1 |
| **Kraft,** Light/Olive Oil | 35 | 3 | 1 |
| **Smart Balance,** Omega | 50 | 5 | 0 |
| **Spectrum,** Light Canola Mayo, | | | |
| Eggless | 35 | 3.5 | 0.5 |
| **Fat Free:** | | | |
| **Kraft:** Original, 1 Tbsp | 10 | 0 | 2 |
| ½ cup, 4 oz | 80 | 0 | 16 |
| **Sugar Free:** | | | |
| **Dukes Mayo,** 1 Tbsp | 100 | 12 | 0 |

### Mayonnaise Style Dressing:
*Per 1 Tbsp, 0.5 oz*

| | C | F | Cb |
|---|---|---|---|
| **Best Foods,** Sandwich Spread | 60 | 5 | 2 |
| **Kraft:** | | | |
| Miracle Whip Dressing: | | | |
| Original | 40 | 3.5 | 1 |
| Light | 20 | 1.5 | 1 |
| Fat Free | 15 | 0 | 3 |
| Mayo: | | | |
| Chipotle | 35 | 3 | 1 |
| Horseradish-Dijon | 35 | 3 | 1 |
| Sandwich Shop, Hot & Spicy | 100 | 11 | 0 |
| **Nasoya,** Egg & Dairy Free: | | | |
| Nayonaise: Regular/Whipped | 40 | 3.5 | 1 |
| Light | 20 | 1.5 | 1 |
| **Sir Kensington's,** Egg/Dairy Free | | | |
| Fabanaise (Vegan Mayo) | 90 | 10 | 0 |

## Quick Guide

### Fresh Fish

**Low Oil:** *Less than 2.5% fat*
**White/Lightly-colored flesh. Examples:**
Cod, Flounder, Haddock, Halibut, Mahi Mahi, Perch, Pike, Pollock, Snapper, Sole, Whiting.

| | C | F | Cb |
|---|---|---|---|
| **Raw,** without bones, 4 oz | 100 | 1 | 0 |
| **Steamed,** broiled, baked, 4 oz | 140 | 1.5 | 0 |
| **Fried:** Lightly floured, 4 oz | 210 | 8 | 3.5 |
| Breaded, 4 oz | 260 | 12 | 8 |
| In Batter, 4 oz | 320 | 16 | 27 |

**Medium Oil:** *2.5-5% fat*
**Lightly-colored flesh. Examples:**
Bluefin Tuna, Catfish, Kingfish, Orange Roughy, Salmon (Pink), Swordfish, Rainbow Trout, Yellowtail.

| | C | F | Cb |
|---|---|---|---|
| **Raw,** without bones, 4 oz | 145 | 7 | 0 |
| **Baked/Broiled,** 4 oz | 195 | 8 | 0 |
| **Fried,** 4 oz | 230 | 11 | 8 |

**High Oil:** *Over 5% fat*
**Darker-colored flesh. Examples:**
Albacore Tuna, Mackerel, Salmon (Atlantic/Chinook/Sockeye), Sardines, Trout.

| | C | F | Cb |
|---|---|---|---|
| **Raw,** without bones, 4 oz | 220 | 14 | 0 |
| **Baked/Broiled,** 4 oz | 275 | 17 | 0 |
| **Fried,** 4 oz | 340 | 23 | 12 |

### Cooking Yields (Fin Fish):
4 oz Raw wt. = 3.5 oz Cooked weight
4 oz Cooked wt. = 5 oz Raw weight

### Calorie & Fat Variations:
The amount of fat/oil in fish varies with the species, season and locality. Within the same fish, fat/oil content is generally higher towards the head.

### Fish & Shellfish

*Edible Weights: (no bones/shell)*

| | C | F | Cb |
|---|---|---|---|
| **Abalone:** Raw, 3 oz | 90 | 0.5 | 5 |
| Fried, 3 oz | 160 | 6 | 10 |
| **Ahi Tuna,** grilled, 6 oz fillet (w/o fat) | 235 | 2 | 0 |
| **Anchovy:** Paste, 1 Tbsp, 0.5 oz | 45 | 3 | 0 |
| Canned in oil, drained, (5), 0.7 oz | 40 | 2 | 0 |
| **Barracuda (Pacific),** raw, 4 oz | 130 | 3 | 0 |
| **Basa/Swai,** raw, 4 oz fillet | 70 | 2 | 0 |
| **Bass:** | | | |
| Sea: Raw, 4.6 oz fillet  | 125 | 2.5 | 0 |
| Baked, 3 oz | 105 | 2 | 0 |
| Striped: Raw, 1 fillet, 5.5 oz | 150 | 3.5 | 0 |
| Baked, 3 oz | 105 | 3 | 0 |
| Freshwater: Raw, 3 oz | 95 | 3 | 0 |
| Baked, 3 oz | 125 | 4 | 0 |

### Fish & Shellfish (Cont)

*Edible Weights: (no bones/shell)*

| | C | F | Cb |
|---|---|---|---|
| **Calamari/Squid:** | | | |
| Raw, 4 oz | 100 | 1.5 | 3.5 |
| Baked, 1 cup | 190 | 6.5 | 5.5 |
| Fried, 3 oz | 150 | 6 | 7 |
| **Catfish:** | | | |
| Farmed: Raw, 1 fillet 5.6 oz | 190 | 9.5 | 0 |
| Baked, 1 fillet 5 oz | 205 | 10 | 0 |
| Wild: Raw, 1 fillet, 5.6 oz | 150 | 4.5 | 0 |
| Baked, 1 fillet, 5 oz | 150 | 4 | 0 |
| Breaded, fried, 1 fillet, 3 oz | 200 | 12 | 7 |
| **Caviar,** black/red, 1 Tbsp, 16g | 40 | 3 | 0.5 |
| **Clams:** Raw (4 large/9 small), 3 oz | 70 | 1 | 3 |
| Breaded, fried (20 small), 6.6 oz | 380 | 21 | 20 |
| Canned, drained, ½ cup, 2.8 oz | 115 | 1 | 0 |
| Steamed (10 small), 3.3 oz | 140 | 2 | 5 |
| **Cod:** | | | |
| Atlantic: Raw, 4 oz | 95 | 1 | 0 |
| Baked, 3 oz | 90 | 1 | 0 |
| Canned, solids & liquid | 90 | 0.5 | 0 |
| Pacific: Raw, 4 oz | 80 | 0.5 | 0 |
| Baked, 3 oz | 70 | 0.5 | 0 |
| **Crab:** | | | |
| Alaska King, 1 leg, cooked, 4.7 oz | 130 | 2 | 0 |
| Blue: Raw, 1 crab, 6 oz | 150 | 1 | 0 |
| Steamed, 3 oz | 70 | 0.5 | 0 |
| Canned, drained, 6.5 oz can | 105 | 0.5 | 0 |
| Dungeness: Raw, 1 crab, 5.8 oz | 140 | 1.5 | 0 |
| Steamed, 4.45 oz | 140 | 1.5 | 0 |
| **Crab Cakes** *(Capt. D's)*, (1), 2.8 oz | 250 | 16 | 16 |
| **Crayfish:** | | | |
| Farmed: Raw, 3 oz | 60 | 1 | 0 |
| Steamed, 3 oz | 75 | 1 | 0 |
| Wild: Raw 3 oz | 65 | 1 | 0 |
| Steamed, 3 oz | 70 | 1 | 0 |
| **Cuttlefish,** raw, 3 oz | 70 | 1 | 1 |
| **Dolphinfish** ~ *See Mahi-Mahi* | | | |
| **Eel:** Raw, 3 oz | 155 | 10 | 0 |
| Baked, 3 oz | 200 | 13 | 0 |
| **Fish & Chips** *(Red Lobster)*, battered, without condiments | 700 | 33 | 61 |
| **Fish Sandwich** *(Burger King)*, without Tartar Sauce | 340 | 9 | 49 |
| **Fish Oil,** 1 Tbsp, 0.5 oz | 125 | 14 | 0 |
| **Flounder/Sole:** | | | |
| Raw, 4 oz | 80 | 2 | 0 |
| Baked, 3 oz | 75 | 2 | 0 |
| **Frozen Fish** ~ *See Pages 114-122* | | | |

| Fish & Shellfish (Cont) | C | F | Cb |
|---|---|---|---|
| *Edible Weights: Without Bones or Shell* | | | |
| **Haddock:** Raw, 4 oz | 85 | 0.5 | 0 |
| Baked, 3 oz | 75 | 0.5 | 0 |
| Smoked, 3 oz | 100 | 1 | 0 |
| **Halibut:** | | | |
| Atlantic: Raw, 4 oz | 105 | 1.5 | 0 |
| Baked, ½ fillet, 5.6 oz | 175 | 2.5 | 0 |
| **Herring:** | | | |
| Atlantic, raw, 4 oz | 180 | 10 | 0 |
| Canned: Plain, drained, 3 oz | 130 | 8 | 0 |
| In Tomato Sauce, 3.5 oz | 140 | 8 | 2 |
| Pickled, 2 pieces, 1 oz | 75 | 5 | 3 |
| Smoked, kippered, 4 oz | 245 | 14 | 0 |
| **Jellyfish:** Raw, 4 oz | 30 | 1 | 0 |
| Dried, Salted, 1 cup, 2 oz | 20 | 1 | 0 |
| **Ling,** raw, 4 oz | 100 | 0.5 | 0 |
| **Lobster,** Northern: | | | |
| 1.5 lb Whole Lobster, edible portion: | | | |
| Raw, 6.3 oz | 140 | 1.5 | 0 |
| Boiled, 5 oz | 140 | 1 | 0 |
| Lobster Salads, average, ½ cup | 220 | 13 | 5 |
| Lobster Newberg, average, ¾ cup | 360 | 20 | 9 |
| Lobster Thermidor, av., 1 serving | 370 | 22 | 15 |
| **Lobster Tail (Rock),** | | | |
| *Red Lobster,* grilled/roasted | 230 | 6 | 2 |
| **Lox,** Regular/Nova, 2 oz | 65 | 2.5 | 0 |
| **Mackerel,** Atlantic: Raw, 4 oz | 230 | 16 | 0 |
| Baked, 3 oz fillet | 225 | 15 | 0 |
| Pacific/Jack: Raw, 4 oz | 180 | 9 | 0 |
| Baked, 3 oz | 170 | 9 | 0 |
| Spanish: Raw, 4 oz | 160 | 7 | 0 |
| Baked, 3 oz | 135 | 5.5 | 0 |
| **Mahi-Mahi/Dolphinfish:** | | | |
| Raw, 4 oz | 95 | 1 | 0 |
| Baked, 4 oz | 125 | 1 | 0 |
| **Monkfish:** Raw, 4 oz | 85 | 1.5 | 0 |
| Baked, 3 oz | 80 | 2 | 0 |
| **Mullet, Striped:** Raw, 4 oz | 135 | 4.5 | 0 |
| Baked, 3 oz | 130 | 4 | 0 |
| **Mussels:** | | | |
| Raw: 4 oz (edible wt) | 100 | 2.5 | 4 |
| 1 cup, 5.3 oz (edible weight) | 130 | 3.5 | 5 |
| Cooked, moist heat, 3 oz | 150 | 4 | 6 |
| **Ocean Perch:** | | | |
| Atlantic: Raw, 4 oz | 90 | 2 | 0 |
| Baked, 3 oz | 80 | 1.5 | 0 |
| **Octopus:** | | | |
| Common: Raw, 4 oz | 95 | 1 | 3 |
| Boiled, 3 oz | 140 | 2 | 4 |
| **Orange Roughy:** | | | |
| Raw, 4 oz | 85 | 1 | 0 |
| Baked, 3 oz | 90 | 1 | 0 |

| Fish & Shellfish (Cont) | C | F | Cb |
|---|---|---|---|
| *Edible Weights: Without Bones or Shell* | | | |
| **Oysters,** Common, Raw, 3 oz | 70 | 2 | 4 |
| Eastern: | | | |
| Farmed: Raw, 6 medium, 3 oz | 50 | 1.5 | 5 |
| Cooked, dry heat, 6 med., 2 oz | 45 | 1.5 | 5 |
| Wild: Raw, 6 medium, 3 oz | 45 | 1.5 | 3 |
| Cooked, dry heat, 6 med., 2 oz | 45 | 1.5 | 3 |
| Breaded & Fried, 6 med., 3 oz | 175 | 11 | 10 |
| Pacific: Raw, 1 medium, 1.8 oz | 40 | 1 | 3 |
| Steamed, 1 medium, 0.8 oz | 40 | 1 | 3 |
| **Perch** ~ *See Ocean Perch* | | | |
| **Pike:** Northern: Raw, 4 oz | 100 | 1 | 0 |
| Baked, 3 oz | 95 | 1 | 0 |
| Walleye: Raw, 4 oz | 105 | 1.5 | 0 |
| Baked, 3 oz | 100 | 1.5 | 0 |
| **Pollock,** Atlantic: Raw, 4 oz | 105 | 1 | 0 |
| Baked, 3 oz | 100 | 1 | 0 |
| **Pompano,** Florida, raw, 4 oz | 185 | 11 | 0 |
| **Red Snapper** ~ *See Snapper* | | | |
| **Roe,** raw, 2 Tbsp, 1 oz | 40 | 2 | 0.5 |
| **Sablefish:** Raw, 4 oz | 220 | 17 | 0 |
| Smoked, 3 oz | 220 | 17 | 0 |
| **Salmon:** | | | |
| Atlantic, Farmed: Raw, 4 oz | 235 | 15 | 0 |
| Baked, 3 oz | 175 | 10 | 0 |
| Steaks: Raw, 7 oz | 410 | 27 | 0 |
| Baked, 6 oz | 365 | 22 | 0 |
| Atlantic, Wild: Raw, 4 oz | 160 | 7 | 0 |
| Baked, 3 oz | 155 | 7 | 0 |
| Steaks: Raw, 7 oz | 280 | 13 | 0 |
| Baked, 6 oz | 310 | 14 | 0 |
| Chinook: Raw, 4 oz | 205 | 12 | 0 |
| Baked, 3 oz | 195 | 11 | 0 |
| Smoked, 3 oz | 100 | 3.5 | 0 |
| King: Raw, 3.5 oz | 185 | 12 | 0 |
| Kippered, 3.5 oz piece | 265 | 16 | 0 |
| Smoked & canned, 3.5 oz | 150 | 6 | 0 |
| Coho: | | | |
| Farmed: Raw, 4 oz | 180 | 8.5 | 0 |
| Baked, 3 oz | 150 | 7 | 0 |
| Wild: Raw, 4 oz | 165 | 6.5 | 0 |
| Steamed, 3 oz | 155 | 6.5 | 0 |
| Pink/Chum: Raw, 4 oz | 145 | 5 | 0 |
| Baked, 3.5 oz | 155 | 5.5 | 0 |
| Canned: Drained solids, 11 oz | 435 | 16 | 0 |
| Without skin & bones, 8.5 oz | 330 | 10 | 0 |
| Sockeye: Raw, 4 oz | 160 | 6.5 | 0 |
| Baked, 3 oz | 145 | 5.5 | 0 |
| Canned, Drained solids, 3 oz | 140 | 6.5 | 0 |
| Smoked, 3.5 oz | 205 | 7.5 | 0 |
| Salmon Cake (1), 3 oz | 240 | 15 | 6 |

## Fish & Shellfish (Cont)

| | C | F | Cb |
|---|---|---|---|
| **Sardines:** *Canned, Average all Brands* | | | |
| Drained of Oil: | | | |
| ¼ cup drained, 2.2 oz | 130 | 9 | 0 |
| 3.75 oz can, drained, 3.3 oz | 190 | 11 | 0 |
| 1 large/2 medium, ⅗", 0.8 oz | 50 | 3 | 0 |
| in Tomato Sauce, 3.8 oz | 150 | 8 | 3 |
| **Sashimi** ~ *See Japanese Foods, Page 171* | | | |
| **Scallops:** Raw, 6 lge/15 small, 3 oz | 65 | 0.5 | 3 |
| Breaded, Fried (6), 5 oz | 385 | 20 | 39 |
| Steamed, 3 oz | 95 | 0.5 | 0 |
| **Sea Bass** ~ *See Bass* | | | |
| **Seafood Salad,** Deli Style, | | | |
| ½ cup, 3.5 oz | 250 | 21 | 11 |
| **Shark:** Raw, 4 oz | 145 | 5 | 0 |
| Baked, 4 oz | 185 | 7 | 0 |
| Batter-dipped, fried, 4 oz | 260 | 16 | 7 |
| **Shrimp:** | | | |
| Raw: Small/Medium (4), 0.8 oz | 15 | 0 | 0 |
| Large (4), 1 oz | 20 | 0 | 0 |
| Breaded & Fried, 4.8 oz | 395 | 24 | 27 |
| Steamed, in shell, 3 oz | 100 | 1.5 | 0 |
| Canned, 1 can, 4.5 oz | 130 | 2 | 0 |
| **Snapper:** Raw, 4 oz | 115 | 1.5 | 0 |
| Baked: 3 oz | 110 | 1.5 | 0 |
| 6 oz fillet | 220 | 3 | 0 |
| **Sole:** Raw, 4 oz | 80 | 2 | 0 |
| Baked, 3 oz | 75 | 2 | 0 |
| **Squid** ~ *see Calamari* | | | |
| **Surimi,** (Imitation Crab), 4 oz | 110 | 0.5 | 17 |
| **Swai/Basa,** raw, 4 oz | 70 | 2 | 0 |
| **Swordfish:** Raw, 4 oz | 165 | 7.5 | 0 |
| Medium Steak, 6 oz | 250 | 11 | 0 |
| Baked: Small Steak, 4 oz | 205 | 7 | 0 |
| Medium Steak, 6 oz | 290 | 13 | 0 |
| **Tilapia:** Raw, 4 oz | 110 | 2 | 0 |
| Baked: 3 oz | 110 | 2.5 | 0 |
| **Trout,** Rainbow: | | | |
| Farmed: Raw, 4 oz | 160 | 7 | 0 |
| Baked, 3 oz | 145 | 6.5 | 0 |
| Wild: Raw, 4 oz | 135 | 4 | 0 |
| Baked, 3 oz | 130 | 5 | 0 |
| **Tuna:** | | | |
| **Raw:** Bluefin, 4 oz | 165 | 5.5 | 0 |
| Skipjack, Yellowfin, av., 4 oz | 120 | 1 | 0 |
| **Baked:** Bluefin, 3 oz | 155 | 5.5 | 0 |
| Skipjack, Yellowfin, av., 3 oz | 110 | 1 | 0 |
| **Canned:** *in Water, drained* | | | |
| Chunk Light: 2 oz | 50 | 1 | 0 |
| 3 oz can | 75 | 1.5 | 1 |
| 5 oz can | 125 | 2.5 | 1.5 |

| **Tuna (Cont):** *in Water, drained (Cont)* | C | F | Cb |
|---|---|---|---|
| Solid White: 2 oz | 60 | 0.5 | 0 |
| 5 oz can | 150 | 1.5 | 0 |
| 7 oz can | 210 | 2 | 0 |
| in Oil, drained: | | | |
| Chunk Light: 2 oz can | 80 | 4 | 0 |
| 5 oz can | 200 | 10 | 0 |
| Solid White: 2 oz can | 90 | 4 | 0 |
| 6 oz can | 270 | 12 | 0 |
| **Whitefish:** Raw, 4 oz | 150 | 6.5 | 0 |
| Baked, 3 oz | 145 | 6.5 | 1 |
| Smoked, 3 oz | 90 | 1 | 0 |
| **Whiting:** Raw, 4 oz | 100 | 1.5 | 0 |
| Baked, 3 oz | 100 | 1.5 | 0 |
| **Yellowtail:** Raw, 4 oz | 165 | 6 | 0 |
| Grilled, 3 oz | 160 | 6 | 0 |

## Other Canned/Packaged Fish

| | C | F | Cb |
|---|---|---|---|
| **Bumble Bee:** *Skinless, Boneless* | | | |
| **Mackerel,** in oil, drained, 1.9 oz | 160 | 15 | 0 |
| **Pink Salmon,** in oil, drained, 2 oz | 60 | 1.5 | 0 |
| **Red Salmon,** in oil, drained, 2.2 oz | 100 | 5 | 0 |
| **Sardines,** in oil, drained, 3 oz | 210 | 15 | 0 |
| **Tuna Ready-To-Eat Kits:** *with Crackers:* | | | |
| Sensations, Tuna Medley: | | | |
| Tom. & Basil, 3 oz can & 3oz Crackers | 150 | 2.5 | 16 |
| Thai Chili, 3 oz can & 3oz Crackers | 180 | 2.5 | 23 |
| **Tuna, Snack on the Run!:** *with Crackers Kit* | | | |
| Tuna Salad, 2.9 oz can, w/- Crackers | 300 | 23 | 18 |
| Tuna, Fat Free w/ Wheat Crackers, | | | |
| 2.9 oz can | 130 | 2.5 | 20 |
| **Tuna, White Albacore:** | | | |
| Pouch, in water, 2 oz | 70 | 1.5 | 0 |
| Solid, in oil, drained, 2 oz | 80 | 2.5 | 0 |
| **Chicken of the Sea:** | | | |
| **Pink Salmon:** Skinless/boneless: 3 oz | 80 | 2 | 0 |
| Traditional, 14.75 oz can, 2.1 oz serve | 90 | 5 | 0 |
| **Sardines,** in oil, smoked, 3.75 oz can | 150 | 10 | 0 |
| **Tuna:** Lunch Solutions, | | | |
| Tuna Salad Cup & Crackers, 3.4 oz | 80 | 0.5 | 7 |
| To-Go-Cups, Tuna Salad, 2.8 oz | 80 | 0.5 | 7 |
| **Starkist:** | | | |
| **Pouch:** *Per 2.6 oz Pouch* | | | |
| Albacore White Tuna in water | 80 | 1.5 | 0 |
| Chunk, Light, Tuna in water | 70 | 0.5 | 0 |
| **Lunch-To-Go Kit,** Chunk Light Tuna | | | |
| with Light Mayo & Crackers, 4 oz | 230 | 9 | 20 |
| **Tuna Creations:** *Per 2.6 oz* | | | |
| Bold Hot Buffalo Style | 70 | 1 | 0 |
| Bold Thai Chili Style | 90 | 1 | 7 |

## Flours & Grains

| | C | F | Cb |
|---|---|---|---|
| **Amaranth Flour** *(Bob's Red Mill)*, ½ cup, 2.2 oz | 220 | 4 | 40 |
| **Arrowroot Flour,** ½ cup, 2.3 oz | 230 | 0 | 56 |
| **Barley:** Grain, regular, ½ cup, 2.6 oz | 255 | 1 | 55 |
| Pearled, raw, 3.5 oz | 350 | 1 | 78 |
| **Buckwheat:** Grain, ½ cup, 3 oz | 290 | 3 | 61 |
| Flour, whole-groat, ½ cup, 2 oz | 200 | 2 | 42 |
| Groats: Roasted, dry, ½ cup, 3 oz | 285 | 2 | 62 |
| Roasted, cooked, 3.5 oz | 80 | 0.5 | 17 |
| **Bulgur:** Dry, ½ cup, 2.5 oz | 240 | 1 | 53 |
| Cooked, ½ cup, 3.2 oz | 75 | 0.5 | 17 |
| **Carob Flour,** ½ cup, 1.8 oz | 115 | 0.5 | 46 |
| **Coconut Flour,** 2 Tbsp, 0.6 oz | 60 | 3.5 | 10 |
| **Corn Kernels,** cooked, av., ½ cup | 80 | 0.5 | 18 |
| **Corn Bran,** ½ cup, 1.3 oz | 85 | 0.5 | 33 |
| **Corn Flour/Masa,** ½ cup, 2 oz | 215 | 2.5 | 43 |
| **Corn Grits:** | | | |
| Dry, ½ cup, 2.8oz | 290 | 1 | 62 |
| Cooked, ½ cup, 4.3 oz | 70 | 0.5 | 15 |
| **Corn Germ,** toasted, ½ cup, 4 oz | 100 | 1.5 | 22 |
| **Cornmeal,** average all varieties: | | | |
| 3 Tbsp, 1 oz | 105 | 0.5 | 22 |
| ½ cup, 2.5 oz | 255 | 1 | 54 |
| Mixes, same as above | 230 | 1 | 48 |
| **Cornstarch:** 1 Tbsp, 0.3 oz | 30 | 0 | 8 |
| ½ cup, 2.3oz | 245 | 0 | 58 |
| **Couscous:** Dry, 1 oz | 110 | 0 | 22 |
| Cooked, 1 cup, 5.5 oz | 175 | 0.5 | 37 |
| **Farina:** Dry, ½ cup, 3 oz | 325 | 0.5 | 69 |
| Cooked, ½ cup, 4 oz | 55 | 0 | 12 |
| **Flaxseed:** Whole, 1 T., 0.3 oz | 45 | 3.5 | 2 |
| Ground, 2 Tbsp, 0.3 oz | 60 | 4.5 | 4 |
| **Garbanzo,** (Chick Pea), ½ cup, 1.6 oz | 180 | 3 | 27 |
| **Gluten Free Flour,** 3 Tbsp | 100 | 0 | 24 |
| **Hemp Flour,** Wholemeal, ½ cup, 3.5 oz | 300 | 10 | 5 |
| **Matzo Meal,** ½ cup, 2.2 oz | 230 | 0.5 | 48 |
| **Millet:** Raw, ½ cup, 3.5 oz | 380 | 4 | 73 |
| Cooked, ½ cup, 3 oz | 105 | 1 | 21 |
| **Oat Bran:** Raw, ⅓ cup, 1 oz | 75 | 2 | 21 |
| Cooked, ½ cup, 3.8 oz | 45 | 1 | 13 |
| **Oats,** Rolled/Oatmeal: | | | |
| Dry/Groats, ½ cup, 1.5 oz | 160 | 3 | 28 |
| Cooked, ½ cup, 4.2 oz | 75 | 1 | 13 |
| **Polenta** ~ *See Cornmeal* | | | |
| **Potato Flour,** ½ cup, 2.8 oz | 285 | 0.5 | 66 |
| **Psyllium Husks,** 1 Tbsp, 0.2 oz | 10 | 0 | 4 |
| **Quinoa:** Dry, ½ cup, 3 oz | 320 | 5 | 59 |
| Cooked, ½ cup, 3.8 oz | 130 | 2 | 24 |
| **Rice Bran,** ½ cup, 2 oz | 180 | 12 | 28 |
| **Rice Flour,** ½ cup, 2.8 oz | 290 | 1 | 63 |

## Flours & Grains (Cont)

| | C | F | Cb |
|---|---|---|---|
| **Rice Polish,** ½ cup, 3.5 oz | 360 | 0.5 | 80 |
| **Rye Flour:** | | | |
| Dark, ½ cup, 2.3 oz | 210 | 2 | 44 |
| Light, ½ cup, 1.8 oz | 190 | 1 | 41 |
| Medium, ½ cup, 1.8 oz | 180 | 1 | 40 |
| **Rye Grain:** ½ cup, 3 oz | 280 | 2 | 59 |
| Flakes, ¼ cup, 1 oz | 100 | 0.5 | 21 |
| **Semolina Flour,** ½ cup, 3 oz | 300 | 1 | 61 |
| **Sorghum,** ½ cup, 3.4 oz | 325 | 3 | 72 |
| **Soy Flour:** | | | |
| Defatted, 1 cup, 3.5 oz | 330 | 1 | 38 |
| Low-Fat, 1 cup, 3 oz | 325 | 6 | 33 |
| Full-Fat, 1 cup, 3 oz | 365 | 17 | 29 |
| **Soy Meal,** defatted, 1 cup, 4.3 oz | 415 | 3 | 49 |
| **Spelt Flour,** ½ cup, 2 oz | 190 | 1 | 41 |
| **Tapioca Pearl:** | | | |
| Dry, ½ cup, 2.7 oz | 270 | 0 | 67 |
| 3 Tbsp, 1 oz | 100 | 0 | 25 |
| **Teff Seed Flour,** 2 oz | 215 | 2 | 42 |
| **Tortilla Flour Mix,** ½ cup, 2 oz | 220 | 6 | 37 |
| **Triticale:** | | | |
| ½ cup, 3.4 oz | 325 | 2 | 70 |
| Flour, wholegrain, ½ cup, 2.3 oz | 220 | 1 | 48 |
| **Wheat Bran,** unprocessed, ½ cup, 1 oz | 65 | 1 | 19 |
| **Wheat Flakes,** ½ cup, 1.5 oz | 160 | 1 | 35 |
| **Wheat Germ:** | | | |
| Raw, ¼ cup, 1 oz | 105 | 3 | 15 |
| Toasted, ¼ cup, 1 oz | 110 | 3 | 14 |
| **Wheat Flour:** | | | |
| White, All Purpose/Self-Rising: | | | |
| 1 level Tbsp, 0.3 oz | 30 | 0 | 6 |
| ½ cup, 2.2 oz | 230 | 0.5 | 48 |
| 1 cup, 4.4 oz | 455 | 1.5 | 95 |
| Whole Wheat, 1 cup, 4.2 oz | 405 | 2 | 87 |

FRUIT TIME

## Fruit ~ Fresh

| | C | F | Cb |
|---|---|---|---|
| *Weights As Purchased* | | | |
| **Apples,** all varieties, average: | | | |
| Whole, with skin: | | | |
| 1 small, 4 oz | 55 | 0 | 14 |
| 1 medium, 5.5 oz | 75 | 0 | 19 |
| 1 large, 8 oz | 110 | 0 | 28 |
| 1 extra large, 11 oz | 145 | 0 | 36 |
| Flesh only, no skin or core: 1 oz | 15 | 0 | 3.5 |
| Slices, 1 cup, 4 oz | 55 | 0 | 14 |
| Candy/Caramel Apple, 1 med., 6.5 oz | 245 | 4 | 54 |
| *Chiquita,* Apple Bites, 14 slices, 5 oz | 80 | 0 | 20 |
| **Apricots:** 1 small, 1.5oz | 20 | 0 | 4 |
| 1 medium, 2 oz | 25 | 0 | 6 |
| 1 large, 3 oz | 40 | 0 | 10 |
| 1 extra large, 4 oz | 50 | 0 | 12 |
| **Asian Pear,** (Nashi Fruit), 1 med., 7 oz | 85 | 0 | 21 |
| **Avocado:** | | | |
| Fuerte (Florida) variety: | | | |
| ¼ medium, 2.7 oz pulp | 90 | 7.5 | 6 |
| ½ medium, 5.4 oz pulp | 180 | 15 | 12 |
| Mashed, 2 Tbsp, 1 oz | 35 | 3 | 2 |
| Hass variety (Californian/Mexican): | | | |
| Cubes, ½ cup, 2.5 oz | 120 | 11 | 6 |
| Mashed: 2 Tbsp, 1 oz | 50 | 4 | 2 |
| ¼ cup, 2 oz | 95 | 8 | 5 |
| Pulp: ¼ medium, 1.5 oz | 70 | 6.5 | 3 |
| ½ medium, 3 oz | 140 | 13 | 7 |
| 1 medium (8.5 oz whole), 6 oz | 280 | 26 | 14 |
| Salad slices (3), 1 oz | 50 | 4 | 2 |

Note: The fat of avocados is heart-healthy. Avocados are very low in carbs ~ most is fiber. This benefits blood sugar and cholesterol levels. Use in place of butter and other high-fat spreads.

| | C | F | Cb |
|---|---|---|---|
| **Banana:** | | | |
| Weight with skin: | | | |
| 1 baby, 3 oz | 50 | 0 | 12 |
| 1 small (5″), 4 oz | 65 | 0 | 16 |
| 1 medium (7″), 5 oz | 80 | 0 | 20 |
| 1 large (8″), 8 oz | 120 | 0 | 30 |
| 1 extra large (9″), 9 oz | 135 | 0 | 34 |
| Flesh only, weight without skin: | | | |
| Mashed, ½ cup, 4 oz | 100 | 0 | 25 |
| Slices, ½ cup, 2.5 oz | 65 | 0 | 16 |
| Green Bananas, weight with skin: | | | |
| 1 medium (7″), 5 oz | 75 | 0 | 18 |
| 1 large (8″), 7 oz | 110 | 0 | 27 |
| **Blackberries,** 1 cup, 5 oz | 60 | 0.5 | 14 |
| **Blueberries:** ¼ cup, 1 oz | 15 | 0 | 4 |
| 1 cup or ½ pint container, 5 oz | 80 | 0 | 20 |
| 1 pint container, 10 oz | 160 | 0 | 40 |

| *Weights As Purchased* | C | F | Cb |
|---|---|---|---|
| **Boysenberries,** 1 cup, 4.5 oz | 60 | 4.5 | 14 |
| **Breadfruit,** ½ cup, 4 oz | 115 | 0 | 30 |
| **Cactus Fruit:** | | | |
| 1 small, 2 oz | 15 | 0 | 4 |
| 1 medium, 5 oz | 40 | 0 | 9 |
| 1 large, 7 oz | 55 | 0 | 13 |
| Pulp, no skin, 1 cup, 5.3 oz | 60 | 0 | 14 |
| **Cantaloupe:** Flesh, without skin, 1 oz | 10 | 0 | 2 |
| Pieces/Balls, 1 cup, 5.5 oz | 55 | 0 | 13 |
| Slices, ½ circle, without rind: | | | |
| 1 thin (buffet), ⅛″, 0.5 oz | 5 | 0 | 1 |
| 1 medium (¼″), 1 oz | 10 | 0 | 2 |
| 1 thick (½″), 2 oz | 20 | 0 | 5 |
| Wedges, length cut, without skin: | | | |
| 1 thin, 1⁄16 medium, 2 oz | 20 | 0 | 5 |
| 1 thick, ⅛ medium, 4 oz | 40 | 0 | 9 |
| Whole, weight with seeds and skin: | | | |
| ½ small, 20 oz | 195 | 1 | 46 |
| ½ medium, 28 oz | 270 | 1.5 | 65 |
| ½ large, 2.5 lb | 370 | 2 | 90 |
| **Cape Gooseberries,** 1 cup, 5 oz | 70 | 1 | 15 |
| **Cherimoya:** Pulp, ½ cup, 3 oz | 60 | 0 | 14 |
| 1 Fruit (11 oz), 8 oz edible | 170 | 1 | 40 |
| **Cherries,** (Red/White), sweet, raw: | | | |
| 6 medium or 4 large, 2 oz | 30 | 0 | 7 |
| 1 cup, 4.5 oz | 75 | 0 | 18 |
| ½ lb quantity | 130 | 0 | 32 |
| Sour, red, raw, 1 cup, 4 oz | 50 | 0 | 12 |
| **Clementine,** 1 medium, 2.6 oz | 35 | 0 | 9 |
| **Coconut,** raw: | | | |
| Young, sweet, | | | |
| Pieces: 1 piece (2″ x 2″), 1.5 oz | 35 | 2 | 4 |
| ½ cup, 3.5 oz | 80 | 5 | 9 |
| Mature, hard, 1 piece (2″x 2″), 1.5 oz | 160 | 15 | 6 |
| **Crabapples,** slices, ½ cup, 2 oz | 40 | 0 | 11 |
| **Cranberries,** | | | |
| fresh, ¼ cup, 1 oz | 25 | 0 | 6.5 |
| **Custard Apple** ~ *See Cherimoya* | | | |
| **Dates:** Medium (1), 0.3 oz | 20 | 0 | 5 |
| Large Medjool (1), 0.5 oz | 40 | 0 | 10 |
| Extra Large Medjool (1), 0.9 oz | 65 | 0 | 16 |
| Chopped, ½ cup, 3 oz | 240 | 0 | 58 |
| **Dragon Fruit,** (Pitahaya): | | | |
| 1 medium, 4″long, 12 oz | 60 | 0 | 12 |
| 1 large, 5″long, 16 oz | 80 | 0 | 18 |
| **Durian,** pulp, 4 oz | 165 | 6 | 31 |
| **Elderberries,** ½ cup, 2.5 oz | 55 | 0.5 | 13 |

| Weights As Purchased | C | F | Cb |
|---|---|---|---|
| **Feijoa,** (Pineapple Guava), 1 medium, 2 oz | 30 | 0.5 | 5.5 |
| **Figs,** green/black: | | | |
| 1 medium, 2 oz | 40 | 0 | 10 |
| 1 large, 3 oz | 60 | 0 | 15 |
| **Gooseberries,** raw, 1 cup, 5 oz | 65 | 1 | 15 |
| **Grapefruit,** all varieties, average: | | | |
| ½ fruit, 10 oz (6 oz flesh) | 55 | 0 | 13 |
| 1 cup sections w/ juice, 8 oz | 75 | 0 | 18 |
| **Grapes:** Average, 1 cup, 5.5 oz | 105 | 0 | 28 |
| 1 small bunch, 4 oz | 80 | 0 | 20 |
| 1 medium bunch, 7 oz | 140 | 0 | 36 |
| 1 large bunch, 16 oz | 315 | 0 | 82 |
| **Granadilla,** pulp, ½ cup, 4 oz | 110 | 0 | 27 |
| **Guanabana,** pulp, ½ cup, 4 oz | 75 | 0 | 19 |
| **Guava,** 1 medium, 4 oz | 80 | 1 | 16 |
| **Honeydew:** | | | |
| 1 slice, ¾" thick, 3 oz | 30 | 0 | 7 |
| 1 wedge, (⅛ of 7" diameter), 12 oz (with rind) | 80 | 0 | 20 |
| Cubes/Balls, 1 cup, 6 oz | 60 | 0 | 14 |
| ½ small (4½ lb whole) | 180 | 0.5 | 42 |
| ½ medium (6 lb whole) | 230 | 1 | 56 |
| **Honey Murcots,** 1 only, 5 oz | 45 | 0 | 11 |
| **Jaboticaba,** 1 cup, 5.5 oz | 55 | 0 | 14 |
| **Jackfruit,** flesh, ⅛, 4 oz | 105 | 0 | 27 |
| **Kiwano,** ½ medium, 5 oz | 35 | 0 | 8 |
| **Kiwifruit:** | | | |
| 1 Medium, 2.7 oz | 45 | 0 | 11 |
| 1 Large, 3.2 oz | 55 | 0 | 13 |
| **Langsat,** Duku, 1 medium, 2 oz | 25 | 0 | 5 |
| **Lemons:** 1 medium, 5oz | 20 | 0 | 4 |
| 1 wedge, 1 oz | 5 | 0 | 1 |
| **Limes,** 1 medium, 2.4 oz | 20 | 0 | 7 |
| **Loganberries,** frozen, ½ cup, 2.5 oz | 40 | 0 | 9 |
| **Longans,** 5 fruit, 0.5oz | 10 | 0 | 2.5 |
| **Loquats,** 4 fruit, 2.3 oz | 30 | 0 | 8 |
| **Lychees,** 4 fruit, 2.3 oz | 30 | 0 | 7 |
| **Mamey Apple,** cubes, 1 cup, 6 oz | 85 | 1 | 20 |
| **Mandarin Orange:** | | | |
| 1 small, 3 oz | 35 | 0 | 9 |
| 1 medium, 4 oz | 45 | 0 | 11 |
| 1 large, 6 oz | 50 | 0 | 13 |
| **Mango:** | | | |
| Slices, ½ cup, 3 oz | 55 | 0 | 14 |
| 1 small mango, 7 oz | 90 | 0.5 | 24 |
| 1 medium: 10 oz | 130 | 0.5 | 34 |
| Side cheek, 4 oz | 60 | 0 | 14 |
| 1 large, 17 oz | 220 | 1 | 58 |
| 1 extra large, 24 oz | 310 | 1.5 | 82 |
| **Marionberries,** 1 cup, 5 oz | 75 | 1 | 15 |

| Weights As Purchased | C | F | Cb |
|---|---|---|---|
| **Melons,** all varieties, average, cubes/balls, 1 cup, 6 oz | 60 | 0 | 14 |
| **Mulberries,** 20 fruit, 1 oz | 15 | 0 | 3 |
| **Nashi Fruit/Asian Pear,** 1 med. 7 oz | 85 | 0 | 21 |
| **Nectarines:** 1 medium, 5oz | 60 | 0 | 14 |
| 1 large, 7 oz | 80 | 0 | 18 |
| **Oheloberries,** ½ cup, 2.5 oz | 20 | 0 | 5 |
| **Olives,** Pickled: Green, 10 lge, 1.5 oz | 60 | 6.5 | 1.5 |
| Ripe, Greek Style, 10 medium, 1 oz | 70 | 6 | 4 |
| Ripe (Black) Californian: | | | |
| 1 small/medium | 5 | 0 | 0.2 |
| 1 large/extra large | 6 | 0.5 | 0.5 |
| 1 jumbo | 7 | 0.5 | 0.5 |
| 1 colossal | 11 | 1 | 0.5 |
| **Oranges,** all varieties, average, weights with skin: | | | |
| 1 small, (2.5" diam.), 5 oz | 45 | 0 | 11 |
| 1 medium (3") 7 oz | 75 | 0 | 18 |
| 1 large, (3.5") 10 oz | 105 | 0 | 25 |
| 1 extra large, (4"), 14 oz | 130 | 0 | 30 |
| Flesh/Pulp only, 1 cup, 6 oz | 85 | 0 | 21 |
| Peel, 1 Tbsp | 0 | 0 | 0 |
| California Navel (3"), 7 oz | 70 | 0 | 17 |
| California Valencia, 1 medium (2¾" diam.) 6 oz | 60 | 0 | 14 |
| Florida Orange, 1 med., 7 oz | 70 | 0 | 17 |
| Sunkist Navel, large, 14 oz | 130 | 0 | 30 |
| **Papaya:** | | | |
| 1" pieces, 1 cup, 5 oz | 60 | 0 | 15 |
| 1 medium, 16 oz | 120 | 0 | 30 |
| Green (unripe), ½ cup, 3.5 oz | 20 | 0 | 5 |
| **Passionfruit:** | | | |
| 1 small, 1.5 oz | 15 | 0 | 3 |
| 1 large, 2.7 oz | 30 | 0 | 6 |
| Pulp, ½ cup, 4 oz | 110 | 0 | 27 |
| **Peaches:** 1 baby/donut, 3 oz | 30 | 0 | 7 |
| 1 small, 5 oz | 50 | 0 | 12 |
| 1 medium, 6 oz | 60 | 0 | 14 |
| 1 large, 7 oz | 70 | 0 | 16 |
| 1 extra large, 9 oz | 90 | 0 | 21 |
| **Pears,** all varieties, average: | | | |
| 1 mini, 2.5 oz | 35 | 0 | 8 |
| 1 small, 5 oz | 75 | 0 | 18 |
| 1 medium, 7 oz | 100 | 0 | 25 |
| 1 large, 9 oz | 130 | 0 | 33 |
| 1 extra large, 12 oz | 170 | 0 | 42 |
| **Pepino,** ½ medium, 4 oz | 20 | 0 | 4 |
| **Persimmons:** Native, 1 oz | 35 | 0 | 9 |
| Japanese (2½"d. x 2½"h), 7 oz | 120 | 0 | 30 |
| Maui, seedless, 1 medium, 5 oz | 100 | 0 | 25 |

| Weights As Purchased | C | F | Cb |
|---|---|---|---|
| **Pineapple,** average all varieties: | | | |
| Weights without skin: | | | |
| 1 thin slice (½"), 2 oz | 30 | 0 | 7 |
| 1 thick slice (¾"), 3 oz | 40 | 0 | 10 |
| 1 cup, chunks, 6 oz | 80 | 0 | 20 |
| Whole fruit, wt with skin: | | | |
| Baby/Mini, 16 oz | 150 | 0 | 39 |
| Medium size, 3 lbs | 450 | 1 | 118 |
| **Canned ~** *See Page 102* | | | |
| **Pitanga,** (Surinam-Cherry) (5), 1.2 oz | 10 | 0 | 2 |
| **Plaintain:** | | | |
| Fresh/Raw, weight with skin: | | | |
| 1 medium, 10 oz | 220 | 0 | 55 |
| Slices, 1 cup, 5 oz | 180 | 0 | 44 |
| Cooked: | | | |
| Mashed, ½ cup, 3.5 oz | 115 | 0 | 30 |
| Slices, 1 cup, 5.5 oz | 180 | 0 | 47 |
| Fried in oil: 10 slices (¼"), 2 oz | 160 | 6 | 26 |
| 1 cup, 4.2 oz | 360 | 14 | 58 |
| **Plums,** all varieties, average: | | | |
| 1 mini/Damson, (1" diam), 0.5 oz | 10 | 0 | 1.5 |
| 1 small (2"), 2.3oz | 30 | 0 | 7 |
| 1 medium (2½"), 3.5 oz | 45 | 0 | 10 |
| 1 large (3"), 5 oz | 60 | 0 | 14 |
| **Plumcot,** 1 medium, 6 oz | 75 | 0 | 18 |
| **Pomegranate:** | | | |
| 1 small (3"), 5.5 oz | 70 | 1 | 15 |
| 1 medium (3½"), 10 oz | 125 | 2 | 27 |
| 1 large (4"), 16 oz | 230 | 3 | 50 |
| Seeds/Arils, ¼ cup, 2 oz | 40 | 1 | 10 |
| **Pomelo,** flesh, ½ cup, 3.5 oz | 35 | 0 | 9 |
| **Prickly Pear ~** *See Cactus Fruit* | | | |
| **Quince,** 1 medium, 3.5 oz | 55 | 0 | 14 |
| **Rambutan/Rambotang,** | | | |
| Red/Yellow, medium, 2 oz | 15 | 0 | 4 |
| **Raspberries:** ½ cup, 2 oz | 30 | 0 | 7 |
| 10 raspberries, 0.8 oz | 10 | 0 | 2 |
| 1 cup, 4.3 oz | 65 | 1 | 15 |
| 1 pint, 11 oz | 160 | 2 | 37 |
| **Sapodilla:** 1 medium, 6 oz | 140 | 2 | 34 |
| Pulp, 1 cup, 8.5 oz | 200 | 2.5 | 45 |
| **Sapote:** | | | |
| Black: 1 medium, 4.5 oz | 60 | 0 | 14 |
| Pulp only, ½ cup, 4 oz | 100 | 1 | 22 |
| Mamey, 1 cup, 6 oz | 220 | 1 | 50 |
| **Satsuma Tangerine,** 1 medium, 3 oz | 45 | 0 | 11 |
| **Soursop,** pulp, 1 cup, 8 oz | 150 | 0.5 | 38 |
| **Starfruit,** (Carambola): | | | |
| 1 medium, (3½" long), 3 oz | 30 | 0 | 6 |
| 1 large (4½"), 4.5 oz | 40 | 0 | 8 |
| **Strawberries:** 1 cup, 5.5 oz | 50 | 0.5 | 12 |
| 6 medium/3 large, 2 oz | 20 | 0 | 4 |
| 1 pint container, heaping, 16 oz | 130 | 1 | 32 |
| Chocolate dipped, 1 large | 45 | 2.5 | 6 |

| Weights As Purchased | C | F | Cb |
|---|---|---|---|
| **Sugar-Apple (Sweetsop),** | | | |
| pulp, ½ cup, 4 oz | 120 | 0 | 28 |
| **Sugar Cane:** | | | |
| Unpeeled, 1 baton (7" long), 4 oz | 30 | 0 | 7 |
| Peeled, 1 small stick (3"), 2 oz | 35 | 0 | 8 |
| **Tamarillo,** 1 medium, 3 oz | 20 | 0 | 3 |
| **Tamarind:** 1 fruit (3"x1") | 5 | 0 | 1.5 |
| Pulp, ½ cup, 2 oz | 140 | 0.5 | 37 |
| **Tangelo:** 1 small, 4 oz | 55 | 0 | 13 |
| 1 medium, 5 oz | 70 | 0 | 17 |
| 1 large, 7 oz | 95 | 0 | 23 |
| **Tangerine,** 1 med., (2½" diam.), 4 oz | 50 | 0 | 13 |
| **Tangor,** 1 medium, 4 oz | 35 | 0 | 7 |
| **Tomatillos:** | | | |
| 3 medium, 3.5 oz | 35 | 0.5 | 6 |
| 1lb (16 oz) quantity | 160 | 2 | 27 |
| **Tomatoes:** | | | |
| 1 small (2¼" diameter), 3 oz | 15 | 0 | 3 |
| 1 medium (2¾"), 5 oz | 25 | 0 | 5 |
| Sliced: 2 thin slices, 1 oz | 5 | 0 | 1 |
| 2 thick (⅜"), 2 oz | 10 | 0 | 2 |
| Wedge, ¼, 1.3 oz | 6 | 0 | 1 |
| 1 large (3½"), 8 oz | 40 | 0.5 | 9 |
| 1 extra large (4"), 12 oz | 60 | 0.5 | 14 |
| Cherry: 4 medium, 2 oz | 10 | 0 | 2 |
| 1 cup, 5 oz | 25 | 0 | 6 |
| Grape, 5 medium, 2 oz | 10 | 0 | 2 |
| Yellow Tear Drop, 3 medium, 1 oz | 5 | 0 | 2 |
| **Canned Tomatoes/Products ~** *See Page 144* | | | |
| **Tree Tomato/Tamarillo,** 3 oz | 20 | 0 | 5 |
| **Ugli Fruit,** Tangelo type, 5 oz | 40 | 0 | 8 |
| **Watermelon:** | | | |
| Flesh only, weights without skin: | | | |
| 1 thin slice (½"), ¼ circle, 3 oz | 25 | 0 | 6 |
| 1 thick slice (1"): ¼ circle, 6 oz | 50 | 0 | 12 |
| ½ circle, 12 oz | 100 | 1 | 24 |
| Buffet Slice, small, thin, 1 oz | 8 | 0 | 2 |
| Cubes or Balls, 1 cup, 5.5 oz | 45 | 0 | 11 |
| Round Seedless Melon, weight with skin: | | | |
| Medium size, 13 lb, (8" diam.): | | | |
| whole melon, 13 lb | 1160 | 5 | 280 |
| wedge, ⅛ whole, 26 oz | 145 | 1 | 35 |
| Mini size, 6 lb, (6.5" diam.): | | | |
| whole melon, 6 lb | 480 | 2.5 | 110 |
| wedge, ⅛ whole, 12 oz | 60 | 0 | 14 |

## Dried Fruit

|  | C | F | Cb |
|---|---|---|---|
| **Apples,** 5 rings, 1 oz | 80 | 0 | 19 |
| **Apricots,** 8 halves, 1 oz | 65 | 0 | 16 |
| **Banana Chips,** ⅓ cup, 1 oz | 180 | 9 | 16 |
| **Banana Flakes,** 4 Tbsp, 1 oz | 80 | 0 | 20 |
| **Cranberries** *(Craisins):* | | | |
| Original, ¼ cup | 130 | 0 | 33 |
| Reduced Sugar, ¼ cup | 100 | 0 | 31 |
| Chocolate Covered, ¼ cup, 2 oz | 180 | 8 | 28 |
| **Dates** ~ *See Dates in Fresh Fruit* | | | |
| **Figs,** 3 medium figs, 1 oz | 90 | 0 | 23 |
| **Goji Berries,** 3 Tbsp, 1 oz | 100 | 0 | 21 |
| **Mango Slices,** 5 pieces, 1.4 oz | 25 | 0 | 6 |
| **Papaya Spears,** 2 pieces, 1.4 oz | 120 | 0 | 30 |
| **Peaches,** 2 halves, 1 oz | 60 | 0 | 15 |
| **Pears,** 3 halves, 2 oz | 140 | 0.5 | 34 |
| **Plums** *(Sunsweet),* (5), 1.4 oz | 100 | 0 | 24 |
| **Prunes/Dried Plums:** | | | |
| with pits, 3 medium, 1 oz | 70 | 0 | 17 |
| without pits, 4 medium, 1 oz | 70 | 0 | 17 |
| Cooked: with sugar, ½ cup, 5 oz | 155 | 0 | 38 |
| without sugar, ½ cup, 4.5 oz | 135 | 0 | 33 |
| **Raisins:** 2 Tbsp, 1 oz pack | 85 | 0 | 22 |
| ½ cup, (unpacked), 2.5 oz | 215 | 0 | 56 |
| **White Mulberries,** 1 oz | 90 | 0.5 | 22 |

## Candied/Glazed Fruit

|  | C | F | Cb |
|---|---|---|---|
| **Apricot,** 1 medium, 1 oz | 70 | 0 | 17 |
| **Cherry,** Maraschino (1) | 8 | 0 | 2 |
| **Citron/Fruit Peel,** 1 oz | 85 | 0 | 20 |
| **Ginger,** 1 oz | 90 | 0 | 21 |
| **Pineapple,** 1 slice, 1.3 oz | 120 | 0 | 29 |
| **Tamarind,** dried, sweetened, 1 oz | 70 | 0 | 17 |

## Fruit Leather Rolls

|  | C | F | Cb |
|---|---|---|---|
| *Betty Crocker:* Fruit By The Foot, | | | |
| 1 roll, 0.8 oz | 80 | 0 | 17 |
| Fruit Gushers, 1 oz | 90 | 1 | 20 |
| Fruit Roll-Ups, 1 roll | 50 | 1 | 12 |
| *Stretch Island,* Leathers, 1 pouch, 0.5 oz | 45 | 0 | 12 |

## Canned/Bottled Fruit

*Solids & Liquids:*
*Per ½ Cup, 4½ oz Unless indicated*

|  | C | F | Cb |
|---|---|---|---|
| **Apricots/Peaches/Pears:** | | | |
| in juice, light | 60 | 0 | 15 |
| in heavy syrup | 105 | 0 | 28 |
| in water/diet | 35 | 0 | 8 |
| **Black/Blueberries:** | | | |
| in heavy syrup | 120 | 0 | 30 |
| in light syrup | 110 | 0 | 26 |

## Canned/Bottled Fruit (Cont)

|  | C | F | Cb |
|---|---|---|---|
| **Cherries,** pitted: | | | |
| in heavy syrup | 105 | 0 | 27 |
| in light syrup | 85 | 0 | 22 |
| in water | 55 | 0 | 15 |
| Maraschino, 1 oz | 50 | 0 | 12 |
| **Fruit Cocktail/Salad:** | | | |
| in heavy syrup | 95 | 0 | 25 |
| in juice, light | 60 | 0 | 16 |
| in water/diet | 35 | 0 | 10 |
| **Gooseberries,** light syrup | 90 | 0 | 24 |
| **Grapefruit,** in light syrup | 75 | 0 | 20 |
| **Lychees,** ½ cup, 4.5 oz | 105 | 0 | 26 |
| **Mixed Fruit:** in fruit juices/light syrup | 70 | 0 | 18 |
| in heavy syrup | 90 | 0 | 24 |
| in water/diet | 40 | 0 | 10 |
| **Pineapple,** all varieties: | | | |
| in heavy syrup, 4.3 oz | 110 | 0 | 26 |
| in own juice, 4 oz | 60 | 0 | 15 |
| **Prunes:** with syrup, 3 oz | 90 | 0 | 23 |
| Stewed in water, ½ cup | 135 | 0 | 35 |

## Fruit Snack Cups

|  | C | F | Cb |
|---|---|---|---|
| **Deli/Take-Out:** Small, 6 oz | 70 | 0 | 16 |
| Large, 12 oz | 140 | 0 | 32 |
| Yogurt and Fruit Cup, 15 oz | 380 | 4.5 | 75 |
| **Del Monte:** | | | |
| **Fruit & Veggie Fusions,** all flav., 4 oz | 70 | 0 | 17 |
| **Fruit Refreshers,** average, 7 oz | 95 | 0 | 24 |
| **Fruit Snack Cups in Gel,** av., 4.5 oz | 80 | 0 | 20 |
| **Light Fruit Cups,** in Gel, av., 4.5 oz | 50 | 0 | 12 |
| **Dole:** | | | |
| **Fruit Bowls In 100% Juice:** *Per 4 oz Container* | | | |
| Diced Pears | 90 | 0 | 22 |
| Mixed Fruit | 80 | 0 | 19 |
| **Fruit in Gel:** *Per 4.3 oz Container* | | | |
| Mixed Fruit, in Black Cherry Gel | 90 | 0 | 24 |
| Average other fruits, in various Gels | 95 | 0 | 24 |

## Apple & Fruit Sauces

|  | C | F | Cb |
|---|---|---|---|
| **Apple Sauce:** | | | |
| Regular/sweetened, 2 Tbsp, 1 oz | 20 | 0 | 6 |
| 4 oz package | 90 | 0 | 22 |
| **Cranberry,** Jellied, ¼ cup | 110 | 0 | 25 |
| **Fruit Sauces & Purees:** | | | |
| All fruit types, average: 2 Tbsp, 1 oz | 25 | 0 | 6 |
| ½ cup, 4 oz | 100 | 0 | 24 |
| **Mott's:** | | | |
| **Apple Sauce:** Orig., sweetened, 4 oz | 90 | 0 | 24 |
| Other Fruit Flavors, sweetened, 4 oz | 90 | 0 | 23 |
| Unsweetened Apple, 3.9 oz | 50 | 0 | 13 |
| **Ocean Spray,** | | | |
| Jellied Cranberry Sce, 3.5 oz | 160 | 0 | 40 |

## Quick Guide    **C**  **F**  **Cb**

### Ice Cream
*Average all Flavors:*

**Regular (10% fat):**
*Examples: Dreyer's Grand, Hood, Friendly's*

| | | C | F | Cb |
|---|---|---|---|---|
| ½ cup, 4 fl.oz |  | 140 | 7 | 16 |
| 1 cup, 8 fl.oz | | 280 | 14 | 32 |
| 1 pint, 16 fl.oz | | 560 | 28 | 64 |

**Rich/Premium (16-17% fat):**
*Examples: Baskin Robbins, Ben & Jerry's, Haagen-Dazs*

| | | | | |
|---|---|---|---|---|
| ½ cup, 4 fl.oz |  | 250 | 16 | 24 |
| 1 cup, 8 fl.oz | | 500 | 32 | 48 |
| 1 pint, 16 fl.oz | | 1000 | 64 | 96 |

**Reduced-Fat/Light (5% fat):**
*Examples: Breyers ½ The Fat, Friendly's Light, Hood Light*

| | | | | |
|---|---|---|---|---|
| ½ cup, 4 fl.oz |  | 140 | 5 | 21 |
| 1 cup, 8 fl.oz | | 280 | 10 | 42 |
| 1 pint, 16 fl.oz | | 560 | 20 | 84 |

**Fat-Free:**
*Example: Breyers*

| | | | | |
|---|---|---|---|---|
| ½ cup, 4 fl.oz | | 90 | 0 | 21 |
| 1 cup, 8 fl.oz | | 180 | 0 | 42 |
| 1 pint, 16 fl.oz | | 360 | 0 | 84 |

**Scoop Shops:**
*Average all Brands*
Add extra for cone (see next column)

| | | | |
|---|---|---|---|
| **Kids,** 3 fl.oz | 125 | 8 | 12 |
| **Regular,** 6 fl.oz | 250 | 16 | 24 |
| **Large,** 9 fl.oz | 375 | 24 | 36 |

**Soft Serve:**
*Average all Brands*

| | | | | |
|---|---|---|---|---|
| **Regular:** ½ cup, 4 fl.oz |  | 255 | 15 | 25 |
| 1 cup, 8 fl.oz | | 510 | 30 | 50 |
| **Light:** ½ cup, 4 fl.oz | | 145 | 3 | 25 |
| 1 cup, 8 fl.oz | | 290 | 6 | 50 |

## Quick Guide

### Frozen Yogurt
*Average all Brands*

| | | | | |
|---|---|---|---|---|
| **Hard:** Low-Fat, ½ cup |  | 110 | 3 | 19 |
| Non-Fat, ½ cup | | 110 | 0 | 24 |
| **Soft:** Low-Fat, ½ cup | | 120 | 4 | 17 |
| Non-Fat, ½ cup | | 100 | 0 | 30 |

**Brands** ~ *See Ice Cream & Novelties Section*

## Quick Guide    **C**  **F**  **Cb**

### Gelato/Ices/Frozen Custard

**Gelato:** *Per ½ Cup*

| | | C | F | Cb |
|---|---|---|---|---|
| Milk base: Vanilla |  | 160 | 6 | 25 |
| Chocolate Hazelnut | | 230 | 15 | 21 |
| Water base, ½ cup | | 100 | 0 | 26 |

**Frozen Custard,** Choc./Vanilla, av:

| | | | |
|---|---|---|---|
| ½ cup | 210 | 11 | 23 |
| Single Scoop, 5 oz wt | 300 | 15 | 38 |
| Double Scoop, 10 oz wt | 600 | 30 | 76 |

**Ice (Milk base):** *Average all flavors*

| | | | |
|---|---|---|---|
| Hard (4% fat), ½ cup | 100 | 3 | 15 |
| Soft Serve (3% fat), ½ cup | 110 | 2 | 19 |
| **Shaved Ice,** average, 12 fl.oz | 160 | 0 | 40 |
| **Sherbet,** average, ½ cup | 110 | 1.5 | 22 |
| **Sorbet,** Fruit, fat free, ½ cup | 70 | 0 | 19 |
| **Fruit Ice Pops** | 80 | 0 | 20 |

### Sundaes

**Baskin Robbins:**

| | | | |
|---|---|---|---|
| **Classic:** Banana Royale | 690 | 28 | 103 |
| Brownie | 810 | 42 | 99 |
| Made with Snickers | 1060 | 43 | 155 |

**Denny's,** Chocolate, 2 scoops,

| | | | |
|---|---|---|---|
| with Caramel Topping & wh. cream | 665 | 33 | 85 |

**Toppings** ~ *See Page 195*

**McDonald's:** *Includes Nut Topping*

**Sundaes:**

| | | | |
|---|---|---|---|
| Hot Caramel | 380 | 12 | 61 |
| Hot Fudge | 380 | 14 | 53 |
| Strawberry | 320 | 10 | 50 |

### Ice Cream Cones & Cups

*Average all Brands*

| | | | |
|---|---|---|---|
| **Wafer Cone/Cup,** average | 20 | 0 | 4 |
| **Sugar Cone,** average | 50 | 0 | 14 |

**Waffle Cone:**

| | | | |
|---|---|---|---|
| Small | 50 | 1 | 10 |
| Large | 90 | 0.5 | 19 |

**Brands:**

| | | | | |
|---|---|---|---|---|
| *Comet,* Sugar Cone |  | 50 | 0 | 11 |
| *Keebler,* Sugar Cone | | 50 | 0 | 10 |
| *Oreo,* Chocolate Cone | | 50 | 1 | 10 |

## Ice Cream ~ Brands    C   F   Cb

**Baskin-Robbins** ~ *See Fast-Foods Section*

**Ben & Jerry's:**

**Scoop Shop Ice Cream:** *Hand Scooped, 3 oz Serving*

| | C | F | Cb |
|---|---|---|---|
| Americone Dream | 240 | 13 | 26 |
| Bourbon Brown Butter | 240 | 13 | 27 |
| Butter Pecan | 250 | 19 | 17 |
| Choc. Chip Cookie Dough | 230 | 13 | 26 |
| Chocolate Fudge Brownie | 220 | 11 | 26 |
| Chunky Monkey | 240 | 15 | 24 |
| Coconut Seven Layer Bar | 250 | 16 | 24 |
| Coffee, Coffee, BuzzBuzzBuzz | 220 | 13 | 23 |
| Mint Chocolate Chunk | 220 | 14 | 22 |
| New York Super Fudge Chunk | 260 | 17 | 24 |
| Salted Caramel Blondie | 220 | 11 | 26 |
| Strawberry Cheesecake | 200 | 12 | 22 |
| Sweet Cream & Cookies | 210 | 12 | 23 |
| Triple Caramel Chunk | 220 | 12 | 26 |

**Ice Cream, 1 Pint Tubs:** *Per ½ Cup*

| | C | F | Cb |
|---|---|---|---|
| Banana Split | 250 | 14 | 28 |
| Cherry Garcia | 260 | 15 | 27 |
| Chubby Hubby | 350 | 21 | 33 |
| Everything But The | 310 | 19 | 29 |
| Milk & Cookies | 280 | 17 | 28 |
| Red Velvet Cake | 260 | 14 | 29 |
| Salted Caramel Almond | 290 | 17 | 28 |
| S'mores | 310 | 16 | 36 |
| Strawberry Cheesecake | 260 | 15 | 28 |
| Truffle Kerfuffle | 340 | 24 | 28 |
| Vanilla Caramel Fudge | 290 | 16 | 33 |
| Vanilla Toffee Bar Crunch | 300 | 20 | 26 |

**Light Ice Cream, 1 Pint Tubs:** *Per ½ Cup*

| | C | F | Cb |
|---|---|---|---|
| Cherry Garcia with a twist | 140 | 4.5 | 24 |
| Chocolate Cookie EnlightenMint | 160 | 7 | 22 |
| Mocha Fudge Brownie | 150 | 3.5 | 27 |
| P.B. Marshmallow Swirl | 160 | 5 | 25 |

**Non Dairy:** *Per ⅔ Cup*

| | C | F | Cb |
|---|---|---|---|
| Choc. Caramel Cluster | 380 | 22 | 40 |
| Choc. Salted 'n Swirled | 320 | 15 | 44 |
| PB & Cookies | 380 | 22 | 41 |

**Fro Yo Frozen Yogurt:** *Per ½ Cup*

| | C | F | Cb |
|---|---|---|---|
| Cherry Garcia | 170 | 3 | 33 |
| Chocolate Fudge Brownie | 180 | 2.5 | 35 |
| Half Baked | 180 | 3 | 36 |
| Pfish Food, 3.6 oz | 250 | 7 | 42 |

## Blue Bunny:    C   F   Cb

**Premium Ice Cream, 1 Pint Cont:** *Per ½ Cup*

| | C | F | Cb |
|---|---|---|---|
| Banana Split, 2.65 oz | 160 | 7 | 23 |
| Bunny Tracks, 2.6 oz | 190 | 11 | 22 |
| Chocolate, 2.3 oz | 130 | 7 | 17 |
| Cookies 'n Cream, 2.3 oz | 150 | 7 | 20 |
| Mint Chocolate Chip, 2.4 oz | 150 | 8 | 18 |

**Sweet Freedom:** *Per ½ Cup*

| | C | F | Cb |
|---|---|---|---|
| Bunny Tracks, 2.5 oz | 140 | 7 | 24 |
| Butter Pecan, 2.54 oz | 110 | 4.5 | 21 |
| Double Strawberry Swirl, 2.53 oz | 90 | 2.5 | 21 |

*Note: Carbohydrate figures include 4-6 g sugar alcohols*

**Frozen Yogurt:** *Per ½ Cup*

| | C | F | Cb |
|---|---|---|---|
| Strawberry Banana | 100 | 2 | 20 |

**Bars/Pops** ~ *See Page 108*

## Breyers:

**Classics:** *Per ½ Cup*

| | C | F | Cb |
|---|---|---|---|
| Choc. varieties, 2.3 oz | 145 | 7.5 | 18 |
| Natural Strawberry, 2.3 oz | 110 | 5 | 14 |
| Vanilla: Extra Creamy, 2.1 oz | 110 | 3 | 18 |
| Other var., av., 2.3 oz | 135 | 7 | 15 |

| | C | F | Cb |
|---|---|---|---|
| **Carb Smart:** Chocolate; Vanilla, 2 oz | 90 | 5 | 12 |
| Peanut Butter, 2.85 oz | 150 | 9 | 17 |

*Note: Carbohydrate figures include 5g sugar alcohol and 4g fiber*

**Cookies & Candy:** *Per ½ Cup*

| | C | F | Cb |
|---|---|---|---|
| Oreo, 2 oz | 130 | 4.5 | 20 |
| Reeses, 2.3 oz | 150 | 6 | 23 |
| Snickers, 2.5 oz | 150 | 6 | 23 |
| 2 in 1, Snickers & M&M's, 2.3 oz | 140 | 5 | 21 |

**Delights:** *Per ⅔ Cup*

| | C | F | Cb |
|---|---|---|---|
| Caramel Brownie; Cookies & Crm, 3.3 oz | 110 | 3.5 | 24 |
| Creamy Chocolate, 3.2 oz | 90 | 2.5 | 22 |

**No Sugar Added:** *Per ½ Cup*

| | C | F | Cb |
|---|---|---|---|
| Butter Pecan, 2 oz | 100 | 5 | 13 |
| Salted Cararmel Swirl, 2 oz | 90 | 4 | 16 |
| Vanilla Choc. Strawberry, 2 oz | 80 | 3 | 13 |

*Note: Carbohydrate figures include 1-6g sugar alcohol and 0-2g fiber*

**Non Dairy:** *Per ½ cup*

| | C | F | Cb |
|---|---|---|---|
| Oreo, 2.15 oz | 140 | 7 | 19 |
| Van. P'nut Butter, 2.2 oz | 140 | 8 | 16 |

**Gelato:** *Per ½ Cup*

| | C | F | Cb |
|---|---|---|---|
| Raspberry Cheesecake, 2.2 oz | 150 | 5 | 25 |
| Vanilla Caramel, 2.8 oz | 180 | 7 | 27 |

**Bruster's:** *Per Dish*

| | C | F | Cb |
|---|---|---|---|
| **Ice Cream:** Banana; Black Raspb., av., 5 oz | 285 | 14 | 37 |
| Butterscotch Ripple, 5 oz | 310 | 15 | 40 |
| Chocolate Mudslide, 5 oz | 340 | 14 | 49 |

**Fat Free, No Added Sugar:**

| | C | F | Cb |
|---|---|---|---|
| Coffee; Sea Salt Caramel, av., 5 oz | 175 | 0 | 36 |
| Fudge Ripple; Mint with Fudge, 5 oz | 200 | 0 | 43 |
| Vanilla; Caramel Swirl, 5 oz | 170 | 0 | 36 |

## Ice Cream ~ Brands (Cont)　**C**　**F**　**Cb**

**Carvel Ice Cream** ~ *See Fast-Foods Section*
**Coldstone Creamery** ~ *See Fast-Foods Section*
**Dairy Queen/Brazier** ~ *See Fast-Foods Section*
**Dannon:**

| | C | F | Cb |
|---|---|---|---|
| **Gelato,** average all flavors, 2.9 oz | 140 | 6 | 20 |
| **Non Dairy Sorbet:** Choc Fudge 2.9 oz | 110 | 0.5 | 25 |
| Average other flavors, 2.9 oz | 85 | 0 | 22 |
| **YoCream Frozen Yogurt**( Yogurt Shops): *Small 3 oz Cup* | | | |
| Premium, Peanut Butter | 120 | 4 | 19 |
| Custard, Vanilla | 170 | 9 | 18 |
| Low Fat: | | | |
| Chocolate Caramel Turtle | 120 | 1.5 | 25 |
| Cake Batter; Dulce De Leche | 110 | 1.5 | 22 |
| Dutch Choc.; French Vanilla, av. | 115 | 2.5 | 20 |
| Fudge Brownie Batter | 110 | 0.5 | 24 |
| No Sugar Added Nonfat: | | | |
| Cheesecake | 80 | 0 | 18 |
| Praline | 90 | 0 | 18 |
| Raspberry | 80 | 0 | 17 |
| Strawberry Banana | 80 | 0 | 18 |

*Note: Carbohydrate figure includes 0-5g sugar alcohol*

**Dippin' Dots:** *Per ½ Cup*

| **Original Dots:** | | | |
|---|---|---|---|
| Banana Split | 160 | 8 | 20 |
| Brownie Batter | 180 | 9 | 22 |
| Cookies 'n Cream | 180 | 10 | 22 |
| Cool Mint Crunch | 190 | 9 | 24 |
| Cotton Candy | 160 | 9 | 18 |
| Strawberry | 160 | 8 | 18 |
| Vanilla | 160 | 9 | 18 |
| **YoDots:** Cookies 'n Cream | 130 | 3 | 25 |
| Cookie Dough | 140 | 2.5 | 26 |
| Strawberry Cheesecake | 100 | 0 | 21 |

**Dreyer's/Edy's:**

| **Classic Ice Cream:** *Per ½ Cup* | | | |
|---|---|---|---|
| Butter Pecan | 150 | 9 | 16 |
| Chocolate; Coffee | 140 | 7 | 16 |
| Chocolate Peanut Butter Cup | 180 | 10 | 18 |
| Mint Choc. Chip; Mocha Alm. Fudge | 160 | 8 | 19 |
| **Nestle:** Toll House Cookie Dough | 160 | 8 | 21 |
| Drumstick Sundae Cone | 170 | 9 | 19 |
| Rocky Road | 160 | 8 | 20 |
| **Slow Churned Triple Filled:** *Per ½ Cup* | | | |
| Chocolate Fudge Cores | 130 | 3 | 22 |
| Creamy Chocolatey Cores | 110 | 2.5 | 20 |
| Rich Caramel Cores | 160 | 5 | 25 |
| **Slow Churned No Sugar Added:** *Per ½ Cup* | | | |
| Butter Pecan | 120 | 5 | 16 |
| Triple Chocolate | 110 | 3.5 | 17 |
| Vanilla Bean | 100 | 3 | 14 |

**Friendly's:**　**C**　**F**　**Cb**

| **Rich & Creamy Ice Cream:** *Per ½ Cup* | | | |
|---|---|---|---|
| Chocolate Chip Cookie Dough | 160 | 8 | 20 |
| Creamy Vanilla Pineapple | 150 | 7 | 19 |
| Forbidden Chocolate | 150 | 8 | 17 |
| French Vanilla | 140 | 7 | 17 |
| Mint Chocolate Chip | 150 | 8 | 17 |
| Peanut Butter Cup | 210 | 12 | 21 |
| **Light:** *Per ½ Cup* | | | |
| Coffee Toffee Crunch | 140 | 5 | 22 |
| **SundaeXtreme:** *Per ½ Cup* | | | |
| Chocolate Fudge Brownie | 150 | 5 | 25 |
| Choc. Chip Cookie Dough | 170 | 6 | 26 |
| Red Velvet Cake | 150 | 5 | 26 |
| **Sherbet,** Watermelon, ½ cup | 130 | 1.5 | 28 |
| **Yogurt Frozen,** | | | |
| Regular, average, ½ cup | 140 | 4.5 | 23 |

**Gelati-da:**

| **Gelato:** *Per ½ Cup, 4 oz* | | | |
|---|---|---|---|
| Amaretto Chocolate | 150 | 4.5 | 23 |
| Choc Mint Milano | 120 | 2.5 | 22 |
| Coffee Fudge Latte | 130 | 2 | 22 |
| Limoncello; Vanilla Marsala, average | 120 | 2.5 | 21 |
| Red Raspberry | 130 | 1.5 | 25 |

**Great Value** *(Walmart):*

| **Ice Cream:** Butter Pecan, ½ cup | 160 | 10 | 15 |
|---|---|---|---|
| Chocolate, ½ cup | 130 | 7 | 17 |
| Chocolate Chip Cookie Dough, ⅔ cup | 210 | 10 | 27 |
| Cookies & Cream, ⅔ cup | 210 | 10 | 27 |
| Mint Choc. Chip, ½ cup | 140 | 8 | 17 |
| Strawberry, ⅔ cup | 150 | 7 | 24 |
| **Sherbet,** av. all flav., ½ cup | 110 | 0 | 26 |

**Haagen-Dazs:**

| **Tubs, Regular:** *Per ½ Cup* | | | |
|---|---|---|---|
| Bourbon Praline Pecan | 380 | 21 | 42 |
| Chocolate Peanut Butter | 330 | 22 | 25 |
| Dulce de Leche | 270 | 16 | 28 |
| White Chocolate Raspberry Truffle | 280 | 16 | 31 |
| **Decadent:** *Per ½ Cup* | | | |
| Honey Salted Caramel Almond | 290 | 18 | 26 |
| Midnight Cookies & Cream | 280 | 16 | 30 |
| **Non Dairy Frozen Dessert:** *Per ½ Cup* | | | |
| Choc. Salted Fudge Truffle | 270 | 11 | 40 |
| Coconut Caramel | 240 | 11 | 34 |
| **Sorbet:** *Per ½ Cup* | | | |
| Mango | 150 | 0 | 38 |
| Raspberry; Lemon, average | 120 | 0 | 31 |

**Healthy Choice,**

| **Greek Frozen Yogurt,** average all varieties, | 105 | 2 | 19 |
|---|---|---|---|

**Bars** ~*See Page 109*

# Ice Cream & Frozen Yogurt

## Ice Cream ~ Brands (Cont)

### Hood:

| | C | F | Cb |
|---|---|---|---|
| **Classic:** *Per ⅔ Cup* | | | |
| Chocolate | 190 | 9 | 25 |
| Classic Trio | 180 | 9 | 23 |
| Coffee Cookies 'N Crm | 200 | 10 | 26 |
| Cookie Dough | 210 | 10 | 28 |
| Creamy Coffee | 180 | 10 | 22 |
| Fudge Twister | 190 | 8 | 27 |
| Golden Vanilla; Patchwork, av. | 190 | 10 | 22 |
| Maple Walnut Flavored | 200 | 11 | 22 |
| **Churned, Light:** *Per ⅔ Cup* | | | |
| Chocolate Chip | 170 | 6 | 26 |
| Coffee | 140 | 4 | 24 |
| Under The Stars | 210 | 10 | 25 |
| Vanilla | 140 | 4 | 24 |
| **Frozen Fat-Free Yogurt:** *Per ⅔ Cup* | | | |
| Chocolate; Strawberry, av. | 130 | 0 | 26 |
| Mocha Fudge | 130 | 0 | 29 |
| Strawberry | 120 | 0 | 25 |

### New England Creamery ~ www.CalorieKing.com

**Jerseymaid** *(Vons): Per ½ Cup*

**Ice Cream:**

| | C | F | Cb |
|---|---|---|---|
| Cookies & Cream | 160 | 8 | 18 |
| Choc Chip; Mint Choc Chip | 150 | 9 | 16 |
| Heavenly Hash | 165 | 9 | 19 |
| Mocha Almond Fudge; Chocolate | 150 | 9 | 16 |
| Neapolitan; Real Vanilla | 140 | 8 | 15 |
| Strawberry | 130 | 6 | 17 |

### Oberweis:

**Super Premium Ice Cream:** *Per ½ Cup*

| | C | F | Cb |
|---|---|---|---|
| Banana Fudge Walnut, 3.1 oz | 250 | 15 | 27 |
| Black Cherry, 3 oz | 220 | 13 | 23 |
| Chocolate Chip, 2.8 oz | 220 | 14 | 20 |
| Cookies & Cream, 2.6 oz | 200 | 13 | 19 |
| Cookie Dough P'nut Butter | 280 | 18 | 27 |
| Espresso Caramel Chip, 3 oz | 240 | 15 | 26 |
| Vanilla, 2.75 oz | 210 | 14 | 18 |

**Oikos** ~ *see Dannon*

### Pinkberry:

**Frozen Yogurt:** *Without Toppings*

| | C | F | Cb |
|---|---|---|---|
| Original: Mini, 3.2 oz wt | 90 | 0 | 19 |
|    Small, 4.9 oz wt | 150 | 0 | 31 |
|    Medium, 8 oz wt | 240 | 0 | 50 |
|    Large, 13 oz wt | 390 | 1 | 81 |
| Chocolate Hazelnut, 8 oz | 360 | 9 | 59 |
| Cookies & Cream, 8 oz | 320 | 4.5 | 59 |
| Passionfruit, 8 oz | 240 | 0 | 50 |
| Peanut Butter, 8 oz | 390 | 16 | 49 |
| Vanilla Latte, 8 oz | 240 | 0 | 47 |

### Red Mango (Stores):

**Frozen Yogurt:** *Without Toppings*

| | C | F | Cb |
|---|---|---|---|
| Fruit Flavors, 5 oz | 150 | 0 | 35 |
| Blueberry Lemonade, 5 oz | 75 | 0 | 20 |
| Choc. Covered Strawberry, 5 oz | 150 | 0 | 30 |
| Dark Chocolate (Ghirardelli), 5 oz | 150 | 0 | 35 |

**Fro-Yo Mashups:** *Per 1 oz without Toppings*

| | | | |
|---|---|---|---|
| Brownie Brittle | 35 | 0.5 | 6 |
| Coffee | 30 | 0.3 | 7 |
| Nutty Nanas | 38 | 0.3 | 7 |
| Peanut Butter | 40 | 1.5 | 6 |
| Salted Caramel; Snickerdoodle | 33 | 0.3 | 7 |

**Bars** ~ *See Page 110*

**Skinny Cow:** *Per ½ cup*

**Ice Cream Tubs, Protein Packed Indulgence:**

| | | | |
|---|---|---|---|
| Chocolate Cake Me Away | 100 | 3 | 13 |
| Fudgetastic Java | 100 | 2.5 | 13 |
| Mint Chip Mash Up | 100 | 3 | 12 |
| Oh Fudge Cookie | 80 | 9 | 49 |
| Oh My! Vanilla Bean | 90 | .5 | 12 |
| Peanut Butter Chocolate | 110 | 3.5 | 12 |
| Rock On! Rocky Road | 100 | 3 | 13 |

**Bars/Sandwiches/Cones** ~ *See Page 110*

**So Delicious:** *Per ⅔ Cup Unless Indicated*

**Frozen Dessert:**

| | | | |
|---|---|---|---|
| **Almond Milk:** Cookies 'N' Cream | 220 | 11 | 30 |
| Mocha Almond Fudge | 240 | 4 | 27 |
| Vanilla, ½ cup | 140 | 8 | 16 |
| **Cashew Milk:** | | | |
| Bananas Foster | 240 | 13 | 29 |
| Dark Chocolate Truffle | 250 | 15 | 30 |
| Salted Caramel Cluster | 250 | 13 | 32 |
| Snickerdoodle | 240 | 11 | 34 |
| **Coconut Milk:** Chocolate | 200 | 11 | 25 |
| Choc. P'Nut Butter Swirl | 300 | 20 | 29 |
| Mocha Almond Fudge | 250 | 15 | 28 |
| No Sugar Added: | | | |
|    Mint Chip | 160 | 11 | 25 |
|    Vanilla Bean | 130 | 9 | 24 |

*Note: Carbohydrate Figure Includes 4-5g Sugar Alcohol*

| | | | |
|---|---|---|---|
| **Oatmilk:** Caramel Apple Crumble | 230 | 10 | 36 |
| Peanut Butter & Raspberry | 250 | 14 | 30 |
| **Soy Milk:** Chocolate Velvet | 170 | 4.5 | 31 |
| Creamy Vanilla | 160 | 4 | 31 |

Ice Cream & Frozen Yogurt

## Ice Cream ~ Brands (Cont)

**Stonyfield Farm:**

| | C | F | Cb |
|---|---|---|---|
| **Frozen Yogurt:** *Per ½ Cup* | | | |
| After Dark Chocolate | 100 | 0 | 22 |
| Creme Caramel | 140 | 1.5 | 27 |
| Gotta Have Vanilla | 100 | 0 | 21 |
| Vanilla Fudge Swirl | 120 | 0 | 26 |

**Stop & Shop** *(Ahold):*

| | C | F | Cb |
|---|---|---|---|
| **Churn Style Ice Cream:** *Per ½ Cup* | | | |
| Chocolate | 100 | 3 | 17 |
| French Vanilla | 110 | 3 | 17 |
| Mint Chocoalte Chip | 110 | 4 | 17 |
| Moose Tracks | 130 | 5 | 17 |
| **Real Ice Cream:** *Per ½ Cup* | | | |
| Black Raspberry | 130 | 6 | 18 |
| Butter Pecan | 160 | 11 | 15 |
| Cafe Au Lait | 130 | 6 | 16 |
| Cherry Vanilla | 140 | 7 | 18 |
| Chocolate | 150 | 8 | 17 |
| Chocolate Moose Tracks | 190 | 11 | 21 |
| Neapolitan | 140 | 7 | 18 |
| Peanut Butter Jumble | 160 | 9 | 18 |

**Tasti D-Lite:**

| | C | F | Cb |
|---|---|---|---|
| **Soft Serve:** *Per 3 oz Wt* | | | |
| Banana | 70 | 1.5 | 14 |
| Birthday Cake | 80 | 1.5 | 14 |
| Black Cherry | 90 | 1.5 | 16 |
| Brownie Batter | 90 | 2 | 16 |
| Butter Pecan | 80 | 1.5 | 16 |
| Cappuccino | 80 | 1.5 | 15 |
| Chocolate Mint | 90 | 1.5 | 18 |
| Cinnamon Crunch | 140 | 3 | 26 |
| Creme Brulee; New York Cheesecake | 90 | 1.5 | 17 |
| Mango | 80 | 1.5 | 16 |
| Mud Pie | 100 | 2 | 19 |
| Nutella Fusion | 110 | 4 | 17 |
| Oreo Mint | 130 | 3 | 22 |
| Peanut Butter | 100 | 4 | 15 |

**Tofutti** *(Milk Free):*

| | C | F | Cb |
|---|---|---|---|
| **Premium Pints:** *Per ½ Cup* | | | |
| Better Pecan | 250 | 15 | 27 |
| Chocolate | 210 | 13 | 20 |
| Vanilla | 210 | 13 | 21 |
| Vanilla Almond Bark | 240 | 15 | 24 |
| Van. Fudge; Wild Berry Supreme, av. | 190 | 9 | 25 |

**TCBY** ~ *See Page 250*

**Turkey Hill:**

| | C | F | Cb |
|---|---|---|---|
| **All Natural:** *Per ⅔ Cup* | | | |
| Belgian Style Choc. | 220 | 11 | 27 |
| Butter Pecan | 240 | 16 | 21 |
| Salted Caramel | 210 | 10 | 28 |
| Raspberry Chocolate Chip | 210 | 11 | 24 |
| **Light,** Moose Tracks, ⅔ c. | 190 | 8 | 26 |
| **No Sugar Added,** | | | |
| Vanilla Bean, ⅔ cup | 100 | 0 | 26 |
| **Premium Ice Cream:** *Per ⅔ Cup* | | | |
| Black Cherry | 170 | 8 | 23 |
| Choco Mint Chip | 200 | 11 | 23 |
| Chocolate Peanut Butter Cup | 230 | 13 | 24 |
| Cookies 'n Cream; Tin Roof Sundae | 200 | 10 | 25 |
| Raspberry Cream Swirl | 170 | 6 | 28 |
| Vanilla Bean | 170 | 9 | 21 |
| Vanilla Chocolate Crunch | 210 | 12 | 25 |
| **Stuff'd,** average all flavors | 195 | 8 | 29 |
| **Frozen Dairy Desserts:** *Per ⅔ Cup* | | | |
| Butter Pecan | 170 | 6 | 24 |
| Pistachio Almond | 160 | 5 | 25 |
| Red Velvet Cake | 190 | 7 | 31 |
| **Sherbet,** Fruit Rainbow, ⅔ cup | 160 | 1.5 | 36 |

**Wawa:**

| | C | F | Cb |
|---|---|---|---|
| **Premium Ice Cream:** *Per ½ Cup* | | | |
| Butter Pecan; Mint Choc. Chip, av. | 180 | 10 | 20 |
| Chocolate; Vanilla Bean, average | 160 | 8 | 20 |
| Cookies & Cream | 180 | 9 | 21 |
| Strawberry Shortcake | 160 | 7 | 22 |

**Wegmans:** *Per ½ Cup Unless Indicated*

| | C | F | Cb |
|---|---|---|---|
| **Organic Premium:** *Per ½ Cup* | | | |
| Chocolate | 270 | 15 | 30 |
| Lemon w/ Blueb. Swirls | 260 | 16 | 24 |
| Mocha Java | 270 | 15 | 28 |
| **Extra Churned,** | | | |
| Cookies & Cream, ½ cup | 130 | 4 | 21 |
| **Light:** *Per ⅔ Cup* | | | |
| Mint Chip | 130 | 4 | 21 |
| Pecan Praline | 170 | 3.5 | 32 |

**Yasso:**

| | C | F | Cb |
|---|---|---|---|
| **Frozen Greek Yogurt Tubs:** *Per ½ Cup* | | | |
| Caramel Pretzelmania | 150 | 3 | 24 |
| Coffee Brownie Break | 130 | 3 | 21 |
| Rolling in the Dough | 130 | 2.5 | 20 |

## Ice Cream Bars & Pops ~ Brands

*Per Bar/Serving Unless indicated* **C** **F** **Cb**

**Ben & Jerry's:**
**Pint Slices:**

| | C | F | Cb |
|---|---|---|---|
| Am. Dream; Choc Chip Cookie Dough | 285 | 18 | 30 |
| Cherry Garcia; Choc Fudge Brownie | 250 | 15 | 27 |
| Coffee Coffee BuzzBuzzBuzz! | 280 | 19 | 26 |
| The Tonight Dough | 290 | 18 | 31 |
| Vanilla Peanut Butter Cup | 300 | 22 | 24 |

**Big Bear** ~ *See Klondike*
**Blue Bunny:**

| | C | F | Cb |
|---|---|---|---|
| **Single Bars:** Chocolate Eclair, 2.8 oz | 210 | 9 | 29 |
| Cookies 'n Cream, 3 oz | 240 | 11 | 33 |
| Heath Bar, 3 oz | 290 | 20 | 26 |
| Nutt'n Better Bar | 270 | 19 | 23 |
| Strawberry Shortcake, 2.8 oz | 200 | 10 | 27 |
| Turtle Bar, 3.5 oz | 360 | 23 | 33 |
| **Snacks,** CMint Choc. Chip, 1.83 oz | 150 | 5 | 24 |
| **Cones, 6 Pack:** | | | |
| Caramel Lovers, 3.4 oz | 310 | 16 | 38 |
| Chocolate Lovers, 3.2 oz | 270 | 12 | 36 |
| Cookies 'n Cream, 3.2 oz | 270 | 13 | 37 |
| **Big Dipper:** Chocolate Lovers, 3 oz | 260 | 12 | 36 |
| Cookies 'n Cream, 3 oz | 260 | 12 | 35 |
| **Ice Cream Sandwiches:** | | | |
| Singles: Chips Galore, 3.4 oz | 310 | 14 | 43 |
| Cookies 'N Cream, 3 oz | 240 | 10 | 37 |
| 8 Pack, Birthday Party, 2.6 oz | 170 | 5 | 30 |
| **Big:** Alaska Bar, 3.25 oz | 250 | 15 | 27 |
| Bopper, Vanilla, 5 oz | 450 | 20 | 63 |
| Sandwich: | | | |
| Double Strawberry, 3.9 oz | 250 | 7 | 42 |
| Mississippi Mud, 4 oz | 280 | 8 | 47 |

**Breyers:**
**Carb Smart, 6 Pack:**

| | C | F | Cb |
|---|---|---|---|
| Almond Bar, 2 oz | 160 | 12 | 13 |
| Fudge Bar, 1.7 oz | 70 | 3 | 11 |
| Smooth Mint Bar, 1.9 oz | 80 | 3 | 12 |
| Vanilla Ice Cream Bar, 2 oz | 150 | 11 | 13 |

*Note: Carbohydrate figure includes 4-5g sugar alcohol*

**Butterfinger** *(Nestle)*,

| | C | F | Cb |
|---|---|---|---|
| **Loaded Ice Cream Bar** | 280 | 17 | 29 |

*Per Bar/Serving Unless indicated* **C** **F** **Cb**

**Cool Classics** *(Krogers):*
**Arctic Blasters:**

| | C | F | Cb |
|---|---|---|---|
| Crispy Bar | 170 | 12 | 15 |
| Fudge Bar | 100 | 1 | 21 |
| Ice Cream Bar | 150 | 10 | 13 |
| Orange Cream | 100 | 2.5 | 18 |
| Strawberry Shortcake | 140 | 8 | 16 |
| Toffee Bar | 160 | 11 | 14 |
| **Icepix:** Grape; Cherry; Orange | 35 | 0 | 8 |
| Honeydew; Watermelon; Cantelope | 35 | 0 | 9 |

**Creamsicles:** *Per Bar*

| | C | F | Cb |
|---|---|---|---|
| **Box of 12,** Orange Cream Pops | 100 | 1.5 | 19 |

**Diana's Bananas:**
**Banana Babies:**

| | C | F | Cb |
|---|---|---|---|
| Milk/Dark Chocolate (1) | 130 | 6 | 18 |
| Milk Choc. & Peanuts (1) | 215 | 13 | 21 |
| **Banana Bites,** (4), 1.5 oz | 100 | 6 | 13 |

**Dove:**
**Single Bars:** *Per 2.6 oz Bar*

| | C | F | Cb |
|---|---|---|---|
| Milk Chocolate Vanilla: | 250 | 16 | 24 |
| And Almonds | 250 | 17 | 21 |
| Caramel Swirl & Cashews | 250 | 16 | 23 |
| Dark Chocolate, Chocolate | 250 | 16 | 26 |
| **Miniatures,** Variety Pack, | | | |
| w/ Milk/Dark Choc.,1 piece | 60 | 4 | 6 |
| **Sorbet Bars:** Dark Chocolate Raspb. | 150 | 8 | 19 |
| Milk Chocolate Strawberry | 150 | 7 | 20 |

**Drumstick** *(Nestlé):*
**Cones:** Banana

| | C | F | Cb |
|---|---|---|---|
| **Cones:** Banana | 290 | 15 | 34 |
| Cookie Dipped Vanilla with Caramel | 310 | 14 | 42 |
| Dipped Butterfinger Chocolate | 270 | 13 | 36 |
| Dulce de Leche | 290 | 13 | 41 |
| Strawberry with Fudge | 300 | 15 | 37 |
| Vanilla Caramel | 300 | 15 | 38 |
| Super Nugget: Van. Fudge | 320 | 17 | 37 |
| **King Size:** Triple Chocolate | 340 | 14 | 50 |
| Vanilla with Choc. Layers | 360 | 16 | 49 |
| **Lil' Drums:** Choc. w/ Choc. Swirls | 130 | 6 | 16 |
| Average other varieties | 110 | 6 | 18 |
| **Simply Dipped:** Mint | 260 | 12 | 37 |
| Vanilla | 260 | 12 | 37 |

## Ice Cream Bars/Pops ~ Brands (Cont)

*Per Bar/Serving*

| | C | F | Cb |
|---|---|---|---|
| Edy's ~ *See Dreyer's* | | | |
| **Eskimo Pie** *(Nestle)*: | | | |
| Milk Chocolate, Vanilla | 150 | 10 | 14 |
| **Fat Boy:** | | | |
| **Sundae On A Stick:** | | | |
| Sea Salt Caramel Pretzel | 270 | 18 | 25 |
| Toffee Crunch | 290 | 21 | 25 |
| Vanilla Nut | 270 | 18 | 25 |
| **Sandwiches:** Chocolate, 3 oz | 210 | 8 | 32 |
| Cookies 'n Cream, 3 oz | 220 | 9 | 34 |
| Mint Chocolate Chip, 3 oz | 230 | 10 | 33 |
| Premium Vanilla | 210 | 8 | 32 |
| S'mores, 3 oz | 230 | 9 | 35 |
| Strawberry, 3 oz | 180 | 7 | 29 |
| Fudge Bar *(Nestle)*, Regular, 2.8 oz | 110 | 2 | 21 |
| **Fudgesicle:** | | | |
| **Fudge Bar:** Original | 100 | 2 | 17 |
| Low Fat | 60 | 1.5 | 12 |
| No Sugar Added | 80 | 1.5 | 19 |
| **Good Humor:** | | | |
| **Dessert Bars, Singles:** | | | |
| Original Vanilla, 2.8 oz | 240 | 15 | 23 |
| Birthday Cake, 2.6 oz | 200 | 10 | 25 |
| Chocolate Eclair, 2 oz | 150 | 7 | 21 |
| Oreo, 1.8 oz | 150 | 8 | 19 |
| Toasted Almond, 2 oz | 160 | 9 | 18 |
| **Cones:** | | | |
| **Single:** Giant King Cone, | | | |
| Choc. & Vanilla, 5 oz | 390 | 22 | 44 |
| King Cone, Vanilla, 2.7 oz | 230 | 14 | 25 |
| **4-Packs:** | | | |
| Oreo Cone, 2.65 oz | 200 | 9 | 29 |
| King Cones, Vanilla, 3 oz | 240 | 12 | 31 |
| **Sandwiches:** | | | |
| **Single:** Giant Neapolitan;Van., 3.6 oz | 220 | 5 | 39 |
| Choc. Chip Cookie, 2.7 oz | 250 | 10 | 40 |
| **Stickless:** *4 or 6-Pack* | | | |
| Reese's PB Dessert Cup, 2.43 oz | 260 | 17 | 25 |
| **Haagen-Dazs:** | | | |
| **Dark Chocolate Bar**, Chocolate | 280 | 20 | 22 |
| **Milk Chocolate Bars:** | | | |
| Coffee & Almond Crunch | 290 | 21 | 22 |
| Vanilla & Almonds | 290 | 21 | 21 |
| Vanilla | 270 | 19 | 22 |
| **Snack Size:** | | | |
| Coffee & Almond Crunch | 190 | 14 | 15 |
| Vanilla & Almonds | 195 | 15 | 13 |
| **Gelato,** Vanilla Caramel Pizzelle | 290 | 19 | 25 |

*Per Bar/Serving*

| | C | F | Cb |
|---|---|---|---|
| **Healthy Choice:** Fudge Bar | 80 | 0.5 | 15 |
| **Smoothie Bars:** | | | |
| Mango Peach | 70 | 0.5 | 14 |
| Raspberry | 80 | 0.5 | 15 |
| Strawberry | 70 | 0.5 | 13 |
| **Hershey's:** | | | |
| **Bars, Gluten Free:** Banjo | 170 | 11 | 17 |
| Fudjo | 120 | 0 | 24 |
| Orange Blossom | 80 | 2.5 | 13 |
| **Cones:** Incredible | 290 | 14 | 38 |
| Moose Tracks | 480 | 28 | 52 |
| P-Nutty | 260 | 15 | 30 |
| Low fat, Cookies & Cream; Crazy, av. | 120 | 1.5 | 25 |
| **Ice Pops**, all flavors | 35 | 0 | 10 |
| **Sandwiches:** | | | |
| Vanilla Ice Cream, 4 oz | 210 | 9 | 30 |
| **Giant:** | | | |
| Andes Creme de Menthe, 6 oz | 350 | 16 | 48 |
| Neapolitan, 6 oz | 280 | 12 | 40 |
| Vanilla, 6 oz | 300 | 12 | 43 |
| **Signature Bars:** Chocolate Eclair | 220 | 10 | 30 |
| Salty Caramel Brownie | 240 | 12 | 30 |
| Strawb. Shortcake | 240 | 11 | 32 |
| **Hood:** | | | |
| **Bars:** Ice Cream Bar | 130 | 7 | 14 |
| Red Sox Sports Bar | 250 | 16 | 26 |
| **Hoodsie:** | | | |
| Cups, Chocolate; Vanilla, 3 oz | 100 | 5 | 12 |
| Sundae Cups, 3 oz | 120 | 5 | 19 |
| **Sandwich:** Av., 2.2 oz | 175 | 6 | 29 |
| Mini's, 1.2 oz | 90 | 3.5 | 14 |
| **Klondike:** | | | |
| **Bars:** | | | |
| **Single,** Orig. Vanilla, 5.5 oz | 300 | 17 | 34 |
| **4-Pack:** | | | |
| Mint Choc. Chip, 2.8 oz | 230 | 14 | 26 |
| **6 Pack:** Cookies & Cream, 2.15 oz | 200 | 10 | 24 |
| Double Chocolate, 3 oz | 240 | 14 | 27 |
| Oreo, Cookies & Cream, 2.57 oz | 250 | 15 | 27 |
| Reeses, PB Cup , 2.75 oz | 250 | 15 | 28 |
| **8-Count Snack Size:** Orig., 1.4 oz | 120 | 7 | 13 |
| English Toffee, 2.6 oz | 230 | 14 | 24 |
| **Choco Taco,** Original, 4 oz | 250 | 12 | 34 |
| **Kandy,** Caramel & Peanuts, 2.7 oz | 250 | 14 | 28 |
| **Sandwiches:** | | | |
| **Single:** Mrs Fields, 3.9 oz | 340 | 12 | 55 |
| Oreo, 4.5 oz | 220 | 7 | 37 |
| **4-Pack:** Mrs Fields, 2.3 oz | 210 | 8 | 34 |
| Oreo, 2.4 oz | 210 | 7 | 35 |
| **6-Pack,** Vanilla, 2.7 oz | 180 | 5 | 31 |

# Ice Cream Bars & Pops

## Ice Cream Bars/Pops ~ Brands (Cont)

*Per Bar/Serving*

| | C | F | Cb |
|---|---|---|---|
| **Luigi's:** *Per 6 fl.oz cup* | | | |
| **Real Italian Ice:** Blue Rasp. Lemon | 130 | 0 | 27 |
| Cherry; Lemon; Strawb. | 100 | 0 | 26 |
| Cherry & Lemon Swirl | 120 | 0 | 30 |
| **M&M's:** | | | |
| **Cone,** Single, 2.6 oz | 250 | 12 | 32 |
| **Sandwiches:** Choc. Ice Cream, 2.9 oz | 240 | 10 | 36 |
| Vanilla Ice Cream, 2.9 oz | 250 | 11 | 35 |
| **Magnum:** | | | |
| **Singles:** Almond | 270 | 18 | 25 |
| Double Caramel | 270 | 17 | 29 |
| **Minis,** Almond | 170 | 11 | 15 |
| **Multipacks:** Dark Chocolate | 240 | 16 | 23 |
| White | 240 | 15 | 24 |
| **Double:** Choc. Hazelnut | 280 | 19 | 26 |
| Raspberry | 260 | 16 | 28 |
| **Non Dairy:** Classic | 230 | 15 | 26 |
| Almond | 255 | 16 | 25 |
| **Minute Maid,** Juice Bars, 2.25 fl.oz | 40 | 0 | 10 |
| **Nestlé:** | | | |
| **Bars:** Crunch | 180 | 11 | 19 |
| Cookies N' Cream | 190 | 12 | 20 |
| Loaded Butterfinger | 280 | 18 | 27 |
| Strawberry Shortcake | 210 | 9 | 31 |
| **Dibs,** Crunch, 4 oz container | 340 | 24 | 30 |
| **Drumsticks ~ See Page 109** | | | |
| **Pops:** Push-Ups | 70 | 1 | 16 |
| Sweetarts | 80 | 0 | 21 |
| **Sandwiches,** Vanilla | 160 | 3.5 | 29 |
| **Popsicle:** Colors (1) | 40 | 0 | 10 |
| Firecracker (1) | 35 | 0 | 9 |
| Marvel Avengers Assemble; Rainbow | 40 | 0 | 10 |
| Scribblers (2) | 60 | 0 | 14 |
| SpongeBob Squarepants Pop-Ups (1) | 70 | 1 | 16 |
| **Reese's** *(Good Humor)*, | | | |
| P'nut Butter Ice Cream Cup, 2.4 oz | 260 | 17 | 25 |
| **Skinny Cow:** *Per Item* | | | |
| **Bars:** Fudge; Chocolate Truffle, av | 105 | 2 | 21 |
| Vanilla Almond Crunch | 190 | 11 | 19 |
| **Candy Bars,** av. all flavors | 155 | 9 | 17 |
| **Cones,** average all flavors | 155 | 3 | 28 |
| **Sandwiches,** all flavors | 180 | 9 | 22 |
| **Snickers:** | | | |
| **Bars:** Milk/Dark Chocolate: 1.7 oz | 180 | 11 | 18 |
| 2.43 oz | 250 | 16 | 26 |
| Mini Bar, 1 piece, 0.9 oz | 90 | 5 | 9 |
| **Cone,** 2.7 oz | 250 | 13 | 31 |
| **Sandwich,** Brownie, 3.3 oz | 300 | 13 | 41 |

*Per Bar/Serving*

| | C | F | Cb |
|---|---|---|---|
| **Snow Cone** *(Wonder)*, av. all, 7 fl.oz | 60 | 0 | 15 |
| **So Delicious** *(Turtle Mountain):* | | | |
| **Almond Based:** | | | |
| **Bars,** Mocha Alm. Fudge | 180 | 13 | 16 |
| **Sandwich,** Vanilla, 1.3 oz | 100 | 4 | 14 |
| **Cashewmilk:** | | | |
| **Dipped Bars:** Dble Choc Delight, 2 oz | 170 | 13 | 16 |
| Salted Caramel Bar, 2 oz | 180 | 13 | 17 |
| **Coconut Milk:** | | | |
| **Dipped Bar:** Coconut Alm., 1.85 oz | 190 | 14 | 15 |
| Vanilla Bean, 1.8 oz | 170 | 12 | 14 |
| **Fudge Bar,** 2 oz | 100 | 6 | 13 |
| **Sandwiches:** | | | |
| Coconut, 1.3 oz | 100 | 4 | 14 |
| Vanilla Bean, 1.3 oz | 100 | 4 | 14 |
| **Tampico,** Freezer Pops, all var., 1.4 oz | 30 | 0 | 7 |
| **Tofutti:** *Per Item* | | | |
| **Bars:** Chocolate Fudge, 1.4 oz | 30 | 0 | 6 |
| Hooray Hooray, 1.4 oz | 120 | 8 | 8 |
| Marry Me, 1.4 oz | 170 | 8 | 22 |
| Totally Fudge Pops | 95 | 1.5 | 19 |
| *Note: Carb figures include 0-7g sugar alcohols* | | | |
| **Cone,** Yours Truly Sundae | 170 | 8 | 22 |
| **Cuties,** average all flavors | 130 | 6 | 18 |
| **Toll House** *(Nestle):* | | | |
| **Chocolate Choc. Chip Cookie** | 220 | 9 | 32 |
| **Vanilla Choc. Chip Cookie** | 380 | 15 | 59 |
| **Turkey Hill:** | | | |
| **Bars:** Vanilla Ice Cream, 3.3 oz | 320 | 23 | 26 |
| **Decadent Delights:** Cherry, 3.2 oz | 380 | 25 | 35 |
| Choc. Covered Strawb., 2.75 oz | 280 | 16 | 31 |
| Coconut, 2.43 oz | 260 | 18 | 21 |
| Triple Chocolate 2.4 oz | 235 | 15 | 21 |
| **Cone,** Vanilla Fudge 3.45 oz | 340 | 19 | 37 |
| **Sandwiches:** Double Decker, 2.54 oz | 200 | 8 | 31 |
| Strawberry Cheesecake, 2.65 oz | 210 | 8 | 33 |
| Vanilla Bean, 2.5 oz | 190 | 7 | 30 |
| **Sundae Cone,** Van. Fudge | 320 | 18 | 33 |
| **Twix,** Ice Cream Bar, 2.43oz | 250 | 14 | 28 |
| **Wegmans:** | | | |
| **Bars:** Fudge, 2.5 oz | 190 | 12 | 16 |
| PB Sundae Crunch, 2.5 oz | 200 | 11 | 22 |
| Vanilla, Choc Coated, 1.9 oz | 160 | 11 | 14 |
| **Sandwiches:** Vanilla, 2.3 oz | 200 | 9 | 24 |
| Light Vanilla, 2.15 oz | 150 | 3 | 29 |
| **Weight Watchers:** *Per Item* | | | |
| **Bars:** Dark Choc. Raspberry | 70 | 2 | 11 |
| English Toffee Crunch | 80 | 3.5 | 11 |
| Giant Bar, Chocolate Fudge | 90 | 1 | 21 |
| **Snack Bars:** Cookies & Cream | 90 | 3 | 15 |
| Divine Triple Chocolate | 90 | 3 | 14 |
| Salted Caramel | 90 | 2.5 | 14 |

## Canned & Packaged Meals ~ Brands

**Amy's:** *Per Serve*

| | C | F | Cb |
|---|---|---|---|
| **Frozen:** | | | |
| **Asian Meals:** | | | |
| Chineese Noodles & Veggies, 9.5 oz | 480 | 21 | 59 |
| Stir-Fry Asian Noodle,10 oz | 300 | 7 | 50 |
| Sweet & Sour Asian Noodle, 8 oz | 310 | 10 | 42 |
| **Bowls:** Asian Dumplings, 8.5 oz | 400 | 13 | 55 |
| Baked Ziti, 9.5 oz | 380 | 13 | 54 |
| Broccoli & Cheddar Bake, 9.5 oz | 420 | 20 | 44 |
| Cheese Lasagna, 10.3 oz | 410 | 16 | 46 |
| Paella, 8.5 oz | 280 | 12 | 35 |
| Pesto Penne w/ Vegetables, 9 oz | 370 | 15 | 46 |
| Pesto Tortellini, 9.5 oz | 450 | 20 | 50 |
| Spinach Ravioli, 8.5 oz | 390 | 10 | 61 |
| Vegan Spinach Ravioli, 8.4 oz | 340 | 8 | 56 |
| **Entrees:** Cheese Enchilada, 4.5 oz | 240 | 14 | 18 |
| Cheese Lasagna, 10.3 oz | 410 | 16 | 46 |
| Macaroni & Cheese, 9 oz | 400 | 16 | 47 |
| Roasted Vegetable Tamale, 10.3 oz | 280 | 7 | 45 |
| **Light & Lean:** Mattar Paneer | 260 | 6 | 42 |
| Spinach Lasagna | 250 | 5 | 40 |
| **Pot Pies:** Broccoli, 7.5 oz | 490 | 29 | 47 |
| Vegetable, 7.5 oz | 440 | 24 | 46 |
| **Snacks:** | | | |
| Cheese & Bean Nachos, 5-6 pcs | 230 | 9 | 29 |
| Swirls: Artichoke & Parmesan (2) | 200 | 11 | 20 |
| Cheddar Jalepeno (2) | 210 | 9 | 25 |
| Mushroom & Cheese; Pesto (2) | 190 | 9 | 20 |
| **Veggie Burger Patties,** Sonoma (1) | 140 | 5 | 18 |
| **Wraps:** | | | |
| Indian Samosa, 5 oz | 250 | 9 | 35 |
| Teriyaki, gluten free, 5.5 oz | 250 | 6 | 38 |
| Tofu Scramble B'fast, gluten free, 5.5 oz | 300 | 13 | 35 |
| **Armour-Star:** | | | |
| Beef Stew, 9 oz | 230 | 12 | 21 |
| Chili with Beans, 7 oz | 380 | 19 | 31 |
| Chili without Beans, 8.5 oz | 400 | 28 | 18 |
| Corned Beef, 2 oz | 120 | 7 | 1 |
| Corned Beef Hash, 7 oz | 420 | 26 | 22 |
| Potted Meat, 1 can, 3 oz | 240 | 22 | 0 |
| **Atkins:** *Per 9 oz Tray/Bowl* | | | |
| **Frozen:** | | | |
| Beef Merlot | 300 | 21 | 9 |
| Chicken & Brocc. Alfredo | 290 | 18 | 10 |
| Chili Con Carne | 330 | 23 | 10 |
| Crustless Chicken Pot Pie | 300 | 19 | 9 |
| Italian Style Pasta Bake | 320 | 18 | 16 |
| Meatloaf w/ Portobello Mshrm Gravy | 330 | 21 | 12 |
| Shrimp Scampi | 290 | 19 | 19 |
| Swedish Meatballs | 390 | 22 | 24 |

**Bagel Bites:** *Per 4 Pieces*

| | C | F | Cb |
|---|---|---|---|
| **Frozen:** | | | |
| Bacon, Egg & Cheese | 190 | 4.5 | 28 |
| Cheese, Sausage & Pepperoni | 200 | 6 | 28 |
| Sausage, Egg & Cheese | 190 | 5 | 28 |
| Supreme | 190 | 5 | 30 |
| Three Cheese | 200 | 5 | 32 |
| **B&M:** | | | |
| **Baked Beans:** *Per ½ cup, 4.6 oz* | | | |
| Original | 160 | 1 | 32 |
| Bacon & Onion | 180 | 1 | 39 |
| Boston's Best | 190 | 1 | 40 |
| Maple Flavor | 160 | 1 | 31 |
| Vegetarian | 160 | 0.5 | 35 |
| **Brown Bread,** Orig., ½ slice, 2 oz | 130 | 0.5 | 28 |
| **Banquet:** | | | |
| **Homestyle Bakes:** *1 Cup, Prepared* | | | |
| Creamy Cheesy Chicken Alfredo | 330 | 15 | 37 |
| Creamy Chicken & Biscuits | 420 | 18 | 53 |
| **Frozen:** | | | |
| Backyard BBQ & Mashed Potato, 8 oz | 290 | 11 | 35 |
| **Chicken:** Fingers, 6.5 oz | 310 | 12 | 33 |
| Fettuccine Chicken Alfredo, 8 oz | 310 | 12 | 38 |
| Chicken Fried Chicken, 10 oz | 330 | 14 | 40 |
| Parmesan, 8.5 oz | 320 | 11 | 41 |
| Strip Meal, 8.9 oz | 440 | 19 | 45 |
| Homestyle Patty, 10 oz | 340 | 17 | 32 |
| Lasagna, with Meat Sauce | 250 | 9 | 31 |
| Mac & Cheese, 8 oz | 240 | 9 | 32 |
| Meatloaf, 11.9 oz | 330 | 11 | 43 |
| Pepper Steak, 10 oz | 320 | 13 | 39 |
| Rigatoni & Italian Sausage, 8 oz | 300 | 12 | 35 |
| Salisbury Steak w/ Mshd Pot., 9.5 oz | 350 | 14 | 44 |
| Spaghetti & Chicken Nuggets, 7 oz | 230 | 7 | 32 |
| Spaghetti & Meatballs, 10 oz | 320 | 14 | 34 |
| Swedish Meaballs, 10.45 oz | 370 | 17 | 39 |
| Turkey, 10 oz | 280 | 11 | 29 |
| **Family:** | | | |
| Gravy & Meat Loaf, 4 oz | 120 | 6 | 9 |
| Salisbury Steak & Gravy, 4.5 oz | 180 | 12 | 11 |
| Zesty Marinara Sce & M'balls, 5 oz | 170 | 10 | 11 |
| **Breakfast Mini Sandwiches:** | | | |
| Chicken & Buttermilk Biscuit (2) | 280 | 13 | 30 |
| Sausage &Buttermilk Biscuit (2) | 330 | 22 | 23 |
| **Pot Pie:** Beef | 380 | 23 | 36 |
| Chicken | 350 | 9 | 33 |
| Chicken & Broccoli | 330 | 18 | 31 |
| Salisbury Steak Deep Dish, 7 oz | 400 | 23 | 40 |
| Turkey | 320 | 18 | 31 |

| Barilla: | **C** | **F** | **Cb** |
|---|---|---|---|
| **Microwaveables:** *Per 9 oz Container* | | | |
| Chicken Alfredo | 610 | 18 | 22 |
| Marinara/Tomato & Basil Penne, av. | 305 | 4 | 62 |
| Sausage & Tomato Rotini | 330 | 5 | 63 |
| **Betty Crocker:** | | | |
| **Bowl Appetit:** *Per Bowl* | | | |
| Herb Chicken Flav. Veggie Rice | 250 | 3 | 51 |
| Pasta Alfredo | 350 | 9 | 55 |
| **Chicken Helper:** *As Packaged* | | | |
| Chicken Fettuccine Alfredo, 1.26 oz | 140 | 1.5 | 28 |
| Chicken Fried Rice, 1.2 oz | 110 | 0 | 24 |
| **Hamburger Helper:** *As Packaged* | | | |
| Bacon Chsebgr; Beef Pasta, av., 1 oz | 95 | 0.5 | 21 |
| Cheesy Enchil.; Crunchy Taco, av., 1.4 oz | 145 | 2 | 29 |
| Del. Beef Strog.; Four Chse Lasag 1 oz | 100 | 1 | 21 |
| Philly Chsesteak, 1.26 oz | 130 | 2 | 25 |
| Potato Stroganoff, 0.9 oz | 90 | 0 | 21 |
| **Potatoes:** *As Packaged* | | | |
| **Casserole:** Cheddar & Bacon, 1 oz | 100 | 0 | 22 |
| Julienne, 0.9 oz | 80 | 0 | 20 |
| Other flavors, 0.9 oz | 90 | 0 | 21 |
| **Mashed Potatoes:** | | | |
| Four Cheese; Loaded,0.8 oz | 90 | 2 | 16 |
| Sour Cream & Chives, 0.8 oz | 80 | 0 | 17 |
| **Tuna Helper:** *As Packaged* | | | |
| Cheesy Pasta; Creamy Pasta, 1.1 oz | 110 | 1 | 21 |
| Crmy Broccoli; Fett. Alfredo, 1.3 oz | 130 | 1 | 26 |
| **Biggest Loser:** | | | |
| **Refrigerated:** | | | |
| **Simply Sensible:** *Per ½ Package* | | | |
| Beef Pot Roast & Gravy | 220 | 5 | 16 |
| Beef Tips & Gravy | 200 | 3.5 | 21 |
| Lasagna | 200 | 5 | 28 |
| Medit.-Style Chicken | 250 | 6 | 36 |
| Zing Chicken | 230 | 1.5 | 38 |
| **Birds Eye:** | | | |
| **Veggie Made:** | | | |
| **Mac & Cheese:** Elbows, | | | |
| w/ Cheddar Cheese Sce, 4 oz | 170 | 5 | 22 |
| Shells w/ White Cheddar Sce, 4 oz | 170 | 5 | 20 |
| **Meals:** Garlic Chicken, 7 oz | 250 | 8 | 29 |
| Chicken Fried Riced Caulif., 7 oz | 120 | 3 | 13 |
| Sweet & Sour Chicken, 8.4 oz | 170 | 1.5 | 28 |
| **Riced:** Original Cauliflower, 2.85 oz | 20 | 0 | 4 |
| Brocc. w/ Chedd. Chse Sce, 3.3 oz | 45 | 1.5 | 4 |
| Chicken Flav. Riced Cauliflower, | | | |
| with Broccoli & Carrots, 4 oz | 45 | 2.5 | 5 |
| **Tots & Fries:** Brocc. & Cheese, 3 oz | 150 | 6 | 20 |
| Broccoli & Potato Fries, 3 oz | 160 | 9 | 21 |
| Cauliflower & Ranch, 3 oz | 150 | 6 | 20 |

| Birds Eye (Cont): | **C** | **F** | **Cb** |
|---|---|---|---|
| **Chef's Favorites:** | | | |
| In Cheese Sauce: Broccoli, 1⅓ cups | 60 | 2.5 | 5 |
| Bruss. Sprouts w/ Bacon, 3.8 oz | 80 | 2.5 | 9 |
| Rstd Pot., Onions & Bacon, 5 oz | 145 | 4 | 23 |
| **Protein Blends:** Asian Style, 7.7 oz | 220 | 4.5 | 36 |
| California Style, 10.8 oz | 350 | 6 | 61 |
| Hawaiian Style, 12.8 oz | 380 | 5 | 72 |
| **Superfood Blends:** Barley & Kale, 10 oz | 240 | 3.5 | 40 |
| Black rice & Edamame, 10 oz | 290 | 4.5 | 48 |
| Chickpea & Spinach, 10 oz | 320 | 7 | 51 |
| Quinoa & Spinach, 10 oz | 310 | 5 | 57 |
| **Voila!:** Alfredo Chicken, 7.5 oz | 230 | 7 | 26 |
| Cheesy Ranch Chicken, 6.7 oz | 190 | 4 | 27 |
| Chkn & Pasta in Parmesan Sce, 9 oz | 370 | 12 | 51 |
| Chicken Florentine, 7.65 oz | 220 | 5 | 28 |
| **Selects:** Beef Lo Mein, 8 oz | 270 | 5 | 42 |
| Mongolian Style Beef, 7.7 oz | 240 | 4.5 | 38 |
| Sausage & Peppers, 8.2 oz | 290 | 14 | 28 |
| Sweet & Sour Chicken, 7.9 oz | 250 | 2 | 46 |
| **Boca:** | | | |
| **Bowls**, average all flavors, 9 oz bowl | 290 | 9 | 42 |
| **Burger Patties:** *Per 2.5 oz Patty* | | | |
| **Original:** All American | 100 | 4 | 6 |
| Original Chik'n | 130 | 4 | 13 |
| Original Turk'y Veggie | 70 | 1 | 6 |
| **Non-GMO Soy:** All American | 110 | 4.5 | 7 |
| Spicy Chik'n Veggie | 130 | 4 | 13 |
| **Chik'n Nuggets**, all flavors (4) | 160 | 5 | 16 |
| **Crumbles**, all flavors, 2 oz | 60 | 0 | 5 |
| **Falafel Bites**, all flavors (4) | 150 | 5 | 23 |
| **Skillet Meal**, Southwestern Taco, 6 oz | 140 | 4 | 20 |
| **Boston Market:** | | | |
| **Frozen Dinners:** *Per Pkg* | | | |
| Beef Steak & Pasta | 380 | 9 | 49 |
| Chicken Parmesan | 500 | 13 | 70 |
| Chicken Pot Pie | 450 | 30 | 35 |
| Country Fried Beef Steak | 520 | 29 | 45 |
| Meatloaf | 440 | 25 | 37 |
| Salisbury Steak | 540 | 31 | 41 |
| Swedish M'balls, 13 oz | 660 | 30 | 67 |
| **Buitoni:** | | | |
| **Refrigerated:** | | | |
| **Ravioli:** Four Cheese, 3.7 oz | 330 | 12 | 42 |
| **Tortellini:** Herb Chckn, 3.9 oz | 330 | 8 | 52 |
| Mixed Cheese, 3.7 oz | 320 | 8 | 47 |
| **Tortelloni**, Sweet Italian Ssg., 4 oz | 350 | 10 | 51 |
| **Other Pasta Dishes** ~ *See Page 133* | | | |
| **Bush's Best:** *Per ½ cup, 4.6 oz* | | | |
| **Baked Beans:** Orig,; Vegetarian, av. | 135 | 0.5 | 29 |
| Black Beans | 105 | 0.5 | 23 |
| Black Eyed Peas | 100 | 1.5 | 17 |
| Dark Red Kidney Beans | 130 | 0 | 24 |
| Garbanzo Beans (Chick Peas) | 120 | 2 | 20 |

# Meals ◆ Entrees ◆ Sides ~ Canned/Packaged  Ⓜ

| Bush's Best (Cont): Per 1/2 Cup, 4.6 oz | C | F | Cb |
|---|---|---|---|
| **Grillin' Beans**, | | | |
| Bourbon & Br. Sugar; Smokehouse | 160 | 0.5 | 33 |
| **Refried Beans**, Traditional, 4.4 oz | 140 | 3 | 21 |
| **Savory Beans**, New Orleans Red | 120 | 1 | 21 |
| **Campbell's:** | | | |
| **Pork & Beans**, 11 oz can, | | | |
| 1/2 cup, 4.6 oz serving | 130 | 0.5 | 27 |
| **Spaghetti O's:** Per 1 Cup | | | |
| Original, 8.9 oz | 170 | 1 | 33 |
| With Meatballs, 8.9 oz | 230 | 7 | 31 |
| With Sliced Franks, 8.9 oz | 220 | 7 | 29 |
| **Chef Boyardee:** | | | |
| **Canned:** Per Cup | | | |
| Beefaroni, 8.8 oz | 240 | 9 | 30 |
| Cheesy Burger Macaroni, 8.9 oz | 180 | 4 | 27 |
| Lasagna; Ma & Cheese, av.,m 8.8 oz | 225 | 8 | 31 |
| **Ravioli:** Per 1 Cup | | | |
| Beef: Regular, 8.7 oz | 220 | 7 | 33 |
| Overstuffed, 9.2 oz | 230 | 5 | 37 |
| Cheese, in Tom. & Meat Sce, 9 oz | 210 | 2 | 40 |
| Chicken, in Tomato Sauce, 8.6 oz | 170 | 1.5 | 33 |
| Ital. Sausage, overstuffed, 9.2 oz | 240 | 6 | 38 |
| **Spaghetti:** with Meatballs, 9 oz | 260 | 11 | 31 |
| Mini Rings & Meatballs, 8.6 oz | 250 | 11 | 29 |
| **Microwaveable:** Per 7.5 oz Cup | | | |
| Beefaroni; Mac & Cheese, av. | 210 | 7.5 | 28 |
| **Ravioli:** Beef | 200 | 7 | 28 |
| Cheese in Tomato & Meat Sauce | 190 | 5 | 28 |
| Mini Micro Beef | 160 | 4 | 25 |
| **Boxed Pizza Maker Kits:** Single Kits | | | |
| Cheese, 1/8 package, 4 oz | 260 | 4 | 47 |
| Pepperoni, 1/8 package, 4 oz | 280 | 8 | 42 |
| Pizza Sauce, w/ Cheese, 1/4 c., 2 oz | 35 | 1.5 | 4 |
| **Dennison's Chili:** Per 15 oz Can | | | |
| **Chili Con Carne:** | | | |
| Original: with Beans | 340 | 14 | 34 |
| without Beans | 260 | 14 | 17 |
| Chunky, with Beans | 330 | 13 | 33 |
| Hot, with Beans | 340 | 14 | 34 |
| Turkey with Beans | 220 | 3.5 | 32 |
| Vegetarian, 99% fat free | 280 | 1.5 | 52 |
| **Devour** ~ See Heinz Page 114 | | | |
| **Dinty Moore** (Hormel): | | | |
| **Big Bowl (Microwave):** Approx. 1/2 of 15 oz Bowl | | | |
| Beef Stew, 7.5 oz | 200 | 10 | 17 |
| Chicken & Dumplings, 7.5 oz | 180 | 5 | 24 |
| Noodles & Chicken, 7.5 oz | 190 | 9 | 20 |
| **Dr. McDougall's:** Per 2 oz Package | | | |
| Asian Noodles, Pad Thai | 200 | 1.5 | 43 |
| Lentil Quinoa Salad | 260 | 3.5 | 46 |
| Sweet Potato Kale Salad | 260 | 3.5 | 48 |

| Eden Organics: | C | F | Cb |
|---|---|---|---|
| Black Beans & Quinoa Chili, 8.8 oz | 200 | 2 | 36 |
| Brown Rice & Pinto Beans, 4.6 oz | 120 | 1 | 24 |
| Curried Rice & Green Lentils, 4.6 oz | 130 | 1 | 21 |
| Kidney Beans & Kamut Chili, 8.8 oz | 240 | 2 | 43 |
| Mexican Rice & Black Beans, 4.6 oz | 110 | 1 | 22 |
| **Farmhouse:** Per 1 Cup Prepared | | | |
| **Pasta:** Fettuccine Alfredo | 460 | 22 | 51 |
| White Cheddar | 380 | 14 | 51 |
| **Rice:** Long Gr., & Wild Herbs & Butter | 250 | 7 | 43 |
| Mexican | 230 | 5 | 42 |
| Roasted Chicken Flavor | 230 | 5 | 44 |
| **French's:** | | | |
| **French Crispy Fried Onions:** | | | |
| Original; White Cheddar:2 Tbsp | 45 | 3.5 | 3 |
| 1/4 cup, 0.5 oz | 90 | 7 | 6 |
| 1 cup, 2 oz | 360 | 28 | 24 |
| **GardenBurger:** | | | |
| **Veggie Burger:** Per 2.5 oz Burger | | | |
| Original | 110 | 3.5 | 17 |
| Black Bean Chipotle | 90 | 3 | 16 |
| Portabella | 90 | 2 | 16 |
| **Garden Lites:** Per Package | | | |
| **Bakes:** Broccoli Cheddar Bake | 200 | 6 | 25 |
| Butternut Squash Souffle | 170 | 1.5 | 36 |
| Roasted Vegetable Bake | 150 | 3 | 24 |
| Spinach | 140 | 3 | 22 |
| **Entrees:** Mac & Cheese, 10 oz | 300 | 11 | 38 |
| Veggie Chili & Cornbread 10 oz | 320 | 10 | 46 |
| **Frittata:** Per Frittata | | | |
| Spinach Egg White, 2 oz | 70 | 4 | 5 |
| Veggie, Bacon & Potato, 2 oz | 80 | 4.5 | 6 |
| **Veggie Cake**, Superfood, 2 oz | 80 | 4 | 8 |
| **Gorton's:** | | | |
| **Frozen:** | | | |
| **Delicious Classics:** | | | |
| **Clams,** Crunchy Breaded, 15 pieces | 210 | 10 | 22 |
| **Flounder:** Crispy Batt. Fillets (2) | 250 | 13 | 25 |
| Crunchy Breaded Fillet (1) | 220 | 9 | 25 |
| **Haddock,** Crispy Batt. Fillets (2) | 250 | 13 | 25 |
| **Pollock:** | | | |
| Beer Battered Tenders (3) | 210 | 11 | 21 |
| Crispy Battered Fillets (2) | 230 | 11 | 23 |
| Fish Sticks (4) | 230 | 10 | 26 |
| **Everyday Gourmet:** | | | |
| **Cod:** Cr. Panko Breadcrumb Fillet (1) | 240 | 12 | 23 |
| Pub Style Beer Batter Fillets (1) | 380 | 24 | 29 |
| **Salmon,** Simply Bake, Rstd Garl Butt. (1) | 140 | 2.5 | 8 |
| **Shrimp,** Breaded Jumbo Butterfly | | | |
| 5 shrimp | 250 | 12 | 25 |
| Seasoned w Seasoning (1) | 130 | 3 | 6 |
| **Tilapia,** Simply Bake w Seasoning (1) | 130 | 3 | 6 |

*continued nex page...*

## Gorton's (Cont):
**Frozen:**
**Golden/IPA Ale Batt.**

| | C | F | Cb |
|---|---|---|---|
| Craft Beer Bites, 5 pcs, 3 oz | 180 | 9 | 16 |
| **Potato Crusted Cod Bites (8)** | 180 | 8 | 17 |

**Smart Solutions:** *Per Fillet*

| | C | F | Cb |
|---|---|---|---|
| **Haddock,** Grilled Fillets (1) | 70 | 1 | 0 |
| **Shrimp,** Black Garlic & Wine Risotto | 380 | 15 | 49 |
| **Tilapia:** Grilled Fillets (1) | 100 | 4 | 1 |
| Lightly Batt. Garl. & Herb Fillets (1) | 180 | 8 | 15 |
| Rstd Garlic & Butter Fillets (1) | 100 | 3 | 1 |

## Great Value *(Walmart)*:
**Frozen:**

| | C | F | Cb |
|---|---|---|---|
| **Breakfast Bowls:**Meat Lovers, 7 oz | 430 | 30 | 14 |
| Sausage & Gravy, 7 oz | 340 | 25 | 14 |
| **Meals:** Beef Stroganoff with Noodles | 380 | 18 | 37 |
| Meatloaf & Mashed Pot., 10 oz | 380 | 21 | 34 |
| Mediterranean Insp. Chicken, 10 oz | 310 | 15 | 26 |
| Rstd Orange Chkn & Veggies, 10 oz | 180 | 4.5 | 18 |
| Spinach Pesto Chkn & Veggies | 240 | 10 | 21 |
| **Steam:** Lemon Herb Chkn, 12 oz | 350 | 6 | 51 |
| Maple Dijon Beef & Vegg., 12 oz | 410 | 10 | 64 |
| Mediterranean Falafel, 12 oz | 310 | 9 | 45 |
| **Skillet Meal**, Shrimp Scampi Linguini, 12 oz | 550 | 23 | 58 |

## Healthy Choice:
**Frozen:**
**Cafe Steamers:**

| | C | F | Cb |
|---|---|---|---|
| Beef Teriyaki, 9.5 oz | 280 | 5 | 42 |
| Chicken & Noodles, 10 oz | 260 | 7 | 31 |
| Crustless Chicken Pot Pie, 9.6 oz | 300 | 6 | 40 |
| General Tso's Spicy Chicken, 10.3 oz | 290 | 3.5 | 47 |
| Grilled Chkn Pesto with Veg., 9.6 oz | 290 | 7 | 36 |
| Sweet & Sour Chicken, 10 oz | 390 | 8 | 65 |
| **Gluten Free:** Beef Merlot, 9.5 oz | 180 | 4 | 20 |
| Cajun Style Chkn & Shrimp, 9.6 oz | 220 | 2.5 | 35 |
| **Vegetarian,** Portab. Spin. Parmesan | 230 | 5 | 38 |
| **Classics:** Chicken Parmig., 11.6 oz | 360 | 12 | 47 |
| Lemon Pepper Fish, 10.7 oz | 290 | 4 | 50 |

**Power Bowls:** *Per Bowl*

| | C | F | Cb |
|---|---|---|---|
| Adobo Chicken | 330 | 8 | 38 |
| Chicken Feta & Farro | 310 | 9 | 34 |
| Cuban Inspired Pork | 340 | 8 | 46 |
| Italian Chicken Sausage & Peppers | 290 | 9 | 36 |
| **Morning:** Pesto Egg Wh. Scramble | 190 | 6 | 21 |
| Unwrapped Burrito Scramble | 170 | 3.5 | 21 |

**Simply Steamers:** *Per Package*

| | C | F | Cb |
|---|---|---|---|
| Beef & Broccoli, 10 oz | 280 | 7 | 32 |
| Beef Chimichurri, 9 oz | 220 | 6 | 24 |
| Chicken & Vegetable Stir Fry, 9.2 oz | 190 | 4 | 15 |
| Gr. Chicken Pesto & Veggies, 9.1 oz | 200 | 5 | 11 |
| Meatball Marinara, 10 oz | 280 | 6 | 36 |

## Heinz:

| | C | F | Cb |
|---|---|---|---|
| **Beans**, Original BBQ, ½ cup, 4.6 oz | 190 | 0.5 | 39 |

**Frozen:**
**Devour Meals:** *Per Package*

| | C | F | Cb |
|---|---|---|---|
| Bacon Topped Turkey w/ Garlic Sce | 410 | 19 | 28 |
| Buffalo Chicken Mac & Cheese | 620 | 31 | 56 |
| Cajun Syle Alfredo w/ Ssg & Chkn | 410 | 19 | 34 |
| Loaded Potato w/ Beef & Bacon | 330 | 14 | 31 |
| Pesto Ravioli w/Spicy Italian Ssg | 670 | 37 | 55 |
| Pulled Chicken Burrito Bowl | 450 | 15 | 47 |
| White Chedd. Mac & Cheese w/ Bacon | 710 | 41 | 54 |
| **Bowls:** Creamy Alfredo Mac & Chse | 350 | 12 | 50 |
| Hot & Melty Nacho Mac & Cheese | 400 | 13 | 60 |
| Sharp Chedd. Mac & Chse w/ bacon | 350 | 10 | 49 |
| **Sandwiches:** Buffalo Chkn Gr. Cheese | 520 | 19 | 60 |
| Philly Cheesesteak Grilled Cheese | 480 | 17 | 62 |
| Smokehouse Angus Beef | 480 | 16 | 61 |
| Sweet & Smoky Pork Grilled Cheese | 510 | 19 | 60 |
| Turkey & Bacon w/ Ranch Gr Chse | 550 | 23 | 59 |

## Hormel:
**Chili with Beans:** *Per 8.7 oz Cup*

| | C | F | Cb |
|---|---|---|---|
| Regular; Hot; Chunky, av. | 265 | 9 | 32 |
| Turkey, 98% Fat-Free | 220 | 3 | 29 |
| Vegetarian, 99% Fat Free | 200 | 1.5 | 35 |

**Chili No Beans:** *Per 8.3 oz Cup*

| | C | F | Cb |
|---|---|---|---|
| Regular | 260 | 14 | 19 |
| Hot; Chunky, average | 255 | 13 | 19 |
| Turkey, 98% Fat-Free | 190 | 3 | 16 |

**Compleats, Comfort Classics:** *Per 7.5 oz Pkg*

| | C | F | Cb |
|---|---|---|---|
| Beefy Mac & Cheese | 230 | 4 | 37 |
| Chicken & Noodles, | 180 | 6 | 20 |
| Dumplings & Chkn | 190 | 3.5 | 32 |
| Noodles & Beef | 170 | 2 | 28 |
| Spaghetti & Meat Sauce | 220 | 6 | 31 |

**Compleats, Homesyle:** *Per Package*

| | C | F | Cb |
|---|---|---|---|
| Beef Pot Roast | 200 | 6 | 20 |
| Chicken Alfredo | 350 | 18 | 30 |
| Chkn Brst, Gravy & Mashed Potatoes | 220 | 4 | 28 |
| Meatloaf, Gravy & Mashed Potatos | 300 | 14 | 28 |
| Salisbury Steak | 300 | 16 | 27 |
| Swedish Meatballs | 280 | 13 | 26 |

**Refrigerated Entrees:** *Per Package*

| | C | F | Cb |
|---|---|---|---|
| H'style Meat Loaf & Tom. Sce, 5 oz | 220 | 9 | 14 |
| Sliced Rstd Turkey Brst & Gravy, 5 oz | 110 | 2.5 | 3 |
| Slow Simm. Beef Tips w/ Gravy, 4.3 oz | 170 | 10 | 3 |
| **Side Dishes:** Bacon Mac & Chse, 8.2 oz | 340 | 11 | 45 |
| Chipotle Chedd. Mac & Chse, 8.2 oz | 340 | 14 | 41 |
| **Tamales:** Beef in Chile Sauce, 7.5 oz | 190 | 9 | 22 |
| Beef, Hot & Spicy in Chile Sce, 7.5 oz | 180 | 8 | 22 |
| Mashed Sweet Potatoes, 5 oz | 170 | 6 | 27 |

| Hot Pockets: | C | F | Cb |
|---|---|---|---|
| **Sandwiches:** *Per Sandwich* | | | |
| **Crispy Buttery Crust:** | | | |
| BBQ Recipe Beef | 320 | 12 | 45 |
| Cheddar Cheeseburger | 290 | 10 | 41 |
| Chicken Broccoli & Cheddar | 280 | 9 | 39 |
| Ham & Cheddar | 270 | 9 | 39 |
| **Crispy Crust:** | | | |
| Five Cheese Pizza | 340 | 16 | 38 |
| Pepperoni Pizza | 330 | 17 | 34 |
| **Croissant Crust:** | | | |
| Chicken Broccoli & Cheddar | 300 | 13 | 36 |
| Hickory Ham & Cheddar | 300 | 13 | 37 |
| Philly Steak & Cheese | 310 | 14 | 37 |
| Breakfast: | | | |
| Bacon, Egg & Chse | 320 | 14 | 37 |
| Sausage, Egg & Cheese | 320 | 15 | 35 |
| **Flaky Crust,** Chicken Pot Pie | 230 | 8 | 31 |
| **High Protein:** | | | |
| Crispy Butter Crust: | | | |
| Chicken Bacon Cheddar Melt | 280 | 10 | 34 |
| Steak & Cheddar | 310 | 13 | 34 |
| Garlic Buttery Crust, | | | |
| Four Meat & Four Cheese Pizza | 310 | 14 | 33 |
| **Pretzel Bread,** Bacon Chedd. Melt | 310 | 12 | 36 |
| **Stuffed Pretzels:** | | | |
| Cheesy Jalapeno | 130 | 3.5 | 19 |
| Chorizo Queso Fundido | 140 | 4.5 | 19 |
| Hungry Jack: | | | |
| **Casserole Potatoes:** *Prepared* | | | |
| Au Gratin | 140 | 4.5 | 24 |
| Cheddar & Bacon | 140 | 4.5 | 24 |
| Cheesy Scalloped | 140 | 4.5 | 24 |
| **Hashbrowns:** *Prepared* | | | |
| Original, ⅓ cup | 100 | 4.5 | 14 |
| Black Pepper & Onions, ¼ cup | 80 | 3 | 13 |
| Cheesy, ½ cup | 140 | 7 | 17 |
| **Mashed Potatoes,** | | | |
| Dry Mix only, ⅓ cup, prepared | 170 | 7 | 24 |
| Hungry Man: | | | |
| **Dinners:** | | | |
| Beer Battered Chicken | 770 | 38 | 73 |
| Bourbon Beef Strips | 500 | 14 | 73 |
| Grilled Beef Patty | 450 | 22 | 39 |
| Salisbury Steak | 580 | 32 | 51 |
| Smokin Backyard Barbeque | 700 | 26 | 92 |
| Spicy Boneless Fried Chicken Patties | 800 | 39 | 82 |
| **Hand Fulls:** *Each* | | | |
| Burstin' Buffalo Chicken (1) | 610 | 28 | 67 |
| Chicken Fajita (1) | 580 | 27 | 68 |
| Fillin' Philly Cheesesteak (1) | 610 | 31 | 64 |
| Wham Bam Ham & Cheese (1) | 640 | 30 | 73 |

| Hungry Man (Cont): | C | F | Cb |
|---|---|---|---|
| **Selects:** *Per Package* | | | |
| Boneless Fried Chicken & Waffles | 800 | 27 | 114 |
| Classic Fried Chicken | 970 | 59 | 59 |
| Mesquite Flav. Classic Fried Chicken | 1050 | 72 | 60 |
| Steak Strips | 420 | 12 | 55 |
| José Olé: | | | |
| **Breakfast Burritos:** | | | |
| Egg & Bacon, 4 oz | 260 | 10 | 30 |
| Egg & Sausage, 4 oz | 240 | 10 | 28 |
| **Burritos:** | | | |
| Chicken Monterey (1) | 270 | 7 | 39 |
| Steak & Cheese (1) | 310 | 11 | 40 |
| Steak & Jalapeno (1) | 280 | 7 | 41 |
| **Chimichangas:** | | | |
| Chicken & Cheese (1) | 330 | 13 | 42 |
| Chipotle Chicken (1) | 330 | 13 | 42 |
| Loaded Beef Nacho (1) | 420 | 25 | 36 |
| Queso Chicken Nacho (1) | 330 | 16 | 33 |
| Steak & Cheese (1) | 310 | 11 | 40 |
| **Dos Tacos:** Seasoned Beef (1) | 280 | 12 | 32 |
| Shredded Chicken (2) | 230 | 9 | 30 |
| **Minis & Bites:** | | | |
| Mini: Chimichangas, | | | |
| Steak & Cheddar (3) | 370 | 20 | 36 |
| Nacho Bites, Chicken & Chse (3) | 220 | 11 | 22 |
| Quesadillas, | | | |
| Chicken & Cheese (3) | 210 | 8 | 25 |
| Tacos: Beef & Cheese (4) | 220 | 11 | 23 |
| Queso Chicken Nacho (5) | 220 | 10 | 24 |
| **Rolled Tacos:** Loaded Beef Nacho (2) | 280 | 14 | 31 |
| Queso Chicken (2) | 270 | 12 | 31 |
| **Taquitos:** Beef, Corn tortillas (3) | 230 | 12 | 26 |
| Beef & Cheese, Flour Tortillas, (2) | 260 | 14 | 26 |
| Chicken, Corn Tortillas, (3) | 200 | 8 | 26 |
| Kashi: | | | |
| **Bowls:** *Per Package* | | | |
| Amaranth Polenta Plantain | 330 | 8 | 56 |
| Black Bean Mango | 310 | 8 | 55 |
| Chimichurri Quinoa | 240 | 7 | 41 |
| Creamy Cashew Noodle | 360 | 14 | 46 |
| Sweet Potato Quinoa | 270 | 6 | 48 |
| **Kid Cuisine:** *Per Meal* | | | |
| Bikini Bottom Chicken Breast Nuggets | 440 | 19 | 55 |
| Bubble Popcorn Chicken | 420 | 13 | 62 |
| Cheese Pizza | 450 | 13 | 68 |
| Friends Forever Mac. & Chse | 380 | 11 | 64 |
| Mini Corn Dogs | 490 | 15 | 75 |
| Oh Buoy Chicken Breast Nuggets | 430 | 19 | 51 |
| Spaghetti with Mini Meatballs | 330 | 7 | 51 |

## Kraft:

| | C | F | Cb |
|---|---|---|---|
| **Macaroni & Cheese:** | | | |
| **Original (7.25 oz Box):** | | | |
| ⅓ box, 2.5 oz (makes 1 cup) | | | |
| As Packaged | 250 | 3 | 47 |
| Prepared, 1 cup | 350 | 13 | 47 |
| **Deluxe:** | | | |
| Orig./4 Cheese/Broccoli/Bacon, average: | | | |
| ¼ box, 3.5 oz (makes 1 cup) | | | |
| As Packaged | 315 | 10 | 42 |
| **Microwave Bowls:** | | | |
| Finding Dory, prepared | 280 | 5 | 51 |
| Average other flavors, | | | |
| mix only, 2 oz | 220 | 4 | 41 |
| **Velveeta:** *Per Container* | | | |
| **Cheesy Bowls:** Bacon Mac & Chse | 330 | 13 | 39 |
| Bean & Rice Burrito | 350 | 9 | 59 |
| Buffalo Style Chkn Mac | 320 | 10 | 36 |
| Chicken Afredo | 300 | 9 | 35 |
| Chicken Chili Cheese Mac | 310 | 10 | 33 |
| Lasagna with Meat Sauce | 340 | 15 | 35 |
| Ultimate Cheeseburger Mac | 360 | 15 | 38 |
| **Shells & Cheese:** Original, 4 oz | 360 | 12 | 49 |
| Bacon, 4 oz | 360 | 14 | 45 |
| Queso Blanco, 4 oz | 360 | 12 | 50 |
| Spicy Chipotle, 4 oz | 370 | 12 | 52 |
| Spicy Jalapeno, 4 oz | 370 | 12 | 51 |

## Kroger:

| | C | F | Cb |
|---|---|---|---|
| **Creamy Mac & Cheese**, 8.8 oz | 400 | 17 | 45 |
| **Rich & Crmy Mac & Cheese**, 2.5 oz | 250 | 2 | 48 |
| **Frozen:** | | | |
| **Meatballs:** *Per 26 oz Package* | | | |
| Flame Broiled, 3 oz | 200 | 13 | 7 |
| Homestyle, 3 oz | 240 | 19 | 6 |
| Italian, 3 oz | 240 | 19 | 6 |
| Swedish Meatballs, 3 oz | 250 | 19 | 7 |
| Turkey, reduced fat, 3 oz | 160 | 9 | 6 |
| **Microwaveable:** *Per Container* | | | |
| 3 Minute Pizza: Cheese | 480 | 18 | 62 |
| Pepperoni | 540 | 25 | 63 |
| Three Meat | 510 | 21 | 64 |
| Beans & Franks in Tomato Sauce | 320 | 13 | 37 |
| Beef Stew | 160 | 8 | 15 |
| Cheeseburger with Bacon | 430 | 21 | 39 |
| **Refrigerated:** | | | |
| Beef Barbacoa, 5 oz | 200 | 10 | 2 |
| Charbr. Boneless Chkn Thighs, | | | |
| with BBQ Sauce, 5 oz | 180 | 1.5 | 17 |
| Chicken Verde w/ chili Sauce, 3.5 oz | 130 | 5 | 1 |
| Pork Burnt Ends in BBQ Sauce, 5 oz | 190 | 3.5 | 21 |

## Lean Cuisine:

| | C | F | Cb |
|---|---|---|---|
| **Comfort:** *Per Complete Meal* | | | |
| Asian-Style Chicken Spring Rolls (3) | 170 | 7 | 19 |
| Baked Chicken | 260 | 8 | 30 |
| Cheddar Bacon Chicken | 220 | 8 | 17 |
| Chicken Club Panini | 350 | 10 | 41 |
| Chicken in Sweet BBQ Sce | 290 | 9 | 30 |
| Chicken Parmesan | 340 | 9 | 46 |
| Chicken Pecan | 370 | 9 | 55 |
| Chicken Ranch Club Flatbread Melt | 370 | 9 | 52 |
| Glazed Chicken | 260 | 4 | 35 |
| Glazed Turkey Tenderloins | 270 | 5 | 41 |
| Herb Roasted Chicken | 160 | 3 | 18 |
| Meatloaf with Mashed Potatoes | 240 | 7 | 25 |
| Philly Steak & Cheese Panini | 330 | 9 | 44 |
| Roasted Turkey Breast | 290 | 4 | 48 |
| Salisbury Steak with Mac & Cheese | 280 | 8 | 28 |
| Steak Portabella | 160 | 5 | 11 |
| **Market Place:** *Per Package* | | | |
| Apple Cranberry Chicken | 280 | 4 | 48 |
| Butternut Squash Ravioli | 260 | 4 | 46 |
| Chicken Cashew Stir Fry | 270 | 2 | 48 |
| Chicken Tikka Masala | 310 | 4 | 51 |
| Chicken with Peanut Sauce | 290 | 7 | 35 |
| Creamy Basil Chicken w/ Tortellini | 240 | 6 | 28 |
| Fiesta Grilled Chicken | 250 | 5 | 33 |
| Garlic Sesame Noodles w/ Beef | 300 | 6 | 46 |
| Mango Chicken with Coconut Rice | 330 | 6 | 50 |
| Moroccan-Style Spiced Beef | 310 | 6 | 47 |
| Mushroom Mezzaluna Ravioli | 270 | 8 | 40 |
| Parmesan Crusted Fish | 290 | 7 | 42 |
| Pomegranate Chicken | 180 | 3 | 20 |
| Sesame Chicken | 330 | 9 | 51 |
| Spicy Beef & Bean Enchilada | 310 | 6 | 50 |
| Spin. Artichoke Ravioli | 280 | 7 | 41 |
| Sweet & Sour Chicken | 300 | 3 | 51 |
| Sweet & Spicy Korean-Style Beef | 320 | 7 | 50 |
| Sweet Sriracha Braised Beef | 180 | 5 | 18 |
| Vermont Mac & Cheese | 250 | 6 | 35 |

| Lean Cuisine (Cont): | C | F | Cb |
|---|---|---|---|
| **Origins** (Meatless)**:** *Per Pkg* | | | |
| Butternut Squash Lasagna | 340 | 6 | 55 |
| Cheese & Bean Enchilada Verde | 290 | 9 | 42 |
| Cheese & Fire Roasted Chile Tamale | 330 | 9 | 55 |
| Coconut Chickpea Curry | 260 | 7 | 38 |
| Farmer's Market Pizza | 320 | 9 | 46 |
| Linguine w/ Ricotta & Spinach | | | |
|    Meatless Meatballs | 280 | 8 | 40 |
| Mushroom & Veg. Shepherd's Pie | 150 | 3 | 25 |
| Ricotta Cheese & Spinach Ravioli | 310 | 7 | 51 |
| Roasted Garlic White Bean Alfredo | 330 | 9 | 50 |
| Sicilian Style Pesto w/ Lentil Pasta | 320 | 8 | 47 |
| Spicy Penne Arrabbiata | 240 | 5 | 40 |
| Tortellini with Red Pepper Sauce | 300 | 8 | 44 |
| Tuscan-Style Vegetable Lasagna | 310 | 7 | 46 |

**Pizzas** ~ *See Page 136*

**Extra Product Listings** ~ *www.CalorieKing.com*

**Lean Pockets:**

| **Sandwiches:** *Per Single Pocket* | | | |
|---|---|---|---|
| **Garlic & Herb Seasoned Crust:** | | | |
|   Caprese; Chicken Parmesan | 250 | 5 | 41 |
|   M'balls & Mozzarella | 280 | 9 | 41 |
|   Pepperponi Pizza | 280 | 8 | 42 |
| **Pretzel Bread:** | | | |
|   Chicken Japalpeno & Cheese | 260 | 7 | 36 |
|   Roasted Turkey, Bacon & Cheese | 270 | 9 | 35 |
|   Uncured Ham & White Cheddar | 270 | 7 | 39 |
| **Seasoned Crust:** | | | |
|   Philly Steak & Cheese | 260 | 7 | 41 |

**Lightlife (Meatless):**

**Frozen:**

| | C | F | Cb |
|---|---|---|---|
| **Gimme Lean Veggie Beef**, 2 oz slice | 60 | 0 | 7 |
| **Smart Deli:** Veggie Bologna, 4 slices | 70 | 1 | 3 |
|   Veggie Ham, 4 slices | 70 | 1 | 4 |
|   Veggie Turkey, 4 slices | 100 | 3.5 | 4 |
| **Smart Ground:** | | | |
|   Original, 1.95 oz | 70 | 0 | 6 |
|   Mexican Crumbles, 1.95 oz | 60 | 0 | 6 |
|   Plant Based, 4 oz | 270 | 17 | 10 |
| **Tempeh:** Original, 3 oz | 140 | 4.5 | 10 |
|   Organic Smoky Strips, 4 slices | 140 | 5 | 10 |

| **Lunchables:** *Per Package* | C | F | Cb |
|---|---|---|---|
| **Chicken Sliders** | 270 | 8 | 42 |
| **Lunch Combinations:** | | | |
|   Asian Style BBQ Chicken | 230 | 11 | 25 |
|   Chicken Dunks | 290 | 10 | 40 |
|   Italian Style Chicken | 230 | 11 | 20 |
|   Turkey & Cheddar with Crackers | 260 | 13 | 22 |
|   Ultimate Nachos | 580 | 27 | 75 |
| **Lunchmakers** *(Armour):* *Per Package* | | | |
| Bologna Cracker Crunchers | 230 | 11 | 22 |
| Chicken Cracker Crunchers | 220 | 10 | 23 |
| Nachos | 210 | 9 | 30 |
| Pepperoni Flav Sausage Pizza | 240 | 10 | 29 |
| Turkey Cracker Crunchers | 220 | 10 | 22 |

**Marie Callender's:**

**Frozen:**

| **Beef:** *Per Container* | C | F | Cb |
|---|---|---|---|
|   Beef Pot Roast | 200 | 4.5 | 26 |
|   Meat Loaf & Gravy | 380 | 13 | 45 |
|   Spaghetti w/ Meat Sce | 540 | 18 | 75 |
|   Salisbury Steak | 400 | 17 | 40 |
|   Slow Roasted Beef | 260 | 9 | 32 |
| **Bowls:** *Per Bowl* | | | |
|   Creamy Vermont Mac & Cheese | 570 | 22 | 71 |
|   Red Chili Grilled Chicken Burrito | 360 | 10 | 44 |
|   Spicy Buffalo Style Chkn Mac & Chse | 540 | 25 | 53 |
|   Sweet & Savory Sesame Chicken | 460 | 14 | 67 |
| **Chicken:** *Per Container* | | | |
|   Cheesy Chicken & Rice | 430 | 14 | 54 |
|   Chicken Parmigiana | 440 | 16 | 51 |
|   Cntry Fried Chkn & Gravy | 560 | 27 | 61 |
|   Roasted Garlic Chicken | 510 | 21 | 56 |
| **Pasta:** *Per Container* | | | |
|   Fettuccini Alfredo & Garlic Bread | 610 | 31 | 59 |
|   Fettuccini, Chicken & Broccoli | 440 | 20 | 38 |
|   Grilled Chicken Alfredo Bake | 460 | 19 | 45 |
| **Pot Pies:** *Per 1 Cup, 7 oz* | | | |
|   Beef | 400 | 21 | 40 |
|   Brocc. & Cheddar Potato | 680 | 40 | 69 |
|   Cheesy Chicken & Bacon | 510 | 32 | 41 |
|   Chicken Corn Chowder | 460 | 28 | 38 |
|   Chili with Beans | 420 | 23 | 43 |
|   Creamy: | | | |
|     Mushroom Chicken | 430 | 25 | 39 |
|     Parmesan Chicken | 430 | 26 | 36 |
|     Turkey | 480 | 28 | 46 |
| **Family size:** *Per 1 Cup* | | | |
|   Chicken, 7 oz | 370 | 21 | 35 |

| Maruchan: | C | F | Cb |
|---|---|---|---|
| **Bowls**, all var., 3.3 oz | 380 | 16 | 50 |
| **Ramen**, Noodle Soup, average all, 3 oz pkg | 380 | 16 | 52 |
| **Instant Lunch**, average, 1 package | 290 | 11 | 39 |
| **Yakisoba:** *Per 4 oz Pkg* | | | |
| Chicken/Teriyaki Beef Flavor, av. | 500 | 18 | 70 |
| Cheddar Cheese Flavor | 540 | 24 | 68 |
| **Michael Angelo's:** | | | |
| **Frozen:** | | | |
| **Calzones:** Meatball (1) | 300 | 10 | 39 |
| Primo Supreme (1) | 330 | 12 | 40 |
| **Gourmet Bowls:** Chicken Cavatappi | 290 | 7 | 37 |
| Gnocchi Alfredo with Bacon | 260 | 10 | 40 |
| Meat Lasagna Bolognese w/ Ssg. | 340 | 14 | 34 |
| **Organic:** Chicken Parmigiana, 10 oz | 310 | 6 | 47 |
| Eggplant Parmigiana, 10 oz | 240 | 12 | 22 |
| Lasagna with Meat Sauce, 10 oz | 370 | 16 | 37 |
| **Signature:** Baked Ziti w/ M'balls, 11 oz | 480 | 20 | 51 |
| Cheesy Pizza Pasta, 10 oz | 390 | 12 | 48 |
| Chicken Alfredo, 11 oz | 340 | 8 | 45 |
| Manicoti w/ Sauce, 11 oz | 400 | 19 | 36 |
| Sausage Lasagna, 11 oz | 470 | 22 | 47 |
| Shrimp Scampi, 10 oz | 580 | 28 | 61 |
| **Minute Rice:** | | | |
| **Ready To Serve:** *Per 4.4 oz Container, Prepared* | | | |
| Brown/Chicken Rice Mix, average | 220 | 3 | 43 |
| Fried/Yellow Rice Mix, average | 220 | 2.5 | 45 |
| **Morningstar Farms (Meatless):** | | | |
| **Breakfast**, Patties, all flavors (1) | 70 | 3 | 3 |
| **Burgers:** | | | |
| Grillers Original (1) | 130 | 5 | 8 |
| Medit. Chickpea (1) | 120 | 4.5 | 13 |
| Spicy Black Bean (1) | 110 | 4.5 | 13 |
| **Chik Patties:** Original (1) | 170 | 7 | 20 |
| Buffalo (1) | 160 | 6 | 19 |
| **Progressive Options:** | | | |
| Indian Veggie Burger (1) | 130 | 8 | 11 |
| White Bean Chili Burger (1) | 150 | 9 | 14 |
| **Veggie Classics:** Buffalo Wings (5) | 200 | 8 | 21 |
| Chik'n Nuggets (4) | 200 | 9 | 20 |
| Parmesan Garlic Wings (5) | 190 | 8 | 19 |
| **Nissin:** | | | |
| **Chow Mein:** *Per 4 oz Package* | | | |
| Chicken/Spicy Chicken Flavor | 500 | 22 | 66 |
| Pad Thai | 560 | 28 | 33 |
| Spicy Chicken Flavor | 500 | 22 | 66 |
| Teriyaki Beef Flavor | 520 | 24 | 64 |
| Shrimp Flavor | 560 | 30 | 64 |
| **Cup Noodles:** Hearty Chicken, 1 pkg | 300 | 12 | 40 |
| Average other flavors, 1 pkg | 290 | 11 | 42 |

| Nissin (Cont): | C | F | Cb |
|---|---|---|---|
| **Cup Noodles (Contd):** | | | |
| **Very Veggie:** Per Pkg | | | |
| Spicy/Soy flavors, av., 2.75 oz | 345 | 11 | 53 |
| Chicken/Beef, 2.75 oz | 330 | 11 | 49 |
| **Old El Paso:** | | | |
| **Dinner Kits:** | | | |
| **Chicken:** Gordita (1) | 310 | 12 | 42 |
| Enchiladas 1½ enchiladas | 400 | 14 | 27 |
| Fajitas, with Peppers & Onions (2) | 330 | 10 | 31 |
| **Ground Beef:** Crunchy Tacos (2) | 250 | 12 | 17 |
| Soft Tacos (2) | 330 | 19 | 30 |
| **Rice & Black Beans,** Burrito (1) | 270 | 10 | 31 |
| **Pasta Roni:** *Per Cup, Prepared* | | | |
| Angel Hair Pasta, with Herbs | 270 | 9 | 38 |
| Butter & Herb Italiano | 300 | 12 | 42 |
| Chicken & Broccoli | 360 | 15 | 47 |
| Chicken Flavor | 300 | 12 | 39 |
| Fettuccine Alfredo | 440 | 24 | 48 |
| Tomato Parmesan | 270 | 9 | 39 |
| White Cheddar & Broccoli | 310 | 13 | 39 |
| **P.F. Chang's:** *Per ½ Package, 11 oz* | | | |
| **Frozen:** | | | |
| **Entrees:** Beef with Broccoli | 310 | 11 | 23 |
| General Chang's Chicken | 370 | 12 | 48 |
| Kung Pao Chicken | 360 | 14 | 35 |
| Mongolian Style Beef | 310 | 7 | 39 |
| Sesame Chicken | 400 | 20 | 34 |
| Sweet & Sour Chicken | 340 | 9 | 51 |
| **Ramen:** Chicken Tonkotsu | 230 | 10 | 20 |
| Veggie Shoyu | 160 | 2 | 28 |
| **Sides**, Vegetable Lo Mein | 270 | 5 | 46 |
| **Prego:** | | | |
| **Ready Meals:** *Per Pouch* | | | |
| Creamy Three Cheese Alfedo Rotini | 370 | 19 | 37 |
| Creamy Tomato Penne | 400 | 15 | 57 |
| Marinara & Italian Sausage Rotini | 350 | 9 | 55 |
| Roasted Tomato & Vegetables Penne | 300 | 4 | 55 |

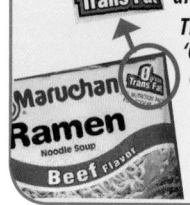

*Most packaged noodle soups are high in calories and fat.*

*Their promotion of 'O Grams Trans Fat' does not make them heart-healthy.*

*They are still high in saturated fat as well as salt/sodium.*

## Rice-A-Roni:

| | C | F | Cb |
|---|---|---|---|
| **Classic Favorites:** *Per Cup, Prepared* | | | |
| Beef | 270 | 5 | 50 |
| Cheddar Broccoli | 350 | 16 | 47 |
| Chkn & Garlic; Mex. Style | 250 | 8 | 41 |
| Rice Pilaf | 310 | 8 | 52 |
| Shells & White Cheddar | 290 | 12 | 39 |
| **Single Serve Cups:** | | | |
| Cheddar Broccoli | 230 | 4.5 | 41 |
| Chicken Flavor | 190 | 1 | 41 |
| Creamy Four Cheese | 240 | 6 | 43 |

## Rosarita:

| | C | F | Cb |
|---|---|---|---|
| Black Beans, 4.5 oz | 110 | 0.5 | 19 |
| Pinto Beans, 4.5 oz | 120 | 0 | 22 |
| **Refried Beans:** | | | |
| Traditional, 4.5 oz | 120 | 2.5 | 18 |
| No Fat, 4.5 oz | 100 | 0 | 18 |
| Restaurant Style, 4.4 oz | 90 | 2.5 | 13 |
| Vegetarian, 4.5 oz | 120 | 2 | 19 |

## Safeway Select (Albertsons):
**Frozen:**

| | C | F | Cb |
|---|---|---|---|
| **Signature Select:** Chkn Enchilada | 300 | 8 | 40 |
| **Classic:** Six Cheese Lasagna | 370 | 10 | 53 |
| Lasagna with Meat Sauce | 450 | 16 | 56 |
| Spaghetti with Meat Sauce | 400 | 9 | 61 |
| **Gourmet Club:** Chicken Enchiladas | 220 | 10 | 22 |
| Mexican Sstyle Lasagna | 390 | 16 | 42 |
| Orange Chicken | 400 | 13 | 56 |
| Shredded Beef Enchilada | 340 | 11 | 47 |
| Triple Cheese Enchilada | 390 | 16 | 49 |

## S & W: *Per ½ Cup*

| | C | F | Cb |
|---|---|---|---|
| **Classic:** Black Beans, 4.6 oz | 120 | 0 | 22 |
| Kidney Beans, 4.6 oz | 110 | 0 | 21 |
| Pinto Beans, 4.6 oz | 100 | 0 | 20 |
| White Beans, 4.6 oz | 100 | 0 | 19 |
| **Flavored:** *Per ½ cup* | | | |
| Indian Style Savory Sides | 150 | 3.5 | 24 |
| New Orleans Style Savory Sides | 160 | 4 | 23 |
| Tuscan Style Savory Sides | 130 | 2 | 21 |

## Seapak ~ *See www.calorieking.com*

## Simply Asia: *Per Container*

| | C | F | Cb |
|---|---|---|---|
| **Japanese:** Ramen Noodles, 2 oz | 200 | 1 | 42 |
| Soba Noodles, 2 oz | 190 | 1 | 40 |
| **Noodle Bowls:** *Per Bowl* | | | |
| Sesame Teriyaki | | | |
| Spicy Mongolian | 430 | 6 | 86 |
| **Street Noodles:** | | | |
| Garlic Basil | 360 | 5 | 74 |
| Kimchi | 360 | 4 | 76 |
| Sesame Ginger | 420 | 4 | 84 |

## Smart Ones (*Weight Watchers*):
**Frozen:**

| | C | F | Cb |
|---|---|---|---|
| **Indulgence:** *Per Package* | | | |
| Chicken Cordon Bleu Orzo | 310 | 6 | 39 |
| Herb Crusted Chicken | 300 | 6 | 40 |
| Portobello Mushroom Risotto | 310 | 10 | 43 |
| **Smartmade:** *Per Package* | | | |
| Black Beans & Cheese over Cilantro Rice | 320 | 6 | 49 |
| Chicken Fried Cauliflower Rice Bowl | 150 | 2.5 | 16 |
| Chicken with Spinach Fettuccine | 220 | 6 | 19 |
| Grilled Sesame Beef & Broccoli | 220 | 5 | 31 |
| Lemon Garlic Chicken Fettuccini | 200 | 4 | 23 |
| Mexican Style Chicken Bowl | 260 | 5 | 33 |
| Mexican Style Pulled Pork Bowl | 320 | 9 | 33 |
| Roasted Turkey & Veggies | 240 | 2.5 | 36 |
| Rosemary Grilled Beef & Veggies | 270 | 8 | 30 |
| White Wome Chicken & Couscous | 190 | 2.5 | 23 |
| **Smart Ones:** *Per Package* | | | |
| Angel Hair Marinara | 200 | 2.5 | 37 |
| Bals. Chkn Margherita | 240 | 4 | 35 |
| Beef & Rice Casserole | 290 | 8 | 41 |
| Brocc. & Chkn Rigatoni | 260 | 4 | 40 |
| Broccoli Cheddar Roasted Potato | 190 | 8 | 21 |
| Canadian Bacon English Muffin | 210 | 6 | 27 |
| Cheese Ravioli, | | | |
| in Mushroom Cream Sauce | 230 | 5 | 35 |
| Cheese Scramble w/ Hash Browns | 210 | 7 | 22 |
| Chicken Enchiladas Suiza | 290 | 6 | 46 |
| Chicken Fettuccini | 300 | 4.5 | 44 |
| Creamy Basil Chicken | 170 | 3.5 | 15 |
| Florentine Ravioli | 210 | 3.5 | 37 |
| Lem. Herb Chkn Picante | 230 | 2.5 | 37 |
| Macaroni & Cheese | 260 | 2 | 50 |
| Meat Sauce Lasagna Bake | 300 | 5 | 51 |
| Pasta Primavera | 210 | 2.5 | 37 |
| Pasta with Ricotta & Spinach | 280 | 6 | 44 |
| Roasted Turkey Breast | 170 | 4 | 17 |
| Santa Fe Rice & Beans | 260 | 6 | 39 |
| Three Cheese Macaroni | 310 | 5 | 50 |
| Three Cheese Ziti Marinara | 300 | 8 | 43 |
| Tuna Noodle Gratin | 270 | 3.5 | 46 |

## Stagg:

| **Chili with Beans, 15 oz Can:** *Per Cup* | C | F | Cb |
|---|---|---|---|
| Classic, 8.7 oz | 290 | 13 | 26 |
| Dynamite Hot, 8.7 oz | 340 | 16 | 33 |
| Laredo, 8.7 oz | 300 | 17 | 23 |
| Silverado, 8.7 oz | 260 | 8 | 30 |

## Stouffer's:

| | C | F | Cb |
|---|---|---|---|
| **Frozen:** | | | |
| **Bowl-Fulls:** *For One* | | | |
| Cheesy Chkn Parmesan | 520 | 16 | 67 |
| Fried Chicken & Mashed Potatoes | 470 | 19 | 51 |
| Slow Roasted Steak & Potatoes | 370 | 15 | 36 |
| Southwest Style Mac & Cheese | 520 | 25 | 47 |
| Spicy Italian Sausage Pasta | 660 | 35 | 63 |
| **Classics:** *For One* | | | |
| Baked Chicken | 240 | 8 | 17 |
| Cheddar Potato Bake | 270 | 17 | 21 |
| Chicken a la King | 360 | 12 | 44 |
| Fettuccini Alfredo | 630 | 35 | 63 |
| Fish Filet with Mac & Cheese | 400 | 19 | 35 |
| Five Cheese Lasagna | 370 | 14 | 39 |
| Green Pepper Steak | 240 | 4 | 32 |
| Macaroni & Cheese | 340 | 16 | 33 |
| Meat Lovers Lasagna | 420 | 19 | 41 |
| Roast Turkey | 270 | 9 | 30 |
| Spagh. w/ Meatballs | 360 | 12 | 45 |
| Tuna Noodle Casserole | 450 | 20 | 45 |
| White Meat Chkn Pot Pie | 590 | 34 | 54 |
| **Chicken Comforts:** *Party Size* | | | |
| Chicken Enchiladas | 280 | 12 | 30 |
| Five Cheese Lasagna | 260 | 8 | 34 |
| Lasagna Italiano | 340 | 12 | 35 |
| Macaroni & Cheese | 350 | 17 | 34 |
| Vegetable Lasagna | 320 | 13 | 35 |
| **Fit Kitchen Protein Bowls:** *Per Package* | | | |
| Bourbon Steak | 280 | 5 | 41 |
| Meatball & Peppers | 360 | 11 | 43 |
| Moroccan Style Chkn | 340 | 4 | 53 |
| Spicy Chicken Chorizo | 360 | 14 | 38 |
| Steak Fajitas | 370 | 9 | 48 |
| Teriyaki Chicken | 325 | 9 | 46 |
| **Simply Crafted:** *Family Size* | | | |
| Five Cheese Lasagna | 230 | 7 | 32 |
| Fettuccine Alfredo with Broccoli | 260 | 7 | 35 |
| Spicy Pomodoro Penne | 260 | 6 | 41 |
| White Cheddar Mac & Cheese | 300 | 7 | 43 |
| **Urban Bistro:** *For One* | | | |
| Aged Asiago Lasagna | 350 | 12 | 40 |
| Beer Glazed Meatballs | 390 | 13 | 40 |
| Cheddar & Goat Cheese Mac | 410 | 16 | 48 |
| Chicken & Cheddar Grits | 240 | 8 | 21 |
| Kentucky Bourbon Glazed Chicken | 280 | 9 | 33 |
| Smoked Gouda & Chorizo Mac | 350 | 13 | 41 |
| Spiced Chicken & Couscous | 320 | 7 | 45 |
| Spiced Tortellini Arrabbiata | 380 | 10 | 56 |

## Swanson:

| | C | F | Cb |
|---|---|---|---|
| **Frozen:** | | | |
| **Dinners:** *Per Package* | | | |
| Chicken Nuggets | 590 | 25 | 71 |
| Chicken Parmigiana | 450 | 23 | 45 |
| Chicken Strips | 480 | 19 | 61 |
| Fried Chicken | 520 | 26 | 54 |
| Meatloaf | 450 | 23 | 46 |
| Rib Style Boneless Pork | 540 | 23 | 71 |
| Salisbury Steak | 450 | 22 | 44 |
| Turkey | 330 | 9 | 45 |
| **Meat Pies:** Beef | 430 | 26 | 37 |
| Chicken | 370 | 20 | 37 |
| Turkeuy | 400 | 23 | 38 |
| **Skillets:** *For Two* | | | |
| Alfredo Chicken | 370 | 12 | 42 |
| Beef Lo Mein | 360 | 6 | 55 |
| Chicken Parmesan | 430 | 14 | 60 |
| Chicken Florentine | 310 | 7 | 40 |
| Creamy Cheddar Chicken | 360 | 8 | 52 |
| Garlic Chicken | 420 | 15 | 51 |
| Garlic Shrimp | 390 | 14 | 49 |
| Teriyaki Chicken | 290 | 2.5 | 51 |
| **Tasty Bite:** | | | |
| **Mains:** *Per ½ Package, 5 oz* | | | |
| Bengal Lentils | 160 | 6 | 20 |
| Bombay Potatoes | 140 | 4 | 22 |
| Channa Masala | 170 | 6 | 23 |
| Coconut Vegetables | 120 | 8 | 10 |
| Jaipur Vegetables | 150 | 10 | 12 |
| Jodhpur Lentils | 130 | 3.5 | 18 |
| Kashmir Spinach | 110 | 7 | 6 |
| Madras Lentils | 150 | 6 | 17 |
| Punjab Eggplant | 100 | 5 | 12 |
| Thai Vegetable Curry | 140 | 9 | 12 |
| **TGI Friday's:** | | | |
| **Angus BBQ Bacon Slider (1)** | 250 | 14 | 21 |
| **Buffalo Style Chicken Wings,** | | | |
| with Sauce, 4.5 oz | 240 | 16 | 10 |
| **Cheddar & Bacon Potato Skins (1)** | 190 | 13 | 15 |
| **Honey BBQ Chicken Wings,** 3 oz | 170 | 11 | 8 |
| **Mozzarella Sticks,** w/ Sauce (1) | 100 | 5 | 10 |
| **Poppers,** | | | |
| Cream Chse Stuffed Jalap. w/ Sce (3) | 240 | 14 | 29 |
| **Thai Kitchen:** | | | |
| **Noodle Carts:** *Per 9.77 oz Tray* | | | |
| Pad Thai | 440 | 2.5 | 98 |
| Thai Peanut | 540 | 12 | 96 |
| **Rice Noodle Soup Bowls,** | | | |
| Spring Onion, 2.4 oz | 130 | 0 | 25 |

| Tofurky: *Per Item* | **C** | **F** | **Cb** |
|---|---|---|---|
| **Plant Based Chick'n:** Barbecue, 3.2 oz | 210 | 6 | 14 |
| Sesame Garlic, 3.2 oz | 210 | 9 | 12 |
| Thai Basil, 3.2 oz | 190 | 7 | 10 |
| **Pockets:** Ham Style & Ched'ar (1) | 290 | 10 | 37 |
| Pepp'roni (1) | 350 | 10 | 49 |
| **Roasts:** Holiday Feast, 5.3 oz | 300 | 10 | 19 |
| With Wild Rice & Stuffing, 5.2 oz | 290 | 10 | 17 |
| Add Gravy, ¼ cup | 40 | 2.5 | 4 |
| **Tempeh:** Original Soy Cake, 3 oz | 170 | 4.5 | 12 |
| Organic Five Grain, 3 oz | 190 | 10 | 15 |
| Sesame Garlic, 3 oz | 130 | 3 | 14 |
| Smoky Maple Bacon, 3 oz | 130 | 1 | 17 |

| Trader Joe's: | | | |
|---|---|---|---|
| **Baked Beans**, Organic, av., ½ cup | 140 | 0 | 29 |
| **Black Beans:** | | | |
| Regular, ½ cup | 110 | 0 | 19 |
| Cuban Style, ½ cup | 100 | 0.5 | 19 |
| Chicken Chili with Beans, 1 cup | 290 | 9 | 32 |
| Pasta, Shells & White Cheddar, 1 cup | 280 | 6 | 47 |
| **Potatoes:** Garlic Mashed, ½ cup | 150 | 7 | 19 |
| Cheddar Cheese Au Gratin, ½ cup | 140 | 5 | 21 |
| Turkey Chili w/ Beans, 1 cup | 240 | 4.5 | 30 |
| **Frozen:** | | | |
| Butter Chicken w/ Basmati Rice, 1 cup | 270 | 8 | 33 |
| Chicken Chow Mein, ⅓ pkg, 6.7 oz | 210 | 2 | 35 |
| Chicken Quesadilla (1), 6 oz | 320 | 16 | 26 |
| Citrus Glazed Chicken with Rice, 8 oz | 270 | 5 | 40 |
| Mac & Cheese: Regular, 1 cup, 7 oz | 360 | 15 | 42 |
| Reduced Guilt, 7 oz | 270 | 6 | 40 |
| **Pies:** Chicken Pot Pie, ½ pie, 8 oz | 360 | 22 | 28 |
| Shepherd's Pie, 1 cup, 8 oz | 170 | 3 | 22 |
| Shrimp Stir Fry, 6.4 oz | 70 | 0.5 | 6 |
| Spaghetti & Beef Meatballs, 1 cup, 9 oz | 380 | 13 | 48 |
| Spicy Beef & Broccoli, 1¾ cups | 430 | 13 | 64 |
| Thai Vegetable Kao Soi, 12.6 oz | 430 | 20 | 55 |
| Vegetable Pad Thai, 10.5 oz tray | 520 | 21 | 74 |

| Tyson: | | | |
|---|---|---|---|
| **Any'tizers Snacks:** | | | |
| **Boneless Chicken Bites:** | | | |
| Buffalo Style, 3 oz | 180 | 9 | 12 |
| Honey BBQ, 3 oz | 210 | 9 | 20 |
| Sriracha, 3 oz | 200 | 11 | 12 |
| Zesty Garlic Parmesan, 2.8 oz | 190 | 9 | 13 |
| Homestyle Chicken Fries (3), 3.2 oz | 230 | 13 | 14 |
| Popcorn Chicken, 3 oz | 170 | 7 | 14 |
| Wings, Tequila Lime flavored, 3 oz | 170 | 11 | 3 |

| Tyson (Cont): | **C** | **F** | **Cb** |
|---|---|---|---|
| **Frozen:** | | | |
| **Beef:** Cntry Fried Steak (1) | 300 | 21 | 15 |
| Hickory Smoked Strips, 3 oz | 120 | 4 | 2 |
| Steak Fingers, 2.5 oz | 250 | 18 | 14 |
| **Breaded Chicken:** Nuggets, 3.2 oz | 270 | 17 | 15 |
| Crispy Strips, 3 oz | 210 | 10 | 17 |
| Fun Nuggets 2.7 oz | 180 | 11 | 10 |
| Honey Batt. Breast Tenders, 3 oz | 210 | 13 | 13 |
| Pizza Nuggets, 3 oz | 250 | 16 | 14 |
| Southern Breast Tenderloins, 3 oz | 180 | 9 | 12 |
| Spicy Breast Patties, 2.7 oz | 200 | 13 | 10 |
| **Dinner Kits:** | | | |
| Four Cheese Chkn & Brocc. Pasta, 9.4 oz | 350 | 15 | 29 |
| Sweet Chiptle Chkn Veggie Hash, 9.1 oz | 270 | 8 | 35 |
| Tomato Herb Chkn Vegge Pasta, 9.4 oz | 270 | 7 | 35 |
| **Grilled Chkn Breasts:** Blackened, 3 oz | 110 | 3 | 1 |
| Breast Fillets, 3.5 oz | 130 | 4.5 | 2 |
| Fajita Strips, 3 oz | 100 | 2 | 2 |
| Oven Roasted, Diced, 3 oz | 100 | 2.5 | 1 |
| Sweet Teriyaki Chicken Fillets, 3 oz | 140 | 6 | 4 |

| Uncle Ben's: | | | |
|---|---|---|---|
| **Flavored Grains:** *Dry Mix Only, as Directed* | | | |
| Average all flavors, 1 cup, cooked | 200 | 0.5 | 42 |
| **Flav. Infusions**, dry mix, av., 1.7 oz | 155 | 0.5 | 34 |
| **Ready Rice:** *Per 1 Cup, Heat & Serve* | | | |
| Brown Jasmin & Edamame | 250 | 5 | 43 |
| Brown Rice & Black Beans | 210 | 3.5 | 37 |
| Butter & Garlic Flavored | 220 | 4 | 41 |
| Cheddar & Broccoli Flav. | 230 | 5 | 41 |
| Creamy Four Cheese Flav. | 220 | 5 | 40 |
| Garden Vegetable | 210 | 2.5 | 42 |
| Jambalaya Flavored | 200 | 2 | 40 |
| Long Grain & Black Beans | 220 | 4.5 | 40 |
| Red Beans & Rice | 210 | 2.5 | 41 |
| Roasted Chicken Flavor | 210 | 3 | 42 |
| Teriyaki Style | 220 | 3 | 42 |

| Van Camp's: | | | |
|---|---|---|---|
| **Baked Beans:** Orig., ½ cup, 4.8 oz | 150 | 0.5 | 30 |
| Bacon, ½ cup, 4.8 oz | 160 | 1 | 30 |
| **Beanee Weenee:** Original, 7.75 oz | 260 | 8 | 33 |
| Barbecue, 7.75oz | 280 | 8 | 39 |
| Smoked Hickory, 7.75 oz | 320 | 8 | 48 |
| **Chili**, with Beans, 9 oz | 410 | 24 | 34 |
| **Pork & Beans**, in Tom. Sce, 4.6 oz | 120 | 1 | 23 |

| Van De Kamp's: | C | F | Cb |
|---|---|---|---|
| **Frozen:** | | | |
| **Fillets:** | | | |
| Beer Battered/Crispy, 3.8 oz | 210 | 10 | 21 |
| Crunchy, 3.8 oz | 240 | 12 | 24 |
| Garlic Herb Cod, 5 oz | 260 | 10 | 26 |
| Lemon Pepper Cod, 5 oz | 260 | 4.5 | 38 |
| **Fish Sticks:** | | | |
| Crunchy, 3.6 oz | 220 | 10 | 20 |
| Nacho, 3 oz | 200 | 10 | 18 |
| Ranch (4), 3 oz | 200 | 10 | 18 |
| **Steam Bags:** Baja Style Cod, 2 cups | 290 | 5 | 38 |
| California Style Salmon, 2 cups | 260 | 7 | 32 |
| Garlic Shrimp, 2 cups | 300 | 8 | 50 |
| Lemon Herb Shrimp, 2 cups | 220 | 4 | 37 |
| **Whole Foods (365):** | | | |
| Chickenless Nuggets, | | | |
| breaded (4), 2.8 oz | 180 | 7 | 16 |
| Meatless Meatballs (4), 2 oz | 110 | 4 | 9 |
| Meatless Burgers (1), 2.5 oz | 120 | 4.5 | 7 |
| Pasta Rings in Tomato Sauce, 1 cup | 150 | 1 | 31 |
| Vegetarian Chili, 1 cup | 130 | 2 | 25 |
| **Worthington/Loma Linda** *(Vegan):* | | | |
| **Big Franks:** 1 link, 1.8 oz | 110 | 6 | 3 |
| Low-fat, 1 link, 1.8 oz | 80 | 2.5 | 3 |
| Burger, 1.94 oz | 70 | 1.5 | 3 |
| Chili, 1 cup, 8.10 oz | 280 | 10 | 25 |
| Choplets, Low Fat, 2 slices, 3.2 oz | 90 | 1 | 4 |
| **Complete Meal Solution:** | | | |
| Chipotle Bowl, 5 oz | 130 | 0 | 23 |
| Hearty Stew, 10 oz | 270 | 2 | 47 |
| Italian Bolognese with Pasta, 5 oz | 130 | 3 | 19 |
| Medit. Tom. & Olive with Pasta, 5 oz | 130 | 3 | 19 |
| Pad Thai, 5 oz | 230 | 5 | 37 |
| Southwest Chunky Stew, 5 oz | 125 | 2 | 19 |
| Thai Red Curry, 5 oz | 130 | 6 | 12 |
| Thai Green Curry, 5 oz | 155 | 5 | 23 |
| Fried Chik'n & Gravy | 140 | 8 | 3 |
| Linketts (1), 1.3 oz | 70 | 4 | 1 |
| Nutolene, 2 slices, 3 oz | 230 | 20 | 2 |
| Saucettes (1), 1.34 oz | 90 | 6 | 1 |
| Swiss Stake with Gravy, 3.25 oz | 120 | 6 | 7 |
| **Tuno:** In Spring Water, 2 oz | 40 | 0 | 2 |
| Lemon Pepper, 2 oz | 55 | 1 | 5 |
| Sesame Ginger, 3 oz | 85 | 1 | 13 |
| Thai Sweet Chili, 3 oz | 90 | 0.5 | 13 |

| Yves Veggie Cuisine *(Meatless):* | C | F | Cb |
|---|---|---|---|
| **Appetizers:** | | | |
| **Balls**, Falafel (3) | 150 | 7 | 17 |
| **Bites:** Broccoli (4) | 80 | 3 | 11 |
| Kale & Quinoa (4) | 80 | 3 | 11 |
| Sweet Pot. & Chickpea (4) | 100 | 3 | 17 |
| **Breakfast:** Veggie Bacon 3 slices | 70 | 0.5 | 3 |
| Veggie Patties (2) | 80 | 2 | 5 |
| **Burger Patties:** | | | |
| Gluten Free Veggie (1) | 110 | 6 | 5 |
| Kale & Root Vegetables (1) | 110 | 6 | 5 |
| **Deli Veggie Slices:** | | | |
| Bologna (3) | 60 | 1 | 2 |
| Ham (5) | 80 | 1 | 5 |
| Pepperoni (10) | 45 | 1 | 3 |
| Salami (5) | 80 | 1 | 5 |
| Turkey (5) | 80 | 1 | 4 |
| **Veggie Dogs:** | | | |
| Good Dog, 1.35 oz | 45 | 1 | 2 |
| Regular (1) | 50 | 0.5 | 2 |
| Jumbo (1), 2.7 oz | 110 | 2 | 4 |
| Tofu (1) | 50 | 1 | 2 |
| **Ground Rounds:** | | | |
| Original Veggie, 1.9 oz | 60 | 0.5 | 5 |
| Garden Veggie Crumble, 1.95 oz | 80 | 1.5 | 9 |
| **Zatarain's:** | | | |
| **New Orleans Style:** *Per Dry Mix Only* | | | |
| Black Beans & Rice, 2.3 oz | 230 | 1 | 47 |
| Boubon Chicken Flav. Rice, 1.6 oz | 160 | 0.5 | 35 |
| Cajun Chicken Flavored Rice, 1.6 oz | 160 | 0.5 | 35 |
| Caribbean Rice Mix, 2.4 oz | 250 | 2 | 53 |
| Jambalaya Mix, 1.6 oz | 160 | 0.5 | 34 |
| Spanish Rice, 1.5 oz | 160 | 0.5 | 33 |
| **Frozen Entrees:** *Per Single Serve* | | | |
| Blackened Chicken Alfredo, 10.5 oz | 500 | 21 | 56 |
| Blackened Chkn w/ Yellow Rice, 10.5 oz | 540 | 17 | 77 |
| Bourbon Chicken Pasta, 10.5 oz | 460 | 17 | 53 |
| Creamy Cajun Style Pasta, 10.5 oz | 420 | 16 | 48 |
| Dirty Rice with Beef & Pork, 10 oz | 430 | 13 | 64 |
| Jambalaya Flavored w/ Ssg, 12 oz | 490 | 10 | 86 |
| Red Beans & Rice w/ Sausage, 12 oz | 540 | 17 | 79 |
| Sausage & Chicken Gumbo w/ Rice, 12 oz | 350 | 13 | 85 |
| Shrimp Alfredo, 10.5 oz | 480 | 20 | 56 |
| Shrimp Scampi with Pasta, 10.5 oz | 350 | 10 | 49 |

Note: Cooking reduces weight of meat by 20-45% due to water and fat losses. Average weight loss is 30%. Actual loss depends on cooking method and cooking time.

Examples:

4 oz raw weight = approx. 3 oz cooked weight

4 oz cooked weight = approx. 5½ oz raw weight

**What 3 oz Cooked Meat Looks Like:**

• Rectangular piece (4" x 2½" x ½" thick)

• Deck of cards (3½" x 2½" x ⅝" thick)

### Quick Guide   C   F   Cb

**Sirloin (Choice Grade):**
**External fat trimmed to ½"**

*Broiled, Edible Portion (no bone)*

**Small/Regular Serving, 3 oz, cooked weight:**
(from 4-4½ oz raw)

| | | | |
|---|---|---|---|
| Lean + external fat (⅛"), 3 oz | 220 | 13 | 0 |
| Lean + marbling, 3 oz | 185 | 9 | 0 |
| Lean only, 3 oz | 160 | 6 | 0 |

(No external fat or marbling)

**Medium Serving, 5 oz, cooked weight:**
(from approximately 7 oz raw)

| | | | |
|---|---|---|---|
| Lean + external fat (⅛"), 5 oz | 365 | 22 | 0 |
| Lean + marbling, 5 oz | 310 | 15 | 0 |
| Lean only, 5 oz | 265 | 10 | 0 |

**Large Serving, 8 oz, cooked weight:**
(from approximately 11-12 oz raw)

| | | | |
|---|---|---|---|
| Lean + external fat (½"), 8 oz | 585 | 36 | 0 |
| Lean + marbling, 8 oz | 500 | 24 | 0 |
| Lean only, 8 oz | 425 | 15 | 0 |

**Extra Large Serving, 12 oz, cooked weight:**
(from approximately 16-17 oz raw)

| | | | |
|---|---|---|---|
| Lean + external fat (⅛"), 12 oz | 875 | 54 | 0 |
| Lean + marbling, 12 oz | 745 | 36 | 0 |
| Lean only, 12 oz | 640 | 22 | 0 |

**Pan Fried:**

Sirloin (Choice), medium serving,

| | | | |
|---|---|---|---|
| Lean + external fat (⅛"), 5 oz | 445 | 30 | 0 |

### Other Steaks   C   F   Cb

**Filet Mignon (Tenderloin):**
**1 Medium steak,** 6 oz raw weight:
Broiled, with ¼" fat trim:

| | | | |
|---|---|---|---|
| Lean + fat (¼"), 4 oz | 360 | 27 | 0 |
| Lean only, 3.5 oz | 230 | 12 | 0 |

**New York/Club Steak:**
**Top Loin/Short Loin:**
1 steak, regular (9.25 raw, ¼" fat):
Broiled: Lean + fat (¼"), 6.3 oz

| | | | |
|---|---|---|---|
| Broiled: Lean + fat (¼"), 6.3 oz | 580 | 43 | 0 |
| Lean + marbling, 5.5 oz | 400 | 25 | 0 |
| Lean only, 5.25 oz | 360 | 20 | 0 |

**Porterhouse Steak:**
**1 Medium, 6 oz raw weight, w/out bone, broiled:**

| | | | |
|---|---|---|---|
| Lean + fat (¼"), 4.3 oz | 410 | 33 | 0 |
| Lean only, 3.5 oz | 210 | 11 | 0 |

1 Large ,12 oz raw weight, without bone, broiled:

| | | | |
|---|---|---|---|
| Lean + fat (¼") 8.5 oz cooked | 820 | 66 | 0 |
| Lean only, 7 oz cooked | 420 | 22 | 0 |

**T-Bone Steak:** *Broiled or Grilled*
**Medium Size:** *8 oz raw weight, without bone*
Approximately 6 oz cooked:

| | | | |
|---|---|---|---|
| Lean + Fat (¼"), 5 oz | 400 | 28 | 0 |
| Lean only, 4 oz | 265 | 12 | 0 |

**Large Size:** *12 oz raw weight*
Approximately 9 oz cooked:

| | | | |
|---|---|---|---|
| Lean + fat (¼"), 7 oz, without bone | 560 | 39 | 0 |
| Lean only, 6 oz, without bone | 400 | 18 | 0 |

**Extra Large Size:** *20 oz raw weight*
Approximately 16 oz cooked:

| | | | |
|---|---|---|---|
| Lean + Fat (¼"), 12 oz, without bone | 960 | 66 | 0 |
| Lean Only, 10 oz, without bone | 660 | 30 | 0 |

**Also See Fast-Foods & Restaurants Section ~**
*Lone Star Steakhouse; Outback Steakhouse*

## Beef – Individual Cuts  **C** **F** **Cb**

### Average All Grades
Edible Weight, Without Bone

**Brisket, whole, braised:**

| | C | F | Cb |
|---|---|---|---|
| Lean + fat (¼" trim), 3 oz | 330 | 27 | 0 |
| Lean + marbling, 3 oz | 250 | 17 | 0 |
| Lean only, 3 oz | 185 | 9 | 0 |

**Chuck Blade, braised:**

| | C | F | Cb |
|---|---|---|---|
| Lean + fat (¼"), 3 oz | 310 | 24 | 0 |
| Lean + marbling, 3 oz | 295 | 22 | 0 |
| Lean only, 3 oz | 245 | 13 | 0 |

**Flank:** Raw, 4 oz

| | C | F | Cb |
|---|---|---|---|
| Flank: Raw, 4 oz | 175 | 8 | 0 |
| Braised, 3 oz | 225 | 14 | 0 |
| Broiled, 3 oz | 155 | 6 | 0 |

**Round, bottom, braised:**

| | C | F | Cb |
|---|---|---|---|
| Lean + marbling, 3 oz | 190 | 7.5 | 0 |
| Lean only, 3 oz | 185 | 6.5 | 0 |

**Round, eye/tip, rstd:**

| | C | F | Cb |
|---|---|---|---|
| Lean + fat (¼"), 3 oz | 205 | 11 | 0 |
| Lean, w/ marbling, 3 oz | 150 | 5 | 0 |

**Round, top:** Per 3 oz, Cooked Weight

| | C | F | Cb |
|---|---|---|---|
| Braised, Lean + fat | 210 | 10 | 0 |
| Lean only | 170 | 4 | 0 |
| Broiled, Lean + fat | 180 | 8 | 0 |
| Lean only | 160 | 5 | 0 |
| Pan-fried, Lean + fat | 235 | 13 | 0 |
| Lean only | 195 | 7 | 0 |

## Beef Ribs

**Back Ribs:** 7" long, visible fat trimmed to ¼"
10.3 oz raw w/ bone or 3.5 oz cooked, braised, w/o bone

| | C | F | Cb |
|---|---|---|---|
| 1 average rib | 410 | 34 | 0 |
| 3 ribs | 1230 | 102 | 0 |

**Short Ribs:** 2½" long, visible fat trimmed to ¼"
6 oz raw with bone or 2.52 oz cooked, braised, w/o bone

| | C | F | Cb |
|---|---|---|---|
| 1 average rib | 320 | 28 | 0 |
| 3 ribs | 960 | 85 | 0 |

## Ground Beef

**Ground Beef, Raw:** Per 4 oz

| | C | F | Cb |
|---|---|---|---|
| 70% lean (30% fat) | 380 | 34 | 0 |
| 75% lean (25% fat) | 335 | 29 | 0 |
| 80% lean (20% fat) | 290 | 23 | 0 |
| 85% lean (15% fat) | 245 | 17 | 0 |
| 90% lean (10% fat) | 200 | 12 | 0 |
| 95% lean (5% fat) | 155 | 6 | 0 |

**Baked/Broiled:**

| | C | F | Cb |
|---|---|---|---|
| Regular (70%), 3 oz | 230 | 16 | 0 |
| Lean (80%), 3 oz | 215 | 14 | 0 |
| Extra lean (90%), 3 oz | 185 | 10 | 0 |

**Pan-Broiled:**

| | C | F | Cb |
|---|---|---|---|
| Regular (70%), 3 oz | 230 | 15 | 0 |
| Lean (80%), 3 oz | 210 | 14 | 0 |
| Extra lean (90%), 3 oz | 195 | 10 | 0 |

**Ground Beef Patties:** Average, 23% Fat

| | C | F | Cb |
|---|---|---|---|
| Raw, 4 oz | 330 | 25 | 0 |
| Broiled, 3 oz (from 4 oz raw) | 250 | 19 | 0 |

## Quick Guide  **C** **F** **Cb**

### Roast Beef
**Round (Eye/Tip, average):** Average All Cuts
**Small/Regular Serving:** 3 oz
(2 thin slices/1 thick slice)

| | C | F | Cb |
|---|---|---|---|
| Lean + fat (⅛" fat trim) | 180 | 9 | 0 |
| Lean only | 145 | 4 | 0 |

**Medium Serving:** 5 oz
(3-4 thin slices)

| | C | F | Cb |
|---|---|---|---|
| Lean + fat (⅛" fat trim) | 300 | 15 | 0 |
| Lean only | 245 | 6.5 | 0 |

**Large Serving, 8 oz:** 3 thick slices

| | C | F | Cb |
|---|---|---|---|
| Lean + fat (⅛" fat trim) | 480 | 24 | 0 |
| Lean only | 385 | 11 | 0 |

**Beef Kebab:** Cooked

| | C | F | Cb |
|---|---|---|---|
| Beef & Veggies, 2 oz | 160 | 10 | 4 |
| If very lean meat | 100 | 4 | 4 |

## Meat Alternatives (Vegan)

**Beyond Meat:**

| | C | F | Cb |
|---|---|---|---|
| Beyond: Burger Patty, 4 oz | 250 | 18 | 3 |
| Crumbles: Beefy, 1.94 oz | 90 | 3 | 3 |
| Fiesty Crumbles, 1.94 oz | 80 | 3 | 1 |
| Grilled Chicken Strips, 3 oz | 130 | 3 | 6 |
| Sausage: Original Brat, 2.9 oz | 190 | 12 | 5 |
| Hot Italian (1), cooked, 2.7 oz | 190 | 12 | 5 |

**Gardein:**

| | C | F | Cb |
|---|---|---|---|
| Beefless: Burger Patty, 3 oz | 130 | 4.5 | 19 |
| Grounds, 2.9 oz | 170 | 5 | 26 |
| Meatballs (3), 3.17 oz | 150 | 7 | 9 |
| Tips, ¾ cup, 3.5 oz | 170 | 7 | 8 |
| Chick'n: BBQ Wings, w/ Sauce, 4.8 oz | 160 | 5 | 17 |
| Crispy Patty (1), 3.1 oz | 170 | 8 | 14 |
| Crispy Golden Nuggets (5), 3 oz | 190 | 8 | 16 |
| Fishless: Golden Filet (2), 3.38 oz | 180 | 12 | 12 |
| Mini Crabless Cakes (3), 2.65 oz | 140 | 6 | 13 |
| Porkless, Sweet & Sour Bites, 2.47 oz | 120 | 3 | 9 |

**Quorn:**

| | C | F | Cb |
|---|---|---|---|
| Meatless: Buffalo Dippes, 3.7 oz | 230 | 10 | 21 |
| Fillets (1), 2.2 oz | 70 | 1 | 7 |
| Fishless Sticks, 3.5 oz | 200 | 8 | 30 |
| Pieces, 3.9 oz | 120 | 3 | 11 |
| Spicy Patties, 2.3 oz | 130 | 5 | 14 |

**Tofurky:**

| | C | F | Cb |
|---|---|---|---|
| Crumbles: Beef Style, 1.94 oz | 90 | 4 | 6 |
| Chorizo, 1.94 oz | 170 | 8 | 6 |
| Feast, 5.3 oz | 300 | 10 | 19 |
| Ham Style Roast, 3.2 oz | 170 | 6 | 8 |
| Roast w/ Wild Rice Stuffing, 5.2 oz | 290 | 10 | 17 |

## Lamb

**C · F · Cb**

**Choice Grade:**

**Leg (Whole), roasted:**

| | C | F | Cb |
|---|---|---|---|
| Lean + fat, 3 oz | 220 | 14 | 0 |
| Lean only, 3 oz | 160 | 7 | 0 |

**Leg (Sirloin Half), roasted:**

| | C | F | Cb |
|---|---|---|---|
| Lean + fat, 3 oz | 250 | 18 | 0 |
| Lean only, 3 oz | 175 | 8 | 0 |

**Leg (Shank Half), roasted:**

| | C | F | Cb |
|---|---|---|---|
| Lean + fat, 3 oz | 190 | 11 | 0 |
| Lean only, 3 oz | 155 | 6 | 0 |

**Loin Chop, broiled:**

1 chop (raw weight, 4.25 oz):

| | C | F | Cb |
|---|---|---|---|
| Lean + fat (2.25 oz edible) | 180 | 12 | 0 |
| Lean only (1.6 oz edible) | 85 | 3.5 | 0 |

**Rib Chop, broiled:**

1 chop (raw wt., 3.5 oz):

| | C | F | Cb |
|---|---|---|---|
| Lean + fat (2.5 oz edible) | 255 | 21 | 0 |
| Lean only (1.75 oz edible) | 105 | 6 | 0 |

**Shoulder (Arm/Blade):**

| | C | F | Cb |
|---|---|---|---|
| Braised: Lean + fat, 3 oz | 295 | 21 | 0 |
| Lean only, 3 oz | 240 | 12 | 0 |
| Broiled: Lean + fat, 3 oz | 240 | 17 | 0 |
| Lean only, 3 oz | 170 | 8 | 0 |
| Roasted: Similar to Broiled | | | |

**Cubed Lamb (Leg/Shoulder):**

For stew or kebab:

| | C | F | Cb |
|---|---|---|---|
| Braised, lean only, 3 oz | 190 | 8 | 0 |
| Broiled, lean only, 3 oz | 160 | 6 | 0 |

## Veal

**Edible Weights:**

**Leg (Top Round):**

| | C | F | Cb |
|---|---|---|---|
| Braised: Lean + fat, 3 oz | 180 | 6 | 0 |
| Lean only, 3 oz | 175 | 5 | 0 |
| Pan-fried, breaded: | | | |
| Lean + fat, 3 oz | 195 | 8 | 9 |
| Lean only, 3 oz | 185 | 6 | 9 |
| Pan-fried, not breaded: | | | |
| Lean + fat, 3 oz | 180 | 7 | 0 |
| Lean only, 3 oz | 155 | 4 | 0 |
| Roasted: Lean + fat, 3 oz | 135 | 4 | 0 |
| Lean only, 3 oz | 130 | 3 | 0 |

## Veal (Cont)

**C · F · Cb**

**Loin Chop:** *1 chop, 7 oz raw weight*

| | C | F | Cb |
|---|---|---|---|
| Braised: Lean + fat, 3 oz | 240 | 15 | 0 |
| Lean only, 3 oz | 190 | 8 | 0 |
| Roasted: Lean + fat, 3 oz | 185 | 11 | 0 |
| Lean only, 3 oz | 150 | 6 | 0 |

**Rib, roasted:** *Lean + fat, 3 oz*

| | C | F | Cb |
|---|---|---|---|
| | 195 | 12 | 0 |
| Lean only, 3 oz | 150 | 7 | 0 |

**Shoulder, Arm/Blade, roasted:**

| | C | F | Cb |
|---|---|---|---|
| Lean + fat, 3 oz | 155 | 7 | 0 |
| Lean only, 3 oz | 140 | 5 | 0 |

**Sirloin, roasted:**

| | C | F | Cb |
|---|---|---|---|
| Lean + fat, 3 oz | 170 | 9 | 0 |
| Lean only, 3 oz | 145 | 6 | 0 |

**Cubed for Stew, braised:**

| | C | F | Cb |
|---|---|---|---|
| Leg/Shoulder, lean only, 3 oz | 160 | 4 | 0 |
| (1 lb raw yields approximately 9.25 oz cooked) | | | |

## Pork

**Fresh Pork:** *Cooked Weight, without bone):*
*4 oz raw weight = approx. 3 oz cooked weight*

**BBQ, Pulled:**

| | C | F | Cb |
|---|---|---|---|
| 2 oz | 90 | 2.5 | 10 |
| 4 oz | 180 | 5 | 20 |
| 8 oz | 360 | 10 | 40 |

**Blade Steak, broiled:**

| | C | F | Cb |
|---|---|---|---|
| Lean + fat, 3 oz | 220 | 15 | 0 |
| Lean only, 3 oz | 190 | 11 | 0 |

**Country Style Ribs, broiled/roasted:**

| | C | F | Cb |
|---|---|---|---|
| Lean + fat, 3 oz | 280 | 22 | 0 |
| Lean only, 3 oz | 210 | 13 | 0 |

**Spareribs, braised:** *Lean & fat, 6 oz*

| | C | F | Cb |
|---|---|---|---|
| (from 1 lb raw weight) | 675 | 52 | 0 |

**Leg (Ham), whole, roasted:**

| | C | F | Cb |
|---|---|---|---|
| Lean + fat, 3 oz | 230 | 15 | 0 |
| Lean only, 3 oz | 180 | 8 | 0 |

**Loin Chops, broiled:** *Average*

(From 1 chop: 5 oz raw weight with bone or 4 oz raw weight, without bone)

| | C | F | Cb |
|---|---|---|---|
| Lean + fat, 3 oz | 200 | 11 | 0 |
| Lean only, 3 oz | 165 | 7 | 0 |

**Loin Roast, roasted:**

| | C | F | Cb |
|---|---|---|---|
| Lean + fat, 3 oz | 210 | 13 | 0 |
| Lean only, 3 oz | 180 | 8 | 0 |

**Rib Chops, (Boneless), broiled:**

| | C | F | Cb |
|---|---|---|---|
| Lean + fat, 3 oz | 220 | 14 | 0 |
| Lean only, 3 oz | 185 | 9 | 0 |

**Rib Roast:**

| | C | F | Cb |
|---|---|---|---|
| Lean + fat, 3 oz | 215 | 13 | 0 |
| Lean only, 3 oz | 180 | 9 | 0 |

## Pork (Cont)    Ⓒ Ⓕ ⒸⒷ

| | C | F | Cb |
|---|---|---|---|
| **Sirloin Chop, broiled:** | | | |
| Lean + fat, 3 oz | 180 | 8 | 0 |
| Lean only, 3 oz | 165 | 6 | 0 |
| **Sirloin Roast, roasted:** | | | |
| Lean + fat, 3 oz | 175 | 8 | 0 |
| Lean only, 3 oz | 170 | 7 | 0 |
| **Tenderloin (Boneless), roasted:** | | | |
| Lean + fat, 3 oz | 125 | 4 | 0 |
| Lean only, 3 oz | 120 | 3 | 0 |
| **Ground Pork:** | | | |
| Raw, average, 1/4 lb, 4 oz | 300 | 24 | 0 |
| Broiled, 3 oz | 250 | 18 | 0 |
| Pan-fried, drained, 3 oz | 260 | 19 | 0 |

## Bacon

| | C | F | Cb |
|---|---|---|---|
| **Raw:** 1 med. slice, 0.75 oz | 95 | 9 | 0 |
| 1 thick slice, 1.3 oz | 175 | 17 | 0 |
| (1 lb raw yields approximately 5 oz cooked) | | | |
| **Broiled/Pan-Fried:** | | | |
| 1 medium slice, 0.3 oz | 40 | 3 | 0 |
| 3 medium slices, 0.8 | 125 | 10 | 0 |
| 2 thin slices, 0.5 oz | 75 | 6 | 0 |
| 1 thick slice, 0.9 oz | 65 | 5 | 0 |
| **Canadian Bacon:** | | | |
| Cooked: 1 slice, 1 oz | 45 | 2 | 0.5 |
| 2 slices, 2 oz | 90 | 4 | 1 |
| **Bacon Bits,** 1 Tbsp, 0.3 oz | 35 | 2 | 0 |
| **Breakfast Strips,** Broiled, 1 sl., 0.4 oz | 50 | 4 | 0 |

## Ham

| | C | F | Cb |
|---|---|---|---|
| **Boneless Ham,** cooked: | | | |
| Regular, (approximately 13% fat): | | | |
| Roasted, 3 oz | 150 | 8 | 0 |
| Extra Lean (5% fat), | | | |
| Roasted, 3 oz | 125 | 5 | 0 |
| **Whole Ham,** cooked: | | | |
| Lean + fat (as purchased) | | | |
| Roasted, 3 oz | 210 | 15 | 0 |
| Lean only, Roasted, 3 oz | 135 | 5 | 0 |
| **Canned Ham:** *Similar to boneless ham* | | | |
| Chopped, canned, 3 oz | 200 | 16 | 0 |
| **Ham Patties,** cooked, (1), 2.3 oz | 220 | 20 | 1 |
| **Ham Steak,** extra lean, 2 oz | 70 | 2.5 | 0 |
| **Lunch Slices ~** *See Deli Meats, Page 128* | | | |

## Game & Other Meats    Ⓒ Ⓕ ⒸⒷ

| | C | F | Cb |
|---|---|---|---|
| **Bison Steak,** | | | |
| lean, 6 oz (raw) | 205 | 4 | 0 |
| **Boar (wild),** roasted, 3 oz | 140 | 4 | 0 |
| **Buffalo Steak,** | | | |
| New West Foods, 4 oz | 70 | 3 | 0 |
| **Caribou,** roasted, 3 oz | 140 | 4 | 0 |
| **Deer/Venison,** roasted 3 oz | 135 | 3 | 0 |
| **Goat (Capretto):** | | | |
| Raw, 3 oz | 95 | 2 | 0 |
| Roasted, 3 oz | 120 | 2.5 | 0 |
| **Ostrich:** | | | |
| *Blackwing Ostrich Meats:* | | | |
| Sausage Patties (2) 2 oz | 60 | 0.5 | 0 |
| Sport Jerky, 0.5 oz piece | 25 | 0 | 0 |
| *New West Foods:* | | | |
| Ground Ostrich, 4 oz | 165 | 7 | 0 |
| Ostrich Steak, 4 oz steak | 130 | 2.5 | 0 |
| **Rabbit:** Roasted, 3 oz | 165 | 7 | 0 |
| Stewed, 1 cup, diced, 5 oz | 290 | 12 | 0 |

## Variety & Organ Meats

| | C | F | Cb |
|---|---|---|---|
| **Brain (Lamb):** Braised, 3 oz | 125 | 9 | 0 |
| Pan-fried, 3 oz | 230 | 19 | 0 |
| **Chitterlings,** pork, simmered, 3 oz | 260 | 25 | 0 |
| **Ears,** pork, simmered, 1 ear, 4 oz | 185 | 12 | 0 |
| **Feet,** Pork: Simmered, 3 oz | 200 | 14 | 0 |
| Cured, pickled, 3 oz | 170 | 14 | 0 |
| *Hormel,* 2 oz | 80 | 6 | 0 |
| **Head Cheese (Pork Snouts/Ears/Vinegar/Spices),** | | | |
| 1 oz slice | 50 | 4 | 0 |
| **Heart,** Beef, braised, 3 oz | 140 | 4 | 0 |
| **Jowl,** pork, raw, 4 oz | 750 | 80 | 0 |
| **Kidneys,** braised, 3 oz | 140 | 5 | 0 |
| **Liver (beef):** Raw, 4 oz | 150 | 4 | 4 |
| Braised, 3 oz | 140 | 4 | 3 |
| Pan-fried, 3 oz | 185 | 7 | 7 |
| **Pancreas,** pork, braised, 3 oz | 185 | 8 | 0 |
| **Pork Cracklins,** 0.5 oz | 80 | 6 | 0 |
| **Pork Hocks,** 1 piece, 6 oz | 340 | 23 | 0 |
| **Scrapple,** pork, 2 oz | 120 | 8 | 8 |
| **Spleen,** pork, braised, 3 oz | 130 | 3 | 0 |
| **Stomach,** pork, raw, 4 oz | 185 | 12 | 0 |
| **Sweetbreads:** | | | |
| Beef./Lamb, cooked, 3 oz | 125 | 9 | 0 |
| **Tail,** pork, simmered, 3 oz | 340 | 31 | 0 |
| **Tongue:** Raised Veal, 3 oz | 170 | 9 | 0 |
| Beef/Lamb/Pork, av., 3 oz | 235 | 17 | 0 |
| **Tripe,** beef, raw, 3 oz | 85 | 3.5 | 0 |

## Quick Guide    C   F   Cb

### Franks & Weiners
*Average All Brands*
**Regular (Pork Mix):** *Per Frank*

| | C | F | Cb |
|---|---|---|---|
| Regular, 1.5 oz | 140 | 13 | 1 |
| Bun Length/Jumbo, 2 oz | 185 | 17 | 2 |
| Extra Long, 2.75 oz | 255 | 24 | 2 |
| Small/Cocktail, each | 30 | 3 | 0.5 |

**Beef Franks:** *Per Frank*

| | | | |
|---|---|---|---|
| Regular, 1.5 oz | 140 | 13 | 2 |
| Bun Length/Jumbo, 2 oz | 175 | 17 | 2.5 |
| $^1/_4$ lb Dog, 4 oz | 375 | 33 | 5 |

### Franks & Weiners

**Ball Park:** *Per 2 oz Frank Unless Indicated*
**Angus Beef:**

| | | | |
|---|---|---|---|
| Original; Bun Size, 2 oz | 170 | 15 | 3 |
| Lean, 1.8 oz | 70 | 5 | 2 |
| **Beef:** Original, Bun Size, 2 oz | 190 | 16 | 4 |
| Deli Style, Regular, 1.8 oz | 150 | 12 | 2 |
| Grillmaster, Hearty, 3 oz | 250 | 21 | 3 |
| Lean, 1.76 oz | 80 | 5 | 2 |
| Park's Finest, 2 oz | 170 | 15 | 2 |
| **Foster Farms,** Chicken; Turkey, 2 oz | 140 | 12 | 1 |

**Hebrew National:** *Per Frank*

| | | | |
|---|---|---|---|
| **Beef:** Regular, 1.7 oz | 150 | 13 | 2 |
| $^1/_4$ Pounder, 4 oz | 350 | 31 | 4 |
| Jumbo, 3 oz | 260 | 23 | 3 |
| 97% Fat-Free, 1.6 oz | 45 | 1 | 2 |
| Bun Length Beef Frank, 2 oz | 170 | 15 | 2 |

**Jennie-O:** *Per Frank*
**Turkey Franks:**

| | | | |
|---|---|---|---|
| 1.2 oz | 70 | 6 | 1 |
| Jumbo, 2 oz | 120 | 10 | 1 |
| Turkey Bratwurst, 3.8 oz | 170 | 10 | 2 |

**Oscar Mayer:** *Per Frank*
**Angus Beef:**

| | | | |
|---|---|---|---|
| Classic, 1.5 oz | 130 | 12 | 1 |
| Bun Length, 1.76 oz | 170 | 15 | 2 |
| **Turkey,** Classic, 1.6 oz | 100 | 7 | 2 |

**Shelton's:** *Per Frank*

| | | | |
|---|---|---|---|
| **Chicken,** uncured, 1.2 oz | 80 | 7 | 0 |
| **Turkey,** Regular, 1.2 oz | 60 | 4.5 | 1 |
| **Zacky Farms,** Chkn; Turkey, av, 2 oz | 115 | 10 | 4 |

## Quick Guide    C   F   Cb

### Fresh Sausages
**Pork/Beef:** *Average All Types*

| | C | F | Cb |
|---|---|---|---|
| **Small:** Raw, 4" link, 1 oz | 85 | 7.5 | 0 |
| Broiled/Pan-fried | 80 | 7 | 0 |
| **Medium:** Raw, 2 oz | 170 | 15 | 0 |
| Broiled/Pan-fried | 165 | 14 | 0 |
| **Large:** Raw, 3 oz | 255 | 22 | 0 |
| Broiled/Pan-fried | 245 | 21 | 0 |
| **Italian:** Raw, 3.2 oz | 315 | 28 | 1 |
| Cooked, 2.4 oz | 230 | 18 | 3 |
| **Chorizo:** Beef Chorizo, 2.5 oz piece | 250 | 23 | 5 |
| Pork Chorizo, 2.5 oz piece | 250 | 23 | 5 |

**Note:** Fat is lost in broiling/pan frying.
Cooked weight = approx. 60-70% raw weight

### Smoked Sausages

*Per Link:*

| | | | |
|---|---|---|---|
| **Butterball,** Turkey, 2 oz | 100 | 6 | 4 |

**Eckrich:**

| | | | |
|---|---|---|---|
| Original (1) | 230 | 18 | 6 |
| Cheddar (1), 2.36 oz | 210 | 18 | 3 |

**Hillshire Farm:**

| | | | |
|---|---|---|---|
| Cheddarwurst, 2 oz | 180 | 16 | 2 |
| Chicken Hardwood, 2 oz | 100 | 7 | 3 |
| Polska Kielbasa, 2 oz | 180 | 16 | 0 |

**Johnsonville** ~ *See CalorieKing.Com*

### Breakfast Sausages/Patties

**Butterball:** *Fully Cooked*

| | | | |
|---|---|---|---|
| **Turkey:** B'fast Sausage Links (3), 2 oz | 90 | 5 | 0 |
| Patties (2), 2 oz | 90 | 5.5 | 0 |

**Jimmy Dean:** *Fully Cooked*
**Heat 'N Serve Sausage Links:**

| | | | |
|---|---|---|---|
| Pork, Regular (3), 1.9 oz | 210 | 19 | 2 |
| Turkey (3), 2 oz | 130 | 8 | 2 |

**Heat 'N Serve Sausage Patties:**

| | | | |
|---|---|---|---|
| Pork, Original (2), 1.8 oz | 200 | 17 | 2 |
| Turkey (2), 1.8 oz | 120 | 8 | 1 |
| **Maple Pork Sausages,** (3), 2.4 oz | 260 | 22 | 3 |
| **Pork Patties,** (2), 2.3 oz | 270 | 24 | 2 |

**Breakfast Sandwiches** ~ *See Page 92*
**Jones Dairy Farm:**
**Golden Brown Sausages:** *Fully Cooked*

| | | | |
|---|---|---|---|
| Mild Pork Sausages (3), 2 oz | 250 | 24 | 1 |
| Maple Pork Sausages (3), 2 oz | 240 | 22 | 2 |

**Vegetarian Patties:**
**Boca** ~ *See Page 117*
**GardenBurger** ~ *See Page 114*

## Bagel, Corn & Hot Dogs  C  F  Cb

### Hot Dogs, Ready-To-Go:
*Includes Ketchup/Relish*

| | C | F | Cb |
|---|---|---|---|
| **Regular,** 1.5 oz frank, 1.5 oz bun | 260 | 15 | 22 |
| **Bun Length,** 2 oz frank, 1.5 oz bun | 290 | 18 | 21 |
| **Jumbo Dog,** 2 oz frank, 2 oz bun | 360 | 20 | 36 |
| **¼ lb Beef Dog,** 2 oz bun | 480 | 15 | 36 |
| **Mile Long Dog,** 2.6 oz dog, 1.5 oz bun | 360 | 24 | 23 |

### Corn Dogs:
| | C | F | Cb |
|---|---|---|---|
| Beef/Pork Frank, average, 2.6 oz | 170 | 10 | 16 |

**Foster Farms:**
**Corn Dogs:**
| | C | F | Cb |
|---|---|---|---|
| Chili Cheese (1), 2.7 oz | 190 | 9 | 21 |
| Honey Crunchy: | | | |
| Regular (1), 2.7 oz | 190 | 9 | 18 |
| Jumbo (1), 4 oz | 280 | 14 | 27 |
| Mini (4), 2.7 oz | 220 | 13 | 19 |

**State Fair:** *Per Dog*
| | C | F | Cb |
|---|---|---|---|
| Beef Corn Dog, 2.7 oz | 230 | 11 | 26 |
| Classic Corn Dog, Reg., 4 oz | 330 | 11 | 34 |
| Mini Classic (5), 3.3 oz | 270 | 14 | 29 |

### Bagel Dogs:
**Hebrew National:**
| | C | F | Cb |
|---|---|---|---|
| **Beef Bagel Dogs,** 4 pieces, 2.75 oz | 240 | 13 | 22 |

**Schwanns,** Bagel Dogs,
| | C | F | Cb |
|---|---|---|---|
| with Cheese, 1 piece, 4.5 oz | 370 | 16 | 40 |

**Vienna Beef:**
| | C | F | Cb |
|---|---|---|---|
| **Bagel Dog:** 5.5 oz | 410 | 19 | 44 |
| 6.5 oz | 490 | 19 | 58 |
| Mini (5), 4.6 oz | 310 | 18 | 31 |

### Hot Dog Toppings/Extras:
| | C | F | Cb |
|---|---|---|---|
| **American Cheese,** 1 slice, 1 oz | 110 | 9 | 1 |
| **Chili Con Carne,** ¼ cup | 50 | 2 | 5.5 |
| **Ketchup,** 1 Tbsp | 15 | 0 | 4 |
| **Mustard,** 1 Tbsp | 20 | 0 | 1 |
| **Onions,** chopped, 1 Tbsp | 5 | 0 | 1 |
| **Pickle Relish,** 1 Tbsp | 20 | 0 | 5 |
| **Sauerkraut,** ½ cup | 20 | 0 | 5 |

## Deli/Lunch Meats & Sausage

**Beef Jerky/Meat Snacks,**
| | C | F | Cb |
|---|---|---|---|
| Berliner (pork/beef), 1 oz | 65 | 5 | 1 |

**Beerwurst (Beef):**
| | C | F | Cb |
|---|---|---|---|
| Small (2¾"diam), ¹⁄₁₆" slice | 20 | 2 | 0 |
| Large (4" diam), ⅛ " slice | 75 | 7 | 0.5 |

**Beerwurst (Pork):**
| | C | F | Cb |
|---|---|---|---|
| Small (2.75"diameter), ¹⁄₁₆" slice | 15 | 1 | 0 |
| Large (4"diameter), ⅛" Slice | 55 | 4 | 0.5 |
| **Blood Sausage,** 1 oz | 100 | 9 | 0.5 |

## Deli/Lunch Meats & Sausages (Cont)

### Bologna:
| | C | F | Cb |
|---|---|---|---|
| Beef Bologna: 1 slice, 1 oz | 90 | 8 | 0 |
| Light, 1 slice, 1 oz | 60 | 4 | 2 |
| *Oscar Mayer:* Regular, 1 oz | 90 | 8 | 1 |
| 98% Fat Free, 1 oz | 40 | 1.5 | 1 |
| Light, 1 slice, 1 oz | 60 | 4 | 1 |
| *Boar's Head,* Ring, 2 oz | 150 | 13 | 1 |
| Pork Bologna: 1 Slice, 1 oz | 65 | 6 | 1 |
| Fat-Free, 1 slice, 1 oz | 20 | 0 | 2 |
| Turkey Bologna, average, 1 oz | 60 | 5 | 0.5 |
| **Bratwurst:** Average, 1 oz | 80 | 7 | 1 |
| *Bob Evan's,* Beer B'wurst, 2.2 oz link | 170 | 14 | 0 |

**Braunschweiger,** (Pork/Liver/Sausage),
| | C | F | Cb |
|---|---|---|---|
| *Oscar Mayer,* 2 oz slice | 190 | 17 | 1 |

**Chicken,** average:
| | C | F | Cb |
|---|---|---|---|
| 1 thick or 2 thin slices, 1 oz | 30 | 1 | 1 |
| 2 oz slice | 60 | 2 | 2 |

*Hillshire Farm,*
| | C | F | Cb |
|---|---|---|---|
| Rotiss. Seasoned Chicken Breast, 2 oz | 50 | 0.5 | 2 |
| **Corned Beef,** average, full fat, 1 oz | 60 | 5 | 0.5 |

**Ham, Sliced:**
| | C | F | Cb |
|---|---|---|---|
| Baked/Broiled, 1 oz slice | 35 | 1 | 1 |
| *Oscar Mayer,* Baked, Lean, | | | |
| 3 slices, 2.3 oz | 80 | 2.5 | 1 |
| Honey/Brown Sugar, av., 1 oz | 35 | 1 | 1 |
| Prosciutto, average, 1 oz | 70 | 5 | 0 |
| **Ham & Cheese Loaf,** average, 1 oz | 70 | 5 | 1 |
| **Italian Sausage,** 2.6 oz | 250 | 20 | 3 |
| **Kielbasa:** Polish Sausage, 2 oz | 65 | 5 | 1 |
| Beef, 2 oz link | 190 | 17 | 1 |
| **Knockwurst,** av., 1 oz | 90 | 8 | 0.5 |
| **Linguica** *(Gaspar's),* 2 oz | 130 | 9 | 1 |
| **Liverwurst,** 1 oz | 65 | 5 | 2 |
| **Liver Pate,** fresh, average, 1 oz | 90 | 8 | 1 |
| **Mortadella,** 1 oz | 105 | 9 | 0 |
| **Olive Loaf:** Average, 1 oz | 70 | 5 | 3 |
| *Oscar Mayer,* 1 oz | 80 | 6 | 1 |
| **Pancetta,** *Boars Head, 1 slice* | 50 | 4.5 | 0 |

## Deli/Lunch Meats & Sausages (Cont)

| | C | F | Cb |
|---|---|---|---|
| **Pastrami (Beef):** | | | |
| *Boar's Head:* | | | |
| 1st cut Brisket, 2 oz | 90 | 4 | 2 |
| Cap-Off Top Round, 2 oz | 80 | 3 | 1 |
| *Hillshire,* Deli Select, | | | |
| Ultra Thin. 2 oz | 60 | 1.5 | 0.5 |
| **Peppered Beef,** 1 oz slice | 40 | 2 | 1 |
| **Pepperoni,** 5 slices, 1 oz | 140 | 13 | 0 |
| **Pickle Loaf,** average, 1 oz | 70 | 5 | 5 |
| **Pickle & Pepper Loaf,** | | | |
| *Boars Head,* 2 oz | 150 | 13 | 2 |
| **Proscuitto/Proscuitti,** av., 1 oz | 70 | 5 | 1 |
| **Roast Beef,** Lean, 1 oz | 40 | 2 | 0 |
| **Salami:** Beef, av., 1 oz | 80 | 7 | 1 |
| *Oscar Mayer,* Hard, 1 slice, 1.8 oz | 100 | 8 | 0.5 |
| Beer Salami, average, 1 oz | 50 | 4 | 0.5 |
| *Oscar Mayer:* Cotto, 1 slice, 1 oz | 70 | 6 | 0.5 |
| Beef Cotto, 1 slice, 1 oz | 60 | 5 | 0.5 |
| Dry, Hard, average, 4 slices, 1 oz | 100 | 8 | 1 |
| Genoa: Average, 1 oz | 100 | 8 | 1 |
| Stick, 1.8 oz | 175 | 14 | 2 |
| *Bridgford,* Italian, 1 oz | 120 | 11 | 0 |
| **SPAM (Hormel):** *Per 2 oz* | | | |
| Classic: 2 oz serving | 180 | 16 | 1 |
| 7 oz can | 630 | 56 | 3.5 |
| 12 oz can | 1080 | 96 | 6 |
| Spam Lite: 2 oz | 110 | 8 | 1 |
| 12 oz can | 660 | 48 | 6 |
| **Other Spam Products:** *Per 2 oz* | | | |
| Hickory Smoked | 180 | 16 | 1 |
| Hot & Spicy | 160 | 16 | 2 |
| Oven Roasted Turkey | 80 | 4.5 | 1 |
| Spam Spresd | 140 | 12 | 1 |
| Spam with Bacon | 180 | 16 | 1 |
| Spam with Cheese | 170 | 15 | 1 |
| 25% Less Sodium | 180 | 16 | 1 |
| **Spam Singles:** *Per 3 oz* | | | |
| Classic, 2.5 oz package | 210 | 18 | 2 |
| Lite, 2.5 oz package | 130 | 9 | 2 |

## Deli/Lunch Meats & Sausages (Cont)

| | C | F | Cb |
|---|---|---|---|
| **Summer Sausage:** | | | |
| *Armour,* Beef, 2 oz | 190 | 17 | 2 |
| *Hillshire Farm,* 2 oz | 190 | 16 | 1 |
| **Treet** *(Armour),* Luncheon Loaf, | | | |
| Original, 2 oz | 140 | 11 | 4 |
| **Turkey,** average: 1 oz slice | 30 | 1 | 0.5 |
| 0.8 oz slice | 22 | 0.5 | 0.5 |
| **Turkey Breast:** | | | |
| *Butterball,* Oven Roasted: | | | |
| 1 slice 1 oz | 30 | 0.5 | 1 |
| Deli Inspirations, | | | |
| Extra Thin Slices, 4 slices, 2 oz | 50 | 1 | 3 |
| *Hillshire,* Deli Select, | | | |
| Oven Roasted, 6 slices, 2 oz | 50 | 0.5 | 2 |
| **Turkey Ham,** 1 slice, 1 oz | 35 | 1.5 | 0.5 |
| **Turkey Loaf,** 1 oz | 30 | 1 | 0.5 |
| **Turkey Pastrami,** 1 oz | 35 | 1.5 | 1 |
| **Turkey Roll,** 1 oz | 40 | 2 | 0.5 |
| **Vegetarian Deli** ~ *See Page 118* | | | |

### Meat Spreads

| | C | F | Cb |
|---|---|---|---|
| **Average All Brands:** | | | |
| Chicken, white meat, 2.1 oz | 140 | 11 | 2 |
| Corned Beef, 2.1 oz | 140 | 11 | 1 |
| Ham, Deviled, 2.1 oz | 180 | 15 | 1 |
| Liverwurst | 160 | 13 | 4 |
| Roast Beef | 130 | 10 | 2 |
| Turkey | 110 | 7 | 2 |
| **Underwood:** *Per 2 oz* | | | |
| Chicken, White Meat | 140 | 11 | 2 |
| Deviled Ham | 180 | 15 | 1 |
| Liverwurst | 160 | 13 | 4 |
| Roast Beef | 130 | 10 | 2 |

### Paté

| | C | F | Cb |
|---|---|---|---|
| **Les Trois Petit Cochons:** *Per 2 oz* | | | |
| **Pate:** de Campagne 2 oz | 240 | 22 | 2 |
| de Canard a l'Orange; Forestier, 2 oz | 210 | 18 | 3 |
| Paysan, 2 oz | 150 | 12 | 2 |
| Rustique, 2 oz | 240 | 22 | 2 |
| Venison, 2 oz | 200 | 16 | 4 |
| Wild Boar, 2 oz | 180 | 15 | 4 |
| **Old Wisconsin Pate,** | | | |
| Braunschweiger, 2 oz | 210 | 18 | 3 |

## Nuts

**C** **F** **Cb**

*Per 1 oz Unless Indicated*

| | C | F | Cb |
|---|---|---|---|
| **Acorns,** raw 1 oz | 110 | 7 | 12 |
| **Almonds:** Dried/Dry Roasted: | | | |
| Whole: 12 medium size, 0.5 oz | 85 | 7.5 | 3 |
| 23-25 medium size, 1 oz | 170 | 15 | 6 |
| ½ cup, 2.5 oz | 420 | 37 | 13 |
| Ground, 1 cup, 3.4 oz | 545 | 47 | 20 |
| Sliced, ½ cup, 1.6 oz | 260 | 22 | 10 |
| Slivered, ½ cup, 2 oz | 310 | 27 | 12 |
| Chocolate Coated (5-6), 1 oz | 150 | 10 | 15 |
| Honey Roasted, 1 oz | 170 | 14 | 8 |
| Oil Roasted (*Blue Diamond*), 1 oz | 170 | 16 | 5 |
| **Brazil Nuts,** 8 medium, 1 oz | 185 | 19 | 3.5 |
| **Cashews,** dry or oil roasted: | | | |
| 14 large/18 med./26 small: 1 oz | 165 | 14 | 9 |
| ½ cup, 2.4 oz | 375 | 31 | 20 |
| Honey Roasted, 1 oz | 165 | 13 | 10 |
| **Chestnuts:** | | | |
| Average, dried, 1 oz | 105 | 1 | 22 |
| Raw/Fresh, 5-6 nuts, 1 oz | 60 | 0 | 13 |
| Canned, water chestnuts, sliced/whole/drained, 1 oz | 30 | 0 | 7 |
| **Coconut, Fresh:** | | | |
| 1 piece, 2"x2"x ½ ", 1 oz | 185 | 18 | 7 |
| Shredded, fresh, ½ cup, 1.4 oz | 140 | 13 | 6 |
| Dried (Desiccated): | | | |
| Sweetened: Shredded, 1 oz | 145 | 10 | 14 |
| Grated, ½ cup, 1.3 oz | 185 | 13 | 18 |
| Unsweetened, 1 oz | 185 | 18 | 7 |
| Cream (canned), ½ cup, 5.2 oz | 285 | 26 | 12 |
| Milk (canned), unsweetened, ¼ cup, 2 fl.oz | 100 | 10 | 3 |
| Water (center liquid), ½ cup, 4.3 oz | 25 | 0 | 4.5 |
| **Filberts or Hazelnuts:** | | | |
| Shelled, 18-20 nuts | 180 | 17 | 4.5 |
| Chopped, ¼ cup, 1 oz | 180 | 18 | 5 |
| Ground, ¼ cup, 0.6 oz | 120 | 12 | 3 |
| **Ginkgo Nuts,** canned, 14 med., 1 oz | 32 | 0.5 | 6.5 |
| **Hickory,** | | | |
| 30 small nuts, 1 oz | 200 | 18 | 5 |
| **Macadamia Nuts,** Shelled: | | | |
| Raw or Dry Roasted, avg: | | | |
| 12 small or 8 med., 1 oz | 200 | 21 | 4 |
| 6-7 large, 1 oz | 200 | 21 | 4 |
| ½ cup, 2.3 oz | 480 | 51 | 10 |
| **Mixed Nuts:** Raw, 18-22 nuts, 1 oz | 170 | 15 | 7 |
| Oil Roasted, all types | 170 | 16 | 6 |
| Sweet Roasts, 26 pieces, 1 oz | 160 | 12 | 10 |
| *Planters,* Dry Roasted/Honey | 160 | 12 | 9 |
| **Nut Toppings,** chopped, 1 Tbsp, 0.3 oz | 40 | 4 | 1.5 |

*Per 1 oz Unless Indicated*

| | C | F | Cb |
|---|---|---|---|
| **Peanuts:** | | | |
| Dry or oil roasted, average: | | | |
| Small handful, 0.5 oz | 85 | 7 | 3 |
| ⅓ cup, 1 oz | 165 | 14 | 6 |
| ½ cup, 2.5 oz | 415 | 35 | 15 |
| 3 oz bag | 500 | 42 | 18 |
| 7 oz bag | 1160 | 98 | 42 |
| Raw: Shelled, 1 oz | 160 | 14 | 4.5 |
| In shell, 1 oz | 115 | 110 | 3 |
| *Planters:* | | | |
| Cocktail, all varieties | 170 | 14 | 5 |
| Honey Roasted | 160 | 13 | 7 |
| Spanish Redskins | 170 | 15 | 4 |
| Sweet N' Crunchy | 140 | 8 | 15 |
| Japanese Style Peanuts, Coated in Crunchy Shell | 150 | 8 | 13 |
| **Pecans,** roasted: | | | |
| 10 halves, 0.5 oz | 95 | 10 | 2 |
| 20 Halves, 1 oz | 195 | 20 | 4 |
| 1 cup, halves, 3.5 oz | 680 | 71 | 14 |
| **Pilinuts,** dried, 1 oz | 215 | 24 | 1 |
| **Pine Nuts,** | | | |
| dried, 1 Tbsp, 0.3 oz | 70 | 7 | 1.5 |
| **Pistachios,** raw: | | | |
| Shelled, 45 nuts, 1 oz | 160 | 13 | 8 |
| Unshelled, 2 oz | 165 | 14 | 7 |
| *Lance,* Roasted, 1.5 oz | 120 | 9 | 6 |
| **Sesame Nut Mix,** 1 oz | 160 | 13 | 9 |
| **Soy Nuts:** Dry Roasted | 130 | 6 | 9 |
| ½ cup, 3 oz | 390 | 18 | 28 |
| *Dr Soy,* Chocolate coated, 1 oz pkg | 140 | 7 | 13 |
| **Trail Mix** (*Planters*): | | | |
| Daybreak, Berry Almond, 1.5 oz | 180 | 7 | 27 |
| Energy Mix, 1.5 oz | 250 | 20 | 14 |
| Fruit & Nut | 140 | 9 | 14 |
| Nut & Chocolate, 1.3oz | 150 | 9 | 14 |
| Nuts, Seeds & Raisins, 1 oz | 160 | 11 | 11 |
| Spicy Nuts & Cajun Sticks | 150 | 11 | 10 |
| Sweet & Nutty, 1 oz | 150 | 9 | 13 |
| **Walnuts,** average all types: | | | |
| 7-10 halves, 0.5 oz | 90 | 9 | 2 |
| 15-20 halves, 1 oz | 175 | 17 | 3 |
| Chopped, ½ cup, 2.2 oz | 380 | 36 | 6 |
| Ground, ¼ cup, 0.7 oz | 130 | 13 | 3 |

### Quick Guide | C | F | Cb

**Peanut Butter:** *Average All Brands*

| | C | F | Cb |
|---|---|---|---|
| 1 level tsp, 0.2 oz | 35 | 3 | 1 |
| 1 level Tbsp, 0.6 oz | 100 | 8.5 | 3.5 |
| 1 oz Quantity | 165 | 14 | 6 |
| ½ cup, 5 oz | 835 | 72 | 29 |

### Peanut Butter ~ Brands

| | C | F | Cb |
|---|---|---|---|
| **Jif:** Regular, all varieties, 2 Tbsp | 190 | 16 | 8 |
| Natural, average all varieties, 2 Tbsp | 185 | 15 | 10 |
| Reduced Fat, all varieties, 2 Tbsp | 190 | 12 | 15 |
| To Go: Crmy/Crunch, av.,1.5 oz cup | 250 | 21 | 11 |
| Chocolate Silk, 1.5 oz cup | 250 | 18 | 18 |
| Whipped: Creamy, 2 Tbsp | 140 | 12 | 6 |
| Chocolate flavored, 2 Tbsp | 150 | 11 | 11 |
| **Laura Scudder's,** Natural, Smooth; Nutty, average, 2 Tbsp | 190 | 16 | 5 |
| **Peter Pan:** | | | |
| **Natural,** Creamy/Crunchy, av., 2 T. | 205 | 17 | 6 |
| **Creamy/Crunchy,** Red.-Fat, 2 Tbsp | 200 | 13 | 14 |
| **Plus Creamy,** 2 Tbsp | 210 | 17 | 7 |
| **Planters,** Creamy/Crunchy, 2 Tbsp | 180 | 15 | 8 |
| **Smucker's,** Goober, Grape/Strawberry, 3 Tbsp. 2 oz | 240 | 13 | 24 |
| **Skippy:** Natural, Creamy/Chunky, 2 T. | 190 | 16 | 6 |
| Reduced Fat, all varieties, 2 Tbsp | 180 | 12 | 15 |
| **PB Bites,** average all, 15 pcs, 1 oz | 160 | 10 | 14 |

### Peanut Butter & Jelly Sandwich

**1 sandwich:** *With 2 oz Bread*

| | C | F | Cb |
|---|---|---|---|
| Thin Spread, 1 Tbsp Peanut Butter + 1 Tbsp Jelly | 310 | 10 | 48 |
| Thick Spread, 2 Tbsp Peanut Butter + 2 Tbsp Jelly | 480 | 19 | 67 |

### Nut & Chocolate Spread

**Nutella:**

| | C | F | Cb |
|---|---|---|---|
| 1 Tbsp, 0.7 oz | 110 | 6 | 11 |
| 2 Tbsp, 1.3 oz | 200 | 11 | 22 |

Note: Nutella contains approx. 50% sugar & 13% hazelnuts

### Other Nut & Seed Butters

*Per 1 Tbsp, 0.5 oz*

| | C | F | Cb |
|---|---|---|---|
| Almond Butter | 100 | 10 | 3.5 |
| Cashew Butter | 95 | 8 | 4.5 |
| Hazelnut Butter; Pecan Butter | 110 | 10 | 2 |
| Pistachio Butter | 90 | 6.5 | 4.5 |
| Sesame Butter (Tahini) | 90 | 8 | 3 |
| Soy Nut Butter | 75 | 5 | 4 |

### Seeds | C | F | Cb

| | C | F | Cb |
|---|---|---|---|
| **Alfalfa Seeds,** sprouted, ½ cup, 0.5 oz | 5 | 0 | 1 |
| **Caraway/Fennel,** 1 tsp | 7 | 0.5 | 1 |
| **Chia Seeds:** 1 Tbsp, 0.4 oz | 45 | 3 | 4 |
| 3 Tbsp, 1 oz | 140 | 8.5 | 12 |
| **Cottonseed Kernels,** roasted, 1 Tbsp | 50 | 3.5 | 2 |
| **Flaxseeds,** 3 Tbsp, 1 oz | 140 | 9 | 9 |
| **Hemp Seeds,** 3 Tbsp, 1 oz | 160 | 14 | 3 |
| **Lotus Seeds,** dried, ½ cup, 0.5 oz | 55 | 0.5 | 10 |
| **Poppy Seeds,** 1 tsp | 15 | 1 | 1 |
| **Pumpkin/Pepita Seeds,** whole: | | | |
| Roasted/Tamari: 1 oz | 150 | 12 | 4 |
| ½ cup, 4 oz | 590 | 48 | 15 |
| Dried (hulled), ¼ cup, 1 oz | 155 | 13 | 5 |
| **Safflower Kernels,** dried, 1 oz | 150 | 11 | 10 |
| **Sesame Seeds:** | | | |
| Dried, 1 Tbsp, 0.3 oz | 50 | 4.5 | 2 |
| Roasted/Toasted, 1 oz | 160 | 14 | 7.5 |
| **Sunflower Kernels/Seeds:** | | | |
| Dried, ¼ cup w/out hulls, 0.3 oz | 200 | 18 | 7 |
| Dry Roasted: 1 Tbsp, 0.3 oz | 45 | 4 | 2 |
| ¼ cup, 1 oz | 165 | 14 | 7 |
| Oil Roasted, ⅓ cup, 1 oz | 170 | 14 | 6.5 |
| **Watermelon Seeds,** dried, ¼ cup, 1 oz | 150 | 13 | 4 |

*Nut eaters are healthier and live longer, say scientists.*

*Nuts are a nutritious source of protein, vitamins, minerals, fiber, healthy fats, and antioxidants.*

*The fat and fiber of nuts can help reduce blood cholesterol. Their protein and fiber also promotes meal satiety (fullness) and reduces hunger levels – of benefit in weight control.*

*Eat nuts instead of high-sugar snacks, candy and soft drinks. Add chopped nuts to breakfast cereals.*

## Quick Guide

| | C | F | Cb |
|---|---|---|---|
| **Pancakes:** | | | |
| **Plain:** *Average All Types* | | | |
| Small (3" diameter), 0.8 oz | 50 | 2 | 6 |
| Medium (4" diameter), 1.3 oz | 85 | 3.5 | 11 |
| Large (6" diameter), 2.5 oz | 175 | 7.5 | 22 |
| *Add Extra for Syrups/Butter* | | | |
| **Pancake Syrup:** Regular, 1 Tbsp | 50 | 0 | 12 |
| ¼ cup, 4 Tbsp | 185 | 0 | 49 |
| Lite, 1 Tbsp | 25 | 0 | 6.5 |
| ¼ cup, 4 Tbsp | 100 | 0 | 27 |
| **Butter/Margarine:** | | | |
| Regular, 1 Tbsp | 100 | 11 | 0 |
| Whipped, 1 Tbsp | 65 | 7.5 | 0 |
| **Waffles:** | | | |
| **Homemade,** 7" waffle, 2.5 oz | 220 | 11 | 25 |
| **Frozen + Toasted,** (4" diam.), 1 oz | 105 | 3 | 16 |

## Pancake Brands

*Prepared as Directed*

| | C | F | Cb |
|---|---|---|---|
| **Aunt Jemima:** *Prepared* | | | |
| **Mixes:** *Makes 4" Pancakes* | | | |
| Original (4) | 250 | 6 | 36 |
| Original Complete (3) | 160 | 1.5 | 32 |
| Buttermilk (4) | 160 | 2.5 | 27 |
| Whole Wheat Blend (3) | 200 | 5 | 30 |
| **Bisquick:** *Prepared with Water* | | | |
| **Pancake/Waffle Mix:** | | | |
| Buttermilk, Complete, Wh. Grain (3) | 210 | 4 | 39 |
| **Hungry Jack:** | | | |
| **Pancake & Waffle Mixes:** *Makes 4" Pancake* | | | |
| Complete Mixes: Just Add Water | | | |
| Chocolate Chip (3) | 190 | 2.5 | 39 |
| Extra Light & Fluffy (3) | 180 | 1 | 38 |
| Wheat Blends (3) | 180 | 1.5 | 39 |
| **Easy Packs:** *Dry Mix Only* | | | |
| Buttermilk, 1.9 oz | 190 | 1 | 39 |
| Chocolate Chip, 1.9 oz | 190 | 2.5 | 39 |
| **Traditional:** *Dry Mix Only* | | | |
| Original, 1.7 oz | 160 | 1 | 34 |
| Buttermilk, 1.7 oz | 160 | 1 | 34 |
| Extra Light & Fluffy, 1.6 oz | 150 | 1 | 32 |
| **Northern Pines,** | | | |
| Premium Mix (3) | 200 | 3.5 | 38 |

## Frozen Breakfasts

| | C | F | Cb |
|---|---|---|---|
| **Eggo** *(Kellogg's):* | | | |
| **Choco-Toast, Chocolatey Chip,** slice (set of 4) | 110 | 4 | 18 |
| **Cinna-Toasts,** Cinnamon Roll slice (set of 4) | 110 | 4 | 18 |
| **French Toast, Thick & Fluffy:** | | | |
| Blueberry, 1 slice | 140 | 2 | 26 |
| Classic | 140 | 2 | 26 |
| **French Toaster Sticks:** | | | |
| Original (2) | 210 | 6 | 35 |
| Cinnamon (2) | 220 | 6 | 38 |
| **Minis Pancakes,** Buttermilk (11) | 270 | 9 | 44 |
| **Pancakes:** | | | |
| Blueberry (3) | 250 | 7 | 42 |
| Chocolate Chip (3) | 260 | 8 | 42 |
| **Bites,** Chocolatey Chip, 1.7 oz pouch | 130 | 3.5 | 24 |
| **Wafflers,** Chocolatey Chip Muffin, 2 wafflers (4 waffle bars) | 250 | 9 | 37 |
| **Pillsbury:** | | | |
| **Pancakes,** | | | |
| Buttermilk; Homestlye, (3) | 230 | 4 | 45 |

## Frozen Waffles

| | C | F | Cb |
|---|---|---|---|
| **Eggo** *(Kellogg's):* | | | |
| Blueberry (2) | 180 | 6 | 29 |
| Chocolatey Chip (2) | 200 | 7 | 32 |
| Strawberry (2) | 180 | 6 | 29 |
| **Nutri-Grain:** | | | |
| Blueberry (2) | 180 | 6 | 30 |
| Whole Wheat , low fat (2) | 140 | 2.5 | 27 |
| **Thick & Fluffy:** Original (1) | 160 | 7 | 22 |
| Cinnamon Brown Sugar (1) | 170 | 7 | 25 |
| **Kashi:** Average (2) | 135 | 5 | 24 |
| Gluten Free, Orig. (2) | 150 | 5 | 26 |
| **Nature's Path:** | | | |
| Ancient Grains (2) | 180 | 6 | 30 |
| Buckwheat Wildberry (2) | 190 | 7 | 33 |
| Chia Plus; Homestyle (2) | 210 | 7 | 34 |
| Dark Chocolate Chip (2) | 220 | 7 | 34 |
| Flax Plus (2) | 200 | 8 | 30 |
| **Van's:** 8 Wh. Grains, Multigrain (2) | 160 | 5 | 29 |
| Homestyle (2) | 190 | 8 | 29 |
| Gluten Free, Apple Cinnamon (2) | 200 | 6 | 35 |
| Mini, Chocolate Chip (12), 3 oz | 210 | 6 | 35 |

### Spaghetti/Pasta

**C** **F** **Cb**

- Pasta includes all shapes and sizes; (e.g. spaghetti, fettuccini, elbows, shells, twists, sheets, cannelloni, linguini, tubes, ziti).
- All regular pasta products have the same cals/fat/carbs on a weight basis.
- 1 oz Dry = approximately 2.5 -3 oz cooked.

### Dry Spaghetti/Pasta

| | C | F | Cb |
|---|---|---|---|
| **1 oz quantity** | 105 | 0.5 | 21 |
| **1lb box/pkg,** 16 oz | 1685 | 7 | 339 |
| **Elbows,** 1 cup, 4 oz | 380 | 2 | 80 |
| **Shells,** small, 1 cup, 3.3 oz | 330 | 1.5 | 69 |
| **Spirals,** 1 cup, 3 oz | 305 | 1.5 | 64 |

### Cooked Spaghetti/Pasta

| | C | F | Cb |
|---|---|---|---|
| **Plain, All Types (no added fat):** | | | |
| Firm/Al Dente (8-10 minutes), 1 oz | 42 | 0.5 | 8.5 |
| Medium (11-13 minutes), 1 oz | 37 | 0.5 | 7.5 |
| Tender (14-20 minutes), 1 oz | 32 | 0.5 | 7 |
| Longer cooking increases water absorbed | | | |
| **Spaghetti:** ½ cup, 2.5 oz | 90 | 0.5 | 18 |
| Medium serving, 1 cup, 5 oz | 225 | 1.5 | 44 |
| Large serving, 2 cups, 10 oz | 450 | 3 | 88 |
| Extra large, 3 cups, 15 oz | 675 | 5 | 132 |
| **Elbows/Spirals,** 1 cup, 5 oz | 220 | 1.5 | 43 |
| **Small Shells,** 1 cup, 4 oz | 180 | 1 | 36 |
| **Protein-fortified:** Dry, 1 c., 3.4 oz | 350 | 2 | 63 |
| Cooked, 1 cup, 5 oz | 230 | 0.5 | 45 |
| **Spinach/Vegetable:** Dry, 1 cup, 3 oz | 310 | 1 | 61 |
| Cooked, 1 cup, 5 oz | 180 | 0.5 | 38 |
| **Whole-wheat:** Dry, 1 cup, 3.8 oz | 365 | 1.5 | 79 |
| Cooked, 1 cup, 5 oz | 175 | 1 | 37 |

### Fresh Pasta (Refrigerated)

**Average All Brands:**

| | C | F | Cb |
|---|---|---|---|
| **Plain/Spinach/Tomato:** | | | |
| As purchased, 4.5 oz | 370 | 3 | 70 |
| Cooked, 1 cup, 5 oz | 185 | 1.5 | 35 |
| **Home-made,** w/o egg, cooked, 1 c. 5 oz | 175 | 1 | 35 |
| **Buitoni:** | | | |
| **Cut Pasta:** | | | |
| Angel Hair, 3 oz | 230 | 2 | 43 |
| Fettuccine/Linguine, 3 oz | 240 | 2 | 45 |
| **House Foods:** | | | |
| **Tofu Shirataki Noodles:** | | | |
| Angel Hair/Fettuccini, | | | |
| Macaroni/Spaghetti, 4 oz | 20 | 0.5 | 3 |
| **Nasoya,** | | | |
| Shirataki Spaghetti, | | | |
| Pasta Zero, ⅔ cup, 4 oz | 15 | 0 | 4 |

### Buitoni: *Per 1 Cup Unless Indicated*

| | C | F | Cb |
|---|---|---|---|
| **Agnolotti,** Mushroom, 3.8 oz | 280 | 10 | 34 |
| **Ravioli,** Four Cheese3.7 oz | 330 | 12 | 42 |
| **Tortellini:** Mixed Cheese, 3.7 oz | 320 | 8 | 47 |
| Spinach Cheese, 3.7 oz | 320 | 7 | 49 |
| **Tortelloni:** Swt Italian Sausage, 4 oz | 350 | 10 | 51 |
| Cheese & Roasted Garlic, 3.7 oz | 280 | 8 | 39 |
| **Other Varieties** ~ *See Page 112* | | | |
| **Pasta Sauces** ~ *See Page 144* | | | |

### Macaroni & Cheese

| | C | F | Cb |
|---|---|---|---|
| **Packaged (Kraft)** ~ *See Page 116* | | | |
| **Restaurant:** *Average* | | | |
| Side Serve, 6 oz | 265 | 13 | 26 |
| Medium serve, 1 cup, 9 oz | 350 | 17 | 34 |
| Large serve, 2 cups, 18 oz | 700 | 34 | 68 |

### Noodles

| | C | F | Cb |
|---|---|---|---|
| **Plain/Egg:** Dry, 1 oz | 110 | 1.5 | 20 |
| 1 cup, 1.4 oz | 145 | 1.5 | 27 |
| **Cooked:** 1 oz | 40 | 0.5 | 7 |
| ½ cup, 2.8 oz | 110 | 1.5 | 20 |
| 1 cup, 5.5 oz | 220 | 3.5 | 40 |
| **Stir-Fried:** 1 cup, 5.5 oz | 270 | 9 | 40 |
| 2 cup serving, 11 oz | 540 | 18 | 80 |
| **Low Carb Noodles,** | | | |
| *Quest Pasta,* 4 oz | 10 | 0 | 3 |
| *Note: Carbs are from glucomannan fiber* | | | |
| **Yolk Free (Cooked):** | | | |
| *Manischewitz,* Yolk Free, 2 oz | 200 | 1 | 41 |
| **Chinese:** Cellophane/Rice, dry, 1 oz | 100 | 0 | 25 |
| Chow Mein/hard, dry, 1 oz | 150 | 9 | 16 |
| **Japanese:** Soba: Dry, 1 oz | 95 | 0.5 | 21 |
| Cooked, 1 cup, 4 oz | 115 | 0.5 | 24 |
| Somen: Dry, 1 oz | 100 | 0.5 | 21 |
| Cooked, 1 cup, 6 oz | 230 | 0.5 | 49 |
| **Japanese Style Pan Fried,** | | | |
| Yaki-Soba (*Maruchan's*), av., 5.6 oz | 260 | 3 | 50 |
| **Ramen Noodles** ~ *See Page 118* | | | |
| **Rice Noodles:** Dry, 3.5 oz | 365 | 0.5 | 83 |
| Cooked, 1 cup, 6.2 oz | 190 | 0.5 | 44 |
| *Yakisoba,* Stir Fry, 3.5 oz | 430 | 6 | 52 |
| *House Foods,* Tofu Shirataki, 4 oz | 20 | 0.5 | 3 |
| *Chikara,* Udon, average, 7.5 oz pkt | 250 | 1 | 52 |
| *Simply Asia/Thai Kitchen* ~ *See Pages 119 & 121* | | | |

### Egg Roll/Won Ton Wrappers

| | C | F | Cb |
|---|---|---|---|
| Egg/Spring Roll (1), 0.8 oz | 65 | 0 | 15 |
| Won Ton Wrapper (1), 0.3 oz | 20 | 0 | 4 |

## Quick Guide ⒸⒻⒸⓑ

**Fruit Pies:** *Average All Brands, 9" Pie*
**Apple; Blueberry; Cherry:**

| | C | F | Cb |
|---|---|---|---|
| Small Serving, | | | |
| ⅛ pie, 4.8 oz | 350 | 16 | 49 |
| Medium Serving, | | | |
| ⅙ pie, 6.5 oz | 465 | 22 | 65 |
| Large Serving | | | |
| ¼ pie, 9.5 oz | 700 | 33 | 98 |
| Whole Pie (9"), 38 oz | 2800 | 131 | 392 |

**Other Pies:** *Per Serving, ⅙ of 9" Pie*

| | C | F | Cb |
|---|---|---|---|
| Chocolate Cream Pie | 345 | 22 | 38 |
| Custard: Egg Pie | 220 | 12 | 22 |
| Coconut Pie | 330 | 18 | 35 |
| Lemon Meringue Pie | 305 | 10 | 53 |
| Peach Pie | 260 | 12 | 39 |
| Pecan Pie | 440 | 23 | 57 |
| Pumpkin Pie | 315 | 14 | 41 |
| Shoo-Fly Pie | 400 | 13 | 70 |

## Dessert/Fruit Pies ~ Brands

**Hostess:**

| | C | F | Cb |
|---|---|---|---|
| Cherry Pie, 4.5 oz | 480 | 20 | 68 |
| Lemon, 4.5 oz | 490 | 22 | 69 |

**Marie Callender's:**

| | C | F | Cb |
|---|---|---|---|
| Key Lime, 4.5 oz | 440 | 19 | 59 |
| Peach Cobbler, 4 oz | 330 | 16 | 43 |
| Pumpkin, 4.5 oz | 360 | 13 | 54 |
| Turtle, 4.7 oz | 560 | 36 | 55 |

**Mrs Smith's:**

| | C | F | Cb |
|---|---|---|---|
| **Cobblers:** Blackberry, 4 oz | 240 | 8 | 38 |
| Peach, 4 oz | 240 | 8 | 39 |
| **Flaky Crust:** *Per ⅛ Pie* | | | |
| Apple, 4.6 oz | 330 | 18 | 41 |
| Cherry, 4.4 oz | 340 | 17 | 43 |
| Peach, 4.6 oz | 330 | 18 | 41 |

**Sara Lee:** *Per Slice*
**Creme Pies:**

| | C | F | Cb |
|---|---|---|---|
| Chocolate, ⅕ pie, 3.9 oz | 440 | 27 | 46 |
| Coconut, ⅙ pie, 4.5 oz | 370 | 20 | 44 |
| Key Lime, ⅕ pie, 4.8 oz | 410 | 17 | 59 |
| **Fruit Pies:** Apple, 4 oz | 300 | 15 | 40 |
| Cherry, 4.27 oz | 330 | 16 | 43 |
| Peach, 4.27 oz | 310 | 15 | 39 |
| Raspberry, 4.27 oz | 340 | 15 | 46 |
| **Seasonal Pies:** Pumpkin, 4.27 oz | 250 | 10 | 37 |
| Sweet Potato, 4.27 oz | 270 | 9 | 43 |

**Tastykake:** Baked Apple Pie (1) — 270 / 11 / 41
Orange Kream-Cicle Pie (1) — 320 / 15 / 42

## Croissants ⒸⒻⒸⓑ

**Average all Brands**

| | C | F | Cb |
|---|---|---|---|
| **Plain/Butter/Cheese:** Mini, 1 oz | 115 | 6 | 13 |
| Small, 1.5 oz | 170 | 9 | 19 |
| Medium, 2 oz | 230 | 12 | 26 |
| Large, 2.5 oz | 290 | 15 | 32 |
| **Sweet Croissants:** | | | |
| Almond Filled, 3 oz | 330 | 18 | 39 |
| Chocolate Filled, 3 oz | 360 | 19 | 43 |
| **Dunkin' Donuts,** Plain Croissant | 340 | 19 | 37 |

**Croissant Sandwiches** ~ *See Page 165*

## Pastry & Pie Crust

| | C | F | Cb |
|---|---|---|---|
| **Pie Crust,** Baked, 9" diameter shell: | | | |
| 1 Pie Shell, 6.5 oz | 970 | 64 | 87 |
| 2-crust Pie, 9", 11.3 oz | 1660 | 109 | 150 |
| **Filo Pastry:** 4 sheets, 2.5 oz | 210 | 2.5 | 40 |
| *Athens,* Phyllo Dough, 5 sheets, 2 oz | 180 | 1 | 36 |
| **Puff:** | | | |
| *Pepperidge Farms:* Sheets, 1.5 oz | 160 | 10 | 16 |
| Bake & Fill Shells, 1.7 oz | 180 | 11 | 18 |
| **Arrowhead Mills,** | | | |
| Graham Cracker Pie Crust, ⅛ of 9" | 110 | 5 | 14 |
| **Keebler:** | | | |
| **Ready Crust:** *Per ⅛ of 9" Crust* | | | |
| Chocolate | 100 | 4.5 | 14 |
| Graham: Regular | 100 | 5 | 14 |
| Reduced Fat | 100 | 3.5 | 15 |
| Shortbread Crust | 100 | 5 | 14 |
| **Marie Callenders,** | | | |
| Pastry Pie Shell,1 oz | 130 | 8 | 13 |
| **Mrs Smith's,** | | | |
| Deep Dish Pie Crust, ⅛ pie, 1 oz | 130 | 8 | 14 |
| **Nabisco:** | | | |
| **Honey Maid,** | | | |
| Graham Cracker Crust,⅛ pie, ¾ oz | 110 | 5 | 14 |
| **Nilla,** Pie Crust, | | | |
| ⅙ of Pie, Crust, 1 oz | 140 | 8 | 18 |
| **Pillsbury,** Pie Crusts, | | | |
| Refrigerated, ⅛, 0.9 oz | 100 | 6 | 12 |
| **Trader Joe's,** Pie Crust, ⅛ pie, 1.2 oz | 190 | 13 | 17 |

## Pie Fillings ~ Canned

**Apple/Blueb./Cherry/Strawb.,** average:

| | C | F | Cb |
|---|---|---|---|
| Sweetened: ⅓ cup, 3.2oz | 90 | 0 | 22 |
| 1 cup, 9.5 oz | 270 | 0 | 66 |
| 1 can, 21 oz | 600 | 0 | 150 |
| Light/Lite, ⅓ cup, 3.2 oz | 60 | 0 | 15 |
| Unsweetened, ⅓ cup, 3.2 oz | 35 | 0 | 8 |
| **Lemon Crm/Creme,** ⅓ cup, 3.2 oz | 130 | 1.5 | 28 |

## Pizzas ~ Ready to Eat

*Figures Based On Pizza Hut Unless Indicated*

### Cheese

*Medium Size (12"):*

| | C | F | Cb |
|---|---|---|---|
| **Hand Tossed Crust:** | | | |
| ⅛ Pizza (1 slice) | 210 | 8 | 26 |
| ½ Pizza (4 slices) | 840 | 32 | 104 |
| Whole Pizza (8 slices) | 1680 | 64 | 208 |
| **Original Pan:** ⅛ Pizza (1 slice) | 240 | 10 | 28 |
| ½ Pizza (4 slices) | 960 | 40 | 112 |
| Whole Pizza (8 slices) | 1920 | 80 | 224 |
| **Thin 'N Crispy Crust:** | | | |
| ⅛ Pizza (1 slice) | 180 | 7 | 22 |
| ½ Pizza (4 slices) | 720 | 28 | 88 |
| Whole Pizza (8 slices) | 1440 | 56 | 176 |

### Ham & Pineapple

*Figures Based On Domino's*
*Medium Size (12"):*

| | C | F | Cb |
|---|---|---|---|
| **Hand Tossed Crust:** | | | |
| ⅛ Pizza (1 slice) | 210 | 6 | 28 |
| ½ Pizza (4 slices) | 840 | 24 | 112 |
| Whole Pizza (8 slices) | 1680 | 48 | 224 |
| **Handmade Pan:** ⅛ Pizza (1 slice) | 290 | 13 | 31 |
| ½ Pizza (4 slices) | 1160 | 52 | 124 |
| Whole Pizza (8 slices) | 2320 | 104 | 248 |
| **Thin Crust:** | | | |
| ⅛ Pizza (1 slice) | 145 | 6.5 | 15 |
| ½ Pizza (4 slices) | 580 | 26 | 60 |
| Whole Pizza (8 slices) | 1160 | 52 | 120 |

### MeatZZA

*Medium Size (12"):*

| | C | F | Cb |
|---|---|---|---|
| **Hand Tossed Crust:** | | | |
| ⅛ Pizza (1 slice) | 270 | 12 | 27 |
| ½ Pizza (4 slices) | 1080 | 48 | 108 |
| Whole Pizza (8 slices) | 2160 | 96 | 216 |
| **Handmade Pan:** ⅛ Pizza (1 slice) | 350 | 19 | 30 |
| ½ Pizza (4 slices) | 1400 | 76 | 120 |
| Whole Pizza (8 slices) | 2800 | 152 | 240 |
| **Thin Crust:** ⅛ Pizza (1 slice) | 215 | 13 | 15 |
| ½ Pizza (4 slices) | 860 | 52 | 60 |
| Whole Pizza (8 slices) | 1720 | 104 | 120 |

## Pepperoni

*Medium Size (12"):*

| | C | F | Cb |
|---|---|---|---|
| **Hand Tossed Crust:** | | | |
| ⅛ Pizza (1 slice) | 220 | 9 | 26 |
| ½ Pizza (4 slices) | 880 | 36 | 104 |
| Whole Pizza (8 slices) | 1760 | 72 | 208 |
| **Handmade Pan:** ⅛ Pizza (1 slice) | 300 | 15 | 29 |
| ½ Pizza (4 slices) | 1200 | 60 | 116 |
| Whole Pizza (8 slices) | 2400 | 120 | 232 |
| **Thin Crust:** ⅛ Pizza (1 slice) | 160 | 9 | 14 |
| ½ Pizza (4 slices) | 640 | 36 | 56 |
| Whole Pizza (8 slices) | 1280 | 72 | 112 |

## Large Pizzas

*Large (14")*

| | C | F | Cb |
|---|---|---|---|
| **Hand Tossed Crust:** | | | |
| **Cheese:** ⅛ Pizza (1 slice) | 290 | 10 | 36 |
| ½ Pizza (4 slices) | 1160 | 40 | 144 |
| **MeatZZA:** ⅛ Pizza (1 slice) | 370 | 17 | 37 |
| ½ Pizza (4 slices) | 1480 | 68 | 148 |
| **Pepperoni:** ⅛ Pizza (1 slice) | 300 | 12 | 35 |
| ½ Pizza (4 slices) | 1200 | 48 | 140 |

## Extra Large, Single Slice

*Figures Based On Sbarro*

| | C | F | Cb |
|---|---|---|---|
| Cheese | 430 | 15 | 51 |
| Ham & Pineapple | 490 | 16 | 60 |
| Sausage | 520 | 24 | 50 |
| X-Treme Pepperoni | 620 | 32 | 53 |

## Individual Personal Pizzas

*Pan (6"): Figures Based On Pizza Hut*

| | C | F | Cb |
|---|---|---|---|
| **Buffalo Chicken** | 640 | 24 | 72 |
| **Cheese** | 600 | 24 | 68 |
| **Pepperoni** | 640 | 28 | 68 |
| **Supreme** | 720 | 36 | 68 |
| **Veggie Lovers** | 560 | 20 | 72 |

*Chicago-Style Deep Dish: Individual*
*Figures Based On Uno Pizzeria*

| | C | F | Cb |
|---|---|---|---|
| **Cheese & Tomato,** 18.8 oz | 1700 | 115 | 110 |
| **Chicago Classic,** 25.8 oz | 2220 | 157 | 112 |
| **Prima Pepperoni,** 18.5 oz | 1720 | 118 | 110 |
| **Sausage& Spinach Alfredo,** 22.7 oz | 1900 | 143 | 79 |

### Frozen Pizzas

| | C | F | Cb |
|---|---|---|---|
| **Amy's:** *Per ⅓ Pizza* | | | |
| Cheese Pizza | 290 | 12 | 33 |
| Margherita | 270 | 12 | 31 |
| Meatless Pepperoni | 340 | 16 | 33 |
| Mushroom & Olive | 260 | 11 | 29 |
| Pesto & Artichoke | 300 | 16 | 34 |
| **Gluten-Free:** Meatless Pepperoni | 320 | 15 | 40 |
| Roasted Vegetable | 320 | 11 | 51 |
| Spinach | 300 | 12 | 36 |
| Vegan Margherita | 290 | 15 | 33 |
| **California Pizza Kitchen:** | | | |
| **Cauliflower:** Artisanal Style Cheese | 270 | 12 | 29 |
| Pepperoni, Mushroom & Sausage | 300 | 15 | 28 |
| **Crispy Thin Crust:** *Per ⅓ Pizza* | | | |
| BBQ Recipe Chicken | 290 | 11 | 33 |
| Four Cheese | 320 | 16 | 29 |
| Margherita | 320 | 17 | 29 |
| Sicilian Recipe | 350 | 17 | 31 |
| Signature Pepperoni | 330 | 17 | 29 |
| The Works | 320 | 17 | 30 |
| **Gluten-Free:** | | | |
| BBQ Recipe Chicken, ½ pizza | 290 | 9 | 37 |
| Margherita, ⅓ pizza | 190 | 8 | 21 |
| **Organic:** Five Cheese & Tomato | 270 | 10 | 33 |
| Mushroom & Green Onion | 250 | 8 | 33 |
| **Celeste:** *Per Pizza* | | | |
| **Pizza For One:** Original 4 Cheese | 380 | 16 | 48 |
| Deluxe | 360 | 15 | 47 |
| Pepperoni | 370 | 16 | 46 |
| Sausage | 370 | 16 | 47 |
| **Daiya** *(Vegan):* | | | |
| Cheese Lovers, ⅓ pizza | 390 | 17 | 54 |
| Meatless Meat Lover's, ¼ pizza | 360 | 16 | 48 |
| Mushroom & Roasted Garlic, ⅓ pizza | 390 | 14 | 58 |
| Pepperoni Style, ⅓ pizza | 470 | 21 | 64 |
| Supreme, ¼ pizza | 340 | 12 | 37 |
| **DiGiorno:** | | | |
| **Cheese Stuffed Crust:** | | | |
| Bacon Cheeseburger, ⅙ pizza | 300 | 11 | 33 |
| Buffalo Style Chkn, ¼ pizza | 370 | 17 | 36 |
| Five Cheese, ⅕ Pizza | 370 | 15 | 42 |
| Pepperoni, ⅕ pizza | 380 | 16 | 42 |
| Three Meat, ⅙ pizza | 300 | 12 | 30 |
| Supreme, ⅙ pizza | 350 | 16 | 35 |
| **Classic Thin Crust,** Supreme, ⅕ pizza | 320 | 15 | 33 |

| **DiGiorno (Cont):** | C | F | Cb |
|---|---|---|---|
| **Original Rising Crust:** *Per ⅙ Pizza* | | | |
| Four Cheese | 290 | 10 | 36 |
| Italian Sausage | 330 | 14 | 36 |
| Spicy Chicken Supreme | 290 | 8 | 36 |
| **Small Pizzas:** *Per ½ Pizza* | | | |
| Cheese Stuffed Crust: | | | |
| Four Cheese | 330 | 15 | 33 |
| Pepperoni | 330 | 16 | 33 |
| Three Meat | 360 | 18 | 34 |
| Traditional Crust: | | | |
| Pepperoni | 365 | 17 | 41 |
| Three Meat | 370 | 17 | 43 |
| **Stuffed Crust:** Better with Bacon | | | |
| ⅕ pizza | 330 | 17 | 27 |
| Supreme, ⅙ pizza | 350 | 16 | 36 |
| **Freschetta:** | | | |
| **Brick Oven:** *Per ⅕ Pizza Unless Indicated* | | | |
| 5 Cheese, ¼ Pizza, 5.2 oz | 370 | 17 | 39 |
| Pepperoni, 4.55 oz | 330 | 17 | 32 |
| Spinach & Roasted M'shrms, 4.5 oz | 270 | 10 | 34 |
| Three Meat, 4.6 oz | 340 | 18 | 32 |
| Supreme, 4.6 oz | 310 | 14 | 33 |
| **Naturally Rising:** *Per ⅙ Pizza Unless Indicated* | | | |
| 4 Cheese Medley, ⅕ Pizza, 5 oz | 370 | 14 | 48 |
| Canada Style Bacon P'apple, 4.5 oz | 290 | 9 | 41 |
| Pepperoni, 4.55 oz | 330 | 13 | 40 |
| Supreme, 5.2 oz | 350 | 15 | 41 |
| **Jeno's:** *Per Pizza* | | | |
| **Crispy 'N Tasty:** | | | |
| Cheese, 5 oz | 310 | 14 | 38 |
| Combination, 5.2 oz | 330 | 16 | 38 |
| Pepperoni, 5 oz | 340 | 17 | 37 |
| Supreme, 5 oz | 310 | 14 | 38 |
| **Kroger:** | | | |
| **Self Rising Crust:** *Per ⅙ pizza* | | | |
| Double Bacon | 300 | 9 | 43 |
| Four Cheese | 300 | 8 | 43 |
| Pepperoni | 320 | 12 | 41 |
| Supreme | 350 | 14 | 43 |
| Three Meat | 340 | 13 | 44 |
| White Chicken | 310 | 11 | 41 |

## Frozen Pizzas (Cont) | C | F | Cb

### Lean Cuisine:

**Comfort Pizzas:** *Per Pkg*

| | C | F | Cb |
|---|---|---|---|
| Four Cheese | 400 | 8 | 64 |
| Pepperoni | 410 | 10 | 59 |
| Supreme | 400 | 10 | 59 |
| Thin Crust BBQ Chicken | 390 | 9 | 55 |
| **Deep Dish:** 3 Meat | 420 | 9 | 63 |
| Spinach & Mushroom | 340 | 7 | 55 |

**Favorites:** *Per Package*

| | C | F | Cb |
|---|---|---|---|
| French Bread Pepperoni | 310 | 7 | 46 |

**Origins:** *Per Package*

| | C | F | Cb |
|---|---|---|---|
| Farmers Market | 320 | 9 | 46 |
| Margherita | 320 | 4 | 55 |

### Red Baron:

**Brick Oven:** *Per ¼ Pizza*

| | C | F | Cb |
|---|---|---|---|
| Cheese Trio, 4.4 oz | 320 | 15 | 34 |
| Meat Trio, 4.6 oz | 320 | 15 | 35 |
| Pepperoni, 4.5 oz | 330 | 17 | 33 |

**Classic Crust:** *Per ¼ Pizza*

| | C | F | Cb |
|---|---|---|---|
| 4 Cheese, 5.25 oz | 380 | 17 | 40 |
| Sausage & Pepp.,4.4 oz | 320 | 16 | 32 |
| Supreme, 4.7 oz | 310 | 15 | 33 |

**Deep Dish Minis:**

| | C | F | Cb |
|---|---|---|---|
| Cheese, 4 pieces, 5.4 oz | 380 | 15 | 48 |
| Pepperoni, 4 pieces, 5.6 oz | 430 | 20 | 48 |

**Deep Dish Singles:** *Per Pizza*

| | C | F | Cb |
|---|---|---|---|
| Hawaiian Style, 5.6 oz | 350 | 14 | 46 |
| Meat-Trio, 5.6 oz | 400 | 18 | 47 |
| Sausage, 5.8 oz | 420 | 20 | 47 |
| **Scrambles:** Bacon, 5.85 oz | 440 | 21 | 45 |
| Sausage, 5.85 oz | 410 | 19 | 46 |

**Thin & Crispy Crust:** *Per ⅓ Pizza*

| | C | F | Cb |
|---|---|---|---|
| 5 Cheese, 5 oz | 350 | 16 | 38 |
| Pepperoni, 5.3 oz | 390 | 20 | 38 |
| Supreme, 4.4 oz | 300 | 15 | 31 |

### Signature Select (Albertsons):

**Rising Crust:** *Per ⅙ Pizza*

| | C | F | Cb |
|---|---|---|---|
| Five Cheese | 340 | 12 | 42 |
| Pepperoni | 380 | 17 | 42 |
| Supreme | 370 | 15 | 43 |

**Ultra Thin Crust:** *Per ⅓ Pizza*

| | C | F | Cb |
|---|---|---|---|
| Pepperoni | 400 | 24 | 26 |
| Supreme | 370 | 21 | 28 |

### Smart Ones (Weight Watchers):

**Savory Italian Recipe Thin Crust:**

| | C | F | Cb |
|---|---|---|---|
| Cheese Pizza, 4.37 oz | 290 | 6 | 42 |
| Pepperoni Pizza, 4.37 oz | 310 | 10 | 39 |

### Stouffer's: | C | F | Cb

**French Bread Pizzas:**

**Two Per Box:**

| | C | F | Cb |
|---|---|---|---|
| Cheese (1) | 360 | 15 | 43 |
| Pepperoni (1) | 410 | 20 | 43 |
| Three Meat (1) | 470 | 25 | 43 |

**Nine Per Box:**

| | C | F | Cb |
|---|---|---|---|
| Pepperoni (1) | 430 | 21 | 44 |

### Tombstone:

**Original:** *Per ¼ Pizza*

| | C | F | Cb |
|---|---|---|---|
| Canadian Bacon | 290 | 11 | 33 |
| Five Cheese | 340 | 15 | 33 |
| Pepperoni | 350 | 17 | 33 |
| Pepperoni & Sausage | 340 | 15 | 34 |

**Brick Oven Thin Crust:**

| | C | F | Cb |
|---|---|---|---|
| Cheese, ⅓ pizza | 330 | 14 | 33 |
| Pepperoni; Supreme, av., ¼ pizza | 305 | 16 | 27 |

**Garlic Bread Crust:**

| | C | F | Cb |
|---|---|---|---|
| Pepperoni, ⅙ pizza | 340 | 15 | 36 |
| Supreme, ⅙ pizza | 320 | 13 | 37 |

### Tony's:

**Pizzeria Style Crust:** *Per ¼ Pizza*

| | C | F | Cb |
|---|---|---|---|
| Cheese, 4.7 oz | 330 | 13 | 41 |
| Meat Trio, 5 oz | 360 | 16 | 41 |
| Pepperoni, 4.7 oz | 330 | 14 | 40 |
| Sausage & Pepperoni, 4.83 oz | 350 | 15 | 41 |
| Supreme, 5.1 oz | 350 | 15 | 41 |

### Totino's:

**Crisp Crust Party Pizza:** *Per ½ Pizza*

| | C | F | Cb |
|---|---|---|---|
| Canadian Bacon | 310 | 14 | 37 |
| Cheese | 310 | 14 | 37 |
| Hamburger | 340 | 16 | 38 |
| Pepperoni & Bacon | 330 | 16 | 37 |
| **Pizza Rolls,** aall flavors, 6 pcs, 3 oz | 210 | 8 | 30 |

### Trader Giotto's:

| | C | F | Cb |
|---|---|---|---|
| Aragula Pizza, 1 sl., 5 oz | 330 | 12 | 38 |
| 3 Cheese Pizza, ⅓ pizza, 4.4 oz | 310 | 9 | 42 |
| Pesto Pizza, ⅓ pizza, 5 oz | 320 | 13 | 38 |
| Pizza 4 Formaggi, 1 sl., 5 oz | 310 | 9 | 42 |
| Pizza Parlanno, ¼ pizza, 4.7 oz | 340 | 16 | 34 |
| Roasted Vege., 1 sl., 5.4 oz | 300 | 11 | 36 |

### Trader Joe's:

| | C | F | Cb |
|---|---|---|---|
| 3 Cheese, ⅓ pizza | 310 | 9 | 42 |
| Ancient Grain, ⅓ pizza | 310 | 16 | 25 |
| BBQ Chicken, ⅓ pizza | 340 | 13 | 39 |
| Organic Woodfired Sicilian, ⅓ pizza | 280 | 12 | 35 |
| Spinach, ⅓ pizza | 300 | 12 | 38 |

| Quick Guide | **C** | **F** | **Cb** |
|---|---|---|---|

### Chicken
From 3lb ready-to-cook chicken
**Breast/Wing Quarter:**

| | | | |
|---|---|---|---|
| **Roasted:** with skin | 300 | 15 | 0 |
| without skin | 185 | 5 | 0 |
| **Fried**, batter dipped | 530 | 30 | 17 |

**Leg Quarter:**
**Thigh & Drumstick:**

| | | | |
|---|---|---|---|
| **Roasted:** with skin | 270 | 16 | 0 |
| without skin | 185 | 8 | 0 |
| **Fried**, batter dipped | 435 | 25 | 15 |

**KFC ~** *See Fast-Foods Section*

| Per 4 oz Edible Portion | | | |
|---|---|---|---|

**Average of Light Meat:** *Per 4 oz without Bone*

| | | | |
|---|---|---|---|
| **Roasted:** with skin | 250 | 12 | 0 |
| without skin | 175 | 4.5 | 0 |
| **Stewed:** with skin | 230 | 12 | 0 |
| without skin | 180 | 4.5 | 0 |
| **Fried:** Batter-dipped, with skin, 4 oz | 315 | 17 | 11 |
| Flour-coated, with skin, 4 oz | 280 | 14 | 2 |

**Average of Dark Meat:** *Per 4 oz without Bone*

| | | | |
|---|---|---|---|
| **Roasted:** with skin | 290 | 18 | 0 |
| without skin | 235 | 11 | 0 |
| **Stewed:** with skin | 265 | 17 | 0 |
| without skin | 220 | 10 | 0 |
| **Fried:** Batter-dipped, with skin, 4 oz | 340 | 21 | 11 |
| Flour-coated, with skin, 4 oz | 325 | 19 | 5 |

| Chicken Parts | | | |
|---|---|---|---|

**Broilers or Fryers:** *Edible Weights (no bone)*
**Breast:** *Per 1/2 Breast*

| | | | |
|---|---|---|---|
| Raw: with skin, 5 oz | 250 | 14 | 0 |
| without skin, 4.25 oz | 140 | 3 | 0 |
| Roasted: with skin, 3.5 oz | 195 | 8 | 0 |
| without skin, 3 oz | 140 | 3 | 0 |
| Stewed: with skin, 4 oz | 200 | 8 | 0 |
| without skin, 3.3 oz | 145 | 3 | 0 |
| Fried: Batter-dipped, w/ skin, 5 oz | 365 | 19 | 13 |
| Flour-coated, with skin, 3.5 oz | 220 | 9 | 2 |

**Drumstick:** *Per Drumstick*

| | | | |
|---|---|---|---|
| Roasted: with skin, 2 oz | 115 | 6 | 0 |
| without skin, 1.5 oz | 75 | 2.5 | 0 |
| Stewed: with skin, 2 oz | 115 | 6 | 0 |
| without skin, 1.5 oz | 80 | 3 | 0 |
| Fried: Batter-dipped, w/ skin, 2.5 oz | 195 | 11 | 6 |
| Flour-coated, with skin, 1.8 oz | 120 | 7 | 1 |

| Chicken Parts (Cont) | **C** | **F** | **Cb** |
|---|---|---|---|

**Broilers or Fryers (Cont):** *Edible Weights (no bone)*
**Thigh Portion:**

| | | | |
|---|---|---|---|
| Raw: with skin, 3.3 oz | | | |
| (4¼ oz with bone) | 200 | 14 | 0 |
| without skin, 2.4 oz | 80 | 3 | 0 |
| Roasted: with skin, 2.3 oz | 155 | 10 | 0 |
| without skin, 2 oz | 110 | 6 | 0 |
| Stewed: with skin, 2.5 oz | 160 | 10 | 0 |
| without skin, 2 oz | 105 | 5 | 0 |
| Fried: Batter-dipped, with skin 3 oz | 240 | 14 | 8 |
| Flour-coated, with skin, 2.3 oz | 165 | 9 | 2 |

**Wing:** *Per Wing, Bone In*

| | | | |
|---|---|---|---|
| Raw Weight, 3.2 oz | | | |
| Raw: with skin | 110 | 8 | 0 |
| without skin | 35 | 1 | 0 |
| Roasted: with skin | 100 | 7 | 0 |
| without skin | 45 | 2 | 0 |
| Fried: Batter-dipped, with skin | 160 | 11 | 5 |
| Flour-coated, with skin | 105 | 7 | 1 |
| Stewed, with skin, 4 oz | 100 | 7 | 0 |

**Buffalo Wings ~** *See Fast-Foods Section*

| | | | |
|---|---|---|---|
| **Neck:** Simmered, with skin | 95 | 7 | 0 |
| without skin | 30 | 2 | 0 |

**Skin Only:** *Skin from 1/2 Chicken*

| | | | |
|---|---|---|---|
| Raw skin, 3 oz | 275 | 26 | 0 |
| Roasted skin, 2 oz | 255 | 23 | 0 |
| Stewed skin, 2.5 oz | 260 | 24 | 0 |
| Fried, flour-coated, 2 oz | 280 | 24 | 5 |
| Fried, batter-dipped, 6.8 oz | 750 | 55 | 44 |

**Roasters:** *Average of Light & Dark Meat*

| | | | |
|---|---|---|---|
| **Roasted:** with skin, 4 oz | 250 | 15 | 0 |
| without skin, 4 oz | 190 | 8 | 0 |
| Dark Meat, without skin | 200 | 10 | 0 |
| Light Meat, without skin | 175 | 5 | 0 |

**Stewing Chicken:** *Per 4 oz, average of Light & Dark Meat*

| | | | |
|---|---|---|---|
| **Stewed:** with skin | 325 | 22 | 0 |
| without skin | 270 | 14 | 0 |
| Dark Meat, without skin | 290 | 17 | 0 |
| Light Meat, without skin | 240 | 9 | 0 |

**Capon Chicken:**

| | | | |
|---|---|---|---|
| **Roasted:** with skin, 4 oz | 260 | 13 | 0 |
| 1/2 Chicken, with skin, 22.5 oz | 1460 | 74 | 0 |

**Chicken Offal & Stuffing:**

| | | | |
|---|---|---|---|
| **Giblets:** Simmered, 1 cup | 230 | 7 | 0.5 |
| Fried, flour-coated, 1 cup | 400 | 20 | 6 |
| **Gizzard**, simmered, 1 cup | 210 | 4 | 0 |
| **Heart**, simmered, 1 cup | 270 | 12 | 0.2 |
| **Liver:** Raw, 4 oz | 130 | 5.5 | 0 |
| Simmered, 1 cup | 215 | 8.5 | 1 |
| **Liver Pate**, fresh, 1 Tbsp, 0.5 oz | 30 | 2 | 1 |
| **Stuffing**, average, 1/2 cup | 180 | 9 | 22 |

# Poultry ~ Chicken ◆ Turkey  (P)

## Chicken Products    C F Cb

**Bumble Bee:**
**Chicken In Water:** *Per 2 oz Drained*
| | | | |
|---|---|---|---|
| Premium White | 70 | 1.5 | 0 |
| Premium Breast | 70 | 1 | 1 |

**Foster Farms:**
| | | | |
|---|---|---|---|
| Chicken Breast Strips, grilled, 3 oz | 100 | 2 | 1 |
| Wings: Chipotle, 3 wings, 3 oz | 190 | 13 | 4 |
| Honey BBQ Glazed, 3 wings, 3 oz | 190 | 11 | 7 |
| Hot 'n' Spicy, 3 wings, 3 oz | 190 | 14 | 1 |

**Tyson:**
**Anytizers, Frozen:**
**Wings:**
| | | | |
|---|---|---|---|
| Hot Wings, Buffalo Style (3) | 190 | 13 | 1 |
| Honey BBQ Seasoned (3) | 190 | 12 | 8 |

**Wyngz, Boneless:**
| | | | |
|---|---|---|---|
| Buffalo Style, 3 pieces, 3 oz | 150 | 7 | 8 |
| Sweet Garlic Glazed, 3 pcs, 2.8 oz | 130 | 5 | 10 |

## Duck, Goose, Quail

**Duck, Roasted:**
| | | | |
|---|---|---|---|
| with skin, 3 oz | 290 | 24 | 0 |
| without skin, 3 oz | 170 | 10 | 0 |
| ½ duck, with skin, 13.5 oz | 1290 | 108 | 0 |
| **Goose:** Roasted with skin, 3 oz | 260 | 19 | 0 |
| without skin, 3 oz | 200 | 11 | 0 |
| **Pheasant**, cooked, 3 oz | 210 | 10 | 0 |
| **Quail**, cooked, 1 whole, 6 oz | 385 | 24 | 0 |

## Turkey

**Fryer-Roasters:** *Per 3 oz Serving*
**Roasted:**
| | | | |
|---|---|---|---|
| Light Meat: with skin | 140 | 4 | 0 |
| without skin | 120 | 1 | 0 |
| Dark Meat: with skin | 155 | 6 | 0 |
| without skin | 140 | 4 | 0 |

**½ of Whole Turkey:** (Approx. 3.3 lbs raw weight without neck and giblets; 1.8 lbs cooked weight)
| | | | |
|---|---|---|---|
| **Roasted:** with skin | 1650 | 74 | 0 |
| without skin | 1125 | 31 | 0 |

**Ground Turkey**, raw: (4 oz raw wt. = 3 oz cooked wt.)
| | | | |
|---|---|---|---|
| 85% lean, regular, 4 oz | 170 | 10 | 0 |
| 93% lean: Average, 4 oz | 160 | 8 | 0 |
| *Jennie-O, 4 oz* | 170 | 8 | 0 |
| *Trader Joe's, 4 oz* | 150 | 8 | 0 |
| 94% lean, | | | |
| *Foster Farms, 4 oz* | 150 | 7 | 0 |
| Breast, no skin, 4 oz | 115 | 1 | 0 |
| Patties: Small, 3 oz | 130 | 7 | 0 |
| Medium, 4 oz | 170 | 7 | 0 |

## Turkey Parts    C F Cb

**Roasted, Edible Weights, without bone:**
**Breast**, (½), (from 17.3 oz raw weight with bone):
| | | | |
|---|---|---|---|
| with skin, 12 oz (no bone) | 525 | 11 | 0 |
| without skin, 10.8 oz | 415 | 2 | 0 |
| **Back** (½): with skin, 4.5 oz | 265 | 13 | 0 |
| without skin, 3.5 oz | 165 | 6 | 0 |

**Leg (Thigh & Drumstick):**
(from 1 lb raw weight with bone)
| | | | |
|---|---|---|---|
| with skin, 8.5 oz (without bone) | 410 | 13 | 0 |
| without skin, 7.8 oz (w/out bone) | 355 | 8.5 | 0 |
| **Wing:** (From 7.3 oz raw weight) | | | |
| with skin, 3 oz (without bone) | 185 | 9 | 0 |
| without skin, 2 oz (w/out bone) | 100 | 2 | 0 |
| **Neck:** Simmered, 1 neck, 9 oz (with bone) | 275 | 11 | 0 |
| **Giblets**, simmered, 1 cup, 5 oz | 240 | 7 | 3 |

## Young Hens (Roasted)

**Light Meat:**
| | | | |
|---|---|---|---|
| with skin, 3 oz | 175 | 8 | 0 |
| without skin, 3 oz | 135 | 3 | 0 |
| **Dark Meat:** with skin, 3 oz | 200 | 11 | 0 |
| without skin, 3 oz | 165 | 7 | 0 |

**Young Toms ~** *Similar to Young Hens*

## Turkey Products

| | | | |
|---|---|---|---|
| **Foster Farms,** Meatballs, cooked, Homestyle (3) | 160 | 9 | 3 |
| **Hormel,** Canned Turkey Breast, in water, 2 oz | 50 | 1 | 0 |
| **Jennie-O:** Bacon, 1 slice, 0.5 oz | 30 | 2.5 | 0 |
| Bratwurst, lean, raw, 1 link, 3.85 oz | 170 | 10 | 2 |
| Burgers, raw, All Natural, White Meat, 5.3 oz | 200 | 10 | 0 |
| Meatballs, Fully Cooked: Italian, 3 oz | 180 | 13 | 2 |
| Home Style, 3 oz | 180 | 13 | 3 |
| **Spam,** Oven Roasted Turkey, 2 oz | 80 | 4.5 | 1 |
| **Trader Joe's,** Italian Turkey Meatloaf, 3 oz | 140 | 8 | 5 |
| **Valley Fresh,** 100% Natural, Canned White Turkey Breast, in water, 2 oz | 50 | 1 | 0 |

## White Rice    C   F   Cb

**Raw:**

| | C | F | Cb |
|---|---|---|---|
| Glutinous, 1 cup, 6.5 oz | 685 | 1 | 151 |
| Long Grain, 1 cup, 6.5 oz | 675 | 1 | 148 |
| Short Grain, 1 cup, 7 oz | 715 | 1 | 158 |
| Wild Rice, 1 cup, 5.5 oz | 570 | 2 | 120 |

**Cooked Rice:** *Boiled/Steamed*

**Short/Medium Grain:**

| | C | F | Cb |
|---|---|---|---|
| ¹/₂ cup, 3.3 oz | 140 | 0 | 30 |
| 1 cup (¹/₂ Pint), 7.2 oz | 265 | 0.5 | 59 |
| 2 cups (1 Pint), 13 oz | 480 | 1 | 106 |
| **Long Grain:** ¹/₂ cup, 2.8 oz | 100 | 0 | 22 |
| 1 cup, 5.5 oz | 205 | 0.5 | 44 |
| **Glutinous/Sticky,** 1 cup, 6 oz | 170 | 0.5 | 37 |
| **Parboiled,** ¹/₂ cup, 3 oz | 105 | 0.5 | 22 |

**Precooked/Instant:**

| | C | F | Cb |
|---|---|---|---|
| Dry, ¹/₂ cup, 3.5 oz | 380 | 1 | 82 |
| Cooked, ¹/₂ cup, 3 oz | 95 | 0.5 | 21 |

**Wild Rice,**

| | C | F | Cb |
|---|---|---|---|
| Cooked, 1 cup, 5.8 oz | 165 | 0.5 | 35 |

## Brown Rice

*Average of Short or Long Grain*

| | C | F | Cb |
|---|---|---|---|
| **Raw/Dry:** ¹/₂ cup, 3.3 oz | 340 | 2.5 | 71 |
| 1 cup, 6.5 oz | 685 | 5.5 | 143 |
| **Cooked:** ¹/₂ cup, 3.5 oz | 110 | 1 | 22 |
| 1 cup, 7 oz | 220 | 2 | 46 |

## Rice Dishes    C   F   Cb

**Chinese Fried Rice:**

| | C | F | Cb |
|---|---|---|---|
| ¹/₂ cup, 2.5 oz | 140 | 4.5 | 21 |
| 1 cup, (¹/₂ Pint), 5 oz | 280 | 9 | 42 |
| 2 cups, (1 Pint), 10 oz | 565 | 18 | 84 |

**Mexican Style Rice:**

| | C | F | Cb |
|---|---|---|---|
| *Taco Time,* Seasoned, 4.6 oz | 200 | 3 | 40 |
| Rice-A-Roni ~ *See Page 119* | | | |
| **Rice with Raisins/Pinenuts,** 1 cup | 400 | 11 | 60 |
| **Rice Pilaf:** Restaurant, 1 cup | 275 | 7.5 | 46 |
| *O'Charley's,* side dish, 1 portion | 160 | 4 | 27 |

**Rice Pudding,**

| | C | F | Cb |
|---|---|---|---|
| *Kozy Shack,* Original, 1 pudding cup | 130 | 2.5 | 24 |
| **Risotto,** 1 cup | 420 | 12 | 70 |
| **Saffron Rice,** 4 oz | 175 | 7 | 25 |
| **Spanish Rice:** 1 cup, 5 oz | 390 | 9 | 72 |
| *El Pollo Loco,* Small, 4.5 oz | 170 | 2.5 | 33 |
| **Sticky Rice,** 1 cup, 5 oz | 155 | 0.5 | 34 |
| **Sushi Rice:** 1 Tbsp | 25 | 0 | 5 |
| 1 cup, 5.2 oz | 390 | 0 | 77 |

**Other Packaged Rice Products:**

Uncle Ben's / Zatarain's ~ *See Page 121*

---

# CalorieKing.com Recipes

See the CalorieKing website for a salubrious selection of healthy recipes – all analyzed for calories, fat, protein, carbohydrate, fiber and sodium.

**Choose from:**
- **Starters/Appetizers**
- **Salads**
- **Entrees: Meat, Fish and Chicken**
- **Vegetarian**
- **Desserts**
- **Cakes, Cookies**
- **Drinks**

*www.CalorieKing.com/recipes*

## HEALTHY RECIPE TIPS

- **Use non-fat milk** in place of whole or 2% milk

- **Use low-fat yogurt** in place of sour cream
- **Skim fat** from surface of soups and casseroles after cooling

- **Add extra vegetables** to soups and hot entrées
- **Cakes/cookies/muffins:** Replace most or all the fat/oil with applesauce and/or prune puree (Example, *Sunsweet Lighter Bake*)

- **Drinks:** Replace sugar with no-calorie sweeteners such as *Equal, Stevia, Splenda* and *Sweet 'N Low*

## Deli Salads

| | **C** | **F** | **Cb** |
|---|---|---|---|
| *Average All Outlets* | | | |
| **Antipasto Salad**, 1/2 cup | 135 | 8 | 13 |
| **3-Bean Salad**, 1/2 cup | 90 | 4.5 | 12 |
| **Bulgur Salad**, 1/2 cup | 70 | 2 | 12 |
| **Caesar Salad**, Classic, 1 cup | 200 | 14 | 15 |
| **Side Salad**, without Dressing | 25 | 0 | 6 |
| **Carrot Raisin:** with Dressing, 1/2 cup | 135 | 12 | 6 |
| without Dressing, 1/2 cup | 20 | 0 | 5 |
| **Chef's Salad:** Regular, w/o Dressing | 620 | 37 | 8 |
| with 2 oz Thousand Island Drssng | 860 | 61 | 8 |
| **Chicken Salad**, 1/2 cup/scoop, 4 oz | 280 | 21 | 2 |
| **Coleslaw:** Traditional, 1/2 cup | 150 | 8 | 18 |
| w/ Low Cal Dressing, 1/2 c. | 50 | 2 | 8 |
| **Corn**, Mexican, 1/2 cup | 240 | 12 | 33 |
| **Cucumber:** Non-Oil Dressing, 1/2 cup | 60 | 0 | 14 |
| with Oil Dressing, 1/2 cup | 140 | 12 | 8 |
| **Eggplant Salad**, 1/2 cup | 75 | 5 | 7 |
| **Fettucini**, with veges, 1/2 cup | 135 | 6 | 16 |
| **Garden Salad**, without Dressing, 1 cup | 10 | 0 | 2 |
| **Greek Salad**, 1 cup | 105 | 8 | 7 |
| **Greek Vegetables**, 1 cup | 110 | 8 | 6 |
| **Lobster Salad**, 1/2 cup, 4 oz | 250 | 21 | 11 |
| **Macaroni Salad**, 1/2 cup, 5 oz | 360 | 26 | 26 |
| **Nicoise**, 1 cup | 450 | 32 | 18 |
| **Pasta Salad**, 1/2 cup | 200 | 11 | 19 |
| **Potato Salad:** Dijon, 3 oz | 120 | 7 | 13 |
| with Mayonnaise, 1/2 cup, 4 oz | 215 | 15 | 17 |
| Lowfat, 1/2 cup | 110 | 1.5 | 21 |
| **Rice Salad**, 1/2 cup | 150 | 10 | 13 |
| **Saffron Rice**, 4 oz | 175 | 7 | 25 |
| **Spinach Salad**, 1 cup | 180 | 13 | 13 |
| **Tabouli**, 1/2 cup | 125 | 7 | 13 |
| **Three Bean Salad**, 1/2 cup | 90 | 4.5 | 12 |
| **Tomato & Mozzarella**, 1/2 cup | 180 | 14 | 10 |
| **Tortellini**, with Basil Pesto, 1/2 cup | 150 | 9 | 15 |
| **Waldorf**, with Mayo, 1/2 cup | 110 | 7 | 12 |
| **Signature Salads:** *Per 6 oz Serving* | | | |
| *(Supplied to Deli's and Institutions)* | | | |
| **Antipasto Salad** | 510 | 50 | 4 |
| **Artichoke Salad,** marinated | 400 | 41 | 8 |
| **California Medley** | 120 | 7 | 15 |
| **Cheese Agnolotti** | 250 | 8 | 23 |
| **Chicken Salad** | 420 | 33 | 11 |
| **Crabmeat Flavored** | 450 | 38 | 20 |
| **Egg Salad** | 300 | 23 | 14 |
| **Fresh Button Mushroom** | 190 | 16 | 6 |

| **Signature Salads** (Cont): *Per 6 oz* | **C** | **F** | **Cb** |
|---|---|---|---|
| **Fresh Button Mushroom** | 190 | 16 | 6 |
| **Ham Salad** | 400 | 32 | 14 |
| **Prima Pasta Salad** | 360 | 30 | 18 |
| **Seafood Pasta Del Mar** | 170 | 10 | 21 |
| **Seafood, Crab & Shrimp** | 420 | 34 | 20 |
| **Shrimp Salad** | 360 | 32 | 8 |
| **Tuna Salad** | 450 | 36 | 14 |

*~ Also See Fast-Foods & Restaurants Section*

## Fresh Salad Packs

*Pre-Packaged (Supermarkets):*

| **Dole:** | | | |
|---|---|---|---|
| **Kits:** *Per 3.5 oz, with Dressing* | | | |
| Caesar: Original | 150 | 12 | 8 |
| Kale | 210 | 15 | 11 |
| Chopped: | | | |
| Chipotle & Cheddar | 120 | 9 | 10 |
| Sesame Asian | 160 | 16 | 13 |
| Southwest | 120 | 9 | 9 |
| **Salad Blends:** *Without Dressing* | | | |
| American; Mediterranean, 3 oz | 15 | 0 | 3 |
| Arugula; Baby Spinach, 3 oz | 20 | 0 | 3 |
| **Fresh Express:** | | | |
| **Complete Salad Kits:** *Per 3 1/2 oz, Prepared* | | | |
| Asian | 120 | 5 | 17 |
| Caesar: Classic | 150 | 12 | 7 |
| Lite | 90 | 6 | 7 |
| Supreme | 160 | 14 | 6 |
| Pear Gorgonzola | 130 | 6 | 17 |
| **Gourmet Cafe:** *Per Package* | | | |
| Chopped Santa Fe | 290 | 19 | 18 |
| Tuscan | 330 | 28 | 9 |
| **Ready Pac:** | | | |
| **Bistro Bowls:** *Per Container, with Dressing* | | | |
| Apple Bleu Pecan, 4.5 oz | 230 | 14 | 23 |
| Caprese, 5 oz | 210 | 17 | 12 |
| Cranb. Walnut, 4.5 oz | 210 | 9 | 26 |
| Kale, Apple Veggie, 5.5 oz | 240 | 13 | 31 |
| Spinach Dijon, 4.76 oz | 280 | 19 | 20 |
| Turkey & Bacon Cobb, 7.3 oz | 290 | 22 | 6 |

## Salad Toppings

| | **C** | **F** | **Cb** |
|---|---|---|---|
| **Bac'n Pieces**, | | | |
| *McCormick*, 1Tbsp, 0.3 oz | 30 | 1 | 2 |
| **Bacon Bits** *(Hormel)*, 1Tbsp | 25 | 1.5 | 0 |
| **Bac-Os, Bits** *(Betty Crocker)*, 1 Tbsp | 30 | 1 | 2 |
| **Chow Mein Noodles**, | | | |
| dry, 1/2 cup | 120 | 7 | 13 |
| **Croutons**, 2 Tbsp, 0.3 oz | 40 | 1 | 7 |
| **Salad Toppins**, | | | |
| *McCormick*, 4 tsp | 35 | 1.5 | 3 |
| **Sunflower Seeds**, 1 Tbsp, 0.3 oz | 45 | 4 | 1.5 |
| **Toasted Sliced Almonds**, 2 T., 0.5 oz | 85 | 7 | 3 |

## Quick Guide  **C** **F** **Cb**

### Salad Dressings
*Average All Brands: Per 2 Tbsp, Approx 1 fl.oz*

| | C | F | Cb |
|---|---|---|---|
| **Balsamic Vinaigrette:** | | | |
| Regular | 90 | 9 | 3 |
| Light, 2 Tbsp | 45 | 4 | 2 |
| Fat Free, 2 Tbsp | 25 | 0 | 6 |
| **Blue Cheese:** Regular, 2 Tbsp | 145 | 15 | 1.5 |
| Regular, ¼ cup, 2 oz | 280 | 30 | 3 |
| Light, 2 Tbsp | 30 | 1 | 4 |
| **Caesar:** Regular, 2 Tbsp | 165 | 17 | 1 |
| Regular, ¼ cup, 2 oz | 310 | 34 | 2 |
| Light, 2 Tbsp | 35 | 1.5 | 5.5 |
| **Coleslaw:** Regular, 2 Tbsp | 125 | 11 | 8 |
| Regular, ¼ cup, 2 oz | 245 | 21 | 15 |
| Light, 2 Tbsp | 110 | 7 | 14 |
| **French:** Regular | 145 | 14 | 5 |
| Regular, ¼ cup, 2 oz | 260 | 25 | 9 |
| Light, 2 Tbsp | 65 | 4 | 9 |
| Fat/Oil-Free, 2 Tbsp | 40 | 0 | 6 |
| **Italian:** Regular, 2 Tbsp | 85 | 8.5 | 3 |
| Regular, ¼ cup, 2 oz | 165 | 16 | 6 |
| Light, 2 Tbsp | 55 | 5.5 | 2 |
| Fat/Oil-Free, 2 Tbas | 15 | 0 | 2.5 |
| **Ranch:** Regular, 2 Tbsp | 145 | 16 | 2 |
| Regular, ¼ cup, 2 oz | 290 | 30 | 4 |
| Light, 2 Tbsp | 60 | 4 | 6.5 |
| Fat-Free, 2 Tbsp | 35 | 0.5 | 8 |
| **Thousand Island:** Reg., 2 T. | 115 | 11 | 4.5 |
| Regular, ¼ cup, 2 oz | 210 | 20 | 9 |
| Light, 2 Tbsp | 60 | 3.5 | 7 |
| Fat-Free, 2 Tbsp | 40 | 0.5 | 10 |

**Enjoy a healthy salad but don't drown it in high-fat salad dressings.**

**Use 'light' dressings to halve the fat and calories.**

## Brands ~ Salad Dressings

| | C | F | Cb |
|---|---|---|---|
| **Annie's Naturals:** *Per 2 Tbsp* | | | |
| **Organic:** Goddess Dressing | 120 | 12 | 2 |
| Green Garlic | 80 | 8 | 2 |
| Papaya Poppy Seed | 90 | 8 | 5 |
| Thousand Island | 90 | 8 | 5 |
| **Vinaigrettes:** | | | |
| Red Wine & Olive Oil | 140 | 14 | 1 |
| Sesame Ginger | 90 | 8 | 4 |
| Shitake & Sesame | 120 | 13 | 1 |
| **Bernstein's:** *Per 2 Tbsp* | | | |
| Creamy Caesar | 120 | 13 | 1 |
| Herb Garden French | 130 | 12 | 6 |
| Italian | 110 | 12 | 1 |
| Restaurant Recipe Italian | 120 | 12 | 1 |
| **Fat-Free**, Cheese & Garlic Italian | 10 | 0 | 2 |
| **Light Fantastic:** Cheese Fantastico | 30 | 1.5 | 3 |
| Roasted Garlic Balsamic | 45 | 3.5 | 3 |
| **Best Foods:** *Per 1 Tbsp Unless Indicated* | | | |
| Dijonnaise, 1 tsp | 5 | 0 | 0 |
| **Mayonnaise:** Real | 100 | 11 | 0 |
| Light | 35 | 3.5 | 1 |
| Low-Fat | 15 | 1 | 2 |
| Canola | 40 | 4 | 1 |
| Olive Oil | 60 | 6 | 1 |
| Mayonesa, Lemom-Lime | 100 | 10 | 0 |
| **Cardini's:** *Per 2 Tbsp* | | | |
| Aged Parmesan Ranch | 150 | 16 | 1 |
| **Caesar:** Original | 140 | 15 | 1 |
| Garlic Lemon | 150 | 16 | 1 |
| Light Caesar | 80 | 8 | 1 |
| Red Jalapeno | 140 | 15 | 1 |
| Three Cheese | 140 | 15 | 1 |
| Honey Mustard | 120 | 11 | 6 |
| Roasted Asian Sesame | 120 | 10 | 6 |
| Vinaigrette, Balsamic: | | | |
| Regular | 100 | 8 | 5 |
| Lite | 50 | 3 | 5 |
| **Great Value** *(Walmart): Per 2 Tbsp* | | | |
| Caesar | 120 | 12 | 2 |
| **Ranch:** Bacon | 140 | 14 | 1 |
| Buttermilk | 110 | 11 | 2 |
| Chipotle | 120 | 13 | 2 |
| Classic | 130 | 14 | 1 |
| Zesty Italian | 60 | 4.5 | 3 |
| **Hampton Creek** *(Vegan): Per 1 Tbsp* | | | |
| **Just Mayo:** | | | |
| Original | 90 | 10 | 0 |
| Chipotle | 60 | 6 | 1 |
| Garlic | 100 | 10 | 0 |
| Sriracha | 90 | 10 | 1 |

# Salad Dressings  S

## Brands ~ Salad Dressings (Cont)

**Hidden Valley:** *Per 2 Tbsp*

| | C | F | Cb |
|---|---|---|---|
| **Greek:** Creamy Caesar; Cucumber Dill | 60 | 5 | 3 |
| Lemon Garlic | 60 | 5 | 4 |
| Ranch | 60 | 5 | 3 |
| **Ranch:** Bacon | 140 | 14 | 1 |
| Buffalo | 110 | 1 | 2 |
| Fiesta Salsa, Light | 60 | 5 | 3 |
| Ranch | 60 | 5 | 3 |
| Southwest Chipotle | 100 | 10 | 2 |
| **Simply Ranch:** Chili Lime | 120 | 12 | 2 |
| Classic Ranch | 110 | 12 | 2 |
| Cucumber Basil | 110 | 12 | 2 |

**Kraft:** *Per 2 Tbsp*

| Regular Dressings: | C | F | Cb |
|---|---|---|---|
| Asian Toasted Sesame | 80 | 6 | 2 |
| Blue Cheese | 120 | 12 | 1 |
| Buttermilk Ranch | 100 | 12 | 1 |
| Catalina Classic | 90 | 6 | 3 |
| Classic Caesar | 110 | 11 | 3 |
| Creamy Balsamic | 90 | 8 | 1 |
| Creamy Italian | 80 | 7 | 1 |
| Cucumber Ranch | 110 | 11 | 1 |
| Honey Mustard | 90 | 6 | 3 |
| Zesty Catalina | 90 | 6 | 3 |
| Zesty Italian | 60 | 4.5 | 1 |
| **Fat Free:** French Style | 45 | 0 | 4 |
| Italian | 15 | 0 | 1 |
| Thousand Island | 50 | 0 | 4 |
| **Lite:** Catalina | 60 | 1 | 4 |
| House Italian | 35 | 1 | 2 |
| Raspberry Vinaigrette | 30 | 1 | 2 |
| Zesty Italian | 25 | 1 | 1 |

**Seven Seas:**

| | C | F | Cb |
|---|---|---|---|
| Green Goddess | 100 | 8 | 2 |
| Viva Italian Anything | 50 | 4.5 | 1 |

**Marie's:** *Per 2 Tbsp*

| Classics: | C | F | Cb |
|---|---|---|---|
| Chunky Blue Cheese | 160 | 17 | 1 |
| Coleslaw | 140 | 13 | 7 |
| Creamy Caesar | 120 | 13 | 1 |
| Creamy Italian Garlic | 180 | 19 | 1 |
| Creamy Ranch | 180 | 19 | 1 |
| Super Blue Cheese | 160 | 17 | 1 |
| Thousand Island | 150 | 15 | 3 |
| **Ranch:** Buttermilk | 150 | 16 | 1 |
| Parmesan | 170 | 19 | 1 |
| **Vinaigrette:** Blue Cheese | 120 | 11 | 4 |
| Garlic Parmesan | 110 | 11 | 2 |
| Mango Chardonnay | 120 | 11 | 6 |
| Mediterranean | 110 | 12 | 2 |
| Rst'd Tomato w/ Parmesan & Basil | 130 | 13 | 2 |

**Marzetti's:** *Per 2 Tbsp*

| | C | F | Cb |
|---|---|---|---|
| **Creamy:** Aged Parm. Ranch | 140 | 14 | 2 |
| Asiago Peppercorn | 130 | 14 | 2 |
| Chunky Blue Cheese | 150 | 15 | 1 |
| Cilantro Avocado | 110 | 12 | 1 |
| Classic Ranch | 160 | 17 | 1 |
| Creamy Caesar | 120 | 12 | 2 |
| Fat Free Sweet & Sour | 45 | 0 | 12 |
| Potato Salad | 160 | 15 | 6 |
| **Light:** Chunky Blue Cheese | 90 | 7 | 4 |
| Classic Ranch | 80 | 8 | 2 |
| Honey French | 80 | 3.5 | 12 |
| Original Slaw | 90 | 7 | 7 |
| Poppyseed | 90 | 5 | 9 |
| Supreme Caesar | 70 | 7 | 2 |
| **Simply Dressed:** Avocado Ranch | 120 | 13 | 1 |
| Blue Cheese | 130 | 14 | 1 |
| Caesar | 120 | 12 | 1 |
| Cucumber Ranch | 80 | 8 | 2 |
| Thousand Island | 130 | 12 | 5 |
| Vinaigrette: Balsamic | 90 | 9 | 4 |
| Champagne | 80 | 8 | 2 |
| Pomegranate | 60 | 4.5 | 6 |

**Newman's Own:** *Per 2 Tbsp*

| | C | F | Cb |
|---|---|---|---|
| **Regular:** Creamy Balsamic | 100 | 8 | 7 |
| Creamy Caesar | 150 | 16 | 1 |
| Family Recipe Italian | 130 | 13 | 1 |
| Honey Dijon Mustard | 140 | 13 | 6 |
| Roasted Garlic | 50 | 4 | 3 |
| **Light:** Balsamic Vinaigrette | 45 | 4 | 2 |
| Caesar | 70 | 6 | 3 |
| Italian | 60 | 6 | 1 |

**Wish-Bone:** *Per 2 Tbsp*

| | C | F | Cb |
|---|---|---|---|
| **Creamy:** Caesar | 180 | 18 | 1 |
| Deluxe French | 120 | 11 | 5 |
| Italian | 110 | 10 | 4 |
| Ranch | 130 | 13 | 2 |
| Russian | 110 | 6 | 14 |
| Thousand Island | 130 | 12 | 5 |
| **Light:** Blue Cheese | 70 | 6 | 2 |
| Creamy Caesar | 70 | 6 | 2 |
| Honey Dijon | 70 | 5 | 6 |
| Italian | 35 | 2.5 | 3 |
| Parmesan Peppercorn Ranch | 60 | 5 | 2 |
| Ranch | 70 | 5 | 4 |
| Thousand Island | 60 | 5 | 4 |
| **Fat-Free:** | | | |
| Chunky Blue Cheese | 30 | 0 | 7 |
| Ranch | 30 | 0 | 6 |
| **Oil & Vinegar:** | | | |
| Balsamic Vinaigrette | 60 | 5 | 3 |
| House Italian | 110 | 10 | 3 |
| Red Wine Vinaigrette | 70 | 5 | 6 |
| Robusto Italian | 80 | 7 | 4 |

### Gravy

| | C | F | Cb |
|---|---|---|---|
| **Homemade Gravy**, average: | | | |
| Thin, little fat, | | | |
| 2 Tbsp, 1 oz | 20 | 1 | 3 |
| Thick: 2 Tbsp, 1.3 oz | 50 | 2 | 9 |
| ¼ cup, 2.5 oz | 100 | 4 | 18 |
| **McCormick:** | | | |
| Brown, 1 Tbsp | 25 | 0.5 | 3 |
| Turkey, 1 Tbsp | 20 | 0.5 | 4 |

### Gravy-In-Jars

| | C | F | Cb |
|---|---|---|---|
| **Boston Market,** | | | |
| Classic Beef, ¼ cup, 2 oz | 30 | 1 | 4 |
| **Campbell's,** | | | |
| Beef/Chicken/Turkey, ¼ cup, 2 oz | 25 | 1 | 3 |
| **Heinz:** *Per ¼ Cup, 2 oz* | | | |
| Homestyle: Bistro Au Jus | 20 | 0.5 | 2 |
| Classic Chicken | 30 | 2 | 3 |
| Pork; Rich Mushroom | 20 | 0.5 | 3 |
| Roasted Turkey | 25 | 1 | 3 |
| Savory Beef | 30 | 1 | 4 |
| **Safeway**, all varieties, ¼ cup, 2 oz | 20 | 0.5 | 4 |

### Tomato Products

| | C | F | Cb |
|---|---|---|---|
| **Whole/Chopped/Crushed/Diced:** | | | |
| Regular: 1 cup, 8.5 oz | 50 | 0 | 10 |
| In Aspic, ½ cup | 50 | 0 | 12 |
| with Green Chili, 1 c., 8.5 oz | 60 | 0 | 16 |
| Stewed, ½ cup, 1.7 oz | 40 | 1.5 | 7 |
| Wedges in Tomato Juice, 1 cup | 70 | 0.5 | 18 |
| Salsa, average, 2 Tbsp, 1 oz | 25 | 0 | 6 |
| **Tomato Ketchup:** | | | |
| Regular: 1 Tbsp, 0.5 oz | 15 | 0 | 4 |
| Single Serve, 1 packet | 10 | 0 | 3 |
| *Heinz*, Simply Heinz | | | |
| 1 Tbsp, 0.5 oz | 15 | 0 | 4 |
| **Tomato Paste:** | | | |
| Regular: 2 Tbsp, 1 oz | 25 | 0 | 6 |
| ¾ cup, 6 oz | 140 | 1 | 32 |
| **Tomato Puree**, ½ cup, 4.5 oz | 50 | 0 | 10 |
| **Tomato Sauce:** | | | |
| Regular, ½ cup, 4.4 oz | 50 | 0 | 11 |
| Spanish Style, ½ cup, 4.3 oz | 40 | 0 | 9 |
| with Mushr., ½ cup, 4.3 oz | 45 | 0 | 10 |
| with Onions, ½ cup, 4.3 oz | 50 | 0 | 12 |
| **Tomato Seasoning**, 3 tsp | 20 | 0 | 4 |
| **Sundried Tomatoes:** | | | |
| Natural, 5-6 pieces, 0.4 oz | 20 | 0 | 5 |
| In Oil, drained, 6 pieces, 0.5 oz | 40 | 2.5 | 4 |

### Sauces ~ Brands

| | C | F | Cb |
|---|---|---|---|
| **A-1:** | | | |
| **Marinades:** *Per Tbsp, ½ oz* | | | |
| Chicago Steakhouse | 20 | 1 | 1 |
| Classic | 15 | 0 | 1 |
| New Orleans Cajun | 25 | 0 | 2 |
| New York Steakhouse | 20 | 0 | 2 |
| **Steak Sauce:** Original | 15 | 0 | 1 |
| Bold & Spicy | 20 | 0 | 1 |
| Cracked Peppercorn | 15 | 0 | 1 |
| Sweet Hickory | 25 | 0 | 2 |
| Thick & Hearty | 25 | 0 | 2 |
| **Barilla:** | | | |
| **Pasta Sauces:** *Per ½ Cup, Unless Indicated* | | | |
| Chunky Traditional | 60 | 1 | 13 |
| Creamy Alfredo | 70 | 6 | 4 |
| Garlic Alfredo | 60 | 5 | 4 |
| Marinara | 70 | 1 | 14 |
| Meat Sauce; Mushroom | 60 | 1 | 13 |
| Sun-Dried Tomato Pesto, ¼ cup | 130 | 10 | 7 |
| Traditional Basil Pesto, ¼ cup | 200 | 19 | 5 |
| **Bertolli:** | | | |
| **Alfredo Sauces:** *Per ¼ Cup* | | | |
| Creamy Basil | 100 | 10 | 2 |
| Four Cheese Rosa | 110 | 10 | 5 |
| Garlic Romano w/ Parmesan | 100 | 10 | 2 |
| **Traditional:** *Per ½ Cup* | | | |
| Five Cheese | 90 | 3.5 | 14 |
| Portobello Mushroom | 70 | 2.5 | 9 |
| Vodka | 150 | 9 | 11 |
| **Buitoni:** | | | |
| **Pasta Sauces:** | | | |
| Alfredo: Regular, ¼ cup | 150 | 14 | 3 |
| Light, ¼ cup | 90 | 6 | 4 |
| Marinara, ½ cup | 70 | 3 | 9 |
| Pesto: with Basil, ¼ cup | 290 | 27 | 5 |
| Reduced Fat, ¼ cup | 230 | 18 | 8 |
| **Bull's-Eye:** *Per 2 Tbsp* | | | |
| **BBQ Sauce:** Original | 50 | 0 | 4 |
| Hickory Smoke | 60 | 0 | 5 |
| **Regional**, average all varieties | 50 | 0 | 4 |
| **Catelli:** *Per ½ Cup* | | | |
| **Pasta**, Garden Select Six Vegetable: | | | |
| Country Mushroom | 70 | 1.5 | 11 |
| Diced Tomato & Basil | 70 | 1 | 12 |
| **Meat Sauce** | 80 | 2.5 | 11 |
| **Pizza Sauce**, all varieties | 60 | 1.5 | 11 |

| Sauces ~ Brands (Cont) | C | F | Cb |
|---|---|---|---|
| **Cento:** | | | |
| Arrabbiata, ½ cup | 60 | 3.5 | 6 |
| Italiano, ¼ cup | 25 | 0 | 6 |
| Marinara, ¼ cup | 60 | 3.5 | 6 |
| Porcini Mushroom Sauce, ½ cup | 80 | 4 | 7 |
| Puttanesca, ½ cup | 70 | 4.5 | 6 |
| Vodka, ½ cup | 100 | 5 | 8 |
| **Classico:** | | | |
| **Alfredo:** *Per ¼ Cup* | | | |
| Creamy | 60 | 4.5 | 3 |
| Roasted Garlic | 60 | 4 | 4 |
| **Family Favorites:** *Per ½ Cup* | | | |
| Meat | 60 | 1 | 10 |
| Parmesan & Romano | 70 | 2 | 10 |
| Traditional | 80 | 2.5 | 13 |
| **Riserva:** Arrabbiata, 4.4 oz | 60 | 1 | 11 |
| Eggplant & Artichoke, 4.4 oz | 60 | 1.5 | 10 |
| Puttanesca | | | |
| **Tomato Cream Sauces:** *Per ½ Cup* | | | |
| Creamy Tomato & Rsd Garlic | 35 | 1.5 | 5 |
| Four Cheese Tomato | 40 | 2 | 5 |
| Spicy Tomato & Parmesan | 40 | 2 | 5 |
| **Contadina:** | | | |
| **Pizza Sauce:** *Per 2.2 oz* | | | |
| Flavored with Pepperoni | 35 | 1 | 6 |
| Original; Four Cheese | 30 | 0.5 | 6 |
| **Tomato Sauce**, average | 20 | 0.5 | 4 |
| **Crosse & Blackwell:** | | | |
| **Meat:** Ham Glaze, 1 Tbsp | 25 | 0 | 7 |
| Mint Meat Sauce, 1 tsp | 5 | 0 | 2 |
| **Seafood:** | | | |
| Cocktail, ¼ cup, 2.5 oz | 90 | 0 | 21 |
| Shrimp Sauce, ¼ cup, 2.5 oz | 90 | 0 | 21 |
| **Dave's Gourmet:** | | | |
| **Pasta Sauces:** *Per ½ cup* | | | |
| Butternut Squash | 100 | 4 | 17 |
| Creamy Parmesan Romano | 120 | 8 | 8 |
| Hearty Marinara | 70 | 3.5 | 9 |
| Red Heirloom | 45 | 1.5 | 7 |
| Rstd Garlic & Sweet Basil | 70 | 4.5 | 8 |
| Spicy Heirloom Marinara | 45 | 1.5 | 7 |
| Wild Mushroom | 80 | 3 | 11 |
| **Del Monte:** | | | |
| **Pasta Sauces:** *Per ½ cup* | | | |
| Four Cheese; Traditional, av. | 60 | 1 | 12 |
| Mushroom | 60 | 1 | 11 |
| Average other varieties | 60 | 1 | 13 |
| **Sloppy Joe Sauce:** *Per ¼ cup* | | | |
| Hickory | 60 | 0 | 14 |
| Original | 60 | 0 | 13 |

| | C | F | Cb |
|---|---|---|---|
| **Emeril's:** | | | |
| **Alfredo**, Four Cheese Sauce, ¼ cup | 60 | 5 | 4 |
| **Pasta Sauces:** *Per ½ Cup* | | | |
| Homestyle Marinara | 90 | 3 | 14 |
| Kicked Up Tomato | 80 | 3.5 | 11 |
| Roasted Gaaahlic | 80 | 3.5 | 12 |
| Roasted Red Pepper | 70 | 3.5 | 9 |
| Vodka Sauce | 110 | 7 | 12 |
| **Francesco Rinaldi:** | | | |
| **Alfredo**, all flavors, ¼ cup | 90 | 8 | 2 |
| **Cheese,** | | | |
| Three Cheese, ½ cup | 70 | 1 | 15 |
| **Garden**, all var., ½ cup | 60 | 1 | 12 |
| **Meat:** Meat Flavored, ½ cup | 70 | 2.5 | 13 |
| Sicilian Family, Sausage, ½ cup | 70 | 2.5 | 11 |
| **Pizza**, ¼ cup | 20 | 0 | 4 |
| **Tomato**, Marinara, ½ cup | 60 | 1 | 12 |
| **French's,** | | | |
| Worcestershire Sauce, 1 tsp | 0 | 0 | 1 |
| **Heinz:** *Per 1 Tbsp* | | | |
| 57 Steak Sauce | 20 | 0 | 4 |
| Chili Sauce | 20 | 0 | 5 |
| Cocktail Sauce, Original, | | | |
| ¼ cup, 2.2 oz | 70 | 0 | 18 |
| Horseradish Sauce | 75 | 6 | 3 |
| Tomato Ketchup: Regular | 20 | 0 | 5 |
| Reduced Sugar | 5 | 0 | 1 |
| Worcestershire Sauce | 5 | 0 | 1 |
| **House of Tsang:** | | | |
| Bangkok Peanut Sce, 1.16 oz | 70 | 5 | 9 |
| Classic Sauce, 0.6 oz | 25 | 0.5 | 5 |
| Ginger Sriracha Sauce, 1.23 oz | 15 | 0 | 4 |
| General Tsao, 0.67 oz | 45 | 0.5 | 10 |
| Green Thai Curry Sauce, 1.1 oz | 60 | 4 | 6 |
| Korean Teriyaki Sauce, 0.67 oz | 35 | 1 | 6 |
| Oyster Flavored Sauce, 0.63 oz | 30 | 0 | 7 |
| Saigon Sizzle Sauce 0.63 oz | 45 | 1 | 8 |
| Sweet & Sour Sauce, 0.63 oz | 35 | 0 | 8 |
| **Hunt's:** | | | |
| BBQ Sauce, Original, 2 Tbsp | 60 | 0 | 16 |
| Hickory & Brown Sugar BBQ Sce, 2 Tbsp | 50 | 0 | 13 |
| **Manwich,** Sloppy Joe Sauce, | | | |
| Original, ¼ cup, 2.3 oz | 35 | 0 | 8 |
| **Pasta Sauce:** *Per ½ Cup* | | | |
| Four Cheese | 60 | 1 | 10 |
| Garlic & Herb | 40 | 1 | 8 |
| Meat Flavor | 60 | 1 | 10 |
| Mushroom | 50 | 0.5 | 10 |
| Traditional | 60 | 1 | 11 |

## Brands (Cont)

| | **C** | **F** | **Cb** |
|---|---|---|---|
| **Kikkoman:** *Per Tablespoon* | | | |
| **Marinade:** Gourmet Teriyaki | 30 | 0 | 7 |
| Honey & Mustard | 30 | 0 | 6 |
| Roasted Garlic & Herbs | 20 | 0 | 4 |
| Toasted Sesame | 40 | 0.5 | 8 |
| **Asian Authentics:** *Per Tbsp, Unless Indicated* | | | |
| Katsu | 20 | 0 | 5 |
| Kotteri Mirin | 50 | 0 | 12 |
| Plum Sauce, 2 Tbsp | 90 | 1 | 21 |
| Sukiyaki | 20 | 0 | 4 |
| Tempura | 5 | 0 | 1 |
| Unagi Sushi Sauce | 40 | 0 | 10 |
| Wasabi Sauce, 1 tsp | 15 | 1 | 1 |
| **Knorr:** | | | |
| **Classic Sauce:** *Per Whole Package* | | | |
| Bernaise, dry mix only | 100 | 0 | 20 |
| Hollandaise, dry mix only | 100 | 0 | 20 |
| **Kraft:** | | | |
| Barbecue Sauce, 2 Tbsp | 60 | 0 | 5 |
| Coleslaw 1.2 oz | 80 | 4.5 | 3 |
| Horseradish, 1 oz | 100 | 9 | 1 |
| Sandwich Spread, 1 Tbsp | 30 | 2 | 1 |
| Tartar, 1 Tbsp | 60 | 5 | 1 |
| **Las Palmas:** *Per ¼ Cup* | | | |
| Green Enchilada Sauce, all varieties, 2 oz | 25 | 1.5 | 3 |
| Red Chili Sauce, | 15 | 0.5 | 3 |
| **La Victoria,** | | | |
| Red/Green Enchilada Sauce, av., 2 oz | 15 | 0.5 | 3 |
| **Lawry's:** | | | |
| **30 Minute Marinade:** *Per Tbsp* | | | |
| Caribbean Jerk | 30 | 0 | 7 |
| Herb & Garlic; Lemon Pepper | 10 | 0 | 2 |
| Mesquite, w/ Lime Juice | 10 | 0 | 2 |
| Sesame Ginger, w/ Mandarin | 30 | 0 | 7 |
| Steak & Chop, w/ Garl. Pepp. | 5 | 0 | 0.5 |
| **Packet Seasonings:** *Dry* | | | |
| Fajitas; Taco, average, 2 tsp | 15 | 0 | 3 |
| Other varieties, average, 2 tsp | 20 | 0 | 4 |
| **Lea & Perrins:** | | | |
| Steak Sauce, Bold, 1 Tbsp | 20 | 0 | 5 |
| Worcestershire Sauce: Original 1 tsp, 5 ml | 5 | 0 | 1 |
| Reduced Sodium | 5 | 0 | 1 |

| | **C** | **F** | **Cb** |
|---|---|---|---|
| **McCormicks:** | | | |
| **Seafood Sauces:** *Per 2 Tbsp* | | | |
| Asian | 50 | 1.5 | 7 |
| Cajun Style | 15 | 0 | 3 |
| Lemon Butter Dill | 100 | 9 | 4 |
| Lemon Herb | 140 | 15 | 0.5 |
| Mediterranean; Santa Fe Style | 20 | 0 | 4 |
| Scampi | 160 | 17 | 2 |
| **Mrs. Dash** | | | |
| **Marinades:** *Per 1 Tbsp* | | | |
| Garlic Herb | 15 | 0 | 3 |
| Lemon Pepper | 10 | 0 | 2 |
| Lime Garlic | 15 | 0 | 3 |
| Sweet Teriyaki | 35 | 0 | 9 |
| **Newman's Own:** *Per ½ Cup* | | | |
| **Pasta Sauce:** Five Cheese | 80 | 2.5 | 11 |
| Marinara; Sockarooni | 70 | 1 | 12 |
| Roasted Garlic | 60 | 1.5 | 11 |
| Tomato & Basil Bombolina | 70 | 2 | 11 |
| Vodka | 140 | 9 | 11 |
| **O Organics** *(Von's):* *Per ½ Cup* | | | |
| Marinara; Roasted Garlic, av. | 60 | 1.5 | 9 |
| Mushroom; Tomato Basil | 50 | 1.5 | 8 |
| **Old El Paso** | | | |
| **Enchilada Sauce:** | | | |
| Green, ¼ cup, 2.15 oz | 25 | 1.5 | 4 |
| Red, ¼ cup, 2.1 oz | 20 | 0 | 4 |
| **Taco Sauce,** all varieties, 1 Tbsp | 5 | 0 | 1 |
| **Pace:** *Per 2 Tbsp* | | | |
| Picante Sauce | 10 | 0 | 2 |
| **Salsa:** Thick & Chunky, av. | 10 | 0 | 3 |
| Fire, Chipotle & Jalapeno | 10 | 0 | 2 |
| Restaurant Style, Peach Mango | 10 | 0 | 3 |
| **Prego:** *Per ½ Cup, Unless Indicated* | | | |
| **Alfredo,** average all varieties, ¼ cup | 70 | 6 | 3 |
| **Classic Italian:** | | | |
| Fresh Mushroom; Traditional | 70 | 1.5 | 12 |
| Marinara | 90 | 5 | 8 |
| Tomato Basil Garlic | 70 | 2.5 | 11 |
| **Farmers Market:** Classic Marinara | 90 | 5 | 9 |
| Four Cheese; Roasted Garlic, av. | 80 | 3.5 | 9 |
| Garden Vegetable | 60 | 2 | 8 |
| Mushroom; Trad. Basil, average | 70 | 2.5 | 9 |
| **Pizza Sauce,** Pizzeria Style, ¼ cup | 35 | 1 | 6 |
| **Pemium Pasta:** Creamy Vodka | 140 | 7 | 15 |
| Italian, with Bacon & Provolone | 100 | 3 | 15 |
| Pesto Marinara | 90 | 3 | 13 |
| Spicy Sausage | 110 | 4 | 15 |
| **Premier Japan,** | | | |
| Hoisin; Teriyaki, 1 Tbsp | 15 | 0 | 3 |

## Brands (Cont)

| Ragu: | C | F | Cb |
|---|---|---|---|
| **Cheesy:** *Per ¼ Cup* | | | |
| Classic Alfredo | 90 | 8 | 2 |
| Creamy Tomato | 90 | 8 | 4 |
| Double Cheddar | 100 | 9 | 2 |
| Four Cheese | 80 | 8 | 2 |
| Light Parmesan Alfredo | 60 | 4 | 2 |
| Roasted Garlic Parmesan | 100 | 9 | 3 |
| Six Cheese | 90 | 2.5 | 14 |
| **Chunky:** *Per ½ Cup* | | | |
| Roasted Garlic | 90 | 2.5 | 14 |
| Average other varieties | 90 | 2.5 | 14 |
| **Homestyle, Thick & Hearty:** *Per ½ Cup* | | | |
| Four Cheese | 90 | 2 | 14 |
| Meat | 90 | 2.5 | 15 |
| Mushroom | 90 | 2.5 | 16 |
| Roasted Garlic | 90 | 2.5 | 15 |
| Rstd Peppers & Garlic | 70 | 1 | 14 |
| Tomato & Basil | 90 | 2.5 | 15 |
| Traditional | 100 | 2.5 | 16 |
| **Old World Style:** *Per ½ Cup* | | | |
| Flavored with Meat | 80 | 2.5 | 10 |
| Marinara | 80 | 2.5 | 11 |
| Traditional | 80 | 2 | 13 |
| **Pizza:** Homemade Style, ¼ cup | 30 | 1 | 5 |
| Quick Sauce, Traditional, ¼ cup | 45 | 1.5 | 6 |
| **Safeway Select:** | | | |
| Salsa, all varieties, average, 2 Tbsp | 15 | 0 | 3 |
| **Select Sauces:** *Per ½ Cup* | | | |
| Arrabbiata | 110 | 8 | 10 |
| Artichoke Pesto | 60 | 2 | 9 |
| Four Cheese | 80 | 3.5 | 11 |
| Marinara | 60 | 2 | 10 |
| Spicy Red Bell Pepper | 50 | 1 | 9 |
| Sundried Tomato & Olive | 60 | 1.5 | 11 |
| Tomato Alfredo; Vodka | 130 | 10 | 9 |
| **Taco Bell,** Creamy Jalapeno Sauce, | | | |
| 1 Tablespoon, 0.5 oz | 70 | 7 | 1 |
| **Tony Roma's:** | | | |
| Bold & Spicy BBQ Sauce, 2 Tbsp | 50 | 0 | 12 |
| Carolina Honeys BBQ Sauce, | | | |
| 2 Tablespoons | 70 | 0 | 18 |
| **Trader Joe's:** | | | |
| BBQ Sauce, | | | |
| Kansas City Style, 2 Tbsp | 60 | 0 | 15 |
| Tomato Basil Marinara, ½ cup | 80 | 4.5 | 10 |
| **Walnut Acres,** | | | |
| Organic Pasta Sauces, | | | |
| average all var., ½ cup, 4.5 oz | 60 | 1 | 11 |

## Seasonings & Flavorings

| | C | F | Cb |
|---|---|---|---|
| **Auromatic Bitters** *(Angostua)*, 1 tsp | 15 | 0 | 4 |
| **Bacon Bits,** average, 1 Tbsp | 35 | 2 | 2 |
| **Bacon Chips** *(Durkee)*, 1 Tbsp | 30 | 1 | 2 |
| **Bac-Os** *(Betty Crocker)*, | | | |
| 1Tbsp | 30 | 1.5 | 2 |
| **Blends** *(Mrs Dash)*, 1 tsp | 0 | 0 | 0 |
| **Butter Buds,** 1 tsp | 5 | 0 | 2 |
| **Flavor Enhancer** *(Accent)*, 1 tsp | 0 | 0 | 0 |
| **Flavor Sprinkles** *(Molly McButter)*, | | | |
| Natural/Cheese, 1 tsp | 5 | 0 | 1 |
| **Garlic Bread Sprinkle,** 1 tsp | 8 | 0.5 | 1 |
| **Garlic Salt,** 1 tsp | 2 | 0 | 0 |
| **Italian Seasoning,** 1 tsp | 4 | 0 | 1 |
| **Lemon Pepper Seasoning,** | | | |
| 1 tsp | 7 | 0 | 1 |
| **Meat Tenderizer,** av., 1 tsp | 7 | 0 | 1 |
| **Salad Crunchies** *(McCormick)*, | | | |
| 1 tsp | 10 | 0.5 | 2 |
| **Salt,** Reg., Sea Salt, Lite Salt | 0 | 0 | 0 |
| **Seasoning** *(Old Bay)*, ¼ tsp | 0 | 0 | 0 |
| **Seasoning Mix** *(Vegit)*, ¼ tsp | 0 | 0 | 0 |
| **Seasoning Mixes,** av., ¼ pkg | 70 | 1 | 9 |
| **Taco Seasoning,** av., ¼ pkg | 30 | 0.5 | 4 |
| **Bragg's,** Liquid Aminos | 0 | 0 | 0 |
| **Old El Paso:** Chili Season. Mix, 1 Tbsp | 8 | 0.5 | 1.5 |
| Cheesy Taco Seasoning Mix, 1 Tbsp | 10 | 0.5 | 2 |
| Taco/Burrito Seasoning Mix, 2 tsp | 15 | 0 | 4 |
| Fajita Seasoning Mix, 1 tsp | 5 | 0 | 1.5 |

## Spices & Herbs

| | C | F | Cb |
|---|---|---|---|
| **Average all types,** 1 tsp | 5 | 0 | 1 |
| **All Purpose,** 1 tsp | 0 | 0 | 0 |
| **Allspice,** ground | 5 | 0 | 1 |
| **Chili Powder** | 8 | 0 | 1 |
| **Cinnamon,** ground | 6 | 0 | 2 |
| **Curry Powder** | 6 | 0 | 1 |
| **Garlic Powder** | 9 | 0 | 2 |
| **Nutmeg,** ground | 12 | 0 | 1 |
| **Onion Powder** | 7 | 0 | 2 |
| **Parsley,** dried | 4 | 0 | 1 |
| **Pepper,** average | 6 | 0 | 1 |
| **Saffron** | 2 | 0 | 0 |
| **Salt-Free Blends,** 1 tsp | 0 | 0 | 0 |
| **Tumeric,** ground | 8 | 0 | 1 |
| **Seeds:** Fenugreek | 12 | 1 | 2 |
| Mustard, Poppyseed | 15 | 1 | 1 |
| Other varieties, average | 7 | 0 | 1 |

## Home-Popped Popcorn    C   F   Cb

| | C | F | Cb |
|---|---|---|---|
| **Popping Corn Kernels**, 2 Tbsp, 1 oz | 110 | 1 | 26 |
| (makes approximately 5 cups) | | | |
| **Air-popped**, without oil: Plain, 1 oz | 110 | 1 | 22 |
| 1 cup, 0.2 oz | 20 | 0 | 5 |
| **Oil-popped:** Plain, 1 oz | 145 | 8 | 16 |
| 1 cup, 0.4 oz | 55 | 3 | 6 |
| **Popcorn Oil**, 1 Tbsp | 120 | 14 | 0 |

## Microwave Popcorn

*Average all Brands: Per 1 Cup Popped, Unless Indicated*

| | C | F | Cb |
|---|---|---|---|
| Butter: Regular, 1 cup | 35 | 2 | 4 |
| Light, 1 cup | 25 | 1 | 4 |
| **Act II Popcorn:** | | | |
| **Butter:** 1 cup | 25 | 1 | 4 |
| 4½ cups, 1 oz | 130 | 6 | 19 |
| **94% Fat-Free Butter:** | | | |
| 1 cup | 20 | 0.5 | 4 |
| 6½ cups, 1 oz | 130 | 2 | 27 |
| **Butter Lovers:** 1 cup | 25 | 1 | 4 |
| 4½ cups, 1 oz | 140 | 7 | 19 |
| **Xreme Butter:** 1 cup | 25 | 1 | 4 |
| 4½ cups | 160 | 9 | 19 |
| **BodyKey** *(Amway)*, Slim Popcorn, Sea Salt, 1 bag | 110 | 7 | 10 |
| **Jolly Time:** | | | |
| **Blast O Butter**, 1 cup | 45 | 3 | 4 |
| **Crispy & Light Butter**, 1 cup | 25 | 1 | 4 |
| **Xtra Butter:** 1 cup | 40 | 2.5 | 4 |
| 4 cups | 160 | 10 | 16 |
| **Newman's Own:** | | | |
| **Butter Flavor**, Microwave: | | | |
| Regular, 3½ cups | 130 | 5 | 18 |
| Light, 3½ cups | 120 | 4 | 19 |
| **Butter Boom**, 3½ cups | 130 | 5 | 18 |
| **Orville Redenbacher's:** *Popped* | | | |
| **Butter:** 4 cups | 170 | 12 | 17 |
| Light, 6 cups | 160 | 6 | 26 |
| Movie Theater Butter, 5 cups | 160 | 10 | 18 |
| Ultimate Butter, 4½ cups | 160 | 9 | 19 |
| **Naturals**, Lime & Salt, 5 cups | 220 | 15 | 21 |
| **Sweet & Savory:** Caramel, 3 cups | 170 | 8 | 26 |
| Cheddar Cheese, 4½ cups | 180 | 14 | 16 |
| **Pop Secret:** *Per Cup* | | | |
| 94% Fat-Free, Butter | 20 | 0 | 3 |
| Double Butter | 40 | 2 | 3 |

## Bagged Popcorn    C   F   Cb

*Average All Brands (Ready-to-Eat)*

| | C | F | Cb |
|---|---|---|---|
| **Regular/Plain:** ½ oz package | 80 | 5 | 8 |
| 1 oz package | 160 | 10 | 16 |
| 4 oz package | 640 | 40 | 64 |
| 2 oz Box (store/airport) | 320 | 16 | 32 |
| 3 oz Bag (9" high x 5" wide) | 480 | 24 | 48 |
| **Caramel Popcorn**, with nuts, 1 cup, 1.5 oz | 230 | 12 | 39 |

## Bagged Popcorn ~ Brands

| | C | F | Cb |
|---|---|---|---|
| **Boston's**, Lite, 3½ cups, 1 oz | 130 | 4.5 | 20 |
| **Cracker Jack:** Original, 1 cup, 2 oz | 240 | 4 | 46 |
| Chocolate & Caramel, 1 cup, 2 oz | 220 | 1 | 50 |
| **Crunch 'N Munch:** | | | |
| **Buttery Toffee:** ⅔ cup, 1.1 oz | 150 | 5 | 24 |
| 1 cup, 1.65 oz | 225 | 7.5 | 36 |
| **Caramel:** ⅔ cup, 1.1 oz | 160 | 7 | 22 |
| 1 cup, 1.65 oz | 240 | 10 | 33 |
| 12 oz box | 1745 | 76 | 240 |
| **Fiddle Faddle:** | | | |
| Average all varieties: 1 oz | 120 | 2 | 24 |
| 1 cup, 2 oz | 240 | 4 | 48 |
| 6 oz box | 720 | 12 | 144 |
| **Popcorn Indiana:** | | | |
| **Kettlecorn,** Original, 2 cups, 1 oz | 130 | 5 | 21 |
| **Popcorn:** | | | |
| Aged White Cheddar, 2.5 cups, 1 oz | 150 | 9 | 14 |
| Chicago Fair, Caramel & Cheese, 1 cup, 1 oz | 140 | 6 | 20 |
| Movie Theater, 2 cups, 1 oz | 160 | 12 | 13 |
| Seasalt, 3.5 cups, 1 oz | 140 | 6 | 17 |
| **Poppycock:** | | | |
| **Bags:** Cashew Lovers, ½ cup, 1 oz | 150 | 6 | 20 |
| Chocolate Lovers, ½ cup, 1.2 oz | 160 | 7 | 22 |
| **Cannisters**, Orig./Pecan Delight, av: | | | |
| ½ cup, 1 oz | 155 | 7 | 20 |
| 1 cup, 2 oz | 310 | 14 | 40 |

## Movie Theater Popcorn

| | C | F | Cb |
|---|---|---|---|
| **Small**, (7 cups): Plain | 385 | 21 | 44 |
| with Butter (3 pumps, 0.8 oz) | 570 | 42 | 44 |
| **Medium**, (15 cups): Plain | 825 | 45 | 94 |
| with Butter (4 pumps, 1 oz) | 1075 | 73 | 94 |
| **Large**, (20 cups): Plain | 1100 | 60 | 124 |
| with Butter (6 pumps, 1.5 oz) | 1485 | 102 | 124 |
| **Butter:** 1 Pump, 0.3 oz | 65 | 7 | 0 |
| 4 Pumps (2 Tbsp), 1 oz | 250 | 28 | 0 |

### Corn & Tortilla Chips   **C** **F** **Cb**

*Average All Brands*

**Corn Chips:**

| | C | F | Cb |
|---|---|---|---|
| Average all types: 1 oz | 150 | 8 | 18 |
| 8 oz bag | 1200 | 64 | 144 |
| *Fritos*, Original, 32 chips, 1 oz | 160 | 10 | 15 |
| **Tortilla Chips:** Average, 1 oz | 140 | 7 | 18 |
| (1 oz = approx. 12 chips or 13 strips) | | | |
| *Doritos:* Original, 1 oz | 140 | 7 | 18 |
|   Nacho Chse; Salsa Verde, av., 1 oz | 140 | 8 | 18 |
| *Popchips:* Chili Limon, 1 oz | 120 | 4 | 19 |
|   Nacho Cheese, 1 oz | 130 | 5 | 18 |
| *Snyder's:* | | | |
|   El Restaurante, all flavors, 1 oz | 150 | 8 | 17 |
|   Yellow Corn/White, av., 1 oz | 135 | 5 | 21 |
| *Tostitos:* | | | |
|   Average all flav., 1 oz | 145 | 7 | 19 |
|   Baked! Scoops, 1 oz | 120 | 3 | 22 |
| *Utz:* Multigrain, 1 oz | 150 | 8 | 16 |
|   Baked, 1 oz | 120 | 2 | 23 |
|   Other flavors, 1 oz | 140 | 8 | 18 |

### Potato Chips/Crisps

*Average All Brands*

**Regular:**

| | C | F | Cb |
|---|---|---|---|
| Plain or flavored, (4 chips) | 30 | 2 | 3 |
| 1 oz package (20 chips) | 150 | 10 | 15 |
| 4 oz quantity | 600 | 40 | 60 |
| 14 oz package | 2100 | 140 | 210 |

### Chips/Crisps ~ Brands

| | C | F | Cb |
|---|---|---|---|
| **Hippeas**, Chick Pea Puffs, | | | |
|   average all flavors, 0.78 oz | 90 | 4 | 11 |
| **Lay's** *(Fritolay):* | | | |
| Classics; Wavy Originals, 1 oz | 160 | 10 | 15 |
|   Kettle Cooked, Original, 1 oz | 150 | 9 | 17 |
| **Pringles:** | | | |
| All Flavors: 1 oz | 150 | 9 | 16 |
|   Large can, 6 oz | 900 | 54 | 96 |
| Stix, To Go Pak, Baked Cheese | 80 | 3 | 10 |
| **Ruffles:** Regular, av. all flavors, 1 oz | 160 | 11 | 15 |
|   Reduced Fat, 1 oz | 140 | 7 | 18 |
| **Simply7**, Hummus/Lentil Chips, | | | |
|   average all flavors, 1 oz | 135 | 5 | 19 |
| **Sun Chips**, Original, 16 crisps, 1 oz | 140 | 6 | 18 |

### Pretzels   **C** **F** **Cb**

*Average All Brands*

**Hard-Baked Pretzels:** *Each*

| | C | F | Cb |
|---|---|---|---|
| 1 oz quantity | 110 | 1 | 23 |
| Sticks, thin, 2¼" (9/oz) | 12 | 0 | 3 |
| Twists, thin, ¼" thick, (5/oz) | 25 | 0 | 5 |
| Dutch (2¾"x 2⅝"), 0.5 oz | 55 | 1 | 11 |
|   *Snyders*, Sourdough, 0.8oz | 100 | 0 | 22 |
| **Soft Pretzel Twists,** average: *Each* | | | |
| Plain: Small, 2 oz | 210 | 2 | 43 |
|   Medium, 4 oz | 390 | 3.5 | 80 |
|   Large, 5 oz | 485 | 4.5 | 100 |
| Big Cheese, 1.8 oz | 130 | 3 | 22 |
| New York Street Vendors, 7 oz | 660 | 6 | 135 |
| *Trader Joe's*, Peanut Butter filled, 1 oz | 140 | 8 | 14 |
| *Snyder's:* Milk Chocolate Dips, 1 oz | 140 | 6 | 19 |
|   White Creme Dips, 1 oz | 130 | 6 | 19 |

### Pretzels ~ Brands

| | C | F | Cb |
|---|---|---|---|
| **Flipz:** Milk Choc, 8 pieces, 1 oz | 130 | 5 | 20 |
|   White Fudge, 7 pcs, 1 oz | 130 | 5 | 20 |
| **Rold Gold** *(Frito-Lay):* | | | |
| Braided Twists, | | | |
|   Honey Wheat (8), 1 oz | 110 | 1 | 24 |
| Pretzel, Sourdough (1) | 90 | 1 | 19 |
| Pretzel Thins (9), 1 oz | 110 | 1 | 23 |
| Rods (3), 1 oz | 110 | 1 | 22 |
| Tiny Twists (18), average, 1 oz | 110 | 0 | 23 |
| Sticks, 1 oz | 100 | 0 | 23 |
| **Snyder's of Hanover:** | | | |
| Butter Snaps (24), 1 oz | 120 | 1 | 25 |
| Choc Dipped Minis, av., 1 oz | 135 | 6 | 20 |
| Gluten Free Pretzel Sticks (30) | 110 | 1.5 | 25 |
| Pieces, average, 1 oz | 140 | 8 | 16 |
| Sticks (28), average, 1 oz | 110 | 1 | 23 |
| Thins (11), 1 oz | 110 | 0 | 23 |
| Twists (7), average,1 oz | 120 | 2 | 24 |
| **Special K,** | | | |
|   Choc. Coated, av., all flavors, 1 oz | 100 | 3.5 | 15 |
| **SuperPretzel:** | | | |
| **6 Count Soft**, Original (1), 2.3 oz | 160 | 1 | 34 |
| Bites (5), 1.9 oz | 140 | 0.5 | 32 |
| Softstix, Cheese (2), 1.76 oz | 130 | 3 | 22 |
| **Utz:** | | | |
| **Pretzels:** Original; Extra Dark, 1 oz | 110 | 1 | 21 |
|   Sourdough, Hard (1) | 90 | 0 | 18 |

## Snacks | C | F | Cb

Note: Actual weight of packaged snacks is usually 5-10% more than label Net Wt. For accuracy, weigh snack and allow extra calories, fat and carbs for any extra weight.

| | C | F | Cb |
|---|---|---|---|
| **Apple Chips** (Seneca), av., 1 oz | 140 | 7 | 20 |
| **Bagel Crisps** (N.Y. Style), 6 crisps, 1 oz | 130 | 6 | 17 |
| **Baguette Chips** (Pillsbury), av., (21) | 130 | 5 | 19 |
| **Banana Chips** (T.Joe's), 13 chips, 1 oz | 160 | 11 | 13 |
| **Beef Jerky** (Jack Link's), av., 1 oz | 80 | 1 | 5 |
| **Beef Sticks** (Slim Jim), Giant, 1 oz | 140 | 11 | 4 |
| *Jack Link's*, Original, 1.5 oz | 160 | 13 | 2 |
| **Beet Chips** (Rhythm), Sea Salt, 1oz | 130 | 4 | 20 |
| *Trader Joes*, 1.3 oz | 140 | 0.5 | 29 |
| **BodyKey** (Amway): | | | |
| Mixed Nuts & Pumpkin Seeds, 1 bag | 200 | 16 | 8 |
| Whole Grain Tortilla Chips, 1 bag | 210 | 11 | 24 |
| **Bugles,** Original; Nacho Cheese, 1 oz | 160 | 9 | 18 |
| **Cheese Balls** (Utz), 1 oz serving | 130 | 7 | 16 |
| **Cheese Bites** (Tr. Joes), 1 oz | 170 | 12 | 0.5 |
| **Cheese Nips,** 1.3 oz package | 170 | 7 | 22 |
| **Cheese Puffs**, average, 1 oz | 160 | 10 | 15 |
| **Cheetos:** | | | |
| Crunchy: Av. all flavors, 1 oz | 155 | 11 | 13 |
| 4 oz package | 640 | 40 | 60 |
| Baked!; Fantastix, av., 1 oz | 130 | 5 | 19 |
| Simply Puffs, Wh. Cheddar, 1 oz | 150 | 9 | 16 |
| **Cheez-It** (Sunshine): | | | |
| **Snack Mix:** Classic, ½ cup, 1 oz | 140 | 4.5 | 20 |
| Double Cheese, ¾ cup, 1 oz | 130 | 5 | 19 |
| Sriracha, ½ cup, 1 oz | 120 | 5 | 17 |
| Sweet & Salty, ½ cup, 1oz | 140 | 5 | 21 |
| **Chester's:** Fries, Flamin' Hot, 1 oz | 150 | 8 | 17 |
| Puffcorn, Cheese, 1 oz | 160 | 11 | 14 |
| **Chex Mix,** (General Mills), | | | |
| Traditional, 1 oz | 120 | 3.5 | 22 |
| **Chicharrones** ~ *See Pork Skins* | | | |
| **Crackers** (Tr. Joes), Mini Edaname (28) | 120 | 2 | 21 |
| **Churros** (Rubio's), Cinnamon, 2 oz | 240 | 13 | 30 |
| **Combo,** Crackers, av., ⅓ cup, 1 oz | 140 | 6 | 18 |
| **Cool Cuts**, Carrot & Ranch, 2.3 oz | 70 | 5 | 5 |
| **Corn Chips** ~ *See Page 149* | | | |
| **Corn Nuts:** Av all flav., 1 oz | 130 | 4.5 | 20 |
| 1.7 oz bag | 210 | 8 | 34 |
| **Corn Puffs/Twists,** (32), 1 oz | 160 | 11 | 15 |
| **Dunkin Stix** (Dolly Madison), (3) | 490 | 25 | 63 |
| **Edamame**, | | | |
| *Seapointe*, Dry Roasted, 1 oz | 130 | 4 | 11 |
| **Fritos:** Corn Chips, all varieties, av., 1oz | 160 | 10 | 15 |
| Flavor Twists, Honey BBQ, 1 oz | 150 | 9 | 16 |

## Snacks (Cont) | C | F | Cb

| | C | F | Cb |
|---|---|---|---|
| **Fruit Snacks** ~ *See Page 102* | | | |
| **Funyuns,** Onion Flavored, 1 oz | 130 | 6 | 16 |
| **Goldfish,** Crackers, av., 1 oz | 140 | 5 | 20 |
| **Gold-n-Chees** (Lance): | | | |
| Snack Crackers, 1.25 oz pkg | 160 | 5 | 25 |
| Snack Mix, 2.25 oz tube | 320 | 17 | 36 |
| **Gripz** (Sunshine), Mighty Tiny (1) | 120 | 6 | 15 |
| **Flamin Hot Peanuts** (Munchies), 1 oz | 180 | 14 | 6 |
| **Kale Chips** (Rhythm), | | | |
| Roasted Garlic & Onion, 1 oz | 160 | 11 | 14 |
| *Trader Joes*, average, 1 oz | 150 | 10 | 9 |
| **Lance,** Sandwich Crackers (6), av. | 200 | 9 | 25 |
| **Munchies** (Frito-Lay), | | | |
| Snack Mix, all flavors, 1 oz | 140 | 7 | 18 |
| **Munchos** (Fritolay), all flavors, 1 oz | 160 | 10 | 16 |
| **Newtons:** | | | |
| Single Serve: 2 oz pkg | 200 | 4 | 40 |
| Fat-Free, 2 oz package | 200 | 0 | 46 |
| **Nutella,** w/ Breadsticks/Pretzels (1) | 270 | 14 | 35 |
| **Nutter Butter,** Sandwich Cookies: | | | |
| 1.87 oz Package | 250 | 10 | 37 |
| Bites, Go-Pak, 3.5 oz | 490 | 21 | 74 |
| **Onion Rings** (T.G.I. Friday), 1 oz | 140 | 7 | 16 |
| **Oreo Cookies,** all Creme Fillings: | | | |
| Double Stuf (2), 1 oz | 140 | 7 | 21 |
| Mini Bite Size: 1 oz | 130 | 6 | 21 |
| Go-Pak, 3.5 oz | 455 | 21 | 74 |
| **Oreo Cakesters,** Golden, Soft, 0.9 oz | 110 | 5 | 16 |
| **Oriental Mix Rice Snacks,** 1 oz | 125 | 3.5 | 21 |
| **Peanut Butter Nuggets,** (10), 1 oz | 140 | 6 | 15 |
| **Pepitas**, dried or roasted, | | | |
| ¼ cup, 1 oz | 155 | 4 | 3 |
| **Pirate's Booty:** | | | |
| Aged White Cheddar, 4 oz | 560 | 24 | 72 |
| Veggie, 4 oz bag | 560 | 28 | 72 |
| **Pita Chips**, (9), average, 1 oz | 130 | 4 | 18 |
| **Plaintain Chips** (Goya), 1 oz | 150 | 8 | 19 |
| **PopCorners**, Butter/Kettle, 1 oz | 125 | 3.5 | 20 |
| **Popcorn** ~ *See Page 148* | | | |
| **Pork Cracklins**, 1 oz | 160 | 12 | 0 |
| **Pork Skins/Rinds:** 1 oz | 160 | 10 | 0 |
| *Baken-ets*, Traditional, 0.5 oz | 80 | 5 | 0 |
| *Mission*, Chiccarones, 4 oz package | 640 | 40 | 0 |
| **Potato Chips** ~ *See Page 149* | | | |
| **Potato Skins** (TGI Friday), | | | |
| all flavors, 16 chips, 1 oz | 140 | 8 | 15 |
| **Puffed Wheat**, | | | |
| *Sabritones*, Chili & Lime, 1 oz | 140 | 8 | 16 |
| **Pretzels** ~ *See Page 149* | | | |

## Snacks (Cont)

| | **C** | **F** | **Cb** |
|---|---|---|---|
| **Rice Cakes:** | | | |
| *Lundberg*, (1), average | 80 | 0.5 | 17 |
| *Quaker:* Plain, lightly salted (1) | 35 | 0 | 7 |
| Chocolate Crunch (1) | 60 | 1 | 12 |
| **Rice Chips**, | | | |
| *Lundberg*, average, 1 oz | 140 | 7 | 18 |
| **Sandwich Crackers:** | | | |
| *Austin,* Cheese Crackers: | | | |
| with Cheddar, 1.4 oz | 190 | 10 | 23 |
| with Peanut Butter, 1.3 oz | 190 | 10 | 23 |
| PB & J Flavored, 1.4 oz | 190 | 8 | 26 |
| *Lance:* Nip Chee, 6 pieces | 190 | 9 | 24 |
| Toasty, 6 pieces | 180 | 9 | 21 |
| Toast Chee, PB, 1.5 oz | 220 | 1 | 25 |
| *Ritz Bits:* Cheese (12), 1 oz Pkg | 150 | 8 | 17 |
| 3 oz Pak | 450 | 25 | 50 |
| P'nut Butter: 1.5 oz pkg | 210 | 11 | 24 |
| Big Bag, 3 oz | 420 | 22 | 48 |
| **Sesame Sticks**, Salted, | | | |
| *SunRidge Farm*, 1 oz | 170 | 12 | 14 |
| **Smart Puffs,** | | | |
| *Pirates Booty*, 1 oz | 140 | 7 | 16 |
| **Soybeans in Pods**, | | | |
| *AFC*, ½ cup, 3.2 oz | 90 | 5 | 3 |
| **Soy Crisps**, average, 1 oz | 120 | 3 | 17 |
| **Soy Nuts:** Dry Roasted, ¼ cup, 1 oz | 130 | 6 | 9 |
| Choc-coated, 1 oz | 140 | 7 | 13 |
| **Sun Chips,** | | | |
| *Fritolay*, average, 1 oz | 140 | 6 | 19 |
| **Takis:** Crunchy Fajitas, 1 oz | 140 | 8 | 16 |
| 4 oz package | 560 | 32 | 64 |
| **Tings** (*Robert's*), 2 oz bag | 300 | 16 | 36 |
| **Toasted Chips (***Ritz***),** av. all, 1 oz | 130 | 5.5 | 20 |
| **Tortilla Chips**, | | | |
| *Garden of Eatin*, Chili & Lime, 1 oz | 140 | 7 | 18 |
| **Trail Mix (Nuts/Seeds/Dried Fruit):** | | | |
| Regular, 3 Tbsp, 1 oz | 140 | 9 | 13 |
| Tropical, 3 Tbsp, 1 oz | 130 | 7 | 16 |
| **Turkey Jerky:** Teriyaki, 1 oz | 80 | 1 | 8 |
| *Trader Joe's*, Original, 1 oz | 60 | 0.5 | 6 |
| **Veggie Crisps**, | | | |
| *Snyder's*, 1 oz | 140 | 6 | 18 |
| **Wheat Thins** (*Nabisco*), av. all, 1 oz | 135 | 5 | 21 |
| **Woats,** Oatsnack, av., ¼ cup, 1 oz | 120 | 5 | 17 |
| **Yogurt Pretzels**, 1.5 oz | 190 | 8 | 28 |
| **Yogurt Raisins**, Vanilla, | | | |
| *Sun-Maid*, 1 oz | 120 | 4.5 | 20 |

## Fruit Snacks

| | **C** | **F** | **Cb** |
|---|---|---|---|
| **Betty Crocker:** Fruit Gushers, 0.9 oz | 90 | 1.5 | 21 |
| Fruit by the Foot, 1 roll, 0.8 oz | 80 | 1 | 17 |
| Fruit Roll Ups, 1 roll, 0.5 oz | 50 | 1 | 11 |
| Fruit Flavored Shapes, | | | |
| all varieties, 0.9 oz | 80 | 0 | 19 |
| **Sunkist:** | | | |
| Fruit Lover's Trail Mix: B'fast Espresso, 1.5 oz | 190 | 9 | 27 |
| Other flavors, 1 oz | 120 | 4 | 20 |
| **Fruit Snack Cups ~ See Page 102** | | | |

## Vending Machines

| | **C** | **F** | **Cb** |
|---|---|---|---|
| **Bugles,** Nacho Cheese, 1 oz | 160 | 9 | 18 |
| **Cheese Balls** (*Utz*), 1 oz | 130 | 7 | 16 |
| **Cheetos,** Crunchy, 1 oz | 150 | 10 | 13 |
| **Cheeze-It,** Snack Mix, 1.5 oz | 195 | 6.5 | 30 |
| **Chester's,** Flamin' Hot Fries, 1 oz | 150 | 8 | 17 |
| **Choc Chip Cookies:** | | | |
| Chips Ahoy, 1.2 oz | 160 | 8 | 22 |
| Famous Amos, (4), 1 oz | 150 | 8 | 18 |
| Grandma's, (1), 1.4 oz | 200 | 10 | 25 |
| **Chocolate Bars:** | | | |
| Hershey's, Milk Choc.,1.6 oz | 220 | 13 | 22 |
| Kit Kat, 1.5 oz | 210 | 11 | 25 |
| Snickers, 1.9 oz bar | 250 | 12 | 33 |
| **Donut**, plain cake, 1.4 oz | 160 | 9 | 18 |
| **Doritos,** av. all flavors, 1 oz | 145 | 8 | 18 |
| **Fritos,** Corn Chips, Orig., 1.8 oz | 280 | 17 | 26 |
| **Fruit Pie**, | | | |
| Hostess, Lemon, 4.5 oz | 510 | 25 | 65 |
| **Granola/Cereal Bars**, av., 1 oz | 140 | 3 | 26 |
| **M & M's:** | | | |
| Milk Chocolate, 1.7 oz | 240 | 10 | 34 |
| Peanuts, 1.8 oz | 250 | 13 | 30 |
| **Oreo Cookies,** 2 oz | 270 | 11 | 41 |
| **Peanut Butter Cups,** | | | |
| Reese's, 1.5 oz | 210 | 12 | 24 |
| **Popcorn**, plain, 1 oz | 160 | 10 | 16 |
| **Pop Chips**, 0.8 oz | 100 | 3 | 16 |
| **Pork Skins**, 1.5 oz | 240 | 15 | 0 |
| **Potato Chips:** 1 oz | 150 | 10 | 15 |
| Baked! (*Ruffles*), Orig.,1 oz | 120 | 3 | 22 |
| **Potato Skins** (*TGI Friday's*), | | | |
| all flavors, 1 oz | 140 | 8 | 15 |
| **Pretzels** (*Snyder's*), Olde Tyme, 1 oz | 120 | 1 | 24 |
| **Raisins**, 0.5 oz package | 45 | 0 | 11 |
| **Rice Krispies Treat** | 90 | 2 | 17 |
| **Skittles,** 2 oz | 230 | 2.5 | 52 |
| **Starburst,** Fruit Chews, Orig., 1.4 oz | 130 | 0 | 31 |
| **Tortilla Chips,** 1 oz | 140 | 7 | 18 |

## Homemade & Restaurant

| Restaurant & Take-Out: Average All Preparations: Per 8 fl.oz | C | F | Cb |
|---|---|---|---|
| Bean Medley | 200 | 3 | 34 |
| Beef Consomme | 30 | 0 | 2 |
| Borscht, with Sour Cream | 130 | 8 | 14 |
| Bouillabaisse | 400 | 15 | 10 |
| Chicken & Corn | 290 | 14 | 20 |
| Chicken & Wild Rice | 80 | 4 | 9 |
| Chicken Consomme | 50 | 0 | 2 |
| Chicken Curry | 180 | 8 | 18 |
| Chicken Jambalaya | 160 | 7 | 8 |
| Chicken Noodle | 80 | 2 | 12 |
| With Chicken | 160 | 4 | 12 |
| Chicken Soup | 80 | 2 | 6 |
| Chili with Beans | 250 | 12 | 25 |
| Clam Chowder | 240 | 15 | 17 |
| Corn & Crab | 120 | 3 | 18 |
| Corn Chowder | 150 | 8 | 16 |
| Cream of Broccoli | 200 | 12 | 20 |
| Cream of Potato | 150 | 6.5 | 17 |
| Cream of Mushroom | 200 | 13 | 15 |
| Fish Chowder | 220 | 15 | 6 |
| French Onion | 420 | 15 | 25 |
| Gazpacho | 50 | 0 | 5 |
| Lentil Soup | 250 | 9 | 28 |
| Lobster Bisque | 320 | 15 | 10 |
| Matzo Ball, with 1 large ball | 180 | 7 | 24 |
| Minestrone | 125 | 2.5 | 20 |
| Mulligatawny | 300 | 15 | 8 |
| Pea & Ham | 240 | 10 | 25 |
| Potato & Bacon | 170 | 7 | 19 |
| Pumpkin, Creamy | 210 | 10 | 26 |
| Shark Fin Soup | 100 | 4 | 8 |
| Spicy Shrimp Soup, 1 bowl | 160 | 7 | 10 |
| Split Pea Soup | 180 | 2.5 | 30 |
| Vegetable (Fat Free) | 75 | 0 | 18 |
| Vegetable Beef | 80 | 2 | 10 |
| Vichyssoise | 200 | 9 | 15 |
| Watercress | 90 | 4 | 13 |

**Other Soups** ~ *See International & Fast-Foods Sections (Arby's, Au Bon Pain, Boston Market, Dunkin' Donuts, Denny's, Schlotzsky's, Sizzler, Souplantation, Sweet Tomatoes, Zoup!)*

**Homemade Soups:** *Calculate calories, fat and carbohydrates from recipe ingredients.*

## Bouillon Cubes & Powders

| Bouillon Cubes: *Average all types* | C | F | Cb |
|---|---|---|---|
| Regular, 1 cube | 5 | 0 | 1 |
| Extra Large, 1 cube | 20 | 1 | 1 |
| **Powders**, average, 1 tsp | 10 | 0 | 1 |
| **Herb-Ox:** | | | |
| Instant Broth & Seasoning, Beef, 1 envelope, 0.14 oz | 5 | 0 | 1 |
| Chicken, 1 envelope, 0.14 oz | 5 | 0 | 1 |

## Soup ~ Brands

**Amy's:**
| Heat & Serve (Organic): *Per 1 Cup, Unless Indicated* | | | |
|---|---|---|---|
| Alphabet | 80 | 0 | 16 |
| Black Bean Vegetable | 140 | 1.5 | 26 |
| Chunky Vegetable | 80 | 1.5 | 13 |
| Carrot Ginger | 200 | 13 | 18 |
| Cream of M'shrm, ³/₄ cup | 150 | 9 | 13 |
| Lentil Vegetable | 160 | 4 | 24 |
| Rustic Italian Vegetable | 190 | 8 | 24 |
| Southwestern Vegetable | 140 | 5 | 20 |
| Split Pea | 110 | 1 | 19 |
| Thai Coconut, ½ can | 160 | 11 | 12 |
| Thai Curry Sweet Pot. Lentil | 280 | 20 | 20 |
| Tuscan Bean & Rice | 160 | 4.5 | 25 |

**Bertoli:** *Per ½ Carton, 12 oz*
| Meal Soups: | | | |
|---|---|---|---|
| Tomato Florentine & Tortellini with Chicken | 420 | 20 | 37 |

**Campbell's:**
| Chunky: *Per Cup, Unless Indicated* | | | |
|---|---|---|---|
| Baked Potato w/ Ched. & Bacon Bits | 190 | 8 | 22 |
| Baked Potato with Steak & Cheese | 190 | 9 | 21 |
| BBQ Seasoned Pork | 170 | 1 | 29 |
| Beef Burrito | 170 | 6 | 19 |
| Beef Rib R'st w/ Pot. & Herbs | 110 | 1.5 | 17 |
| Beer-n-Cheese, with Beef & Bacon | 200 | 9 | 22 |
| Chicken Corn Chowder | 180 | 8 | 20 |
| Chipotle Chicken & Corn Chowder | 180 | 8 | 20 |
| Classic Chicken Noodle | 120 | 3 | 14 |
| Creamy Chkn & Dumplings | 170 | 9 | 14 |
| Fajita Chkn w/ Rice & Beans | 130 | 1 | 23 |
| Grilled Chicken & Sausage Gumbo | 140 | 3.5 | 21 |
| Kickin' Buffalo-Style Chicken | 150 | 7 | 15 |
| Mushroom Swiss Burger | 160 | 7 | 16 |
| Philly-Style Cheesesteak | 170 | 9 | 14 |
| **Hearty:** Beef Barley | 140 | 1 | 24 |
| Chicken with Vegetables | 80 | 1 | 13 |
| Cheeseburger Soup | 200 | 12 | 15 |
| Italian Style Wedding | 110 | 2.5 | 16 |

## Campbell's (Cont):

**Condensed Soup:** *Per ½ Cup, 4 fl.oz*

| | **C** | **F** | **Cb** |
|---|---|---|---|
| Broccoli Cheese | 100 | 5 | 11 |
| Beef Noodle | 70 | 1.5 | 9 |
| Beef with Vege & Barley | 100 | 1 | 18 |
| Cheddar Cheese | 100 | 5 | 14 |
| Chicken Gumbo | 70 | 1.5 | 12 |
| Cream of Asparagus | 100 | 7 | 8 |
| Cream of Celery | 100 | 7 | 8 |
| Cream of Mushr'm with Rstd Garlic | 90 | 6 | 9 |
| Cream of Onion | 100 | 6 | 10 |
| Green Pea | 180 | 3 | 28 |
| Old Fashioned Tom. Rice | 125 | 1.5 | 25 |
| Tomato | 90 | 0 | 20 |
| **25% Less Sodium:** Chicken Noodle | 60 | 1.5 | 9 |
| Cream of Mushroom | 100 | 7 | 8 |
| **98% Fat Free:** Broccoli Cheese | 80 | 2 | 12 |
| Cream of Celery | 60 | 2.5 | 9 |
| Cream of Mushroom | 60 | 2 | 9 |

**Soup on the Go:** *Per Container*

| | | | |
|---|---|---|---|
| Cheesy Chicken Tortilla | 100 | 4 | 13 |
| Cheesy Potato with Bacon Flav. | 130 | 6 | 16 |
| Classic Tomato | 140 | 0.5 | 32 |
| Creamy Tomato | 230 | 10 | 30 |
| Creamy Tomato Parmesan Bisque | 230 | 8 | 35 |

**Healthy Request:** *Per ½ cup, Unless Indicated*

| | | | |
|---|---|---|---|
| Cheddar Cheese | 60 | 1 | 12 |
| Cream of Chicken | 70 | 2.5 | 9 |
| New England Chowder, 1 cup | 130 | 3 | 21 |
| Savory Vegetable, 1 cup | 110 | 0.5 | 22 |
| Tomato | 90 | 1.5 | 17 |
| Tuscan-Style Lentil | 140 | 0.5 | 25 |
| Vegetable | 90 | 1 | 19 |

**Homestyle:** *Per Cup*

| | | | |
|---|---|---|---|
| Butternut Squash Bisque | 130 | 5 | 18 |
| Chicken Noodle | 90 | 2.5 | 10 |
| Creamy Chicken & Herb Dumplings | 160 | 9 | 14 |
| Creamy Gouda Bisque with Chicken | 190 | 11 | 16 |
| Creole-Style Chicken w/ Beans & Rice | 130 | 3 | 18 |
| Italian Style Wedding | 120 | 3.5 | 15 |
| Mexican-Style Chkn Tortilla | 130 | 2 | 20 |
| Potato Broccoli Cheese | 170 | 10 | 16 |
| Southwest-Style White Chicken Chili | 130 | 2 | 20 |
| Vegetable Medley | 90 | 0.5 | 18 |
| **Light:** Baked Pot. w/ Bacon & Cheddar | 100 | 3 | 15 |
| Chicken & Dumplings | 90 | 2.5 | 12 |
| Creamy Chicken Alfredo | 90 | 2 | 12 |
| New England Clam Chowder | 100 | 1.5 | 16 |

## Campbell's (Cont):

**Slow Kettle Style:** *Per Container*

| | **C** | **F** | **Cb** |
|---|---|---|---|
| Baked Potato with Smoked Bacon | 390 | 26 | 33 |
| Braised Beef Stew | 300 | 9 | 34 |
| Creamy Broccoli Cheddar Bisque | 340 | 25 | 22 |
| Fiesta Chicken Lime Tortilla w/ Chkn | 190 | 3 | 28 |
| Kickin' Crab & Sweet Corn Chowder | 440 | 27 | 37 |
| Portobello Mushr'm & Madeira Bisque | 420 | 31 | 29 |
| Roasted Red Pepper & Gouda Bisque | 300 | 16 | 32 |
| Tomato & Sweet Basil Bisque | 510 | 28 | 58 |
| Vegetarian Black Bean | 420 | 3 | 77 |

## Health Valley Organics: *Per Cup*

**40% Less Sodium:**

| | | | |
|---|---|---|---|
| Chicken Noodle | 80 | 2 | 11 |
| Garden Vegetable | 90 | 0 | 18 |
| **Creamed:** | | | |
| Cream of Chicken | 120 | 3 | 17 |
| Cream of Mushroom | 90 | 1.5 | 16 |
| **No Salt Added:** | | | |
| Chicken & Rice | 100 | 1.5 | 19 |
| Chicken Noodle | 80 | 2 | 13 |
| Lentil | 150 | 1.5 | 27 |
| Minestrone | 100 | 2 | 18 |
| Split Pea | 160 | 2.5 | 26 |
| Tomato | 110 | 2 | 22 |
| Vegetable | 90 | 2 | 15 |

## Healthy Choice:

**Canned:** *Per Cup*

| | | | |
|---|---|---|---|
| Chicken & Dumplings | 150 | 3 | 22 |
| Chicken Noodle | 90 | 0.5 | 12 |
| Chicken with Rice | 110 | 3 | 15 |
| Country Vegetable | 110 | 0.5 | 21 |
| Vegetable Beef | 130 | 1.5 | 20 |

## Imagine:

**Broths, Organic:** *Per Cup*

| | | | |
|---|---|---|---|
| Beef Flavor | 20 | 1 | 2 |
| Free Range Chicken | 20 | 0.5 | 2 |
| Vegetable | 20 | 0 | 4 |
| Vegetarian, No-Chicken | 15 | 0 | 2 |

**Chunky Style, Organic:** *Per Cup*

| | | | |
|---|---|---|---|
| Chicken & Dumplings | 120 | 4.5 | 16 |
| Ginger Miso | 70 | 1.5 | 11 |
| Italian Style Wedding | 150 | 4.5 | 20 |
| Italian Vegetables & Beans | 130 | 1.5 | 25 |
| Loaded Baked Potato | 120 | 5 | 18 |
| Potato Quinoa & Spinach | 120 | 3.5 | 19 |
| Soy-Ginger Chicken & Edamame | 80 | 2 | 10 |
| White Bean & Kale | 110 | 1 | 21 |

*Continued Nex Page...*

## Imagine (Cont):

**Creamy:** *Per 8 fl.oz Cup*

| | C | F | Cb |
|---|---|---|---|
| Butternut Squash | 100 | 1.5 | 21 |
| Cauliflower & Potato | 70 | 1 | 14 |
| Garden Tomato | 80 | 1 | 16 |
| Potato Leek | 90 | 2.5 | 14 |
| Portobello Mushroom | 80 | 2.5 | 12 |
| Tomato; Tomato Basil | 80 | 1 | 15 |

**Kettle Cuisine:** *Per 8 fl.oz Cup*

| | C | F | Cb |
|---|---|---|---|
| Albondigas Meatball Soup | 170 | 7 | 17 |
| Beef, Barley & Vegetable | 110 | 2 | 14 |
| Broccoli Cheddar | 320 | 24 | 15 |
| Buffalo Chicken | 250 | 15 | 14 |
| Carrot Ginger | 110 | 4 | 18 |
| Chicken Tortilla | 120 | 3 | 15 |
| Chipotle Sweet Potato | 140 | 7 | 20 |
| Classic Gazpacho | 60 | 1 | 10 |
| Cream of Crab | 290 | 22 | 15 |
| Hot Honey & Butternut Squash | 140 | 4 | 26 |
| Lobster Bisque | 270 | 18 | 18 |
| Manhattan Clam Chowder | 120 | 3 | 16 |
| Minestrone | 80 | 2 | 14 |
| North Atlantic Haddock Chowder | 260 | 17 | 14 |
| Portuguese Kale with Linguica | 200 | 7 | 21 |
| **Organic:** Chickpea & Chicken | 210 | 6 | 25 |
| Tomato Cheddar | 250 | 16 | 14 |

## Knorr:

**Cubes:** *Per ½ Cube, 1 Cup, Prepared*

| | C | F | Cb |
|---|---|---|---|
| Beef; Chicken, average | 15 | 1.5 | 1 |
| Vegetable | 20 | 1 | 1 |

**Homestyle Stock:** *Per 1 Tsp*

| | C | F | Cb |
|---|---|---|---|
| Beef | 10 | 0.5 | 1 |
| Chicken | 10 | 1 | 0.5 |

## Lipton:

**Cup-a-Soup:** *Per Envelope*

| | C | F | Cb |
|---|---|---|---|
| Chkn Noodle, White Meat | 50 | 1 | 8 |
| Cream of Chicken | 70 | 1.5 | 12 |

**Recipe Secrets:** *Per 1 Tbsp Dry Mix*

| | C | F | Cb |
|---|---|---|---|
| Onion | 20 | 0 | 4 |
| Onion Mushroom | 35 | 0 | 7 |
| Savory Herb with Garlic | 35 | 0 | 6 |

## Manischewitz:

**Canned:** *Per 1 cup*

| | C | F | Cb |
|---|---|---|---|
| Broth, Chicken | 15 | 0 | 2 |
| Chicken Noodle | 180 | 2 | 20 |

**Glass Jar:** *Per 1 Cup*

| | C | F | Cb |
|---|---|---|---|
| Matzo Ball | 120 | 5 | 15 |
| Reduced Sodium | 130 | 6 | 17 |
| Matzo Ball in Broth | 180 | 8 | 23 |
| Reduced Sodium | 180 | 8 | 21 |

## Maruchan:

**Instant Lunch,**

| | C | F | Cb |
|---|---|---|---|
| average all flavors, 1 pkg | 290 | 12 | 38 |
| **Ramen,** all flavors, 1 pkg, 3 oz | 380 | 14 | 52 |

## Nissin:

**Souper Meal:** *Per ½ of 4.3 oz Ctn*

| | C | F | Cb |
|---|---|---|---|
| Chicken Flavor, with Veggie Medley | 280 | 13 | 37 |
| Picante Shrimp Flavor, Hot & Spicy | 290 | 13 | 37 |
| **Top Ramen,** all flavors, 3 oz pkg | 380 | 14 | 53 |

## Pacific Foods:

**Condensed:** *Per ½ Cup*

| | C | F | Cb |
|---|---|---|---|
| Cream of Chicken | 90 | 3.5 | 10 |
| Cream of Mushroom | 80 | 3.5 | 10 |

**Hearty Organic:** *Per 1 Cup*

| | C | F | Cb |
|---|---|---|---|
| Butternut Squash Bisque | 120 | 3 | 22 |
| Cashew Carrot Ginger Bisque | 140 | 6 | 22 |
| Coconut Curry | 200 | 9 | 28 |
| Poblano Pepper & Corn Chowder | 180 | 9 | 22 |
| Rosemary Potato Chowder | 170 | 8 | 22 |
| Santa Fe Style Chicken | 140 | 2.5 | 22 |
| Spicy Black Bean & Kale | 120 | 0 | 24 |
| Split Pea & Uncured Ham | 160 | 2 | 26 |
| Vegetable Quinoa | 110 | 2 | 20 |

## Progresso:

**Broths:** Beef, 1 cup

| | C | F | Cb |
|---|---|---|---|
| Beef, 1 cup | 20 | 0 | 3 |
| Chicken, 1 cup | 10 | 0 | 1 |
| Vegetable, 1 cup | 5 | 0 | 1 |

**Rich & Hearty:** *Per Cup*

| | C | F | Cb |
|---|---|---|---|
| Beef Pot Roast w/ Country Vegetables | 110 | 1.5 | 17 |
| Chicken & Homestyle Noodles | 100 | 2 | 14 |
| Creamy Roasted Chicken Wild Rice | 120 | 4.5 | 15 |
| Creamy Roasted Vegetable | 140 | 6 | 19 |
| Hearty Chicken Pot Pie | 150 | 5 | 21 |
| Lentil & Andouille Sausage | 210 | 11 | 22 |
| Minestrone w/ Italian Sausage | 150 | 5 | 17 |
| New England Clam Chowder | 180 | 8 | 22 |
| Tomato Florentine w/ Italian Sausage | 160 | 6 | 20 |

**Traditional:** *Per 1 Cup*

| | C | F | Cb |
|---|---|---|---|
| Cheese Tortellini | 100 | 1 | 20 |
| Chickarina | 110 | 4 | 12 |
| Chicken & Sausage Gumbo | 110 | 2.5 | 17 |
| Italian-Style Wedding | 120 | 4 | 15 |
| Manhattan Clam Chowder | 100 | 2 | 17 |
| Steak Burger & Country Vegetables | 130 | 4 | 17 |

**Vegetable Classic:** *Per 1 Cup*

| | C | F | Cb |
|---|---|---|---|
| Creamy Mushroom | 150 | 10 | 11 |
| Green Split Pea | 160 | 2.5 | 29 |
| Minestrone | 100 | 2 | 20 |
| Southwestern-Style Corn | 110 | 2 | 20 |

**Light:** *Per 1 cup*

| | C | F | Cb |
|---|---|---|---|
| Beef Pot Roast | 80 | 1.5 | 12 |
| Broccoli Cheese | 120 | 6 | 11 |
| Chicken Noodle | 70 | 1 | 9 |
| Vegetable | 70 | 0 | 15 |

| Safeway (Vons): | C | F | Cb |
|---|---|---|---|
| **Signature Soups:** *Per Cup* | | | |
| Baked Potato w/ Bacon | 400 | 27 | 26 |
| Bella Minestrone | 350 | 8 | 60 |
| Chicken & White Bean Chili | 160 | 2 | 21 |
| Stompin' Steak Chili with Beans | 230 | 7 | 22 |
| Thai-Style Chicken Coconut Curry | 300 | 20 | 23 |
| **Swanson:** | | | |
| **Broth:** *Per 8 fl.oz Cup* | | | |
| Beef | 15 | 0 | 1 |
| Chicken | 10 | 0.5 | 1 |
| Organic Chicken | 15 | 0.5 | 1 |
| Vegetable | 10 | 0 | 2 |
| Crafted: Parmesan Brodo | 20 | 0.5 | 1 |
| Roasted Chicken Broth | 30 | 0 | 1 |
| Infused: Beef | 15 | 0.5 | 2 |
| Thai Ginger | 30 | 0.5 | 5 |
| Tuscan Chicken | 20 | 0.5 | 2 |
| **Tabatchnick:** | | | |
| **Frozen:** | | | |
| **Dairy:** *Per 7.5 oz Pouch* | | | |
| Corn Chowder | 130 | 4.5 | 21 |
| Cream of Mushroom | 100 | 5 | 11 |
| New England Potato | 130 | 4.5 | 20 |
| **Gluten Free:** *Per 7.5 oz Pouch* | | | |
| Balsamic Tomato & Rice | 110 | 3.5 | 18 |
| Southwest Bean | 220 | 5 | 36 |
| Split Pea | 140 | 0 | 34 |
| Wilderness Wild Rice | 90 | 0.5 | 19 |
| **Low Sodium:** *Per 7 .5oz Pouch* | | | |
| Barley & Mushroom | 80 | 1 | 17 |
| Split Pea | 140 | 0 | 34 |
| Vegetable | 90 | 1.5 | 17 |
| **Meat:** *Per 7.5 oz Pouch* | | | |
| Frenchman's Onion | 60 | 1.5 | 11 |
| Wilderness Wild Rice | 90 | 0.5 | 19 |
| **Pareve:** *Per 7.5 oz Pouch* | | | |
| Black Bean | 220 | 2.5 | 39 |
| Minestrone | 110 | 1.5 | 20 |
| **Shelf Stable:** *Per ⅔ Cup, 5.3 fl.oz* | | | |
| **Broth:** Classic Chicken | 5 | 0 | 0 |
| Other Chicken Flavors | 10 | 0 | 1 |
| Gourmet Beef | 5 | 0 | 0 |
| **Soup,** Creamy Tomato | 70 | 2 | 14 |
| **Thai Kitchen:** | | | |
| **Rice Noodle Soup Bowls:** *Per Bowl* | | | |
| Hot and Sour Rice Noodle | 250 | 4 | 51 |
| Lemongrass & Chili | 250 | 3.5 | 52 |
| Roasted Garlic | 250 | 3 | 52 |
| Spring Onion | 260 | 4.5 | 50 |
| Thai Ginger | 260 | 3 | 52 |

| Trader Joe's: | C | F | Cb |
|---|---|---|---|
| **28 fl.oz Cans:** *Per Cup* | | | |
| Chunky, Low Fat: | | | |
| Lentil with Vegetables | 140 | 3 | 21 |
| Minestrone | 110 | 2.5 | 19 |
| **14.5 oz Cans:** *Per Cup* | | | |
| Organic: Black Bean | 140 | 1.5 | 26 |
| Lentil Vegetable | 160 | 4 | 24 |
| Split Pea | 100 | 0 | 19 |
| **10.75 oz Can,** | | | |
| Low Sodium, Minestrone | 200 | 4 | 37 |
| **15 oz Can,** | | | |
| Low Fat, Chicken Noodle, 1 cup | 90 | 1 | 14 |
| **32 fl oz. Cartons:** *Per Cup* | | | |
| Butternut Squash | 90 | 2 | 16 |
| Carrot & Ginger | 80 | 1 | 17 |
| Creamy Corn & Rstd Pepper | 110 | 2 | 23 |
| Latin Style Black Bean | 70 | 1 | 12 |
| Sweet Potato Bisque | 130 | 1 | 28 |
| Organic: Butternut Squash | 70 | 0 | 17 |
| Tomato & Rstd Red Pepper | 100 | 3.5 | 15 |
| Low Sodium, Creamy Tomato | 90 | 3.5 | 15 |
| **17.6 fl.oz Cartons:** *Per Cup* | | | |
| Beef, Barley with Veggies | 100 | 0.5 | 16 |
| Chicken Noodle with Veggies | 100 | 1 | 16 |
| **Ramen Soups:** *Per 43g Container* | | | |
| Chicken | 180 | 4 | 29 |
| Miso | 180 | 3 | 31 |
| **Whole Foods:** *Per Cup* | | | |
| **365 Organic:** | | | |
| Chicken Noodle | 100 | 1.5 | 12 |
| Lentil | 70 | 0 | 15 |
| Minestrone | 140 | 1.5 | 23 |
| Southwestern Black Bean | 120 | 1 | 23 |
| Tomato Basil | 90 | 2 | 16 |
| **Wolfgang Puck:** *Per Cup* | | | |
| **Organic:** | | | |
| Butternut Squash | 140 | 11 | 10 |
| Chicken & Dumplings | 140 | 7 | 14 |
| Classic Minestrone | 120 | 2.5 | 20 |
| Corn Chowder | 210 | 13 | 20 |
| Free Range Chkn with Rice | 110 | 4 | 15 |
| New Engl. Clam Chowder | 150 | 7 | 18 |
| Signature Tortilla | 140 | 3.5 | 21 |
| Thick Hearty Lentil & Veggie | 160 | 1 | 29 |
| Thick Hearty Garden Vegetable | 120 | 4 | 20 |
| Tomato Basil Bisque | 150 | 6 | 21 |

## Soybean Products | C | F | Cb

| | C | F | Cb |
|---|---|---|---|
| **Cheeses (Soy)** ~ *See Page 78* | | | |
| **Miso Soy Bean Paste:** | | | |
| *Cold Mountain:* Light Yellow, 1 tsp | 10 | 0 | 1 |
| Mellow Red, 1 tsp | 15 | 0 | 3 |
| Red, 1 tsp | 10 | 0 | 1 |
| **Miso Soup (dry mix):** | | | |
| 1 Tbsp., dry mix | 35 | 1 | 5 |
| 1 cup, prepared | 35 | 1 | 5 |
| **Natto,** $\frac{1}{2}$ cup, 3 oz | 160 | 7 | 14 |
| **Okara (Tofu fiber residue),** $\frac{1}{2}$ C., 2 oz | 47 | 1 | 8 |
| **Tempeh:** 1 piece, 3 oz | 180 | 8 | 12 |
| Fried, 3 oz | 250 | 14 | 14 |
| **Seitan** *(Westsoy)*, Strips, 3 oz | 120 | 2 | 4 |
| **Soybean Protein** *(TVP)*, 1 oz | 95 | 0 | 8 |
| **Soy Bean Paste,** 1 tsp | 10 | 0 | 2 |
| **Soy Beans** ~ *See Page 160* | | | |
| **Soy Drinks** ~ *See Page 49* | | | |

## Tofu ~ Brands

| | C | F | Cb |
|---|---|---|---|
| **Azumaya Tofu:** | | | |
| Extra Firm; Firm, av., 3 oz | 70 | 4 | 2 |
| Soft (Silken), 3.2 oz | 45 | 2 | 1 |
| **House Foods:** *Per 3 oz* | | | |
| **Premium:** Firm | 70 | 4 | 2 |
| Extra Firm | 80 | 4.5 | 2 |
| Grilled, Super Firm | 80 | 4.5 | 3 |
| Medium Firm | 60 | 3 | 2 |
| Soft (Silken) | 60 | 3 | 2 |
| **Omega 3 Tofu,** Extra Firm | 80 | 5 | 1 |
| **Organic Tofu:** Firm | 70 | 4 | 2 |
| Extra Firm | 70 | 3.5 | 2 |
| **Tofu Cutlets:** Organic | 130 | 8 | 3 |
| Savory; Spicy Garlic, average | 155 | 8 | 7 |
| Teriyaki | 170 | 8 | 9 |
| **Mori-Nu Tofu:** | | | |
| **Extra Firm,** 3 oz, 1" slice | 50 | 2 | 1 |
| **Firm:** 3 oz, 1" slice | 50 | 2.5 | 2 |
| Lite, 3 oz, 1" slice | 30 | 1 | 1 |
| **Organic,** Silken, 3 oz, 1" slice | 45 | 2 | 1 |
| **Soft,** 3 oz, 1" slice | 45 | 2.5 | 1 |
| **Nasoya:** (Organic): Extra Firm, 3 oz | 80 | 4 | 3 |
| Firm, 3 oz | 70 | 3.5 | 2 |
| Silken, 3.2 oz | 45 | 2 | 1 |
| Sprouted: Super Firm, 3.2 oz | 140 | 8 | 3 |
| Cubed, 3 oz | 100 | 5 | 3 |
| **Tofubaked:** | | | |
| Sesame Ginger, 2 oz | 90 | 5 | 2 |
| Teriyaki, 2 oz | 80 | 4.5 | 2 |
| **Toss'ables:** Balsamic Vinaig., 3 oz | 150 | 8 | 6 |
| Garlic & Herb, 3 oz | 150 | 8 | 5 |

## Supplements | C | F | Cb

| | C | F | Cb |
|---|---|---|---|
| **Aloe Vera Juice,** undiluted, 2 fl.oz | 5 | 0 | 1 |
| Flakes, 1 heaping Tbsp, 0.3 oz | 30 | 0.5 | 4 |
| Powder, 1 heaping Tbsp, 0.5 oz | 50 | 0.5 | 6 |
| Tablets, 2 tabs | 4 | 0 | 0.5 |
| **Calcium Chews:** *CVS,* 1 chew | 20 | 0 | 3 |
| *Trader Joe's,* Chocolate,1 chew | 20 | 1 | 3 |
| **Cod Liver Oil,** 1 Tbsp | 125 | 13 | 0 |
| *Fiber Choice,* 2 tabs | 15 | 0 | 4 |
| **Fiber,** | | | |
| *Fibersure,* 1 heaping tsp | 25 | 0 | 6 |
| **Fish Oil Capsules,** (1), av. | 10 | 1 | 0 |
| **Flax Oil:** | | | |
| Capsules (2) | 10 | 1 | 0 |
| *Barlean's,* softgels (3) | 110 | 11 | 0 |
| **Garlic Tablets/Capsules,** each | 3 | 0 | 0 |
| **Glowelle:** | | | |
| Beauty Drink, 8 fl.oz | 100 | 0 | 24 |
| Powder Stick (1) | 50 | 0 | 12 |
| **Lecithin Granules,** 1 Tbsp | 55 | 4 | 0.5 |
| *Metamucil,* Powder: | | | |
| Orange (Smooth Texture), 1 rounded Tbsp | 45 | 0 | 12 |
| Sugar-Free, 1 rounded tsp | 20 | 0 | 5 |
| Pink Lemonade, Sugar-Free, 1 rounded tsp | 20 | 0 | 5 |
| **Capsules:** Heart & Digestive (6) | 10 | 0 | 3 |
| Strong Bones (5) | 10 | 0 | 3 |
| **Meta,** Fiber Wafers (2) | 100 | 4.5 | 16 |
| **Protein,** Powders, av., 1 oz | 100 | 0.5 | 0 |
| **Seaweed:** Dried, 1 oz | 85 | 0.5 | 22 |
| Soaked, drained, 1 oz | 15 | 0.5 | 3 |
| **Spirulina,** 1 tablet | 2 | 0 | 0.5 |
| **Vitamins/Minerals:** Tabs/Caps (1) | 2 | 0 | 0 |
| Vitamin E Capsules, each | 5 | 0.5 | 0 |
| **Viactiv Chews,** Choc. (1) | 20 | 0.5 | 4 |

## Cough & Pharmaceutical

| | C | F | Cb |
|---|---|---|---|
| **Antacids:** Av., 1 tablet | 4 | 0 | 1 |
| Liquid, 1 Tbsp | 6 | 0 | 1 |
| **Antacid Sodium Counts** ~ *See Page 280* | | | |
| **Cough/Cold Syrups:** | | | |
| Regular: With sugar, 1 Tbsp | 35 | 0 | 9 |
| With alcohol, 1 Tbsp | 46 | 0 | 9 |
| *Diabetic Tussin,* Sugar Free, 1 T. | 0 | 0 | 0 |
| **Cough Drops/Lozenges** ~ *See Page 75* | | | |
| *Sudafed,* Syrup 1 tsp | 14 | 0 | 3 |
| *Tylenol,* Liquid: Child, 1 tsp | 17 | 0 | 4 |
| Extra Strength, 1 tsp | 11 | 0 | 3 |

## Sugar

| | **C** | **F** | **Cb** |
|---|---|---|---|
| **White Sugar, granulated:** | | | |
| 1 level teaspoon, 4g | 15 | 0 | 4 |
| 1 heaping teaspoon, 6g | 25 | 0 | 6 |
| 1 Tablespoon, 12g | 50 | 0 | 12 |
| 1 ounce, 1 oz | 110 | 0 | 28 |
| 1 cup, 7 oz | 775 | 0 | 200 |
| 1 lb (16 oz) | 1760 | 0 | 454 |
| Single Portion Packages: | | | |
| 1 stick | 15 | 0 | 4 |
| 1 packet | 15 | 0 | 4 |
| 1 cube | 10 | 0 | 2.5 |
| **Brown Sugar:** 1 Tbsp | 50 | 0 | 13 |
| 1 ounce, 1 oz | 110 | 0 | 28 |
| 1 cup, not packed, 5 oz | 550 | 0 | 140 |
| 1 cup, packed, 7.8 oz | 835 | 0 | 216 |
| **Powdered Sugar:** | | | |
| Sifted, 1 cup, 3.5 oz | 390 | 0 | 100 |
| Unsifted, 1 cup, 4¼ oz | 470 | 0 | 120 |
| **Coconut Palm Sugar**, 1 tsp, 4g | 15 | 0 | 4 |
| **Dextrose**, 1 tsp | 12 | 0 | 3 |
| **Fructose**, powder, 1 tsp | 12 | 0 | 3 |
| **Glucose Powder**, 1 oz | 110 | 0 | 27 |
| **Glucose Tablets**, (1) | 20 | 0 | 5 |
| **Palm Sugar**, 3 Tbsp | 45 | 0 | 11 |
| **Piloncillo**, (Brown Sugar), 3oz | 325 | 0 | 81 |
| **Turbinado Sugar**, 2 Tbsp, 1 oz | 110 | 0 | 27 |

## Sugar Substitutes

| | | | |
|---|---|---|---|
| **Agave**, 1 Tbsp, 0.7 oz | 60 | 0 | 16 |
| **DiabetiSweet**, 1 teaspoon | 9 | 0 | 4.5 |
| *Note: Carb figure includes 4.5 g sugar alcohol* | | | |
| **Domino**, Light, ½ tsp | 5 | 0 | 2 |
| **Equal:** Tablet (2) | 0 | 0 | 0 |
| Granular, 1 tsp | 0 | 0 | 0 |
| Packet (1) | 0 | 0 | 0 |
| **Next**, 1 packet | 0 | 0 | 0 |
| **Nectresse**, 1 packet | 0 | 0 | 0 |
| **NutraSweet**, 1 tsp | 0 | 0 | 0 |
| **Splenda**, Granulated No Calorie Sweetener: | | | |
| 1 tsp | 0 | 0 | 0 |
| 1 cup | 95 | 0 | 24 |
| Packets, all flavors | 0 | 0 | 0 |
| Sugar Blend, Orig/Brown, ½ cup | 385 | 0 | 96 |
| **Stevia**, single serving | 0 | 0 | 0 |
| **Sugar Twin**, 1 packet | 0 | 0 | 0 |
| **Sweet 'N Low**, 1 packet | 0 | 0 | 0 |
| **Truvia**, 1 packet | 0 | 0 | 0 |
| **Walgreens**, Wal-Sweet, 1 packet | 0 | 0 | 0 |
| **Whey Low**, 1 tsp | 4 | 0 | 1 |

## Syrups, Molasses, Agave

**Syrups· Plain:** *Average All Brands (Corn/Rice/Maple/Pancake/Sundae/Waffle) Includes Aunt Jemima, Cary's, Karo, Hershey's, Hungry Jack, IHOP, Log Cabin, Mrs Butterworth's*

| | **C** | **F** | **Cb** |
|---|---|---|---|
| **Regular/Dark/Light Color:** | | | |
| 1 Tbsp, 0.5 fl.oz | 55 | 0 | 14 |
| ¼ cup (4 Tbsp) | 220 | 0 | 55 |
| Single Portion, 1.5 oz pkg | 170 | 0 | 42 |
| **Lite**, 1Tbsp, 1 oz | 25 | 0 | 6 |
| **Sugar-Free:** 2 Tbsp, 1 oz | 18 | 0 | 5 |
| *Maple Grove*, Cozy Cottage, 2 Tbsp | 10 | 0 | 3 |
| *IHOP*, 4 Tbsp, 2 oz | 20 | 0 | 7 |
| **Fruit Syrups**, *(IHOP)*, ¼ cup, 2 oz | 200 | 0 | 52 |
| **Honey Cream Syrup**, ¼ cup, 2 oz | 220 | 0 | 55 |
| **Molasses:** Dark/Light: 1 T, 0.7 oz | 60 | 0 | 15 |
| 1 cup, 12 oz | 975 | 0.5 | 252 |
| **Blackstrap**, 1 Tbsp, 0.8 oz | 47 | 0 | 13 |
| **Agave Nectar**, av. all flavors, | | | |
| 1 Tablespoon, 0.8 oz | 60 | 0 | 15 |

## Flavored Syrups/Ice Cream Toppings

| | | | |
|---|---|---|---|
| **Hershey's:** *Per 2 Tbsp* | | | |
| Double Chocolate, | 105 | 0 | 26 |
| Other Flavors, average | 90 | 0 | 23 |
| Lite | 45 | 0 | 12 |
| **Smuckers:** *Per 2 Tbsp* | | | |
| **Magic Shell**, average all flavors | 220 | 17 | 16 |
| **Spoonables:** Reg., average all flavors | 115 | 1 | 28 |
| Sugar Free: Caramel; Hot Fudge | 90 | 0 | 24 |
| Strawberry | 30 | 0 | 9 |
| *Note: Carb figures include 8g-17g sugar alcohol* | | | |
| **Sundae Syrups:** Regular, av. all flavors | 105 | 0 | 25 |
| Sugar Free, average all flavors | 90 | 0 | 24 |
| *Note: Carb figures includes 15g sugar alcohol* | | | |

## Honey, Jam, Preserves

***Average all Brands***

| | | | |
|---|---|---|---|
| **Honey:** 1 tsp, 0.23 oz | 20 | 0 | 5.5 |
| 1 Tbsp, 0.7 oz | 60 | 0 | 17 |
| 1 oz | 85 | 0 | 24 |
| ½ cup, 6 oz | 515 | 0 | 145 |
| Single Portion, 0.5 oz package | 45 | 0 | 12 |
| **Jams/Jellies/Marmalade/Preserves:** | | | |
| Regular: 1 tsp, 0.3 oz | 20 | 0 | 5 |
| 1 Tbsp, 0.8 oz | 55 | 0 | 14 |
| 1 ounce, 1 oz | 80 | 0 | 20 |
| Single Portion, 0.5 oz pkg | 40 | 0 | 11 |
| **Apple/Fruit Butters**, 1 T., 0.6 oz | 20 | 0 | 6 |
| **Fruit Spreads:** Regular, 1 tsp | 15 | 0 | 4 |
| Low Sugar, 1 tsp | 8 | 0 | 2 |
| **Jelly:** Regular, average, 1 tsp | 18 | 0 | 4.5 |
| Imitation, Low Calorie, 1 tsp | 4 | 0 | 1 |

| Vegetables | C | F | Cb |
|---|---|---|---|
| **Alfalfa Sprouts**, ¹/₂ cup, 0.5 oz | 5 | 0 | 0.5 |
| **Artichokes**, Globe/French: | | | |
| 1 medium, 4.5 oz | 60 | 0 | 13 |
| 1 large, 5.7 oz | 75 | 0 | 17 |
| **Artichoke Heart**, plain, 2 pieces | 15 | 0 | 3 |
| **Asparagus**, raw/frozen: | | | |
| Cuts & Tips, ¹/₂ cup, 4.3 oz | 20 | 0 | 3 |
| Spears, 3 medium | 10 | 0 | 2 |
| **Bamboo Shoots**, cooked, ¹/₂ cup, 2 oz | 7 | 0 | 1 |
| **Beans**, Green/Snap/String: | | | |
| 10 beans (4" long), 2 oz | 20 | 0 | 4 |
| Pieces, ¹/₂ cup, 3 oz | 30 | 0 | 7 |
| Dried Beans (Kidney, Brown, Lima, Navy, Pinto, White): | | | |
| Raw: 2 Tbsp, 1 oz | 95 | 0.5 | 18 |
| 1 cup, 7 oz | 665 | 3 | 126 |
| Cooked: 1 oz | 35 | 0 | 7 |
| ¹/₂ cup, 3 oz | 105 | 0 | 21 |
| **Bean Sprouts**, average, ¹/₂ cup, 2 oz | 15 | 0 | 3.5 |
| **Beets (Beetroot):** | | | |
| Raw, 1 beet (2" diam.), 4 oz | 35 | 0 | 8 |
| Cooked, 1 cup, slices, 3 oz | 35 | 0 | 8 |
| **Canned ~ See Page 161** | | | |
| **Beet Greens**, cooked, ¹/₂ cup, 2.5 oz | 20 | 0 | 4 |
| **Bell Pepper ~ See Peppers** | | | |
| **Bitter Melon/Gourd**, 1 cup, 1.5 oz | 15 | 0 | 1.5 |
| **Blackeye Peas**, cooked, ¹/₂ cup, 3 oz | 100 | 0.5 | 18 |
| **Bok Choy (Chinese Chard)**, | | | |
| cooked, 3 oz | 10 | 0 | 1.5 |
| **Breadfruit**, ¹/₄ small fruit, 3 oz | 100 | 0 | 26 |
| **Broadbeans (Fava Beans):** | | | |
| Green, raw, (in pod): 4 pods | | | |
| (3.5 oz with shells, 1.2 oz beans) | 30 | 0 | 6 |
| 1 cup beans, without shell, 4.5 oz | 110 | 1 | 22 |
| Mature Seeds: Raw, 1 cup, 5.3 oz | 510 | 2.5 | 87 |
| Cooked, 1 cup, 3 oz | 95 | 0 | 17 |
| **Broccoflower**, ¹/₅ head, 3.5 oz | 35 | 0 | 7 |
| **Broccoli:** Raw, chopped,1 cup, 3 oz | 30 | 0 | 6 |
| 3 Florets, 2.5 oz | 25 | 0 | 5 |
| 1 Spear (5" long), 1.oz | 10 | 0 | 2 |
| 1 Whole: Medium, 14 oz | 135 | 1.5 | 26 |
| Large, 21 oz | 205 | 2 | 40 |
| 1 Head (no stalk), 11 oz | 105 | 1 | 21 |
| 1 Stalk, small (5" long), 5.3 oz | 50 | 0.5 | 10 |
| **Brocco Sprouts**, ¹/₂ cup, 1 oz | 15 | 0 | 2 |
| **Brussels Sprouts:** | | | |
| Cooked, ¹/₂ cup, 2.8 oz | 30 | 0.5 | 6 |
| 2 Sprouts, 1.5 oz | 15 | 0 | 3 |
| **Butterbeans**, cooked, ¹/₂ cup, 3 oz | 90 | 0 | 16 |
| **Cabbage**, average other flavors: | | | |
| Raw: 1 leaf, large, 1 oz | 5 | 0 | 2 |
| Shredded, 1 cup, 2.5 oz | 15 | 0 | 4 |
| ¹/₂ large head (7" diam), 22 oz | 150 | 1 | 35 |
| Cooked, shredded, ¹/₂ cup, 2.5 oz | 15 | 0.5 | 3.5 |

| Vegetables (Cont) | C | F | Cb |
|---|---|---|---|
| **Cactus Leaf (Nopales):** | | | |
| 1 leaf, 4.5 oz | 20 | 0 | 4 |
| 1 cup (slices), 3 oz | 15 | 0 | 3 |
| **Carrots**, regular thick variety: | | | |
| 1 small, 4 oz | 45 | 0 | 11 |
| 1 medium, 6 oz | 70 | 0 | 16 |
| 1 large, 8 oz | 95 | 0 | 22 |
| Chopped, 1 cup, 4.5 oz | 50 | 0 | 12 |
| Grated, 1 cup, 4 oz | 45 | 0 | 11 |
| Slices, 1 cup, 4.5 oz | 50 | 0 | 12 |
| Sticks (4"), 4-5, 1.5 oz | 20 | 0 | 4 |
| Long thin variety, 1 medium, 2.2 oz | 25 | 0 | 6 |
| Baby: Snack size, 3 medium, 1 oz | 10 | 0 | 2.5 |
| Snack Pack, 3 oz | 30 | 0 | 7 |
| **Cassava**, raw, 1 cup, 2.5 oz | 330 | 0.5 | 78 |
| **Cauliflower**, raw: | | | |
| Pieces, 1 cup, 3.5 oz | 25 | 0 | 5 |
| ¹/₂ medium head, 10 oz | 70 | 0 | 15 |
| Cooked, 3 florets, 2 oz | 10 | 0 | 2 |
| **Celeriac**, ¹/₂ cup, raw, 2.8 oz | 35 | 0 | 7 |
| **Celery:** 1 large stalk, 11", 2.2 oz | 10 | 0 | 2 |
| 4 Strips, thin sticks, 0.5 oz | 5 | 0 | 1 |
| Chopped, 1 cup, 3.5 oz | 15 | 0 | 3 |
| **Chard (Swiss)**, ¹/₂ cup, cooked, 3 oz | 20 | 0 | 3.5 |
| **Chayote Squash:** | | | |
| 1 medium, 7 oz | 40 | 0 | 9 |
| Pieces, 1 cup, 4.5 oz | 25 | 0 | 6 |
| **Chickpeas**, (Garbanzo Beans): | | | |
| Dry, 1 cup, 7 oz | 730 | 12 | 121 |
| Cooked, 1 cup, 5.8 oz | 270 | 4 | 45 |
| **Chicory Greens**, 1 cup, 1 oz | 7 | 0 | 1.5 |
| **Chili Peppers ~ See Peppers** | | | |
| **Chinese Long Bean**, slices, 1 cup, 3.2 oz | 45 | 0 | 8 |
| **Chives**, chopped, 1 Tbsp | 1 | 0 | 0 |
| **Choy Sum**, 3 oz | 15 | 0 | 3 |
| **Cilantro**, (Coriander), 1 cup | 5 | 0 | 0.5 |
| **Collards**, cooked, ¹/₂ cup, 3 oz | 25 | 0 | 5 |
| **Corn**, Yellow/White: | | | |
| Raw: Kernels, 1 cup, 3 oz | 80 | 0.5 | 19 |
| Ear (5"x 1³/₄"), 5.5 oz | 155 | 1 | 37 |
| Cooked: Kernels, ¹/₂ cup, 3 oz | 77 | 0.5 | 18 |
| Cob, small, 2.3 oz | 60 | 0.5 | 14 |
| Ear, large, 5.5 oz | 120 | 1 | 28 |
| **Cress**, garden, raw, 1 cup, 1.8 oz | 15 | 0 | 3 |
| **Cucumber**, average other flavors: | | | |
| Slices, ¹/₂ cup, 2 oz | 10 | 0 | 2 |
| Green, 1 medium (9"), 11 oz | 45 | 0 | 11 |
| Persian, 1 medium (8"), 6 oz | 25 | 0 | 5 |
| **Daikon Radish**, ¹/₂ cup, slices, 2 oz | 9 | 0 | 2 |
| **Dandelion Greens**, raw, ¹/₂ cup, 1 oz | 10 | 0 | 2.5 |
| **Edamame**, (Immature green soybeans): | | | |
| Shelled, ¹/₂ cup, 2.6 oz | 110 | 5 | 8 |
| With shells, 10 pods, 1.3 oz | 30 | 1 | 3 |

| Vegetables (Cont) | C | F | Cb |
|---|---|---|---|
| **Eggplant**, raw: 4 oz | 30 | 0 | 7 |
| ¹/₂ cup, 1" pieces, 1.5 oz | 10 | 0 | 2 |
| 1 slice, fried, 1 oz | 75 | 4 | 10 |
| **Endive**, Belgian/French: Raw, | | | |
| 1 medium head (6"), 2.5 oz | 12 | 0 | 3 |
| **Fennel**, 1 cup, sliced, 3 oz | 25 | 0 | 7 |
| **Gai Choy Cabbage**, cooked, 1 cup, 6 oz | 20 | 0 | 3 |
| **Gai Lan**, (Chinese Kale), cooked, 1 cup | 35 | 0.5 | 7 |
| **Garbanzo Beans ~** *See Chick Peas* | | | |
| **Garlic**, 1 clove | 4 | 0 | 1 |
| **Ginger:** ¹/₄ cup slices, 1 oz | 20 | 0 | 5 |
| Crystallized (sugared), 7 pieces, 1.5 oz | 130 | 0 | 35 |
| **Horseradish**, raw, 1 pod, 0.5 oz | 5 | 0 | 1 |
| **Jerusalem Artichoke**, raw, ¹/₂ cup | 55 | 0 | 13 |
| **Jicama**, raw, sliced, ¹/₂ cup, 2.3 oz | 25 | 0 | 6 |
| **Kale**, 1 cup, chopped, 2.5 oz | 35 | 0.5 | 7 |
| **Kalettes**, 1 cup, 2 oz | 30 | 0 | 4 |
| **Kohlrabi**, cooked, ¹/₂ cup, 1.8 oz | 17 | 0 | 5 |
| **Leek**, cooked, 1 whole, 4.5 oz | 40 | 0 | 9 |
| **Lentils**, green/brown: Dry, 1 oz | 100 | 0.5 | 17 |
| 1 cup, 6.8 oz | 675 | 3 | 115 |
| Cooked, ¹/₂ cup, 3.5 oz | 115 | 0.5 | 20 |
| **Lettuce:** 1 cup, chopped/shredded, 2 oz | 7 | 0 | 1 |
| Butterhead, 2 leaves, 0.5 oz | 2 | 0 | 0.5 |
| Cos/Romaine, shredded, 1 cup | 10 | 0 | 2 |
| Iceberg: 1 outer leaf, 0.5 oz | 2 | 0 | 0.5 |
| 1 medium head, 16 oz | 75 | 1 | 16 |
| **Lima Beans**, baby, cooked, ¹/₂ cup, 3 oz | 105 | 0 | 20 |
| **Lotus Root**, cooked, 10 slices, 3 oz | 60 | 0 | 14 |
| **Mung Bean Sprouts**, ¹/₂ cup, 2 oz | 15 | 0 | 3 |
| **Mushrooms**, average all varieties: | | | |
| Raw, diced/siced, 1 cup, 3 oz | 20 | 0 | 3 |
| Pieces, 1 cup, 1.3 oz | 8 | 0 | 1 |
| Fried/Sauteed, 6 oz | 220 | 16 | 10 |
| Grilled, pieces, ¹/₂ cup, 2.5 oz | 20 | 0.5 | 4 |
| Shitake, dried, 1 oz package | 90 | 0 | 22 |
| **Mustard Greens**, raw, ¹/₂ cup, 1 oz | 7 | 0 | 2 |
| **Okra:** Raw, 8 pods, 4 oz | 30 | 0 | 7 |
| Cooked, ¹/₂ cup, 2.8 oz | 20 | 0 | 4 |
| **Onions**, Raw: 1 small, 2.5 oz | 30 | 0 | 7 |
| 1 medium, 4 oz | 50 | 0 | 11 |
| 1 large, 5.5 oz | 65 | 0 | 15 |
| 1 jumbo, 16 oz | 190 | 0.5 | 46 |
| Chopped: ¹/₂ cup, 3 oz | 35 | 0 | 8 |
| 1 Tbsp, 0.4 oz | 5 | 0 | 1 |
| Slices: 1 cup, 4 oz | 50 | 0 | 12 |
| 1 medium slice (¹/₈"), 0.5 oz | 5 | 0 | 1 |
| 1 large slice (¹/₄"), 1.3 oz | 15 | 0 | 4 |
| Flakes, dried ¹/₄ cup, 0.5 oz | 50 | 0 | 12 |
| Rings, breaded & fried, 2 rings | 80 | 5 | 9 |
| Scallions, ¹/₂ cup, 2 oz | 15 | 0 | 3 |
| Spring, chopped, ¹/₂ cup, 2 oz | 15 | 0 | 3 |

| Vegetables (Cont) | C | F | Cb |
|---|---|---|---|
| **Parsley**, chopped, ¹/₂ cup, 1 oz | 10 | 0 | 2 |
| **Parsnip:** 1 medium, 4 oz | 85 | 0 | 20 |
| Cooked, slices, ¹/₂ cup, 2.8 oz | 55 | 0 | 13 |
| **Peas:** Green, raw, ¹/₄ cup, 1.5 oz | 30 | 0 | 5 |
| With pods, 0.5 lb | 70 | 0 | 13 |
| Snow Peas, 10 pods, 1.2 oz | 15 | 0 | 3 |
| Split: Dry, hulled, 1 oz | 100 | 0.5 | 17 |
| Cooked, 1 cup, 7 oz | 230 | 1 | 42 |
| **Peppers:** | | | |
| Sweet, 1 medium, 4.2 oz | 30 | 0 | 7 |
| Bell: 1 medium, 4.2 oz | 30 | 0 | 7 |
| raw, chopped, ¹/₂ cup, 2.5 oz | 20 | 0 | 5 |
| 2 rings (5" diam. x ¹/₄" thick) | 3 | 0 | 1 |
| Chili: Green/Red, 1.5 oz | 20 | 0 | 5 |
| Habanero, 1 only, 0.3 oz | 10 | 0 | 2 |
| **Pigeon Peas**, cooked, ¹/₂ cup, 3 oz | 95 | 1 | 17 |
| **Pimientos**, 3 medium, 3.5 oz | 25 | 0 | 5 |
| **Poi**, ¹/₂ cup, 4.2 oz | 135 | 0 | 33 |
| **Potatoes:** | | | |
| **Raw** (with skin): | | | |
| 1 baby, 2 oz | 45 | 0 | 10 |
| 1 small, 6 oz | 135 | 0 | 30 |
| 1 medium, 8 oz | 180 | 0 | 40 |
| 1 large, 12 oz | 270 | 0 | 60 |
| 1 extra large, 16 oz | 360 | 0 | 80 |
| **Baked**, (no added fat), 1 medium: | | | |
| Plain: With skin, 7 oz (cooked wt) | 185 | 0 | 42 |
| Without skin, 5.5 oz (cooked wt) | 145 | 0 | 34 |
| With Skin/Toppings: | | | |
| With 2 tsp fat | 255 | 8 | 42 |
| With Grated Cheese, 1 oz | 300 | 9 | 42 |
| With Plain Yogurt, 2 Tbsp | 220 | 2 | 45 |
| With Sour Crm & Chives, 2 Tbsp | 240 | 5 | 43 |
| **Mashed:** | | | |
| With milk plus fat, ¹/₂ cup, 4 oz | 120 | 4.5 | 18 |
| KFC Style without gravy, 4 oz | 90 | 3 | 15 |
| Loaded (fat/cream/cheese/bacon): | | | |
| Side serving, 6 oz | 180 | 9 | 22 |
| Large serving, 12 oz | 360 | 18 | 44 |
| **Roasted,** with oil: | | | |
| Whole, 1 small, 3 oz | 140 | 5 | 20 |
| Diced, 1 cup, 5 oz | 180 | 8 | 30 |
| **Potato Skins**, baked w/ cheese topping, | | | |
| ¹/₂ whole, 4 oz | 240 | 13 | 22 |
| **French Fries:** Small serving, 2.6 oz | 250 | 13 | 30 |
| Medium serving, 4 oz | 380 | 20 | 47 |
| Frozen, uncooked, 18 fries, 4 oz | 165 | 5.5 | 28 |
| Oven-heated, 18 fries, 4 oz | 165 | 5.5 | 28 |
| Take-Out, 1 cup, 5 oz | 440 | 25 | 60 |
| **Au Gratin**, ¹/₂ cup, 4.3 oz | 160 | 9 | 14 |
| **Scalloped,** 8.5 oz | 220 | 9 | 26 |

## Vegetables (Cont)    C   F   Cb

| | C | F | Cb |
|---|---|---|---|
| **Pumpkin:** | | | |
| Raw, 1" cubes, 1 cup, 4 oz | 30 | 0 | 7 |
| Cooked: | | | |
| Baked, without fat, 4 oz | 90 | 7 | 9 |
| Mashed: 1 scoop, 2 oz | 10 | 0 | 2 |
| 1/2 cup, 4.3 oz | 25 | 0 | 6 |
| Pumpkin Flowers, 1 cup, 1.2 oz | 5 | 0 | 1 |
| **Purslane:** Cooked, 1/2 cup, 2 oz | 10 | 0 | 2 |
| Raw, 1" cubes, 1 cup, 1.5 oz | 5 | 0 | 1.5 |
| **Radicchio:** 2 leaves, 0.5 oz | 5 | 0 | 1 |
| Shredded, 1 cup, 1.5 oz | 20 | 0 | 4 |
| **Radishes:** 1 small | 0 | 0 | 0 |
| 10 medium/5 large, 1.6 oz | 5 | 0 | 1 |
| Slices, 1/2 cup, 2 oz | 10 | 0 | 2 |
| **Rhubarb,** raw, 1/2 cup, 2 oz | 15 | 0 | 3 |
| **Rutabaga,** cubes, cooked, 1/2 cup, 3 oz | 30 | 0 | 7 |
| **Salsify,** cooked, slices, 1/2 cup, 2.5 oz | 50 | 0 | 11 |
| **Sauerkraut,** 1/2 cup, 2.5 oz | 15 | 0 | 3 |
| **Seaweed:** Dried, 1 oz | 5 | 0 | 2 |
| Soaked, drained, 1 oz | 15 | 0 | 4 |
| Nori/Laver, dried, 6 sheets, 0.5 oz | 35 | 0 | 5 |
| **Shallots,** chopped, 1 Tbsp, 0.5 oz | 5 | 0 | 1 |
| **Sorrel,** raw, 1/2 cup, 4 oz | 20 | 0 | 4 |
| **Soybeans:** Dry, 1/2 cup, 3.3 oz | 390 | 18 | 28 |
| Mature, dry, 1 oz | 120 | 5.5 | 9 |
| Cooked, 1/2 cup, 3 oz | 150 | 7.5 | 8 |
| **Soy Products/Tofu/Tempeh ~** *See Page 156* | | | |
| **Spinach:** Cooked, 1/2 cup, 3 oz | 20 | 0 | 4 |
| Creamed, average, 1/2 cup, 4.5 oz | 190 | 15 | 8 |
| Raw: 3 leaves, 1 cup, 1 oz | 7 | 0 | 1 |
| 1 Bunch, 12 oz | 80 | 1.5 | 12 |
| **Squash:** | | | |
| Summer: Raw, 1/2 cup, 2.5 oz | 10 | 0 | 2 |
| Cooked, slices, 1/2 cup, 3 oz | 15 | 0 | 3 |
| Winter, cooked: | | | |
| Acorn: Cubes, 1/2 cup, 3.5 oz | 35 | 0 | 9 |
| 1/2 medium (10 oz raw weight) | 115 | 0 | 30 |
| Butternut: Cubes, 1/2 cup, 3.5 oz | 40 | 0 | 10 |
| 1/4 medium (9 oz raw weight) | 115 | 0 | 30 |
| Spaghetti, 1/2 cup, 1.8 oz | 15 | 0 | 3 |
| **Succotash,** cooked, 1/2 cup, 3.3 oz | 110 | 1 | 23 |
| **Sweetcorn ~** *See Corn* | | | |
| **Sweet Potatoes:** | | | |
| Cooked with skin (w/o fat), | | | |
| 1 medium, 4 oz | 105 | 0 | 24 |
| Without skin, mashed, 1/2 cup, 5.5 oz | 125 | 0 | 29 |
| Fries (Alexia, Julienne syle), | | | |
| approximately 12 pieces, 3 oz | 140 | 5 | 24 |

## Vegetables (Cont)    C   F   Cb

| | C | F | Cb |
|---|---|---|---|
| **Swiss Chard,** cooked, chopped, 1 c., 6 oz | 35 | 0 | 7 |
| **Taro,** cooked, 1/2 cup, 2.3 oz | 95 | 0 | 23 |
| **Tomatoes:** 1 small (2 1/4" diam.), 3 oz | 15 | 0 | 3 |
| 1 medium (2 3/4" diameter), 5 oz | 25 | 0 | 5 |
| 1 large (3 1/2" diameter), 8 oz | 40 | 0.5 | 9 |
| 1 extra lge (4" diam.), 12 oz | 60 | 0.5 | 14 |
| Chopped, 1 cup, 6.5 oz | 35 | 0.5 | 7 |
| **Tomatillo:** 1 medium, 1.2 oz | 10 | 0 | 2 |
| 1 lb quantity for recipe | 135 | 4.5 | 27 |
| **Turnip:** Cooked, 1/2 cup, 2.8 oz | 15 | 0 | 4 |
| Greens, cooked, 1/2 cup, 2.5 oz | 15 | 0 | 3 |
| **Water Chestnuts:** 5-6 nuts, 1 oz | 56 | 0 | 13 |
| Raw, slices, 1/2 cup, 2.3 oz | 60 | 0 | 15 |
| Canned, 1 oz | 15 | 0 | 3 |
| **Watercress,** 10 sprigs, 1 oz | 3 | 0 | 0.5 |
| **Yams:** Cooked, steamed, 1/2 cup, 2.5 oz | 80 | 0 | 19 |
| Baked: | | | |
| 1 medium (6") 8 oz | 265 | 0.5 | 63 |
| 1 large (9") 12 oz | 400 | 0.5 | 94 |
| **Yardlong Bean,** 1 pod, 0.5 oz | 5 | 0 | 1 |
| **Yucca Root,** raw, 1/2 cup, 3.5 oz | 165 | 0 | 39 |
| **Zucchini:** Raw, 1 medium, 7 oz | 30 | 0.5 | 7 |
| 1 large, 12 oz | 60 | 1 | 12 |
| Cooked, slices, | | | |
| 1/2 cup, 3 oz | 15 | 0 | 4 |

## Frozen Vegetables

| | C | F | Cb |
|---|---|---|---|
| **Birds Eye:** | | | |
| **Flavor Full:** Buffalo Cauliflower, 3.3 oz | 50 | 2 | 7 |
| Ranch: Broccoli, 3 oz | 50 | 1.5 | 5 |
| Cauliflower, 3.3 oz | 50 | 2 | 6 |
| Salt & Vinegar Potatoes, 3.9 oz | 150 | 4 | 25 |
| Steakhouse Green Beans, 3 oz | 60 | 2.5 | 6 |
| Teriyaki Broccoli, 3 oz | 50 | 1.5 | 7 |
| **Steamfresh:** Asparagus Spears (6) | 20 | 0 | 3 |
| Chopped Kale, 3.1 oz | 25 | 0 | 4 |
| Cut Green Beans, 3 oz | 30 | 0 | 5 |
| **Mixtures:** Brocc. Cauliflower, 3 oz | 25 | 0 | 4 |
| California Blend, 2.7 oz | 25 | 0 | 4 |
| Stir-Fry: Broccoli, 3.6 oz | 40 | 0 | 7 |
| Oriental, 4 oz | 60 | 0 | 11 |
| Sugar Snap, 3.4 oz | 40 | 0 | 7.5 |
| Sweet Peas, 3.2 oz | 70 | 0 | 12 |
| Unshelled Edamame, 2.6 oz | 90 | 3 | 9 |

# Vegetables & Legumes Ⓥ

## Frozen Vegetables (Cont) | C | F | Cb

**Green Giant:**

| | C | F | Cb |
|---|---|---|---|
| **Mashed Cauliflowe:** Original, 4.2 oz | 80 | 5 | 7 |
| Cheddar & Bacon, 4.2 oz | 90 | 6 | 6 |
| Riced Cauliflower/with Brocc., 3 oz | 20 | 0 | 4 |
| **Roasted Veggies:** Broccoli, 3 oz | 30 | 0 | 6 |
| Brussels Sprouts, 3 oz | 30 | 0 | 6 |
| Carrots, 3 oz | 30 | 0.5 | 7 |
| Cauliflower, 3 oz | 20 | 0 | 3 |
| Corn, 3 oz | 120 | 1.5 | 25 |
| **Sautes:** | | | |
| **Fire Roasted,** Prepared: | | | |
| Corn, Peppers & Onions, 1/2 cup | 80 | 0.5 | 16 |
| Root Veggies w/ Red Onions, 2/3 c. | 60 | 0 | 14 |
| Tri color Peppers, 1/3 cup | 25 | 0 | 5 |
| Zucchini, Carrots & Onions, 1/3 cup | 20 | 0 | 4 |
| **Kits:** Herb B'Nut Squash Medley, 4.3 oz | 35 | 1 | 7 |
| Chipotle Harvest, 1 cup prepared | 280 | 3 | 25 |
| Thai Coconut, 1 cup prepared | 210 | 4 | 18 |
| **Steamers:** Corn Niblets, 3 oz | 90 | 1 | 19 |
| Backyard Gr. Potatoes, 1/2 cup prep. | 110 | 3 | 20 |
| Creamed Spinach, 3.8 oz | 70 | 2 | 9 |
| **Veggie Tots:** Broccoli & Cheese, 3 oz | 130 | 6 | 14 |
| Brocolli; Cauliflower, 3 oz | 110 | 4.5 | 15 |

**Ore-Ida:** *Per 3 oz Unless Indicated*

**Fries:**

| | C | F | Cb |
|---|---|---|---|
| Bold & Crispy:  Chili Cheese Crinkle | 160 | 7 | 22 |
| Garlic Black Pepper Steakhouse | 180 | 8 | 25 |
| Zesties, Seasoned | 180 | 7.5 | 26 |
| Zesty, Seasoned Curly | 185 | 9 | 24 |
| Classic: Golden Crinkles | 120 | 4.5 | 19 |
| Golden | 130 | 3.5 | 21 |
| Steak | 110 | 3 | 19 |
| Extra Crispy Easy, Golden Crinkles | 170 | 6 | 25 |
| Extra Crispy: Fast Food Fries | 150 | 6 | 24 |
| Golden Crinkles | 160 | 7 | 22 |
| Seasoned Crinkles | 150 | 6 | 22 |
| Premium: Crispers | 230 | 14 | 23 |
| Country Style French | 130 | 4.5 | 20 |
| Golden Twirls | 150 | 6 | 23 |
| Texas Crispers | 150 | 7 | 20 |
| **Hash Browns:** Golden Patties (1) | 140 | 8 | 15 |
| Potatoes O'Brien | 60 | 0 | 13 |
| Shredded Hash Browns Pattie (1) | 70 | 0 | 16 |
| **Mashed Potato Bites:** | | | |
| Four Cheese, 2.5 oz | 180 | 10 | 18 |
| Loaded Baked, 2.5 oz | 170 | 10 | 18 |
| **Onion:** Chopped, 3 oz | 20 | 0 | 5 |
| Gourmet Rings, 2.7 oz | 185 | 9 | 24 |
| Onion Ringers, 3 oz | 180 | 10 | 21 |
| **Steam n' Mash:** Cut Russet, 3.5 oz | 70 | 0 | 16 |
| **Tater Tots**, Reg., Crispy Crowns,av. | 165 | 9 | 20 |

## Canned/Bottled | C | F | Cb

*Solids & Liquid*

| | C | F | Cb |
|---|---|---|---|
| **Artichoke Hearts:** | | | |
| *Fancifoods:* Plain, 1 oz (1) | 8 | 0 | 1 |
| Marinated, 1/4 bottle, 1 oz | 25 | 1.5 | 2 |
| **Asparagus:** Drained, 3 spears | 10 | 0 | 1.5 |
| Pieces, 1/2 cup, 4.3 oz | 25 | 0.5 | 3 |
| **Bamboo Shoots,** 1 cup, 4.5 oz | 25 | 0 | 4 |
| **Bean Salad,** 1/2 cup, 4.4 oz | 90 | 0 | 20 |
| **Beans:** Baked, 1/2 cup, 4.5 oz | 120 | 0.5 | 27 |
| Butter, 1/2 cup, 4.5 oz | 90 | 0 | 16 |
| Green, 1/2 cup, 2.5 oz | 15 | 0 | 3 |
| Italian, 1/2 cup, 4.5 oz | 30 | 0 | 6 |
| Kidney, 1/2 cup 3.5 oz | 105 | 0.5 | 19 |
| Lima, 1/2 cup, 4.5 oz | 80 | 0 | 15 |
| Pinto, 1/2 cup, 4.5 oz | 105 | 1 | 19 |
| **Beets:** Sliced, 1/2 cup, 3 oz | 25 | 0 | 6 |
| Crinkle/Pickled, 1/2 cup | 80 | 0 | 20 |
| **Carrots:** Sliced, 1/2 cup, 2.5 oz | 20 | 0 | 4 |
| *Del Monte,* Honey Glazed, 1/2 cup | 75 | 0 | 18 |
| **Corn:** Kernels, 1/2 cup, 4.5 oz | 80 | 0.5 | 18 |
| Creamed style, 1/2 cup, 4.5 oz | 90 | 0.5 | 23 |
| **Garbanzo/Chick Peas,** 1/2 c, 4.2 oz | 145 | 1.5 | 27 |
| **Hearts of Palm,** (1), 1.2 oz | 7 | 0 | 1 |
| **Mushrooms:** 1/2 cup, 2.5 oz | 20 | 0 | 4 |
| In Butter Sauce, 2 oz | 20 | 1 | 2 |
| **Onions:** Cocktail (1) | 0 | 0 | 0 |
| Pickled, 1 medium, 0.5 oz | 10 | 0 | 2 |
| **Peas,** 1/2 cup, 3.4 oz | 60 | 0.5 | 10 |
| **Peppers:** Hot Chili, Jalapeno (1), 1 oz | 5 | 0 | 1 |
| Red/Green, 1 oz | 5 | 0 | 1 |
| Sweet, undrained, 2.5 oz | 13 | 0 | 3 |
| Jalapeno, with liquid, | | | |
| 1/2 cup chopped | 20 | 0.5 | 3 |
| Fried, drained, 2 Tbsp, 1 oz | 60 | 5 | 3 |
| **Salsa,** average all varieties, 2 Tbsp | 10 | 0 | 2 |
| **Sauerkraut,** drained, 1 cup, 5 oz | 25 | 0 | 6 |
| **Spinach,** 1/2 cup, 3.5 oz | 25 | 0.5 | 3.5 |
| **Succotash:** Cream Style, 1/2 cup | 100 | 0.5 | 23 |
| w/ whole kernels, undrained, 1/2 cup | 80 | 0.5 | 18 |
| **Sweetcorn** ~ *See Corn* | | | |
| **Sweet Potato,** 1/2 cup, 3.5 oz | 90 | 0 | 24 |
| **Tomatoes,** Sundried: Nat., 5-6 pieces | 20 | 0 | 5 |
| In Oil, drained, 6 pieces, 0.5 oz | 40 | 2.5 | 4 |
| **Tomato Products** ~ *See Page 144* | | | |
| **Vegetables,** mixed, 1/2 cup, 4 oz | 45 | 0 | 8 |
| **Yams:** In Light Syrup, 1/2 cup, 4 oz | 105 | 0 | 25 |
| Candied, 1/2 cup, 5 oz | 170 | 0 | 46 |
| **Zucchini,** in Tomato Sauce, 1/2 cup, 4 oz | 30 | 0 | 8 |

Updated Nutrition Data ~ www.CalorieKing.com
Persons with Diabetes ~ See Disclaimer (Page 22)

161

## Quick Guide    **C** **F** **Cb**

**Yogurt:** *Average All Brands: Per 8 oz Container*

| | C | F | Cb |
|---|---|---|---|
| **Plain Yogurt:** Whole | 140 | 8 | 10 |
| Low-Fat | 145 | 3.5 | 16 |
| Fat-Free | 125 | 0.5 | 17 |
| **Fruit Flavored:** Whole | 225 | 8 | 32 |
| Low-Fat | 230 | 3 | 43 |
| Fat-Free, regular | 215 | 0.5 | 43 |
| Fat-Free, no sugar added | 80 | 0 | 15 |

**Yogurt Parfait/Deli Cups:**

**With Fruit Pieces:** ($^2/_3$ Yogurt + $^1/_3$ Fruit)

| | C | F | Cb |
|---|---|---|---|
| Small, 8 oz cup | 140 | 3 | 20 |
| Large, 12 oz cup | 210 | 4.5 | 30 |

**With Fruit + Granola:**

| | C | F | Cb |
|---|---|---|---|
| Small, 8 oz cup (+ 0.75 oz Granola) | 235 | 7 | 30 |
| Large, 12 oz cup (+ 1.3 oz Granola) | 400 | 13 | 58 |

## Yogurt ~ Brands

**Activia:**

| | C | F | Cb |
|---|---|---|---|
| **4 oz Containers:** Fiber with Fruit, av. | 100 | 1.5 | 19 |
| Fruit/Fusion, average all flavors | 90 | 2 | 15 |
| Lactose Free, average | 100 | 2 | 16 |
| Light, nonfat, all flavors | 60 | 0 | 10 |
| **Probiotic:** Fruit flavors, av. | 90 | 1.5 | 16 |
| Fruit On Bottom | 90 | 2 | 15 |
| Fruit with Cereal | 100 | 1.5 | 19 |
| Lactose Free, Fruit Flav., av., | 90 | 2 | 16 |
| Light Fruit Flavors, average, 4 oz | 60 | 0 | 10 |
| **Greek, nonfat, 5.3 oz Ctn:** | | | |
| Regular, average all flavors | 125 | 0 | 20 |
| Probiotic: Blueberry, non fat, 5.3 oz | 150 | 0 | 18 |
| Other flavors, 5.3 oz | 125 | 0 | 19 |

**Axelrod:**

| | C | F | Cb |
|---|---|---|---|
| **32 oz Ctn:** Regular Plain, 8 oz | 160 | 8 | 15 |
| Fat Free, Plain, 8 oz | 130 | 0 | 19 |
| **6 oz Containers:** | | | |
| Low Fat, Fruit flavors, av. | 180 | 1.5 | 36 |
| NonFat Vanilla | 90 | 0 | 17 |

**Brown Cow:**

**Cream Top, On The Bottom:** *Per 5.3 oz Ctn*

| | C | F | Cb |
|---|---|---|---|
| Whole Milk: Apricot Mango | 150 | 5 | 22 |
| Chocolate | 170 | 5 | 26 |
| Fruit Flavors, average | 160 | 5 | 24 |

**Cream Top:** *Per 5.3 oz Ctn*

| | C | F | Cb |
|---|---|---|---|
| Whole Milk: Plain | 110 | 6 | 9 |
| Cherry Vanilla | 160 | 5 | 25 |
| Coffee; Vanilla | 150 | 6 | 18 |
| Specialties Flavors | 150 | 5 | 22 |

**Cabot:** *Per 8 oz Serving*    **C** **F** **Cb**

**Greek Style, 32 oz Ctn:**

| | C | F | Cb |
|---|---|---|---|
| Plain | 310 | 22 | 12 |
| Lowfat (2%): Plain | 180 | 5 | 12 |
| Strawberry; Van. Bean, av. | 240 | 4 | 35 |
| Triple Cream, Vanilla Bean | 350 | 17 | 35 |
| **Nonfat,** Plain | 110 | 0 | 18 |

**Chobani Greek Yogurt:** *Per 5.3 oz Unless Indicated*

| | C | F | Cb |
|---|---|---|---|
| **Blended:** Coconut | 140 | 4.5 | 15 |
| Mixed Berry | 140 | 2.5 | 18 |
| **Coconut Based:** Plain, slightly swt | 130 | 8 | 16 |
| Other flavors | 145 | 7 | 20 |
| **Creamy Blended,** average | 150 | 4.5 | 16 |
| **Flip:** Almond Coco Loco | 230 | 10 | 23 |
| Coffee Brownie Bliss | 180 | 4 | 25 |
| **Fruit On The Bottom:** | | | |
| Apricot; Mango; Strawb Banana, av. | 130 | 2.5 | 18 |
| Strawberry/Blueb./Back Cherry, av. | 115 | 0 | 17 |
| **Gimmies,** average all flavors, 4 oz | 145 | 4 | 20 |
| **Less Sugar:** *Per 4.5 oz Ctn* | | | |
| Honey Pistachio/Van. Mocha, av. | 140 | 4 | 16 |
| Mango Coconut | 160 | 7 | 13 |
| Wild Blueb./Madag. Van. Cinnamon | 120 | 2.5 | 11 |
| **Nut Butter,** average all flavors, 5.3 oz | 165 | 7 | 15 |
| **Plain, 32 oz Ctn::** Lowfat, 8 oz | 130 | 3.5 | 7 |
| Nonfat, 8 oz | 90 | 0 | 6 |
| Whole Milk, 8 oz | 170 | 9 | 7 |

**Dannon:**

**Activia ~** *See Activia*

| | C | F | Cb |
|---|---|---|---|
| **Creamy,** Strawberry, 4 oz | 70 | 0 | 14 |
| **Fruit On The Bottom,** av, 5.3 oz | 130 | 1.5 | 25 |
| **Lowfat:** Plain, 6 oz | 100 | 2.5 | 12 |
| Coffee; Vanilla, 6 oz | 140 | 2 | 24 |
| **Plain, 32 oz Ctn:** Lowat, 8 oz | 150 | 3.5 | 19 |
| Nonfat, 8 oz | 120 | 0 | 18 |
| Whole Milk, 8 oz | 150 | 8 | 11 |
| **Whole Milk,** all flav., 5.3 oz | 140 | 4.5 | 20 |

**Fage Greek Yogurt:**

| | C | F | Cb |
|---|---|---|---|
| **Total:** Plain 5% Milk Fat, 7 oz | 190 | 10 | 6 |
| Plain, 2% Milk Fat, 7 oz | 140 | 4 | 6 |
| Plain, 0% Milk Fat, 6oz | 90 | 0 | 5 |
| **Total Split Cups:** *Per 5.3 oz* | | | |
| 5% Milk Fat: Fruit Flav., av. | 150 | 6 | 13 |
| Honey | 210 | 6 | 29 |
| 2% Milk Fat: Fruit Flavors | 120 | 2.5 | 13 |
| Honey | 190 | 2.5 | 29 |
| 0% Milk Fat, Fruit Flavors | 105 | 0 | 14 |

## Yogurt Brands (Cont)

| | C | F | Cb |
|---|---|---|---|
| **Great Value** (Walmart): | | | |
| **Greek, Fat Free:** | | | |
| 32 oz Ctn: Plain, 6 oz | 90 | 0 | 7 |
| Vanilla, 6 oz | 90 | 0 | 10 |
| **Greek Non Fat Light:** Per 5.3 oz Ctn | | | |
| Banana Cream; Peach; Vanilla | 80 | 0 | 9 |
| Strawberry | 120 | 0 | 19 |
| **Original, 32 Oz Ctn:** | | | |
| Strawberry Banana; Vanilla, 6 oz | 130 | 1.5 | 26 |
| **Kemps:** | | | |
| **5 lb Containers:** | | | |
| **Lowfat:** Plain, Sweeetened, 6 oz | 120 | 2 | 15 |
| **Nonfat:** Raspberry, 6 oz | 130 | 0 | 27 |
| Strawberry; Blueberry, 6 oz | 120 | 0 | 26 |
| Vanilla, 6 oz | 130 | 0 | 28 |
| **Kroger,** CarbMaster, all flavors, 6 oz | 70 | 1.5 | 5 |
| **La Yogurt:** Per 6 oz Container | | | |
| **Low Fat:** Orig., Fruit Flavors, av. | 155 | 1.5 | 30 |
| Rich & Creamy, Fruit Flav., av. | 180 | 1.5 | 33 |
| **LALA:** | | | |
| **32 oz Tubs,** Plain, 6 oz | 110 | 1.5 | 14 |
| **Singles,** Fruit Flav., av., 6 oz | 160 | 1.5 | 30 |
| **Lucerne:** | | | |
| **Greek Nonfat,** Plain, 8 oz | 130 | 0 | 14 |
| **Low-Fat,** Mixed Berry, 6 oz | 140 | 2 | 26 |
| **Light Nonfat,** Blueberry, 6 oz | 100 | 0 | 18 |
| **Fat Free,** Plain, 6 oz | 90 | 0 | 16 |
| **Mountain High:** Per 8 oz | | | |
| **32 oz Containers:** | | | |
| Whole Milk Original: Plain | 170 | 7 | 15 |
| Strawberry; Vanilla | 200 | 7 | 28 |
| Lowfat: Plain | 130 | 2.5 | 16 |
| Vanilla | 170 | 2.5 | 28 |
| Fat Free: Plain | 110 | 0 | 16 |
| Vanilla | 160 | 0 | 28 |
| **Nancy's:** | | | |
| **Natural Whole Milk:** Per 8 oz | | | |
| Fruit On Top, average | 225 | 5 | 39 |
| Honey | 170 | 8 | 17 |
| **Nonfat Fruit On Top:** Raspberry, 8 oz | 170 | 0 | 32 |
| Strawberry, 8 oz | 160 | 0 | 30 |
| Other Fruit Flavors, average, 8 oz | 150 | 0 | 27 |
| **Fruit on Bottom,** av., 8 oz | 145 | 0 | 27 |
| **Organic:** Grass Fed, Vanilla, 6 oz | 140 | 6 | 15 |
| Greek: Plain, 6 oz | 160 | 6 | 7 |
| Honey, 6 oz | 180 | 6 | 12 |
| Lowfat, Plain, 8 oz | 150 | 3 | 16 |
| Nonfat: Plain, 8 oz | 120 | 0 | 17 |
| Maple; Vanilla, 6 oz | 120 | 0 | 21 |
| Whole Milk, Plain, 8 oz | 180 | 8 | 16 |

| | C | F | Cb |
|---|---|---|---|
| **Oikos** (Dannon): | | | |
| **Crunch:** Vanilla Almond, 5 oz | 180 | 7 | 18 |
| Other Flavors, av., 5 oz | 170 | 3 | 25 |
| **Nonfat,** Plain, 5.3 oz | 80 | 0 | 6 |
| **Oh! Double Cream,** av. all flav., 5.3 oz | 215 | 11 | 23 |
| **Protein,** av. all flavors, 5 oz | 155 | 1.5 | 19 |
| **Triple Zero Greek,** all flavors, 5.3 oz | 120 | 0 | 14 |
| **Whole Milk,** av. all flav., 5.3 oz | 160 | 4 | 20 |
| **0 Organics** (Vons): Greek, Vanilla, 6 oz | 130 | 0 | 15 |
| Whole Milk: Plain, 6 oz | 130 | 6 | 11 |
| Vanilla, 6 oz | 160 | 6 | 22 |
| **Siggi's:** | | | |
| **Skyr:** Per 5.3 oz Unless Indicated | | | |
| **0%:** Plain | 90 | 0 | 6 |
| All Flavors, average | 110 | 0 | 13 |
| **2%:** Coconut | 170 | 5 | 16 |
| Fruit Flavors, average | 140 | 2.5 | 14 |
| **4%:** Fruit flavors, 4.4 oz | 130 | 4.5 | 11 |
| Fruit, no added sugar, av., 4.4 oz | 115 | 4 | 8 |
| **Simple Sides,** av. all flavors, 5.3 oz | 200 | 8 | 18 |
| **Triple Cream,** Vanilla Flav., av., 4 oz | 200 | 8 | 17 |
| **Silk:** Per 5.3 oz Containers | | | |
| **Almond Yogurt:** Plain | 180 | 13 | 10 |
| Fruit flavors, average | 180 | 11 | 18 |
| Vanilla | 200 | 11 | 21 |
| **Oat Yeah,** Vanilla | 80 | 0 | 17 |
| **Soy Yogurt:** Fruit flavors, av | 140 | 3.5 | 21 |
| Vanilla | 140 | 3.5 | 20 |
| **So Delicious:** | | | |
| **Coconut Milk:** Plain, 8 oz | 170 | 7 | 25 |
| Blueberry, 5.3 oz | 140 | 4 | 24 |
| Chocolate, 5.3 oz | 150 | 5 | 27 |
| Vanilla, 5.3 oz | 130 | 4 | 22 |
| Unsweetened, Plain; Vanilla, 8 oz | 110 | 7 | 11 |
| **Oatmilk,** av, all flavors, 5.3 oz | 75 | 0 | 16 |
| **Stonyfield Organic:** | | | |
| **Dairy Free** (Soy): | | | |
| Fruit Flav., 5.3 oz | 150 | 2.5 | 26 |
| Vanilla | 130 | 2.5 | 20 |
| **Fruit On The Bottom:** | | | |
| Blueberry On The Bottom, 5.3 oz | 90 | 0 | 17 |
| Chocolate Underground, 5.3 oz | 120 | 0 | 22 |
| **0% Fat,** Plain, 5.3 oz | 70 | 0 | 10 |
| **Low Fat:** Plain, 8 oz | 110 | 2 | 14 |
| Strawberry, 5.3 oz | 100 | 1.5 | 16 |
| Vanilla | 150 | 2 | 25 |
| **Whole Milk:** Strawb.; Vanilla, 5.3 oz | 140 | 5 | 18 |
| **32 oz Ctn:** Plain, 1 cup 8 oz | 160 | 9 | 12 |
| Maple, 8 oz | 200 | 8 | 24 |
| **Greek,** Plain, 5.3 oz | 130 | 5 | 6 |
| **Pouch,** Strawb. Beet Berry, 3.5 oz | 100 | 3 | 12 |
| **Yobaby,** Apple; Blueberry, 4oz | 100 | 4 | 12 |

# Y Yogurt

## Yogurt Brands (Cont) — C F Cb

| Trader Joe's: | C | F | Cb |
|---|---|---|---|
| **Organic:** Greek, Nonfat, Plain | 80 | 0 | 6 |
| Whole Milk, Strawb., 5.3 oz | 150 | 5 | 17 |
| Lowfat, av. all flavors, 6 oz | 150 | 2.5 | 26 |
| Nonfat, plain, 6 oz | 80 | 0 | 6 |
| **Greek, Lowfat (2%):** | | | |
| Almond Butter coconut, 5.3 oz | 170 | 6 | 16 |
| Plain, 1 cup, 8 oz | 120 | 0 | 7 |
| **Greek, Whole Milk:** | | | |
| 5.3 oz Cups, av. all flavors | 180 | 6 | 18 |
| 16 oz Ctn: Plain, 1 cup, 8 oz | 280 | 22 | 12 |
| **Greek Low Fat Mix-Ins:** | | | |
| Coconut & Almond Granola, 5.3 oz | 190 | 5 | 21 |
| Vanilla & Pretzel, 5.3 oz | 180 | 3.5 | 27 |
| **Icelandic Style:** | | | |
| Non Fat: Plain, 8 oz | 130 | 0 | 10 |
| Strawberry, 8 oz | 190 | 0 | 26 |
| **Low Fat:** | | | |
| Vanilla with Almonds, 4.6 oz | 160 | 7 | 20 |
| Prestirred, Strawberry, 8 oz | 220 | 3 | 40 |
| **European Style:** | | | |
| Organic, Plain: Whole Milk, 1 cup, 8 oz | 170 | 7 | 14 |
| Nonfat, 1 up, 8 oz | 120 | 0 | 17 |
| **Voskos:** | | | |
| **Greek:** | | | |
| 2x Protein (0%), Exotic Fig, 5.3 oz | 160 | 0 | 28 |
| Real Fruit: Fruit Flavors, av., 6 oz | 140 | 0 | 19 |
| Coconut Cream, 6 oz | 160 | 0 | 22 |
| 16 oz Tubs: Orig. Plain, 8 oz | 280 | 20 | 15 |
| Nonfat Vanilla, 8 oz | 200 | 0 | 30 |
| **Wallaby Organic:** | | | |
| **Aussie Creme**, average, 5.3 oz | 215 | 11 | 2 |
| **Lowfat Greek**, Plain, 5.3 oz | 100 | 2 | 7 |
| **Whole Milk Greek**, Fruit Flav., 5.3 oz | 170 | 6 | 19 |
| **Wegmans:** | | | |
| **Fruit On The Bottom, Lowfat:** | | | |
| Blueberry; Cherry Vanilla, 6 oz | 160 | 2 | 29 |
| Average other Fruit Flavors, 6 oz | 175 | 2 | 34 |
| **Greek**, Organic Non-Fat: Plain, 5.3 oz | 100 | 0 | 6 |
| Fruit flavors, av., 5.3 oz | 125 | 0 | 18 |
| Vanilla, 5.3 oz | 110 | 0 | 13 |
| **Whole Foods (365):** | | | |
| **32 oz Ctn, Plain:** Whole Milk, 8oz | 160 | 9 | 13 |
| Low-Fat, 8 oz | 120 | 2 | 15 |
| Fat-Free, 8 oz | 120 | 0 | 17 |
| **6 oz Ctn:** Blueb. Lemon | 160 | 1.5 | 31 |
| Peach Melba | 140 | 1 | 27 |
| **Greek**, 0% Nonfat, Plain, 6 oz | 80 | 0 | 5 |
| **YoCrunch:** *Per 4 oz Container* | | | |
| **Lowfat Vanilla Yogurt:** | | | |
| Chips Ahoy; Twix, av. | 185 | 4 | 32 |
| M&M's; Oreo, av. | 125 | 3 | 22 |

## Yogurt Brands (Cont) — C F Cb

| Yoplait: | C | F | Cb |
|---|---|---|---|
| **Original:** All flavors, 6 oz | 155 | 2 | 28 |
| Multipack, all flavors, 6 oz | 150 | 2 | 26 |
| **32 Container:** | | | |
| Plain, nonfat, 8 oz | 130 | 0 | 20 |
| Average Fruit Flavors, 8 oz | 200 | 1.5 | 41 |
| **Light,** 6 oz cup, all flavors | 90 | 0 | 16 |
| **Lactose Free,** av. all flavors, 6 oz | 150 | 2 | 26 |
| **FruitSide,** all flavors, 5.3 oz | 160 | 4 | 25 |
| **Greek 100 Protein,** av. all flav., 5.3 oz | 100 | 0 | 11 |
| **Go-Gurt:** Tube, 2 oz | 50 | 0.5 | 10 |
| Dunkers, av., 2.2 oz tray | 125 | 3 | 23 |
| Characters, all flavors, 2 oz tube | 50 | 0.5 | 10 |
| **Snack Size,** Blueb. Strawb. Banana, 4 oz | 100 | 1 | 21 |
| **Whips!:** | | | |
| Regular: Coconut Crème, 4 oz | 150 | 4 | 24 |
| Chocolate, Vanilla Crème, 4 oz | 160 | 4 | 25 |
| Sea Salt Caramel, 4 oz | 160 | 4 | 27 |
| Average other flavors, 4 oz | 140 | 2 | 25 |
| Greek 100, all flavors, 4 oz | 100 | 0 | 15 |
| **YQ (Ultra-Filtered):** Plain, 5.3 oz | 100 | 3 | 2 |
| Coconut, 5.3 oz | 120 | 2.5 | 9 |
| Other Flavors, 5.3 oz | 130 | 2.5 | 12 |

## Yogurt Drinks & Probiotics

| Dannon: | C | F | Cb |
|---|---|---|---|
| **Activia Probiotics:** | | | |
| Dailies, all flavors, 3.15 fl.oz | 70 | 1.5 | 12 |
| Drinks, av. all flavors, 7 fl oz | 165 | 3 | 28 |
| Smoothies, av. all flavors, 7 fl.oz | 135 | 4 | 18 |
| **DanActive Dailies,** all flav., 3.1 fl.oz | 70 | 1 | 11 |
| **Danimals Smoothies,** | | | |
| average all flavors, 3.1 fl.oz | 50 | 0 | 11 |
| **Light & Fit,** all flavors, 7 fl.oz | 90 | 0 | 14 |
| **Glen Oaks,** av. all flav., 8 fl.oz | 150 | 2.5 | 27 |
| **Lifeway Kefir:** | | | |
| **Biokefir,** all flavors, 3.5 fl.oz | 60 | 0 | 10 |
| **Organic Whole Milk:** Plain, 8 fl.oz | 160 | 8 | 12 |
| Other Flavors, 8 fl.oz | 190 | 8 | 20 |
| **Organic Lowfat:** Plain, 8 fl.oz | 110 | 2 | 12 |
| Other flavors, 8 fl.oz | 140 | 2 | 20 |
| **Plantiful:** Plain, 8 fl.oz | 90 | 1 | 9 |
| Other Flavors, 8 fl.oz | 110 | 1 | 14 |
| **Probugs,** 3.5 fl.oz | 80 | 3 | 11 |
| **Stonyfield:** | | | |
| **Smoothies: Low Fat,** av., 6 oz | 110 | 1.5 | 17 |
| 10 oz bottle, average | 180 | 3 | 29 |
| **Whole Milk,** Strawberry, 6 oz | 160 | 7 | 18 |
| **Yakult:** Regular, 2.7 fl.oz bottle | 50 | 0 | 12 |
| **Light,** 2.7 fl.oz | 30 | 0 | 6 |

## Cafeteria-Style Foods | **C** | **F** | **Cb**

*Average All Preparations:*

| | C | F | Cb |
|---|---|---|---|
| **Beef Stroganoff**, 5 oz | 195 | 13 | 7 |
| **Beef Stroganoff**, with 4 oz noodles | 350 | 14 | 36 |
| **Chicken Lasagna**, 1 piece | 300 | 11 | 32 |
| **Chicken Chop Suey**, with 4 oz rice | 245 | 4 | 37 |
| **Deep Dish Burrito**, 7 oz | 265 | 13 | 20 |
| **Ground Beef Casserole**, 2 scps, 6 oz | 245 | 13 | 17 |
| **Italian Meat Sce**, for Spaghetti, 5 oz | 150 | 9 | 9 |
| with 5 oz Spaghetti | 350 | 10 | 49 |
| **Lasagna**, 1 piece | 275 | 11 | 25 |
| **Meatloaf**, 3 oz | 205 | 13 | 4 |
| **Ranch Beans**, 2 scoops, 6 oz | 350 | 11 | 45 |
| **Red Beans & Rice**, 7 oz | 280 | 9 | 37 |
| **Scalloped Potato/Ham**, 2 scoops, 6 oz | 160 | 6 | 20 |
| **Stuffed Shells in Sauce**, (1) | 105 | 3 | 17 |
| **Swedish Meatballs**, (3) | 205 | 12 | 9 |
| **Sweet & Sour Pork/Rice**, 9 oz | 240 | 3 | 40 |
| **Swiss Steak**, w/ Mushroom Gravy, 6 oz | 280 | 11 | 4 |
| **Tator Tot Casserole**, 2 scoops, 6 oz | 260 | 15 | 20 |
| **Tenderloin Tips/Mshrm Gravy:** 5 oz | 210 | 13 | 3 |
| With 5 oz noodles | 395 | 15 | 38 |
| **Tuna Noodle Casserole**, 2 scoops, 6 oz | 180 | 6 | 17 |
| **Turkey Tetrazzini**, 2 scoops, 6 oz | 195 | 7 | 17 |
| **Vegetable Lasagna**, 1 piece | 250 | 13 | 21 |

### Croissants

| | C | F | Cb |
|---|---|---|---|
| **Unfilled**, medium 1.5 oz | 180 | 10 | 21 |
| **Filled:** With Ham (2 oz), garnish | 280 | 14 | 24 |
| With Ham (2 oz), Cheese (2 oz) | 470 | 30 | 20 |
| With Chick (2 oz) Cheese (2 oz) | 470 | 30 | 20 |
| With Turkey/Ham/Cheese (2 oz ea.) | 580 | 36 | 20 |
| *Au Bon Pain:* Ham & Cheese | 390 | 21 | 35 |
| Spinach & Cheese | 290 | 17 | 28 |

**7-Eleven** ~ *See Page 236*

### Bagels

| | C | F | Cb |
|---|---|---|---|
| **Plain:** Large, 4 oz (without filling) | 320 | 2 | 65 |
| With 2 oz Cream Cheese | 500 | 27 | 54 |
| With 2 oz Lox (Smoked Salmon) | 400 | 4 | 65 |

**Also see Bagels Section** ~ *Page 54*
**Fast-Foods Restaurants** ~ *Page 175*
**Au Bon Pain** ~ *Page 179*
**Bruegger's** ~ *Page 185*
**Einstein Bros Bagels** ~ *Page 199*

## Sandwiches | **C** | **F** | **Cb**

*No Spreads Unless Indicated:*
*Includes 2 Slices Bread ~ 3 oz*

| | C | F | Cb |
|---|---|---|---|
| **BLT**, (5 strips Bacon, 2 Tbsp Mayo) | 600 | 40 | 46 |
| **Breaded Chicken & Garnish** | 540 | 28 | 46 |
| **Chicken Salad**, with Mayo., 5 oz | 580 | 30 | 49 |
| **Chopped Liver, Egg Mayonnaise** | 630 | 25 | 44 |
| **Corned Beef with Mustard**, 5 oz | 560 | 28 | 44 |
| **Egg Salad**, with Mayonnaise | 570 | 29 | 49 |
| **Egg Salad Club**, with Bacon & Mayo, | 780 | 53 | 49 |
| **Grilled Cheese**, (3 oz) | 540 | 30 | 44 |
| **Ham**, (4 oz), Cheese (4 oz), & Mayo. | 910 | 56 | 44 |
| **Lobster Salad**, (4 oz), w/ Mayo. | 530 | 25 | 45 |
| **Overstuffed Tuna Salad**, (7 oz) | 870 | 39 | 75 |
| **Philly Cheese Steak Sandwich** | 550 | 23 | 42 |
| **Reuben**, (6 oz Beef/Pastrami, | | | |
| 2 oz Cheese, 2 Tbsp Dressing) | 920 | 60 | 28 |
| **Roast Beef**, (4 oz), with Mustard | 460 | 12 | 45 |
| **Roast Pork**, (4 oz), with Apple Sauce | 500 | 16 | 55 |
| **Shrimp Salad Club**, w/ Bacon & Mayo | 800 | 57 | 48 |
| **Sloppy Joe with Sauce**, (7 oz) | 600 | 30 | 45 |
| **Steak Sandwich**, (5 oz cooked) | 680 | 32 | 41 |
| **Triple Cheese Melt**, (4 oz) | 720 | 45 | 46 |
| **Tuna Salad**, (5 oz), with Mayonnaise | 610 | 30 | 49 |
| **Turkey Breast**, (5 oz), w/ Mayo. | 460 | 18 | 44 |
| **Turkey Breast**, (5 oz,) with Mustard | 360 | 7 | 44 |
| **Turkey Club**, with Bacon & Mayo. | 830 | 38 | 31 |
| **Vegetarian**, with Avocado & Cheese | 820 | 49 | 72 |

**7-Eleven** ~ *Page 236*
**Schlotzsky's** ~ *Page 237*
**Subway** ~ *Page 245*

### Wraps & Roll-Ups

*Average All Types*
**Meat/Chicken/Fish/Veggie:**

| | C | F | Cb |
|---|---|---|---|
| Small, approximately 9 oz | 500 | 25 | 48 |
| Regular, approximately 15 oz | 830 | 40 | 80 |
| Large, approximately 22 oz | 1400 | 70 | 134 |

**Fast-Foods Restaurants** ~ *Page 175*
**Au Bon Pain** ~ *Page 179*
**Sonic Drive-In** ~ *Page 241*
**Subway** ~ *Page 245*
**WAWA** ~ *Page 254*

## Fair & Carnival Foods  **C**  **E**  **CP**

**Barbeque Chicken/Meats:**

| | C | E | CP |
|---|---|---|---|
| **Chicken**, ½ chicken, 15 oz | 740 | 24 | 34 |
| **Grilled Chicken Pita**, with dressing | 680 | 19 | 82 |
| **Teriyaki Chicken**, on stick, w/ dress. | 250 | 6 | 4 |
| **Pork Ribs**, 18 oz | 1360 | 68 | 21 |
| **Turkey Leg:** Regular, 19 oz | 1135 | 54 | 0 |
| Caveman (2lb Turkey Leg, with 1lb Bacon) | 2360 | 177 | 3 |
| **Bacon:** Fried, on-a-stick, with syrup | 230 | 16 | 5 |
| Choc-covered Bacon, 4.5 oz dish | 640 | 43 | 30 |
| **Beef Stew over Rice**, 2 cups | 440 | 14 | 61 |
| **Butter Balls**, deep fried, 4 Balls | 460 | 38 | 24 |
| **Cheese Curds**, Breaded & fried, *Culver's*, 6.7 oz | 670 | 38 | 54 |
| **Corn Dogs:** Regular, 4 oz | 250 | 14 | 23 |
| Jumbo, 6 oz | 375 | 21 | 36 |
| Pretzel-Wrapped Dog | 300 | 16 | 30 |
| Papa Pup, on-a-stick | 400 | 24 | 32 |
| Pronto Pup, on-a-stick | 170 | 9 | 16 |
| **Corn On The Cob**, 8″ (1), 16 oz | 200 | 1 | 42 |

**Finger Foods:**

| | C | E | CP |
|---|---|---|---|
| **Artichoke**, fried, 9 pieces | 250 | 14 | 24 |
| **Chicken Nuggets**, (6) | 340 | 17 | 26 |
| **Chicken Strips**, (4), 4.5 oz | 445 | 21 | 33 |
| **Onion Rings**, 3 rings | 310 | 13 | 40 |
| **Onion Flower** | 1320 | 72 | 140 |
| **Shrimp**, Fried, 10-12 pieces, 5 oz | 555 | 30 | 36 |
| **Spam**, deep-fried in batter, 2 pieces | 330 | 24 | 18 |

**Gator:**

| | C | E | CP |
|---|---|---|---|
| **Big Gator**, Nuggets/Hushpuppies | 550 | 31 | 54 |
| **Stick Gator**, 1 sausage | 250 | 20 | 4 |

**Greek:**

| | C | E | CP |
|---|---|---|---|
| **Baklava**, 2″ square | 245 | 13 | 32 |
| **Falafel**, 11.6 oz | 660 | 27 | 85 |
| **Greek Salad**, 14 oz | 520 | 48 | 17 |
| **Gyro**, 7.5″, 12 oz | 680 | 40 | 55 |
| **Spanakopita**, 8 oz | 200 | 7.5 | 23 |

**Hamburgers:**

| | C | E | CP |
|---|---|---|---|
| ⅓ **Pound Burger**, 7.5 oz | 670 | 41 | 26 |
| **Cheeseburger**, 6 oz | 550 | 36 | 25 |

**Hot Dogs:** *With Bun*

| | C | E | CP |
|---|---|---|---|
| **Regular:** No extras | 215 | 14 | 28 |
| With Chili, 6 oz | 450 | 32 | 32 |
| With Chili & Cheese, 7.3 oz | 500 | 36 | 31 |
| ⅓ **Pound Hot Dog** | 550 | 41 | 31 |
| **Foot Long Hot Dog** | 470 | 26 | 41 |
| **Jumbo**, Bratwurst/Kielbasa, average | 800 | 60 | 28 |

## Fair & Carnival Foods (Cont)

**Mexican:**  **C**  **F**  **Cb**

| | C | F | Cb |
|---|---|---|---|
| **Burrito**, with Bean/Beef, 17 oz | 1100 | 41 | 104 |
| **Carne Asada**, 14.5 oz | 820 | 44 | 58 |
| **Cheese Quesadilla**, 1.8 oz | 480 | 27 | 40 |
| **Chicken Taco**, 3.3 oz | 210 | 12 | 16 |
| **Fish Taco**, 5 oz | 270 | 13 | 31 |
| **Jalapeno Pepper**, choc-covered (3) | 270 | 15 | 31 |
| **Nachos with Cheese**, 9″ plate | 860 | 59 | 70 |
| **Tamale**, 3.5 oz | 180 | 8 | 21 |
| **Taquito**, 5 oz | 370 | 17 | 43 |

**Pizza:**

| | C | F | Cb |
|---|---|---|---|
| **Pizza Bread**, Pepperoni, ½ loaf, 12 oz | 1115 | 32 | 151 |
| **Pizza on-a-stick**, 1 piece | 535 | 28 | 55 |
| **Personal Pizza:** *Per 7″* | | | |
| Cheese | 670 | 24 | 80 |
| Pepperoni | 795 | 35 | 80 |
| Ham & Pineapple | 800 | 31 | 87 |

**Potatoes & Fries:**

| | C | F | Cb |
|---|---|---|---|
| **Australian Battered Potatoes** | 1290 | 66 | 155 |
| **Baked Potato**, 14 oz | 435 | 0.5 | 100 |
| **Fries:** French, 7 oz | 560 | 24 | 79 |
| Cheese Fries, 10 oz | 645 | 38 | 62 |
| Chili Fries, 10 oz | 700 | 36 | 83 |
| Curly Fries, 7 oz | 620 | 30 | 78 |
| Jamaican Jerk Fries, 7 oz | 640 | 34 | 77 |
| **Sweet Potato**, baked, 14 oz | 405 | 0.5 | 97 |
| **Tornado**, on-a-stick | 210 | 15 | 18 |

**Salads/Sides:**

| | C | F | Cb |
|---|---|---|---|
| **Chili**, 1 cup | 280 | 11 | 24 |
| **Cole Slaw**, 5 oz | 350 | 21 | 37 |
| **Pickle**, whole (6″) | 30 | 0 | 8 |
| **Potato Salad**, 5 oz | 290 | 15 | 35 |

**Sandwiches:** *7½″ Roll*

| | C | F | Cb |
|---|---|---|---|
| **Ham**, 11 oz | 645 | 39 | 47 |
| **Hot Pastrami**, 9 oz | 760 | 17 | 62 |
| **Roast Beef**, 11 oz | 620 | 36 | 46 |
| **Philadelphia Cheese Steak**, 13 oz | 680 | 36 | 49 |
| **Turkey**, 11 oz | 665 | 24 | 65 |

**Drinks:**

| | C | F | Cb |
|---|---|---|---|
| **Icee**, 16 fl.oz | 235 | 0 | 59 |
| **Shakes**, average, 16 fl.oz | 690 | 33 | 85 |
| **Slushies:** Horchata, 16 fl.oz | 280 | 8 | 50 |
| Lemonade, 18 fl.oz | 210 | 0 | 52 |
| Orange Julius, 20 fl.oz | 490 | 10 | 96 |
| Strawberry Julius, 20 fl.oz | 430 | 0 | 98 |
| **Soft Frozen Lemonade**, 12 fl.oz | 300 | 0 | 78 |
| **Smoothies**, Berry Flavors, 16 fl.oz | 350 | 1 | 80 |

## Fair & Carnival Foods (Cont)

| | C | F | Cb |
|---|---|---|---|
| **Cakes, Pastries:** | | | |
| **Funnel Cake,** Plain (1) | 760 | 44 | 80 |
| **Toppings:** | | | |
| Apple Cinnamon, 2 oz | 85 | 3 | 16 |
| Cinnamon & Sugar, 2 tsp | 40 | 0 | 10 |
| Strawberry & Cream, 2 oz | 70 | 0 | 16 |
| **Cheesecake on-a-stick,** 6 oz | 655 | 47 | 56 |
| **Churro,** (1), 9", 1.6 oz | 170 | 8 | 22 |
| **Cream Puff,** 4.3 oz | 500 | 43 | 22 |
| **Fried Twinkie,** (1) | 420 | 34 | 45 |
| **Puff-on-a-Stick,** (4), 8.6 oz | 995 | 86 | 44 |
| **Strawberry Crepe,** 4.3 oz | 280 | 14 | 36 |
| **Twinkie Dog,** (Sundae) | 500 | 14 | 89 |
| **Candied Apple,** 7 oz | 330 | 0 | 80 |
| **Cookies:** | | | |
| **Sweet Martha,** (1), 0.8 oz | 90 | 4 | 14 |
| **Deep Fried: Oreos,** tray (5) | 890 | 48 | 108 |
| Cookie Dough on stick, 3 pieces | 670 | 32 | 89 |
| **Cotton Candy:** | | | |
| Small, 1 oz | 110 | 0 | 27 |
| Large, 2.3 oz | 250 | 0 | 62 |
| Family Size, 5.5 oz | 610 | 0 | 151 |
| **Dirt Dessert,** 1 cup, 9.3 oz | 405 | 12 | 69 |
| **Donuts,** Jumbo Twist, (1), 7.5 oz | 905 | 49 | 109 |
| **Fried Dough/FryBread:** | | | |
| **Plain:** 7", 3.7 oz | 390 | 19 | 47 |
| 9", 4³/₄ oz | 510 | 25 | 61 |
| **Toppings:** Cinnamon Sugar, 2 tsp | 40 | 0 | 10 |
| Butterscotch; Caramel, 2 Tbsp | 115 | 0 | 29 |
| Hot Fudge, average, 2 Tbsp | 110 | 4 | 22 |
| Cheese Powder, 2 tsp | 70 | 3 | 2 |
| Honey, 1 Tbsp, 0.8 oz | 65 | 0 | 17 |
| **Fudge,** 1.5 oz | 200 | 11 | 25 |
| **Ice Cream & Frozen Treats:** | | | |
| **Deep-fried Klondike Bar,** w/ syrup | 430 | 16 | 18 |
| **Dippin' Dots Ice Cream,** 6 oz cup | 380 | 20 | 46 |
| **Frozen Banana,** choc. coated, 5 oz | 240 | 4 | 53 |
| **Frozen Yogurt,** in sugar cone, 14 oz | 475 | 2 | 94 |
| **Ice Cream:** Small, sugar cone, 10 oz | 775 | 42 | 83 |
| Large, sugar cone, 14 oz | 935 | 54 | 96 |
| **Sherbet,** 8 oz | 270 | 4 | 59 |
| **Snow Cone,** with 3 oz syrup | 270 | 0 | 68 |
| **Strawberry,** Choc. Dipped, 1 piece | 125 | 7 | 15 |
| **Popcorn:** | | | |
| **Plain:** Small, 3 oz | 450 | 24 | 48 |
| Large, 6 oz | 900 | 48 | 96 |
| **Kettle Corn:** Small, 5 oz | 600 | 15 | 110 |
| Large, 10 oz | 1200 | 30 | 220 |
| **Pretzels,** Soft, 4.5 oz | 340 | 2 | 70 |
| **S'more,** on stick | 275 | 16 | 27 |

## Stadium Foods

| | C | F | Cb |
|---|---|---|---|
| **Burgers:** | | | |
| **Bacon Burger,** 8.3 oz | 470 | 25 | 34 |
| **Cheeseburger,** 8.3 oz | 450 | 23 | 33 |
| **Hamburger,** 7.8 oz | 400 | 19 | 33 |
| **French Fries,** 6.4 oz | 470 | 34 | 39 |
| **Fruit Cup,** 6 oz | 80 | 0 | 20 |
| **Hot Dogs:** | | | |
| **Chili Dog,** 7.7 oz | 520 | 29 | 45 |
| **Hot Dog,** 6.4 oz | 465 | 21 | 50 |
| **Jumbo Dog,** 6 oz | 440 | 25 | 38 |
| **Kraut Dog with Sauerkraut ,** 7.8 oz | 490 | 27 | 41 |
| **Individual Pan Pizza** (6"): *Per Pizza* | | | |
| **BBQ Chicken** | 630 | 24 | 71 |
| **Cheese** | 630 | 27 | 71 |
| **Pepperoni** | 660 | 30 | 70 |
| **Nachos,** 40 chips, with 4 oz cheese | 1100 | 59 | 132 |
| **Sandwiches:** | | | |
| **Chicken:** With Bacon, 8.3 oz | 530 | 31 | 41 |
| With Cheese, 8.3 oz | 510 | 29 | 40 |
| Without Cheese, 7.7 oz | 460 | 25 | 40 |
| **Polish Sausage Sandwich,** 7 oz | 565 | 33 | 46 |
| **Snacks:** | | | |
| **Brownie,** 2.5" x 4.5" | 360 | 18 | 44 |
| **Cheese Sauce,** 1.3 oz | 100 | 8 | 4 |
| ***Cheetos,*** 2.8 oz package | 440 | 28 | 42 |
| **Chocolate Chip Cookie,** 2.3 oz | 280 | 12 | 40 |
| **Churro,** (1), 10", 2 oz | 210 | 10 | 26 |
| ***Doritos,*** Nacho, 2.8 oz package | 390 | 20 | 48 |
| **King Size Candy:** | | | |
| *Butterfinger,* 3.8 oz | 480 | 18 | 75 |
| *Nestle Crunch,* 2.8 oz | 390 | 21 | 85 |
| ***Lay's,*** Chips, 2.8 oz package | 440 | 28 | 42 |
| **Peanuts,** in shell, 8 oz | 930 | 80 | 24 |
| **Popcorn:** Small (9 cup size) | 575 | 35 | 56 |
| Large (15 cup size) | 950 | 58 | 93 |
| **Pretzel,** Soft, Reg., 5.5 oz | 490 | 3.5 | 101 |
| **Red Vines,** 5 oz box | 500 | 0 | 117 |
| **Snow Cone:** With 3 oz syrup | 270 | 0 | 68 |
| With 6 oz syrup | 540 | 0 | 136 |
| **Beverages:** | | | |
| **Orange Juice,** 12 fl.oz | 180 | 0 | 2 |
| **Beer:** | | | |
| *Heineken,* 16 fl.oz | 200 | 0 | 16 |
| *Miller:* Draft, 16 fl.oz | 195 | 0 | 17 |
| Lite, 16 fl.oz | 125 | 16 | 4 |
| *Jack Daniels,* Punch, 12 fl.oz | 235 | 0 | 34 |
| **Wine,** White, 9 fl.oz | 190 | 0 | 6 |
| **Soda,** (with ¹/₂ ice), average: | | | |
| 20 fl.oz | 160 | 0 | 40 |
| 32 fl.oz | 260 | 0 | 65 |
| ***Starbuck's,*** Coffee, Frappuccino, 9.5 fl.oz | 200 | 3 | 37 |

# Restaurant & International Foods

## Asian & Chinese Dishes | C | F | Cb

**Appetizers:**
| | C | F | Cb |
|---|---|---|---|
| **Crab Cake,** 2.3 oz | 125 | 10 | 1 |
| **Dumplings:** *Per Dumpling* | | | |
| Pork: Steamed | 80 | 4.5 | 5 |
| Fried | 90 | 6 | 5 |
| Vegetable, steamed | 35 | 1 | 5 |
| **Egg Rolls,** Mini, 3 rolls | 100 | 3 | 11 |
| **Spring Roll:** | | | |
| Small, 1.5 oz | 85 | 4 | 9 |
| Medium, 3 oz | 170 | 8 | 17 |
| Large, 5 oz | 290 | 15 | 29 |
| **Wonton,** 1 only | 75 | 4 | 5 |
| **Soup:** Egg Flower, bowl 12 oz | 90 | 2 | 16 |
| Hot & Sour Soup, bowl 12 oz | 110 | 3.5 | 14 |
| **Rice:** Plain,1 cup, 6.5 oz | 320 | 2 | 66 |
| 2 Cups, 13 oz | 640 | 4 | 132 |
| Fried: 1 cup, 5 oz | 365 | 11 | 55 |
| Large dish, 16 oz | 950 | 28 | 67 |
| **Noodles,** Chinese Egg, cooked, 1 cup | 200 | 4 | 37 |

**Entrees & Mains:** *Per Serving*
| | C | F | Cb |
|---|---|---|---|
| **Almond Chicken,** 6 oz | 270 | 10 | 21 |
| **BBQ Pork,** 5.5oz | 440 | 23 | 15 |
| **Beef in Black Bean Sauce,** 8.5 oz | 390 | 17 | 17 |
| **Broccoli Beef,** 6 oz | 370 | 21 | 13 |
| **Chicken & Broccoli,** 5.5 oz | 160 | 8 | 10 |
| **Chicken Skewers,** 3 oz | 210 | 9 | 18 |
| **Chop Suey:** | | | |
| Chicken, 5 oz | 140 | 9 | 2 |
| Pork, 5 oz | 170 | 12 | 3 |
| **Chow Mein,** Beef/Chicken, 8 oz | 390 | 12 | 59 |
| **Crab Puff/Rangoon,** 1 dumpling | 190 | 11 | 13 |
| **Crispy Fried Chicken,** 8 oz | 485 | 33 | 12 |
| **Egg Drop Soup:** With Noodles, 1 cup | 110 | 3 | 16 |
| Without Noodles, 1 cup | 60 | 3 | 4 |
| **Egg Foo Yung with Sauce,** 1 cup | 270 | 15 | 16 |
| **Kung Pao Chicken,** 5.5 oz | 240 | 15 | 12 |
| **Lemon Chicken,** 5 oz | 525 | 21 | 57 |
| **Lo Mein,** stir-fried, 8 oz | 705 | 42 | 49 |
| **Omelet,** Chicken/Shrimp, 16 oz | 990 | 82 | 10 |
| **Orange Chicken,** 5.5 oz | 500 | 27 | 42 |
| **Steamed Whole Fish,** | | | |
| $^1/_2$ Sockeye Salmon | 646 | 36 | 23 |
| **Sweet & Sour:** | | | |
| Fish, 20 oz | 1160 | 58 | 106 |
| Pork, 5.5 oz | 400 | 23 | 35 |
| **Vegetable Combo,** with oil, 6 oz | 367 | 5 | 66 |
| **Vegetables,** Steamed, without oil, 6 oz | 135 | 1 | 29 |
| **Sauces:** Mandarin Sauce 1.5 oz | 70 | 0 | 17 |
| Potsticker Sauce, 1.5 oz | 35 | 0 | 8 |
| **Bubble Tea,** average, 12 fl oz | 280 | 0.5 | 68 |
| **Fortune Cookie,** each | 32 | 0.5 | 7 |

## Cajun & Creole | C | F | Cb

| | C | F | Cb |
|---|---|---|---|
| **Alligator,** cooked, 4 oz | 160 | 2 | 0 |
| **Baked Herb Chicken,** 1 serving | 850 | 53 | 2 |
| **Bouillabaisse** | 400 | 15 | 10 |
| **Cajun Fried Turkey,** 1 serving | 630 | 25 | 0 |
| **Cocktail Sauce,** 2 Tbsp | 30 | 0 | 6 |
| **Couche-Couche,** $^1/_2$ cup | 80 | 0 | 17 |
| **Crawfish Bisque,** 1 serving | 500 | 10 | 10 |
| **Crawfish,** cooked, 2 oz | 45 | 0.5 | 0 |
| **Creole Jambalaya,** | | | |
| 1 serving | 550 | 30 | 15 |
| **Frog Legs,** steamed (2) | 45 | 0 | 0 |
| **Guinea Fowl,** flesh, 4 oz, cooked | 160 | 4 | 0 |
| **Hogshead Cheese,** $^1/_4$ cup | 80 | 5.5 | 0 |
| **Jambalaya,** Shrimp & Crabmeat | 520 | 14 | 12 |
| **Red Beans & Rice,** 1 serving | 400 | 17 | 52 |
| **Roasted Quail,** with Bacon, on Toast | 550 | 25 | 15 |
| **Remoulade Sauce,** 2 Tbsp, 1 oz | 110 | 11 | 2 |
| **Shrimp Creole,** 1 serving | 450 | 20 | 10 |
| **Stuffed Smothered Steak,** | | | |
| with 1 cup Rice | 890 | 50 | 50 |
| **Turtle,** cooked, 3 oz | 120 | 3 | 0 |

## Canadian Foods | C | F | Cb

| | C | F | Cb |
|---|---|---|---|
| **Bagels,** Montreal-Style: | | | |
| Plain, 100g/3.5 oz | 300 | 2 | 60 |
| Poppyseed, 100g/3.5 oz | 310 | 4 | 58 |
| Sesame, 100g/3.5 oz | 320 | 6 | 56 |
| **Bannock:** Plain 33g/1.2 oz | 120 | 3 | 20 |
| With currants/raisins, 85g/3 oz | 215 | 9 | 32 |
| **Meals:** | | | |
| **Baked Beans in Maple Syrup,** | | | |
| 1 cup, 250g/8.8 oz | 320 | 1 | 62 |
| **Donnairs** (*Pizza Delight*): | | | |
| Famous, regular, 250g/8.8 oz | 510 | 21 | 60 |
| Super, regular, 310g/11 oz | 685 | 34 | 62 |
| **Poutine:** | | | |
| *A&W,* 330g/12 oz | 610 | 33 | 58 |
| *Boston Pizza,* regular, 400g/14 oz | 610 | 30 | 67 |
| *Burger King,* Classic, 330g/11.6 oz | 680 | 36 | 72 |
| *Harvey's,* 240g/8.5 oz | 730 | 41 | 63 |
| *McDonald's,* 1 serving | 510 | 29 | 44 |
| *Swiss Chalet,* | | | |
| Chalet -Style, 340g/12 oz | 150 | 12 | 195 |
| **Shish Taouk:** | | | |
| Chicken: 1 skewer, 200g/7 oz | 270 | 25 | 9 |
| Wrap, 455g/16 oz | 1150 | 12 | 195 |
| **Tassot:** | | | |
| Beef, 283g/10 oz | 430 | 28 | 12 |
| Goat, 100g/3.5 oz | 360 | 36 | 9 |
| **Toutiere,** 170g/6oz | 600 | 42 | 35 |

## Canadian (Cont)

| | C | F | Cb |
|---|---|---|---|
| **Pastries:** | | | |
| **Beaver Tails:** | | | |
| Cheese & Garlic, 80g/2.8 oz | 390 | 30 | 28 |
| Cinnamon & Sugar, 80g/2.8 oz | 315 | 13 | 30 |
| **Butter Tart**, mini, 1 tart | 120 | 3 | 16 |
| **May West,** | | | |
| Original, 54g/1.9 oz | 240 | 11 | 34 |
| **Nanaimo Bar**, 56g/2 oz | 270 | 16 | 30 |
| **Snacks:** Maple Syrup Taffy, 40g/1.4 oz | 130 | 0 | 33 |
| Potato Chips: Dill Pickle Flav., 40g | 160 | 10 | 15 |
| Ketchup Flavor, 50g/1.8 oz | 260 | 16 | 26 |

## French Foods

| | C | F | Cb |
|---|---|---|---|
| **Blanquette d'Agneau,** (Lamb Stew) | 800 | 30 | 17 |
| **Brioche,** 1 cake | 280 | 14 | 34 |
| **Bouillabaisse** | 400 | 15 | 10 |
| **Coq au Vin,** leg/thigh | 700 | 28 | 31 |
| **Coquilles St. Jacques** | 320 | 13 | 36 |
| **Crème Brulée,** 1 serving | 460 | 40 | 21 |
| **Baguette,** 3 slices, 2.2 oz | 150 | 1 | 35 |
| **Creme Caramel,** (Caramel Custard) | 260 | 10 | 38 |
| **Crepe Suzette,** 1x6" crepe with sauce | 220 | 10 | 13 |
| **Duck a l'Orange,** ¼ duck, 22 oz | 970 | 44 | 19 |
| **Escargot,** (Snails), in garlic butter (6) | 200 | 10 | 4 |
| **Frog Legs,** fried, 4 medium pairs | 400 | 20 | 10 |
| **Lamb Noisettes,** fried, 2 chops | 500 | 40 | 1 |
| **Potage Creme Crecy,** (Carrot Soup) | 360 | 18 | 14 |
| **Salade Nicoise,** (Tuna/Olives/Vegs) | 450 | 13 | 14 |
| **Veal Cordon Bleu,** (Veal/Ham) | 650 | 25 | 18 |
| **Vichyssoise,** (Potato /Leek Soup), 1 c. | 200 | 9 | 15 |
| **Baguette & French Stick ~** *Page 54* | | | |

## German Foods

| | C | F | Cb |
|---|---|---|---|
| **Beef:** Goulash with Veggies | 520 | 20 | 46 |
| Weiner Schnitzel, 1 medium | 750 | 35 | 38 |
| **Chicken:** Fried, Viennese-style | 530 | 20 | 28 |
| Livers with Apple/Onion, 6 oz | 460 | 28 | 10 |
| **Herring,** pickled: Rollmops, 4 oz | 260 | 16 | 3 |
| With Sour Cream, 4 oz | 310 | 20 | 3 |
| **Pork,** Sauerbraten (Pot Roast) | 650 | 35 | 15 |
| **Sausage:** Bratwurst, grilled, 6 oz | 450 | 37 | 2 |
| Hot Sausage Curry | 300 | 7 | 6 |
| **Cakes:** | | | |
| **Black Forest,** 1 slice | 380 | 16 | 30 |
| **Bavarian Bread Dumpling,** 3 small | 330 | 10 | 28 |
| **Kugelhupf Cake,** 1 large slice, 4 oz | 400 | 23 | 40 |
| **Torte:** Linzer (Almond/Raspb. Jam) | 430 | 18 | 58 |
| Sacher (Chocolate/Apricot Jam) | 260 | 12 | 23 |

## Greek Foods

| | C | F | Cb |
|---|---|---|---|
| **Baklava Pastry:** Small | 240 | 13 | 32 |
| Large, 3.8 oz | 400 | 21 | 45 |
| **Calamari,** deep fried, 1 cup | 300 | 13 | 17 |
| **Chicken Kebob Plate** | 345 | 13 | 8 |
| **Dolmades,** 2 rolls, 6 oz | 200 | 5 | 13 |
| **Galactobureko,** 1 only | | | |
| (Filo, Custard, Pastry in Syrup) | 360 | 15 | 48 |
| **Greek Chicken Salad** | 400 | 18 | 9 |
| **Gyros:** 6" Pita, 8 oz | 475 | 32 | 35 |
| 7½" Pita, 12 oz | 680 | 40 | 55 |
| **Hummus & Pita,** 4 oz | 260 | 12 | 30 |
| **Kataifi,** (Filo, Nut, Pastry in Syrup) | 350 | 11 | 56 |
| **Moussaka:** Small serving, 8 oz | 350 | 22 | 22 |
| Large serving, 16 oz | 700 | 44 | 44 |
| **Soup,** Avgolemono (Egg & Lemon with Chicken & Rice), 1 cup | 85 | 6 | 5 |
| **Souvlaki,** (Lamb), each, 2 oz | 120 | 6 | 1 |
| **Stuffed Tomatoes,** (2) | 250 | 12 | 17 |
| **Taramosalata,** 1 T., 0.5 oz | 40 | 3 | 2 |
| **Tyropita,** (Filo/Egg/Cheese Pastry) | 350 | 26 | 31 |

## Hawaiian

| | C | F | Cb |
|---|---|---|---|
| **Ahi Tuna,** grilled w/o fat, 6 oz fillet | 220 | 2 | 0 |
| **Chicken Long Rice,** 1 cup, 7 oz | 240 | 14 | 12 |
| **Gyoza,** 1 only | 55 | 2 | 6 |
| **Haupia,** (Coconut Pudd.), 1 pce, (4"x 2½") | 120 | 6 | 17 |
| **Hawaiian Sweet Bread,** ½ slice, 2 oz | 180 | 4.5 | 29 |
| **Kalua:** Chicken, 4 oz | 280 | 16 | 0 |
| Pork, 4 oz | 350 | 24 | 0 |
| **Kim Chee,** (pickled cabbage), ½ cup, 4 oz | 20 | 0 | 5 |
| **Kulolo,** (Taro Pudding), 1 slice | 125 | 5 | 19 |
| **Lau Lau:** | | | |
| Chicken (1), 7 oz | 280 | 21 | 3 |
| Pork (1), 7 oz | 320 | 26 | 5 |
| **Loco Moco,** (rice/burger/egg/gravy) | 650 | 27 | 63 |
| **Lomi Salmon,** ¼ cup, 4 oz | 20 | 1 | 2 |
| **Malasadas,** (Donut), 2 oz | 240 | 13 | 26 |
| **Manapua,** (Char Siu Pork Bun), 2.3 oz | 180 | 8 | 25 |
| **Poi,** (mashed cooked taro), 1 cup., 8.5 oz | 270 | 0.5 | 65 |
| **Poke,** average all types, 3 oz | 90 | 1 | 0 |
| **Portuguese Sausage,** 2 oz | 180 | 15 | 2 |
| **Potato Salad,** ½ cup, 5 oz | 170 | 10 | 17 |
| **Shave Ice,** *(Matsumoto)*, all flavors: | | | |
| With Ice Cream, 1 large | 300 | 4 | 64 |
| With Beans, 1 large | 290 | 0 | 72 |
| **Spam Musubi:** | | | |
| With Regular Spam | 265 | 11 | 34 |
| (4 oz rice+1.3 oz Spam/7-Eleven Hawaii) | | | |
| Homemade, w/ Lite Spam (50% less fat) | 220 | 5 | 34 |
| **Taro Pancake Mix,** ⅓ cup (makes 2) | 140 | 2 | 26 |

# Restaurant & International Foods

## Hawaiian (Cont) — **C** **F** **Cb**

**Plate Lunches:**

| | C | F | Cb |
|---|---|---|---|
| **Chicken Katsu**, (9 oz:) With Rice | 1110 | 48 | 108 |
| + Macaroni Salad, ³/₄ cup | 1360 | 68 | 123 |
| or Tossed Salad + 2 T. French Dress. | 1240 | 61 | 111 |
| **Hamburger**, (5 oz): With Rice | 710 | 24 | 81 |
| Gravy + Macaroni Salad | 1135 | 49 | 112 |
| **Mahi Mahi**, (7 oz): With Rice | 650 | 12 | 90 |
| + Macaroni Salad + Tartar Sce | 1150 | 58 | 109 |
| or Macaroni Salad, w/o Tartar ce | 935 | 34 | 108 |
| or Tossed Salad + 3 Tbsp Fr. Dress. | 815 | 27 | 96 |
| or Tossed Salad, without dressing | 670 | 12 | 93 |
| **Teri Beef, (5 oz):** With 2 scoops Rice | 790 | 23 | 94 |
| + Macaroni Salad, ³/₄ cup | 1095 | 47 | 113 |
| or Tossed Salad, without dressing | 800 | 23 | 95 |

## Indian & Pakistani

*Per Serving, Meat dishes allow 4 oz meat/serving*

| | C | F | Cb |
|---|---|---|---|
| **Aloo Samosa**, each | 155 | 12 | 12 |
| **Alu Gosht Kari**, (Meat/Potato Curry) | 600 | 40 | 23 |
| **Chicken Korma** | 500 | 35 | 6 |
| **Chicken Pilaf** | 700 | 53 | 50 |
| **Chicken Tikka** | 260 | 16 | 2 |
| **Chicken Vindaloo** | 400 | 20 | 8 |
| **Chapati/Roti**, 7" diameter, 1 piece | 60 | 0.5 | 11 |
| **Dahl**, (Lentil Puree): | | | |
| 1 cup, without oil | 230 | 1 | 37 |
| 1 Tbsp Tadka (oil topping) | 120 | 13 | 0 |
| **Dhakla**, (Lentil Dish), 1" square, 1 oz | 105 | 5 | 13 |
| **Dhansak**, ½ cup | 105 | 3.5 | 11 |
| **Gosht Kari** | 460 | 25 | 17 |
| **Lamb Pilaf** | 520 | 35 | 40 |
| **Lassi**, (Sweet or Mango), 1 cup, 8 oz | 160 | 4 | 24 |
| **Masala Gosht**, (Beef/Tomato/Gravy) | 400 | 25 | 18 |
| **Mulligatawney Soup** | 300 | 15 | 8 |
| **Murgh Tikka**, 1 cup | 300 | 4 | 7 |
| **Naan Flatbread**, 2 oz | 160 | 3.5 | 29 |
| **Pappadum**, 1 large/2 small | 50 | 3 | 5 |
| **Pesrattu**, (Lentil Crepe), 9", 2.6 oz | 130 | 5 | 15 |
| **Pork Vindaloo Curry**, without Rice | 620 | 47 | 3 |
| **Rajmah**, 1 cup | 225 | 5 | 35 |
| **Rogan Josh**, | | | |
| without Rice/Potatoes | 500 | 30 | 3 |
| **Shahi Korma**, (Braised Lamb) | 430 | 28 | 3 |
| **Tandoori Chicken:** | | | |
| Breast | 260 | 13 | 5 |
| Leg/Thigh portion | 300 | 17 | 6 |

## Italian Dishes — **C** **F** **Cb**

**Entrees:**

| | C | F | Cb |
|---|---|---|---|
| **Baked Ziti:** Small | 370 | 27 | 32 |
| Regular | 575 | 42 | 49 |
| **Breadstick** , 2 oz piece | 120 | 2.5 | 25 |
| **Broccoli Fettucine Alfredo**, regular | 815 | 23 | 125 |
| **Bruschetta**, 2 slices | 380 | 17 | 53 |
| **Calzones**, av. all varieties | 840 | 34 | 101 |
| **Cannelloni**, 1 tube, 6 oz | 280 | 15 | 18 |
| **Cheese Breadstick**, 2.4 oz piece | 180 | 8 | 20 |
| **Cheese Ravioli**, with sauce | 495 | 17 | 65 |
| **Chicken Alfredo** | 775 | 29 | 82 |
| **Chicken Parmigiana**, 11 oz | 520 | 22 | 16 |
| **Chicken Scallopine**, dinner | 1110 | 71 | 68 |
| **Eggplant Parmigiana** | 900 | 39 | 78 |
| **Fettucine Alfredo:** Lunch, 9 oz | 885 | 65 | 63 |
| Dinner, 15 oz | 1475 | 108 | 104 |
| **Linquine & Seafood**, dinner | 1130 | 71 | 79 |
| **Manicotti Formaggio** | 800 | 38 | 57 |
| **Meat Lasagne:** | | | |
| Small, 10 oz | 440 | 23 | 39 |
| Large, 16 oz | 700 | 36 | 60 |
| **Meat Ravioli** | 725 | 22 | 102 |
| **Minestrone Soup**, 1 bowl | 110 | 2 | 18 |
| **Penne Rustica:** Lunch | 1300 | 71 | 76 |
| Dinner | 1540 | 80 | 101 |
| **Ravioli**, over-stuffed, average | 990 | 67 | 57 |
| **Panini Sandwich:** | | | |
| Chicken, 16 oz | 900 | 38 | 81 |
| Meats, average, 18 oz | 940 | 39 | 81 |
| Vegetarian, 15 oz | 750 | 31 | 83 |
| **Pizza, Ready-To-Eat** ~ *See Page 135* | | | |
| **Spaghetti & Meatballs:** | | | |
| With Tomato Sauce: Kids | 500 | 20 | 58 |
| Medium/Lunch | 1080 | 63 | 89 |
| Large/Dinner | 1430 | 81 | 119 |
| With Meat Sauce: Kids | 550 | 25 | 56 |
| Medium/Lunch | 1300 | 79 | 84 |
| Large/Dinner | 1700 | 103 | 110 |
| **Veal Marsala**, dinner | 1320 | 66 | 132 |
| **Veal Parmigiana**, dinner | 1270 | 65 | 116 |
| **Vegetable Primavera** | 610 | 8 | 116 |
| **Salad,** | | | |
| Caprese , 11 oz | 445 | 34 | 10 |
| **Desserts:** | | | |
| **Gelato:** Vanilla (Milk Base), ¹/₂ cup | 200 | 15 | 18 |
| Choc. Hazelnut (Milk), ¹/₂ cup | 370 | 29 | 26 |
| Water Base, ¹/₂ cup | 100 | 0 | 25 |
| **Lemon Ice,** | 180 | 0 | 45 |
| **Tiramisu**, 1 piece, 5 oz | 400 | 29 | 30 |
| **Further listings** ~ *See Fast-Foods Section* | | | |

## Japanese

| | C | F | Cb |
|---|---|---|---|
| **Sashimi:** (Sliced Raw Seafood/Beef) | | | |
| Ika (Squid), 4 oz | 105 | 2 | 0 |
| Hamachi (Yellowtail), 4 oz | 165 | 6 | 0 |
| Maguro (Yellowfin Tuna), 4 oz | 120 | 1 | 0 |
| Niku (Beef), 5 oz | 200 | 10 | 0 |
| Saba (Mackerel), 4 oz | 160 | 7 | 0 |
| Suzuki (Sea Bass), 4 oz | 110 | 0.5 | 0 |
| Tako (Octopus), 4 oz | 95 | 1 | 0 |
| **Sushi Rice:** Cooked, 1 Tbsp | 25 | 0 | 5 |
| 1 cup, 5.3 oz | 380 | 3 | 82 |
| **Sushi (Maki) Rolls:** *Per Piece* | | | |
| Average all types (California Rolls; Cream Cheese with Crab; Eel; Salmon; Shrimp; Tuna; Yellowtail; Vegetable) | | | |
| Small (1.2" diam. x 1.2" high), 0.8 oz | 25 | 0.5 | 3.5 |
| Medium (1¼" diam. x 1¼" high), 1.6 oz | 50 | 1 | 7 |
| Large (2¼" diam. x ⅞" high), 2 oz | 60 | 1.5 | 9 |
| **Sushi Packs:** *Per Pack* | | | |
| Average all types: 6 large pieces | 370 | 5 | 55 |
| 9 medium pieces | 360 | 6 | 60 |
| 12 small pieces | 265 | 3 | 45 |
| Futomaki (thick roll), 6 pieces | 380 | 5 | 72 |
| Hand Roll (Cone), 4 oz | 120 | 2 | 18 |
| Inari (rice filled soybean pocket), 4 pces | 420 | 9 | 73 |
| **Sushi-Nigiri,** (fish on rice), | | | |
| average all varieties, 1 piece | 70 | 0.5 | 12 |
| **Sushi Plate**, Assorted: 6 pieces | 420 | 3 | 36 |
| Combination (Sushi & Sushi Rolls) 2 Sushi + 6 small & 3 medium rolls | 400 | 7 | 72 |
| **Dipping Sauces:** Average, 2 Tbsp | 30 | 0 | 7 |
| Ginger Vinegar Dressing, 2 Tbsp | 20 | 0 | 5 |
| **Edamame:** (young green soybeans): | | | |
| Boiled beans (no pods), 4 oz | 160 | 7 | 12 |
| Steamed (in pods), 4 oz | 60 | 3 | 5 |
| **Katsu-don,** Pork with Rice | 1100 | 39 | 141 |
| **Miso Soup,** with Tofu pieces, 1 cup | 85 | 3 | 11 |
| **Sake Wine,** (16% alcohol), 3 fl.oz | 115 | 0 | 7 |
| **Seaweed Salad,** 1.5 oz | 20 | 2 | 0 |
| **Sukiyaki,** (Beef/Tofu/Veggies), 8 oz | 400 | 24 | 32 |
| **Tempura:** | | | |
| 3 large shrimp & veggies | 320 | 18 | 25 |
| 1 shrimp only | 60 | 4 | 3 |
| **Teppan Yaki,** (Steak, Seafood & Veggies), 10 oz serving | 470 | 30 | 15 |
| **Teriyaki:** Beef, 4 oz | 350 | 25 | 4 |
| Chicken, 4 oz | 260 | 9 | 7 |
| Salmon, medium, 6 oz | 270 | 8 | 3 |
| **Yakatori,** 1 skewer, 2.5 oz | 140 | 5 | 1 |

## Kosher/Deli Foods

| | C | F | Cb |
|---|---|---|---|
| **Bagel/Bialy,** 1 small, 2 oz | 160 | 2 | 32 |
| **Beiglach,** (Cheese Knish) | 350 | 17 | 35 |
| **Blintzes:** Average, 1 only | 120 | 1 | 25 |
| With Sour Cream & Preserves | 370 | 10 | 30 |
| **Borscht,** (Without Sour Cream): 1 cup | 85 | 3 | 14 |
| Diet/Reduced Calorie, 1 cup | 30 | 1 | 7 |
| **Cabbage Rolls,** (meat/rice), 5 oz | 170 | 6 | 21 |
| **Chicken Broth:** 1 cup | 80 | 8 | 0 |
| With vegetables | 100 | 8 | 5 |
| With noodles | 150 | 9 | 16 |
| Lowfat, plain, 1 cup | 25 | 1 | 0 |
| **Cholent,** 1 medium serving, 1 cup | 350 | 16 | 48 |
| **Chopped Liver:** 1 serving, 3 oz | 110 | 6 | 5 |
| With Egg Salad, ¼ cup | 100 | 7 | 3 |
| **Farfel,** dry, ½ cup | 90 | 0.5 | 21 |
| **Gefilte Fish Balls:** | | | |
| Regular, 1 | 55 | 2 | 4 |
| With Jelled Broth | 80 | 2 | 6 |
| Cocktail size, 1 oz | 30 | 1 | 2 |
| Sweet: Medium, 2 oz | 65 | 2 | 4 |
| With Jelled Broth | 95 | 2 | 9 |
| **Hallah,** (Yeast Bread), 1 slice, 1 oz | 85 | 2 | 14 |
| **Herring:** Smoked, 2 oz | 120 | 8 | 0 |
| In Sour Cream, 2 oz | 150 | 10 | 0 |
| **Kasha,** cooked, ½ cup | 100 | 0.5 | 20 |
| **Kipfel,** (Vanilla/Almdond Cookie), 1 pce | 60 | 2 | 7 |
| **Knaidlach** ~ *See Matzo Balls* | | | |
| **Knish:** Kasha/Potato, 1 only | 130 | 4 | 22 |
| Cheese, 1 only | 350 | 17 | 35 |
| **Kreplach,** beef, 1 piece | 40 | 1 | 6 |
| **Kugel,** potato/noodle, 1 serving | 300 | 20 | 25 |
| **Latkes,** (Potato Pancake): 2 oz | 200 | 11 | 22 |
| 3 Latkes w/ Sour Cran Apple Sauce | 750 | 25 | 95 |
| **Lochshen:** Plain, 1 cup | 130 | 2 | 26 |
| Pudding, 1 cup | 380 | 13 | 48 |
| **Lox,** (Smoked Salmon), 2 oz | 65 | 2 | 0 |
| **Mandelbrot,** (Almond Bread), 1 slice, ¼" thick | 45 | 2 | 5 |
| **Matzo,** 1 oz board | 110 | 0.5 | 21 |
| **Matzo Balls:** 2 small, or 1 large, 2" | 90 | 3 | 12 |
| Extra large ball, 3" | 180 | 6 | 24 |
| **Matzo Ball Soup:** | | | |
| Cup w/ 2 small or 1 large ball | 150 | 5 | 27 |
| Bowl w/ Chkn & Noodles | 325 | 13 | 34 |
| *Jerry's Deli,* large bowl | 560 | 17 | 56 |
| **NY Cheesecake,** 4 oz | 350 | 24 | 26 |
| **Pierogi,** potato/cheese, 1 piece | 90 | 4 | 11 |
| **Reuben S'wich,** w/ ½ lb Corned Beef | 920 | 60 | 28 |
| **Schmaltz,** (Rend'd Chicken Fat), 1 T. | 90 | 10 | 0 |

## Korean Food

| | C | F | Cb |
|---|---|---|---|
| **Bibimbab**, (Veg. & Beef on Rice), 1 cup | 565 | 15 | 89 |
| **Bulgogi**, (Barbeque Beef), 3.5 oz | 325 | 12 | 15 |
| **Galbi (Short Ribs)**, 16 oz | 975 | 61 | 16 |
| **Gujeolpan**, (Pancake with Meat & Vegetables), 1 cup with 1 pancake | 340 | 11 | 39 |
| **Japchae**, (Noodle w/ Veggies & Meat), 1¼ cups | 365 | 19 | 34 |
| **Sides:** | | | |
| **Kimchee**, (Cabbage Relish), ½ cup | 30 | 0 | 6 |
| **Namool**, (Assorted Vegetables), 1 cup | 125 | 6.5 | 9 |
| **Soups:** *Per Serving* | | | |
| **Muguk**, (Radish & Chive Soup), 6 oz | 105 | 7 | 6 |
| **Samgyetang**, (Ginseng Chkn Soup): | | | |
| Without Chicken Skin, 1 cup | 520 | 11 | 60 |
| With Chicken Skin, 1 cup | 725 | 35 | 60 |
| **Yuk Gae Jang**, (Spicy Beef Soup), 1¼ cups | 180 | 13 | 5 |

## Lebanese/Middle East

| | C | F | Cb |
|---|---|---|---|
| **Baba Ghannouj**, 2 Tbsp, 1 oz | 70 | 6 | 2 |
| **Baklava**, (Pastry, Nuts, Syrup), 1 pastry, 1³⁄₄ oz | 245 | 18 | 18 |
| **Cabbage Rolls,** (Cabb. Leaf, Meat, Rice), 1 roll, 3 oz | 100 | 3 | 12 |
| **Cous Cous,** (Semolina, Milk, Fruit, Nuts), 1 cup | 400 | 21 | 43 |
| **Falafel**, (Chick Pea Fritter), Fried, 1 medium, 1 oz | 60 | 4 | 4 |
| **Hummus**, ¼ cup, 2.2 oz | 105 | 3 | 5 |
| **Fried Kibbi**, (Wheat, Meat Pinenuts), 1 piece, 3 oz | 180 | 8 | 15 |
| **Kafta**, (Ground Lamb, Ssge on Skewer), 1 skewer, 1.5 ozoz | 85 | 5 | 2 |
| **Kibbeh Naye**, (raw Lamb, Bulgur & Spice) 1 cup, 9 oz | 450 | 18 | 28 |
| **Lebanese Omelet**, 1 serving, 4 oz (Egg, Spinach, Pinenuts, Onion) | 200 | 12 | 13 |
| **Pilaf**, (Rice, Onion, Raisins, Apr., Spice) 1 cup | 400 | 11 | 60 |
| **Shawourma**, (Spit-Roast Beef), 4 oz serving | 280 | 15 | 2 |
| **Shish Kabob**, 1 stick, 2.5 oz | 130 | 7 | 2 |
| **Spinach Pie**, 1 piece, 3.5 oz | 290 | 21 | 20 |
| **Sweet Almond Sanbusak**, (Pastry, Almonds, Spices), 1 piece | 200 | 15 | 11 |
| **Tabouli**, 1 serving, 4 oz | 125 | 7 | 13 |
| **Tahini Sauce**, average, 1 Tbsp | 90 | 8 | 2 |

## Mexican Food

| | C | F | Cb |
|---|---|---|---|
| **Burritos** *(Taco Bell):* Bean | 370 | 10 | 56 |
| Supreme Beef | 420 | 16 | 53 |
| **Chili**, plain, ¼ cup | 90 | 6 | 8 |
| **Chili con Carne:** With Beans, 1 cup | 310 | 17 | 15 |
| Without Beans, 1 cup | 370 | 28 | 10 |
| **Chimichangas**, Beef, 5 oz | 400 | 19 | 43 |
| **Chorizo Sausage**, 2 oz | 265 | 23 | 0 |
| **Churro**, (1), 1.5 oz | 150 | 8 | 18 |
| **Corn Chips**, ½ cup, 1 oz | 160 | 10 | 17 |
| **Enchilada**, average | 330 | 10 | 49 |
| **Fajitas**, Chicken | 200 | 7 | 20 |
| **Guacamole**, average, 2 Tbsp, 1 oz | 45 | 4 | 2 |
| **Horchata:** *(Don Jose)*, 1 cup, 8 fl.oz | 140 | 4 | 25 |
| *Cacique*, 1 pint bottle, 16 fl.oz | 320 | 7 | 62 |
| **Margarita**, with 1.5 oz Tequila | 160 | 0 | 6 |
| **Masa**, (Pre-mixed for Tamales), 1 oz | 80 | 5 | 9 |
| **Menudo:** | | | |
| With Hominy, 1 cup | 240 | 9 | 19 |
| Without Hominy, 1 cup | 170 | 9 | 2 |
| **Nachos:** With cheese, peppers, 1 portion, 6-8 nachos, 7 oz | 600 | 33 | 60 |
| With cheese, beans, beef, peppers, 1 portion, 6-8 nachos, 9 oz | 570 | 31 | 56 |
| *Del Taco:* Regular, 4 oz | 300 | 19 | 30 |
| Macho Nachos, 17 oz | 1000 | 56 | 94 |
| *Taco Bell,* BellGrande®, 10.8 oz | 780 | 40 | 84 |
| **Nopal Cactus Salad**, 1 cup | 130 | 9 | 11 |
| **Papas Fritas**, (1), 6 oz | 325 | 18 | 40 |
| **Piloncillo**, (Brown Sugar): | | | |
| 1 Tbsp, 0.5 oz | 50 | 0 | 13 |
| Cone, small, 3", 3 oz | 325 | 0 | 81 |
| **Quesadilla**, Cheese | 490 | 28 | 39 |
| **Queso Fresco**, ¼ cup | 80 | 4.5 | 8 |
| **Refried Beans**, ¾ cup, 6 oz | 160 | 3 | 26 |
| **Rice Pudding**, (Arroz Con Leche), 4 oz | 140 | 3 | 24 |
| **Soup**, Black Bean, 1 bowl | 200 | 3 | 34 |
| **Tacos** *(Taco Bell):* | | | |
| Crunchy: Regular | 170 | 10 | 12 |
| Supreme | 200 | 12 | 15 |
| Soft: Crispy Potato | 270 | 13 | 31 |
| Grilled Steak | 250 | 14 | 19 |
| Taco Salad with Salsa | 840 | 52 | 85 |
| **Taco Sauce**, average, ¼ cup | 15 | 0 | 3 |
| **Taco Shell**, regular | 50 | 2 | 8 |
| **Tamales**, Beef/Chicken, av. 4.5 oz | 250 | 11 | 27 |
| **Taquitos**, Beef & Cheese, 4.5 oz | 330 | 15 | 36 |
| **Tostada** (*Taco Bell*) | 250 | 10 | 29 |
| **Tortilla**, Corn, 6" diameter | 70 | 1 | 14 |
| **Tortilla Chips**, 1 oz | 150 | 8 | 18 |
| **Soup**, Black Bean, 1 bowl | 200 | 3 | 34 |

*Extra Food Listings ~ See Fast Food Section*
*(Examples: Del Taco, Taco Bell, Taco Cabana, Taco Time)*

## Mexican (Cont)

| | **C** | **F** | **Cb** |
|---|---|---|---|
| **Breads:** | | | |
| **Bolillos**, 1 roll, 3.5 oz | 240 | 4 | 42 |
| **Mexican Cornbread**, 4" square | 210 | 11 | 19 |
| **Pan de Leche**, 1 roll, 1.3 oz | 110 | 2.5 | 20 |
| **Telera**, 2 oz | 150 | 1.5 | 19 |
| **Cakes, Cookies, Pastries Pan Dulce:** | | | |
| **Banderilla,** 1 piece | 140 | 10 | 8 |
| **Bigotes,** 7" | 570 | 22 | 44 |
| **Capirotada**, (Bread Pudding), 10 oz | 810 | 38 | 107 |
| **Cinnamon Cookies**, 2 | 125 | 8 | 13 |
| **Concha**, av. all varieties: | | | |
| Small (3" diameter), 2.5 oz | 250 | 8 | 38 |
| Medium (4" diameter), 3.5 oz | 350 | 11 | 53 |
| Large (5" diameter), 5.5 oz | 550 | 18 | 84 |
| **Cream Puff**, with Custard, 4.3 oz | 255 | 14 | 25 |
| **Cuernos**, (Horns), 3 oz | 340 | 17 | 41 |
| **Donut**, large, 4", 3.5 oz | 440 | 21 | 58 |
| **Elotes**, 3.5 oz | 450 | 24 | 51 |
| **Empanadas**, average all varieties: | | | |
| Medium, 3 oz | 300 | 14 | 42 |
| Large, 4 oz | 400 | 19 | 56 |
| **Fiesta Cookie**, (1), 2.3 oz | 280 | 8 | 47 |
| **Galletas Mixtas:** | | | |
| Small, 1 oz | 100 | 2.5 | 16 |
| Medium, 2 oz | 200 | 5 | 32 |
| Large, 3 oz | 300 | 7.5 | 48 |
| **Guayaba**, 3.3 oz | 360 | 14 | 53 |
| **Jelly Roll**, (1), 3.3 oz | 240 | 4 | 46 |
| **Mantecadites**, 4.5 oz | 670 | 42 | 64 |
| **Mini Cupcake**, (1), 1.8 oz | 180 | 8 | 25 |
| **Muffins/Nino Enbuelto**, large, 6 oz | 465 | 11 | 48 |
| **Nuez**, 3.3 oz | 380 | 17 | 52 |
| **Ojo de Buey**, 4 oz | 360 | 15 | 55 |
| **Orejas**, 1 medium, 3 oz | 310 | 15 | 38 |
| **Pan Dulce**, 1 bun | 330 | 10 | 45 |
| **Panquecitos**, 2.5 oz | 260 | 11 | 36 |
| **Piedras**, 4 oz | 470 | 15 | 76 |
| **Polvorones:** Small, 1.5 oz | 180 | 9 | 24 |
| 1 large, 3 oz | 370 | 18 | 48 |
| **Pound Cakes**, mini, 3.5 oz | 380 | 16 | 52 |
| **Puerquitos**, 3.5 oz | 350 | 12 | 55 |
| **Rebanadas**, 3.5 oz | 390 | 18 | 51 |
| **Roles De Canela**, (Cinn. Roll), 4.5 oz | 490 | 15 | 81 |
| **Roscas**, 1 piece, 2.8 oz | 360 | 18 | 44 |
| **Semitas** (Bimbo), 1 piece, 2.2 oz | 210 | 6 | 33 |
| **Sopapillas**, (flaky pastry puffs): 1 piece | 100 | 7 | 10 |
| With Honey & Cream | 200 | 14 | 18 |
| **Strawberry Crema Roll**, 2.5 oz slice | 240 | 5 | 45 |
| **Extra Food Listings** ~ See CalorieKing.com | | | |

## Polish

| | **C** | **F** | **Cb** |
|---|---|---|---|
| **Cabbage Rolls**, w/ Sour Cream, 2 small | 220 | 10 | 30 |
| **Chicken Casserole**, w/ Mshrms, 1 cup | 520 | 27 | 5 |
| **Kielbasa**, (Sausages, Onions, fried), 2 large | 350 | 28 | 2 |
| **Meatballs**, in sour cream, 3 x 1½" balls | 300 | 16 | 11 |
| **Pierogi**, Fruit/Vegetables, 3" ball | 80 | 2 | 15 |
| **Pork Goulash**, (Pork/Vegetable Stew) | 550 | 21 | 38 |
| **Pot Roast**, with Vegetables | 630 | 21 | 28 |

## Soul Foods

| | **C** | **F** | **Cb** |
|---|---|---|---|
| **Breakfast Sausage**, fried, 2 patties | 250 | 17 | 0 |
| **Brunswick Stew**, 1 cup, 8.5 oz | 320 | 14 | 19 |
| **Cornbread**, homemade, 3 oz | 200 | 7.5 | 28 |
| **Fatback**, 0.5 oz | 110 | 11 | 0 |
| **Ham Hock**, pickled, 3 oz | 200 | 12 | 0 |
| **Hog Maw**, 1 oz | 70 | 4.5 | 0 |
| **Hominy**, cooked, ¾ cup | 110 | 0.5 | 25 |
| **Hush Puppies**, 5 pieces | 260 | 12 | 35 |
| **Kale**, cooked, ½ cup | 20 | 0.5 | 4 |
| **Opossum**, roasted, without bone, 3 oz | 190 | 9 | 0 |
| **Oxtail**, cooked, without bone, 2 oz | 85 | 4.5 | 0 |
| **Pig's Ear**, ¼ ear | 50 | 3 | 0 |
| **Pig's Foot**, ½ foot | 70 | 4.5 | 0 |
| **Pig's Tail**, ⅓ tail | 115 | 10 | 0 |
| **Poke Salad**, cooked, ½ cup | 16 | 0.5 | 3 |
| **Pork Brains**, braised, 3 oz | 115 | 8 | 0 |
| **Pork Chitterlings**, simmered, 3 oz | 260 | 25 | 0 |
| **Pork Cracklings**, 0.5 oz | 80 | 6 | 0 |
| **Pork Neck Bones**, cooked, no bone, 2 oz | 100 | 4.5 | 0 |
| **Pork Skin**, 1 cup | 70 | 4.5 | 0 |
| **Pork Tongue**, ⅓ tongue | 75 | 5.5 | 0 |
| **Sousemeat**, 1 oz | 60 | 4.5 | 0 |
| **Succotash**, ½ cup | 80 | 1 | 17 |
| **Sweet Potato Pie**, ⅛ of 9" pie | 250 | 12 | 34 |
| **Tripe**, 2 oz | 55 | 2 | 0 |
| **Vienna Sausage:** | | | |
| 2 small, 1 oz | 90 | 8 | 1 |
| 1 small, 0.5 oz | 45 | 4 | 0.5 |

OLD McDONALDS FARM
128  FOR PEOPLE WHO WANT BETTER
Brooklyn

# Restaurant & International Foods

## Spanish

| | C | F | Cb |
|---|---|---|---|
| **Arroz Abanda,** (Fish with Rice) | 340 | 8 | 31 |
| **Arroz Con Pollo,** (Rice/Chkn Salad) | 500 | 23 | 50 |
| **Clams Marinara,** 8 clams | 330 | 16 | 22 |
| **Cochifrito,** (Lamb with Lemon/Garlic) | 650 | 25 | 5 |
| **Cochinillo Asado,** | | | |
| (Rst Suckling Pig), 2 slices | 300 | 15 | 3 |
| **Cocido Madrileno,** | | | |
| (Madrid-Style Boiled Dinner) | 450 | 27 | 18 |
| **Flan de Leche,** (Caramel Custard) | 325 | 9 | 52 |
| **Fritadera de Ternera,** (Sauteed Veal) | 450 | 27 | 2 |
| **Gazpacho,** 1 bowl | 60 | 0 | 15 |
| **Mole Poblano,** ¹/₂ cup | 205 | 14 | 16 |
| **Paella a la Valenciana,** | | | |
| (Chicken & Shellfish Rice) | 900 | 42 | 70 |
| **Pollo a la Espanola,** (Chicken) | 475 | 30 | 4 |
| **Ternera al Jerez,** (Veal with Sherry) | 660 | 29 | 6 |
| **Zarzuela,** (Fish & Shellfish Medley) | 530 | 27 | 40 |

## Thai Foods

| | C | F | Cb |
|---|---|---|---|
| **Appetizers:** Satay Pork, 1 oz | 100 | 4 | 2 |
| Spring Roll, 1.3 oz | 110 | 6 | 13 |
| **Soups,** Tom Yam (Hot & Sour): | | | |
| Spicy Shrimp/Seafood: | | | |
| 1 cup | 100 | 4 | 6 |
| 1 bowl | 160 | 7 | 10 |
| Vegetarian, 1 cup | 50 | 0 | 11 |
| **Curries:** Chicken with Ginger, 1 cup | 390 | 34 | 4 |
| Thick Red Curry with Beef, 1 cup | 600 | 50 | 7 |
| Thai Chicken Curry, 1 cup | 340 | 23 | 4 |
| Massaman Curry, 1 cup | 680 | 57 | 8 |
| Green Curry with Pork, 1 cup | 480 | 44 | 5 |
| **Pad Thai,** large serving, 18 oz | 990 | 38 | 125 |
| **Fish:** Steamed with Spicy Thai Sce | 450 | 8 | 46 |
| Crispy Fried, 5 oz | 290 | 15 | 9 |
| **Spicy Chicken,** stir-fry | 450 | 22 | 14 |
| **Spicy Garlic Tofu,** stir-fry | 340 | 18 | 18 |
| **Sticky Thai Rice:** Plain 1 cup, 6 oz | 170 | 0.5 | 36 |
| With Coconut & Sesame Seeds, 1 cup | 880 | 28 | 120 |
| **Stir-fried Rice Noodles,** 1 cup 5.5 oz | 270 | 9 | 40 |
| **Stir-fried Vegetables,** 1 cup | 100 | 3 | 18 |
| **Salads:** Green Papaya Salad | 160 | 0 | 40 |
| Spicy Prawn, 9 shrimp | 170 | 3 | 15 |
| Thai Beef Salad, 1 serving | 260 | 9 | 15 |
| Thai Chicken, 1 serving | 330 | 9 | 17 |
| Thai Noodle, 1 serving | 410 | 13 | 45 |
| **Satay Chicken & Peanut Sauce,** | | | |
| 1 satay stick | 390 | 24 | 20 |
| **Sauce,** Peanut Satay, | | | |
| ¹/₂ cup, 4 oz | 160 | 10 | 13 |

## Vietnamese

| | C | F | Cb |
|---|---|---|---|
| **Banh Cuon,** (Steam Rice w/ Pork), 1 roll | 105 | 7 | 8 |
| **Bo Nuong,** (Beef Satay), 2 sticks | 265 | 9 | 4 |
| **Bo Xao Dau Phong,** | | | |
| (Ginger Beef with Onion, Fish Sce) | 750 | 30 | 10 |
| **Ca Chien Gung,** (Whole Snapper/Ginger) | 600 | 16 | 6 |
| **Canh Chay,** (Vegetable/Tofu Soup) | 80 | 3 | 13 |
| **Cari Chicken,** 1 cup | 475 | 29 | 16 |
| **Cari Chicken,** with Rice Noodle, | | | |
| 1 cup curry & 1 cup noodles | 660 | 29 | 60 |
| **Cari Chicken,** with Steamed Rice, | | | |
| 1 cup curry & 1 cup rice | 650 | 29 | 55 |
| **Cuu Xao Lan,** (Curried Lamb and | | | |
| Veggies in Coconut) | 900 | 40 | 80 |
| **Ga Chien,** (Crisp Chick + Plum Sauce) | 900 | 40 | 105 |
| **Ga Nuong,** (Chicken Satay + Sauce) | 240 | 10 | 4 |
| **Ga Xao Rau,** (Marinated Chicken | | | |
| Braised with Vegetables) | 800 | 26 | 100 |
| **Gio Lua,** (Lean Pork Pie), ⅛ of pie | 245 | 12 | 0 |
| **Goi Cuon,** (Cold Spring Rolls), 1 roll | 60 | 1 | 7 |
| **Rau Cai Xao Chay,** (Stir Fried Veggies) | 400 | 15 | 65 |
| **Thit Bo Vien,** (Beef Balls), 6 balls | 225 | 14 | 2 |
| **Thit Heo Goi Baup Cai,** | | | |
| (Spicy Cabb. Rolls with Pork), 1 roll | 200 | 7 | 11 |
| **Soup:** *Per Bowl, ½ Cup* | | | |
| Bun Bo Hue, (Hot & Spicy Soup): | | | |
| Without Pork Feet | 340 | 9 | 35 |
| With Pork Feet | 830 | 45 | 35 |
| Chicken & Rice Noodle Soup | 400 | 3 | 55 |
| Pho Bo, (Beef Noodle Soup) | 410 | 7 | 59 |
| Pho Ga, (Chicken Noodle Soup) | 460 | 6 | 58 |
| Pho Tai, (Rare Beef & Noodle Soup) | 440 | 7 | 73 |
| **Salad,** Goi Du Du, | | | |
| (Green Papaya), ¹/₂ cup | 155 | 3 | 29 |
| **Sauce,** Nuoc Cham (Hot Sauce) | 5 | 0 | 1 |

## Gourmet & Miscellaneous

| | C | F | Cb |
|---|---|---|---|
| **Ants Eggs/Larvae,** 1 Tbsp | 20 | 0 | 0 |
| **Ants,** chocolate coated, 3 Tbsp | 140 | 7 | 2 |
| **Bee Maggots,** canned, 3 Tbsp | 65 | 2 | 0 |
| **Caviar,** black/red, 1 Tbsp | 40 | 3 | 0 |
| **Caterpillars,** canned, 2 oz | 60 | 2 | 0 |
| **Frog Legs,** fried, 1 pair (large) | 125 | 7 | 0 |
| **Haggis,** boiled, 4 oz | 350 | 24 | 22 |
| **Locusts,** roasted, 1 oz | 35 | 1 | 0 |
| **Silkworms,** raw, 1 oz | 60 | 2 | 0 |
| **Snails in garlic butter,** 6 large | 200 | 10 | 4 |
| **Snake,** roasted, 4 oz | 160 | 6 | 0 |

©2020 Allan Borushek

*Nutritional data is based on U.S. outlets*

### For More Restaurants & Full Nutritional Data
~ See CalorieKing.com

| | | | | | | | |
|---|---|---|---|---|---|---|---|
| A&W; Applebees | 176 | Haagen-Dazs; Hardee's | 204 | Red Robin | 232 |
| Arby's | 177 | Hissho Sushi | 205 | Roly Poly | 233 |
| Atlanta Bread Co | 178 | Hot Dog on a Stick | 205 | Round Table Pizza | 233 |
| Au Bon Pain; Auntie Anne's | 179 | Hungry Howie's Pizza | 206 | Rubio's Coastal Grill | 234 |
| Back Yard Burgers | 179 | IHOP; In-N-Out Burger | 206 | Ruby Tuesday | 234 |
| Baja Fresh; Baskin Robbins | 180 | Jack in the Box; Jack's | 207 | Runza | 235 |
| Big Apple Bagels | 181 | Jamba Juice | 208 | Saladworks | 236 |
| Biggby Coffee | 181 | Jersey Mike's Subs | 208 | Sandella's | 237 |
| BJ's Restaurant; Blimpie | 182 | Jimmy John's | 209 | Sarku Japan; Schlotzsky's | 237 |
| Bob Evans | 183 | Johnny Rockets | 209 | Shake Shack; Shakey's | 238 |
| Bojangles; Boston Market | 184 | KFC | 210 | Shari's; Sheetz | 239 |
| Boston Pizza | 184 | Krispy Kreme; Krystal | 211 | Sizzler; Skyline Chili | 240 |
| Bruegger's; Burgerville | 185 | LaRosa's Pizzeria | 212 | Smoothie King | 241 |
| Burger King | 186 | La Salsa Mexican | 212 | Snappy Tomato | 241 |
| Captain D's Seafood | 187 | Little Caesars; Long John Silver's | 213 | Sonic Drive-In | 241 |
| Caribou Coffee; Carl's Jr. | 187 | Macaroni Grill; Manhattan Bagel | 214 | Souplantation | 242 |
| Carvel | 188 | Marie Callender's; Max & Erma's | 215 | Southern Tsunami | 242 |
| Charley's Grilled Subs | 188 | McAlister's Deli | 216 | Starbucks | 243 |
| Cheesecake Factory | 188 | McDonald's; Mellow Mushroom | 216 | Steak Escape | 244 |
| Chick-fil-A; Chili's | 189 | Mimi's Cafe | 218 | Steak 'n Shake | 245 |
| Chipotle; Chuck E. Cheese | 190 | Mr. Goodcents; Mr. Hero | 218 | Subway | 245 |
| Church's Chicken; Cici's Pizza | 190 | Mrs Fields Cookies | 219 | Swiss Chalet | 246 |
| Cinnabon | 190 | My Favorite Muffin | 219 | Taco Bell | 247 |
| Claim Jumper | 191 | Nathan's Famous; Ninety Nine | 219 | Taco Cabana; Taco Del Mar | 248 |
| Cold Stone Creamery | 191 | Noodles & Company | 220 | Taco John's; Taco Mayo | 249 |
| Costco Food Court; Cousins Subs | 191 | O'Charley's | 220 | Taco Time; TCBY | 250 |
| Culver's | 192 | Old Spaghetti Factory | 221 | TGI Friday's; Thundercloud Subs | 251 |
| Dairy Queen; D'Angelo's | 192 | Olive Garden; On the Border | 221 | Tim Hortons | 252 |
| Daphne's Greek Cafe | 193 | Orange Julius | 221 | T.J. Cinnamons | 251 |
| Davanni's | 193 | Outback Steakhouse | 222 | Togo's | 252 |
| Del Taco; Denny's | 194 | Panera Bread | 223 | Tropical Smoothie Cafe | 253 |
| Dippin' Dots | 196 | Papa Gino's; Papa John's | 224 | Tubby's | 253 |
| Domino's; Donatos Pizza | 196 | Papa Murphy's | 224 | Uno Pizzeria & Grill | 253 |
| Eat 'N Park | 198 | Pei Wei Asian Diner | 224 | Villa Fresh Italian | 254 |
| Edo Japan; Einstein Bros | 199 | Perkins | 225 | Vocelli Pizza | 254 |
| El Pollo Loco | 200 | Peter Piper Pizza; P.F. Chang's | 226 | Wahoo's Fish Taco; WAWA | 254 |
| Fatburger; Fazoli's | 200 | Pizza Hut | 227 | Wendy's | 255 |
| Firehouse Subs | 201 | Pizza Ranch | 228 | Whataburger; White Castle | 256 |
| Five Guys; Flame Broiler | 201 | Popeye's; Port of Subs | 228 | Wienerschnitzel; Winchell's | 257 |
| Freshens | 201 | Pret A Manger | 229 | WingStreet; Woody's Bar-B-Q | 257 |
| Godfather's Pizza | 202 | Pretzelmaker | 230 | Yard House | 258 |
| Golden Corral; Gold Star Chili | 202 | Quiznos Subs | 230 | Yoshinoya | 258 |
| Great American Bagel Co | 203 | Rally's/Checkers; Ranch One | 231 | Zaxby's | 258 |
| Great Steak; Green Burrito | 203 | Red Hot & Blue; Red Lobster | 231 | | |

## A&W® (Sept '19)

| | | | |
|---|---|---|---|
| *Burgers:* Cheeseburger | 400 | 21 | 39 |
| Double Cheeseburger | 455 | 26 | 40 |
| Hamburger | 340 | 16 | 39 |
| Bacon Cheeseburger: Original | 440 | 25 | 41 |
| Double | 645 | 41 | 42 |
| Papa Burger | 550 | 33 | 43 |
| *Sandwiches:* | | | |
| Crispy Chicken | 550 | 25 | 52 |
| Fish | 575 | 29 | 58 |
| Grilled Chicken Club | 490 | 22 | 40 |
| Hand-Breaded: Chicken Tender Club | 565 | 20 | 51 |
| Chicken Tender Sandwich | 475 | 13 | 51 |
| *Chicken Tenders,* breaded, 3 pcs | 260 | 9 | 5 |
| *Corn Dog Nuggets,* 10 pieces | 350 | 17 | 40 |
| *Hot Dogs:* Plain | 310 | 19 | 23 |
| Coney Chili Dog | 340 | 20 | 26 |
| Coney Cheese Dog | 380 | 23 | 28 |
| Footlong Hotdog | 460 | 34 | 21 |
| *Fries:* | | | |
| Chili Cheese Fries, 7 oz | 410 | 17 | 52 |
| **French Fries:** | | | |
| Small/Kids, 2.5 oz | 200 | 8 | 29 |
| Regular, 4 oz | 310 | 13 | 45 |
| Large, 5.5 oz | 430 | 17 | 61 |
| Onion Rings, 7-9 rings | 350 | 16 | 45 |
| *Dipping Sauces:* Per 1.25 oz | | | |
| BBQ | 90 | 0 | 22 |
| Honey Mustard | 140 | 11 | 10 |
| Papas, Regular/Spicy | 170 | 15 | 8 |
| Spicy Ketchup | 60 | 0 | 15 |
| *A & W Root Beer:* Small, 16 fl.oz | 220 | 0 | 58 |
| Regular, 20 fl.oz | 270 | 0 | 72 |
| Large, 32 fl.oz | 440 | 0 | 116 |
| *Famous Floats:* | | | |
| **A&W Root Beer Float:** | | | |
| 16 oz Cup | 330 | 5 | 70 |
| 20 oz Cup | 350 | 5 | 77 |
| 32 oz Cup | 640 | 10 | 136 |
| **Diet Root Beer,** 16 oz | 170 | 5 | 30 |
| *Freeze:* | | | |
| **A&W Root Beer:** 16 oz | 370 | 8 | 68 |
| 32 oz | 820 | 18 | 150 |
| **Diet Root Beer,** 16 oz | 260 | 8 | 39 |
| *Polar Swirls:* Oreo/M&M's, av. 12 oz | 605 | 23 | 92 |
| Reese's, 12 oz | 615 | 29 | 82 |
| *Shakes:* | | | |
| **Chocolate/Vanilla,** av., 16 oz | 590 | 18 | 97 |
| **Strawberry,** 16 oz | 670 | 29 | 90 |
| *Soft Serve:* Includes Cone | | | |
| Small, 4 oz | 200 | 5 | 32 |
| Regular, 5.5 oz | 260 | 7 | 41 |
| *Sundaes:* Choc./Strawberry, av. | 310 | 8 | 50 |
| Caramel/Hot Fudge, av. | 345 | 10 | 54 |

## Applebees® (Sept '19)

| | C | F | Cb |
|---|---|---|---|
| *Appetizers:* As Served | | | |
| Boneless Wings, plain | 660 | 22 | 49 |
| Dressings: Bleu Cheese | 220 | 22 | 3 |
| Buttermilk Ranch | 180 | 18 | 3 |
| Sauces: Honey BBQ | 220 | 0 | 54 |
| Sweet Asian Chili | 250 | 2 | 55 |
| Brew Pub Pretzels & Beer Chse Dip | 1200 | 48 | 154 |
| Brisket Quesadillas | 1020 | 68 | 59 |
| Chipotle Lime Chicken Quesadillas | 960 | 62 | 59 |
| Chips & Salsa | 620 | 27 | 85 |
| Crunchy Onion Rings | 1250 | 56 | 173 |
| Mozzarella Sticks | 850 | 43 | 77 |
| Neighborhood Nachos | 1970 | 126 | 124 |
| Spinach & Artichoke Dip | 940 | 57 | 88 |
| *Burgers:* Without Sides | | | |
| Brunch | 1220 | 80 | 64 |
| Classic | 770 | 48 | 44 |
| Quesadilla | 1280 | 91 | 47 |
| Triple Bacon | 1140 | 78 | 48 |
| Whisky Bacon | 1260 | 82 | 70 |
| *Chicken:* As Served, without Choice of Extra Sides | | | |
| Bourbon Street Chicken & Shrimp | 610 | 26 | 42 |
| Cedar Grilled Lemon Chicken | 600 | 25 | 51 |
| Chicken Tenders Platter | 1450 | 80 | 132 |
| Chicken Wonton Stir Fry | 790 | 20 | 104 |
| Classic Chicken Parmesan | 1370 | 57 | 136 |
| Fiesta Lime Chicken | 11920 | 58 | 110 |
| Grilled Chicken Breast | 190 | 4 | 1 |
| Sweet & Savory Grilled Chicken | 590 | 25 | 49 |
| *Fajitas:* Loaded Chicken | 1560 | 78 | 135 |
| Loaded Shrimp | 1440 | 75 | 136 |
| Loaded Sirloin Steak | 1660 | 89 | 137 |
| *Handhelds:* Without Sides | | | |
| BBQ Brisket Tacos | 1160 | 66 | 104 |
| Chicken Fajita Rollup | 1060 | 65 | 63 |
| Clubhouse Grille S'wch | 1040 | 60 | 77 |
| Grilled Chicken Bacon Wrap | 770 | 27 | 73 |
| *Pasta:* As Served | | | |
| Breadsticks with Alfredo Sauce | 1580 | 95 | 137 |
| Brocc. Alfredo w/ Grilled Chicken | 1290 | 76 | 79 |
| Three Cheese Chicken Penne | 1190 | 69 | 73 |
| *Seafood:* As Served, without Choice of Extra Sides | | | |
| Cedar Salmon with Glaze | 370 | 12 | 27 |
| Double Crunch Shrimp | 1170 | 50 | 144 |
| Shrimp Wonton Stir Fry | 680 | 17 | 105 |

Updated Nutrition Data ~ www.CalorieKing.com
Persons with Diabetes ~ See Disclaimer (Page 22)

# Applebees® cont... (Sept '19)

| *Steaks & Ribs: W/out Sauce or Sides* | **C** | **F** | **Cb** |
|---|---|---|---|
| 6 oz USDA Sirloin | 200 | 7 | 1 |
| 8 oz USDA Sirloin | 270 | 10 | 1 |
| **Bourbon Street Steak** | 650 | 32 | 41 |
| **Double Glazed Baby Back Ribs:** | | | |
| Full Rack | 850 | 64 | 1 |
| Half Rack | 430 | 32 | 0 |
| **Riblets:** Plate | 900 | 50 | 61 |
| Platter | 1290 | 74 | 75 |
| **Shrimp & Parmesan Sirloin:** 6 oz | 490 | 32 | 6 |
| 8 oz | 560 | 34 | 6 |
| *Ribs Sauce:* | | | |
| **Honey BBQ/Texas Style BBQ, av:** | | | |
| Full Rack | 155 | 1 | 36 |
| Half Rack | 75 | 0.5 | 18 |
| *Ribs Toppers:* Grilled Onions | 45 | 2.5 | 5 |
| Crispy Onion Tanglers | 170 | 12 | 14 |
| Sauteed Garlic Mushrooms | 170 | 15 | 6 |
| Shrimp 'n Parm Toppers | 290 | 24 | 5 |
| *Salads: Per Regular, with Dressing, without Bread* | | | |
| Caesar with Grilled Chicken | 780 | 55 | 26 |
| Crispy Chicken Tender | 1180 | 79 | 70 |
| Fiesta Chicken Chopped | 850 | 45 | 75 |
| Oriental Grilled Chicken | 1290 | 83 | 89 |
| Southwestern Steak Salad | 960 | 64 | 57 |
| Tuscan Garden Shrimp | 530 | 36 | 26 |
| *Fries & Sides:* Baked Potato | 460 | 30 | 41 |
| Loaded | 530 | 35 | 42 |
| Caesar Side Salad | 220 | 18 | 11 |
| Classic Fries | 430 | 20 | 57 |
| Four-Cheese Mac & Cheese | 480 | 28 | 35 |
| Garlic Mashed Potatoes | 250 | 11 | 35 |
| Garlic Mashed Potatoes, loaded | 440 | 27 | 37 |
| Garlicky Green Beans | 180 | 14 | 11 |
| House Salad without dressing | 120 | 6 | 12 |
| Onion Rings | 510 | 28 | 60 |
| Steamed Broccoli | 100 | 8 | 6 |
| *Soup:* Broccoli Cheese | 280 | 22 | 12 |
| Chicken Tortilla | 160 | 7 | 17 |
| French Onion | 340 | 20 | 22 |
| Loaded Potato | 410 | 35 | 13 |
| New England Clam Chowder | 190 | 13 | 12 |
| Portsmouth Clam Chowder | 160 | 7 | 18 |
| Tomato Basil | 180 | 11 | 16 |
| *Desserts:* Blue Ribbon Brownie | 1400 | 61 | 196 |
| Chocolate Chip Cookie Sundae | 1290 | 62 | 173 |
| Hot Fudge Sundae Shooter | 350 | 18 | 44 |
| Southern Apple Fritter | 1260 | 69 | 150 |
| Triple Choc. Meltdown | 1000 | 54 | 118 |

# Arby's® (Sept '19)

| *Sandwiches:* | **C** | **F** | **Cb** |
|---|---|---|---|
| **Beef 'n Cheddar:** Classic | 450 | 20 | 45 |
| Double | 630 | 32 | 48 |
| ½ Pound | 740 | 39 | 48 |
| **Roast Beef:** Classic | 360 | 14 | 37 |
| Double | 510 | 24 | 38 |
| ½ Pound | 610 | 30 | 38 |
| **Buttermilk Chicken:** | | | |
| Buffalo Chicken | 500 | 23 | 49 |
| Chicken Bacon & Swiss | 610 | 30 | 51 |
| Chicken Cordon Bleu | 660 | 34 | 49 |
| Crispy Chicken | 510 | 25 | 48 |
| **Signature:** Loaded Italian | 680 | 40 | 49 |
| Reuben | 680 | 31 | 62 |
| Roast Beef Gyro | 550 | 29 | 48 |
| Smokehouse Brisket | 600 | 35 | 42 |
| Turkey Gyro | 470 | 20 | 48 |
| **Turkey:** | | | |
| Grand Turkey Club | 480 | 23 | 38 |
| Roast Turkey & Swiss | 710 | 28 | 79 |
| Roast Turkey, Ranch & Bacon | 800 | 34 | 79 |
| **Wraps:** Roast Turkey & Swiss | 520 | 27 | 39 |
| Roast Turkey, Ranch & Bacon | 620 | 34 | 39 |
| *Sliders:* Buffalo Chicken | 290 | 13 | 31 |
| Chicken Tender 'n Cheese | 290 | 12 | 30 |
| Ham 'n Cheese | 230 | 9 | 22 |
| Jalapeno Roast Beef 'n Cheese | 240 | 11 | 21 |
| Roast Beef 'n Cheese | 240 | 11 | 21 |
| *Chicken Tenders:* 3 pieces | 360 | 17 | 28 |
| 5 pieces | 600 | 28 | 47 |
| *Dipping Sauces:* Buffalo, 1 oz | 10 | 1 | 2 |
| Honey Mustard, 1 oz | 140 | 13 | 5 |
| Ranch, 1 oz | 100 | 11 | 2 |
| *Curly Fries:* Small, 4.5 oz | 410 | 22 | 49 |
| Medium, 6 oz | 550 | 29 | 65 |
| Large, 7 oz | 650 | 35 | 77 |
| *Loaded Curly Fries,* 8 oz | 670 | 44 | 57 |
| *Sides: Without Sauce* | | | |
| **Jalapeno Bites:** | | | |
| 5 pieces | 290 | 17 | 31 |
| 8 pieces | 470 | 27 | 50 |
| **Mozzarella Sticks:** 4 pieces | 440 | 23 | 37 |
| 6 pieces | 650 | 35 | 56 |
| **Potato Cakes:** 3 pcs | 370 | 21 | 35 |
| 4 pieces | 490 | 28 | 46 |
| **Steakhouse Onion Rings,** 5 rings | 420 | 21 | 52 |

*continued next page...*

## Arby's® cont... (Sept '19)

*Salads:* Without Dressing

| | | C | F | Cb |
|---|---|---|---|---|
| **Chopped Farmhouse:** | | | | |
| Crispy Chicken | | 430 | 24 | 26 |
| Roast Turkey | | 240 | 13 | 9 |
| **Chopped Side Salad** | | 70 | 5 | 4 |

*Dressings:* Per 1.5 oz Packet

| | C | F | Cb |
|---|---|---|---|
| Balsamic Vinaigrette | 130 | 12 | 4 |
| Buttermilk Ranch | 210 | 22 | 2 |
| Dijon Honey Mustard | 180 | 16 | 8 |
| Light Italian | 20 | 1 | 2 |
| *Kids Menu:* Chicken Tenders (2) | 240 | 11 | 19 |
| Chicken Tender 'N Cheese Slider | 290 | 12 | 30 |
| Curly Fries | 250 | 13 | 29 |
| Ham 'n Cheese Slider | 230 | 9 | 22 |
| Pizza Slider | 300 | 17 | 22 |
| Roast Beef 'n Cheese Slider | 240 | 11 | 21 |

*Breakfast:* Per Serving

| | C | F | Cb |
|---|---|---|---|
| **Biscuits:** Bacon, Egg & Cheese | 480 | 29 | 38 |
| Ham, Egg & Cheese | 470 | 25 | 39 |
| Sausage, Egg & Cheese | 640 | 45 | 39 |
| **Croissants:** Bacon, Egg & Cheese | 440 | 27 | 29 |
| Ham, Egg & Cheese | 420 | 23 | 30 |
| Sausage, Egg & Cheese | 590 | 44 | 30 |
| **Sourdoughs:** | | | |
| Bacon, Egg & Cheese | 490 | 23 | 46 |
| Ham, Egg & Cheese | 470 | 19 | 47 |
| Sausage, Egg & Cheese | 640 | 39 | 47 |
| **Wraps:** Bacon, Egg & Cheese | 500 | 27 | 42 |
| Ham, Egg & Cheese | 440 | 22 | 42 |
| Sausage, Egg & Cheese | 630 | 41 | 42 |
| *Sauces:* Arby's, 0.5 oz | 15 | 0 | 3 |
| Bronco Berry, 1 oz | 60 | 0 | 15 |
| Cheddar Cheese, 1.5 oz | 50 | 3.5 | 4 |
| Horsey, 0.5 oz | 60 | 5 | 3 |
| Marinara, 1 oz | 20 | 0 | 4 |
| Spicy Three Pepper, 0.5 oz | 25 | 1 | 3 |
| Tangy BBQ, 1 oz | 40 | 0 | 9 |
| *Desserts:* Apple Turnover | 430 | 18 | 65 |
| Cherry Turnover | 390 | 13 | 65 |
| Salted Caramel & Chocolate Cookie | 430 | 18 | 65 |
| *Iced Tea,* Unsweetened, small cup | 5 | 0 | 1 |
| *Juice,* Capri Sun Fruit Juice, 6.5 oz | 80 | 0 | 21 |

*Shakes:* Per Medium

| | C | F | Cb |
|---|---|---|---|
| Jamocha; Ultimate Choc. | 755 | 23 | 125 |
| Vanilla | 630 | 23 | 95 |

## Atlanta Bread Co® (Sept '19)

*Breakfast Bagel Sandwiches:*

| | C | F | Cb |
|---|---|---|---|
| Egg & Cheese | 525 | 17 | 69 |
| Egg, Cheese & Ham | 505 | 13 | 69 |
| Egg, Cheese & Turkey Sausage | 500 | 14 | 68 |
| *Side,* Breakfast Potatoes | 170 | 9 | 20 |
| *Paninis:* Chicken Pesto | 735 | 30 | 76 |
| Cuban | 845 | 41 | 75 |
| Steakhouse | 725 | 33 | 68 |
| *Sandwiches:* Chicken Salad | 745 | 42 | 57 |
| Grilled Triple Cheese | 640 | 36 | 55 |
| Roast Beef | 475 | 16 | 52 |
| Roasted Turkey | 510 | 16 | 58 |
| Veggie | 480 | 18 | 60 |

*Salads:* Per Full Size, with Dressing, without Bread

| | C | F | Cb |
|---|---|---|---|
| Balsamic Blue | 605 | 44 | 40 |
| Caesar | 790 | 55 | 60 |
| Chopstix Chicken | 855 | 46 | 80 |
| Cobb | 730 | 17 | 32 |
| Greek | 700 | 51 | 40 |
| *Sides,* Black Beans & Corn | 190 | 9 | 24 |

## Au Bon Pain® (Sept '19)

*Bagels:* Per Bagel

| | C | F | Cb |
|---|---|---|---|
| Asiago Cheese, 3.6 oz | 300 | 7 | 45 |
| Cinnamon Raisin, 3.1 oz | 240 | 0.5 | 52 |
| Everything, 3.2 oz | 240 | 1.5 | 50 |
| Honey Sprouted Grain, 3.6 oz | 250 | 1.5 | 53 |
| Plain Bagel, 3.1 oz | 230 | 1 | 49 |
| Sesame Seed Bagel, 3.2 oz | 250 | 2.5 | 50 |
| Whole Wheat Skinny , 1.6 oz | 90 | 1 | 21 |

*Breakfast Sandwiches:*

| | C | F | Cb |
|---|---|---|---|
| 2 Eggs on a Bagel | 380 | 11 | 50 |
| with Bacon | 430 | 15 | 50 |
| with Bacon & Cheese | 480 | 20 | 51 |
| Egg Whites On Skinny Wheat Bagel: | | | |
| Cheddar | 210 | 7 | 22 |
| Cheddar & Avocado | 360 | 23 | 25 |
| Smoked Salmon Wasabi | 370 | 9 | 54 |
| *Fruit Cup,* large, 12 oz | 140 | 0.5 | 36 |

*Yogurt Parfait:*

| | C | F | Cb |
|---|---|---|---|
| Blueb. Yogurt & Wild Blueb. 10.2 oz | 380 | 10 | 68 |
| Greek Van. Yog. & Wild Blueb., 10.2 oz | 340 | 8 | 47 |
| Greek Van. Yog. & Strawberry,11.3 oz | 340 | 8 | 48 |
| *Oatmeal,* Classic Medium, 12 oz | 260 | 5 | 47 |

*Sandwiches:* Per Whole Sandwich

| | C | F | Cb |
|---|---|---|---|
| **Cafe:** Extra Bacon BLT | 530 | 24 | 57 |
| Prime Roast Beef | 620 | 20 | 74 |
| Tuna Salad | 480 | 12 | 59 |
| **Signature:** 2 Tomato Caprese | 560 | 27 | 57 |
| Toasted Chicken & Avocado | 660 | 29 | 61 |

**178**

## Au Bon Pain® cont... (Sept '19)

### Harvest Hot Bowls:

| | C | F | Cb |
|---|---|---|---|
| Mayan Chicken | 550 | 10 | 84 |
| Mediterranean Chicken | 700 | 27 | 76 |
| Roasted Vegetarian | 640 | 72 | 75 |
| Teriyaki Steak | 650 | 11 | 98 |

### Soups: Per 12 fl.oz

| | | | |
|---|---|---|---|
| Chicken Florentine | 280 | 15 | 27 |
| Chicken Noodle | 120 | 2.5 | 15 |
| Clam Chowder | 350 | 20 | 32 |
| French Onion | 110 | 5 | 15 |
| Harvest Pumpkin | 230 | 13 | 24 |
| Lemon Orzo Chicken | 230 | 12 | 20 |
| Lobster & Corn Bisque | 280 | 16 | 25 |
| Potato Leek | 290 | 21 | 22 |
| Vegetarian Beef & Barley | 160 | 3 | 22 |

### Salads: Without Dressing

| | | | |
|---|---|---|---|
| Chicken Caesar Asiago | 290 | 9 | 21 |
| Chicken Cobb, w/ Avocado | 460 | 25 | 17 |
| Harvest Turkey | 380 | 15 | 32 |
| Vegetarian Deluxe | 260 | 13 | 26 |
| Dressings: Bals. Vinaigrette, 1.5 oz | 80 | 7 | 5 |
| Caesar, 1.5 oz | 190 | 19 | 3 |
| Ranch, 1.5 oz | 180 | 19 | 4 |

### Cake, Cookies, Croissants, Danish, Dessert:

| | | | |
|---|---|---|---|
| **Cake,** Iced Carrot, 4.2 oz | 430 | 23 | 52 |
| **Cinnamon Swirl Roll,** 5.2 oz | 550 | 25 | 76 |
| **Cookies:** | | | |
| Chocolate Chip, 2.8 oz | 370 | 18 | 54 |
| Oatmeal Raisin, 2.2 oz | 290 | 11 | 46 |
| **Croissants:** Almond, 4 oz | 500 | 31 | 47 |
| Apple & Cinn., 3.4 oz | 220 | 8 | 35 |
| Chocolate, 4 oz | 470 | 25 | 55 |
| Plain, 2.4 oz | 280 | 16 | 28 |
| **Danish:** | | | |
| Raspb. Almond, 4.9 oz | 500 | 22 | 66 |
| Sweet Cheese, 4.7 oz | 410 | 20 | 50 |
| **Muffins:** Blueberry, 4.9 oz | 480 | 25 | 59 |
| Double Choc. Chunk, 4.7 oz | 580 | 30 | 66 |
| Raisin Bran, 4.7 oz | 430 | 12 | 75 |
| **Palmier,** 2.6 oz | 380 | 20 | 46 |

### Beverages:

| | | | |
|---|---|---|---|
| Caffe Latte, 16 fl.oz | 140 | 7 | 12 |
| Caramel Macchiato, 16 fl.oz | 270 | 8 | 41 |
| Hot Chocolate, 16 fl.oz | 350 | 12 | 51 |
| Raspberry Iced Tea, 24 fl.oz | 180 | 0 | 50 |
| Strawberry Banana Smoothie, 16 fl.oz | 290 | 0 | 68 |

*For Complete Items ~ See CalorieKing.com*

## Auntie Anne's® (Sept '19)

### Pretzels: With Butter

| | C | F | Cb |
|---|---|---|---|
| Cinnamon Sugar | 470 | 12 | 84 |
| Jalapeno | 330 | 5 | 63 |
| Original | 340 | 5 | 65 |
| Pepperoni | 480 | 16 | 65 |
| Roasted Garlic & Parm. | 380 | 8 | 68 |
| Sour Cream & Onion | 380 | 8 | 68 |
| Sweet Almond | 390 | 6 | 74 |

### Dipping Sauces:

| | | | |
|---|---|---|---|
| Caramel, 1.5 oz | 130 | 3 | 23 |
| Cheese, 1.4 oz | 90 | 8 | 2 |
| Hot Salsa, 1.4 oz | 90 | 8 | 2 |
| Light Cream Cheese, 1.25 oz | 80 | 6 | 1 |
| Marinara, 2 oz | 45 | 1 | 7 |
| Melted Cheese, 2 oz | 150 | 12 | 6 |
| Sweet Glaze, 1.4 oz | 130 | 0 | 32 |
| Sweet Mustard, 1.25 oz | 60 | 2 | 10 |

### Pretzel Dogs: Original

| | | | |
|---|---|---|---|
| | 360 | 20 | 33 |
| Cheese | 370 | 20 | 33 |
| Jalapeno & Cheese | 370 | 20 | 34 |
| Jumbo | 610 | 29 | 67 |
| Mini Pretzel Dogs (8) | 510 | 29 | 45 |

### Beverages: Per 16 fl.oz

| | | | |
|---|---|---|---|
| **Frozen Lemonade Mixer,** | | | |
| Blue Raspberry; Strawberry, av. | 235 | 0 | 60 |

## Back Yard Burgers® (Sept '19)

### Black Angus Burgers: On White Bun

| | C | F | Cb |
|---|---|---|---|
| **Back Yard:** Without Cheese | | | |
| Classic Burger | 580 | 28 | 48 |
| Double Classic | 860 | 46 | 48 |
| Black Jack Burger | 660 | 38 | 43 |
| Black & Bleu Burger | 760 | 46 | 45 |
| Chipotle Burger | 810 | 48 | 55 |
| Mushroom Swiss Burger | 660 | 37 | 43 |

### Chicken Sandwiches: On White Bun

| | | | |
|---|---|---|---|
| Blackened Chicken, w/out cheese | 610 | 27 | 49 |
| Black Jack Chicken Club | 700 | 37 | 46 |
| Grilled Chicken, w/out cheese | 450 | 12 | 45 |
| Hawaiian Chicken, w/out cheese | 520 | 12 | 63 |

### Specialties:

| | | | |
|---|---|---|---|
| Breaded Chicken Tender Basket, | | | |
| w/o Toppings, Chse, Sce or Bread | 540 | 36 | 27 |
| Veggie Burger, without cheese | 420 | 11 | 67 |

### Turkey Burgers: On White Bun

| | | | |
|---|---|---|---|
| Classic, w/out cheese | 530 | 28 | 41 |
| Club | 650 | 38 | 42 |
| Wild | 600 | 34 | 43 |

*continued next page ...*

# Fast - Foods & *Restaurants*

## Back Yard Burgers® cont... (Sept '19)

*Fries:*

| | C | F | Cb |
|---|---|---|---|
| **Chili Cheese Fries,** seasoned, reg. | 790 | 59 | 52 |
| **Seasoned Fries:** Regular, 4.5 oz | 480 | 36 | 38 |
| Large, 6 oz | 640 | 47 | 50 |
| **Sweet Potato Fries,** regular, 6 oz | 450 | 29 | 40 |
| **Waffle Fries:** Reg., 6 oz | 820 | 56 | 66 |
| Large, 8 oz | 1100 | 75 | 88 |
| *Sides:* Back Yard Chili | 310 | 18 | 15 |
| Creamy Coleslaw | 200 | 16 | 15 |
| Loaded Baked Potato | 420 | 21 | 45 |
| Panko Onion Rings, regular, 4 oz | 340 | 13 | 47 |
| *Salads: Without Dressing* | | | |
| **Back Yard Salad:** w. Grilled Chicken | 350 | 10 | 21 |
| with Blackened Chicken | 450 | 21 | 22 |
| Cranberry Pecan Grilled Chicken | 660 | 30 | 52 |
| Side Salad | 140 | 6 | 14 |
| *Dressings:* Bleu Cheese | 220 | 24 | 1 |
| Gorgonzola Vinaigrette | 170 | 15 | 6 |
| Honey Mustard | 200 | 20 | 7 |
| Ranch, Homestyle | 150 | 16 | 1 |
| *Dessert/Cobblers:* Apple/Cherry | 390 | 16 | 58 |
| Apple/Cherry Cobbler A La Mode | 540 | 24 | 78 |
| *Ice Cream,* A La Carte | 150 | 8 | 20 |
| *Milk Shakes: With Whole Milk & Whipped Topping* | | | |
| Chocolate: Vanilla, average | 750 | 35 | 98 |
| Chocolate Oreo | 850 | 40 | 115 |
| Peanut Butter | 830 | 51 | 79 |

## Baja Fresh® (Sept '19)

*Baja Bowls: With Black Beans*

| | C | F | Cb |
|---|---|---|---|
| Carnitas | 680 | 18 | 92 |
| Chicken | 700 | 20 | 82 |
| Shrimp | 660 | 20 | 83 |
| Steak | 690 | 22 | 82 |
| Veggie | 540 | 14 | 90 |
| *Burritos: With Standard Components* | | | |
| **Baja:** with Carnitas | 800 | 41 | 63 |
| with Chicken | 820 | 46 | 53 |
| with Steak | 810 | 45 | 53 |
| **Bean & Cheese:** *With Pinto Beans* | | | |
| Carnitas | 1060 | 40 | 113 |
| Chicken | 1080 | 44 | 103 |
| Steak | 1070 | 44 | 103 |
| **Mexicano:** *With Black Beans* | | | |
| Chicken | 800 | 27 | 94 |
| Steak | 790 | 26 | 94 |
| **Ultimo:** Carnitas | 950 | 45 | 88 |
| Chicken | 970 | 50 | 78 |
| Steak | 960 | 50 | 78 |
| *Nachos: Regular Size, with Black Beans* | | | |
| Carnitas | 1110 | 56 | 106 |
| Cheese | 1020 | 54 | 100 |
| Chicken | 1150 | 60 | 101 |

## Baja Fresh® cont... (Sept '19)

*Fajitas: With Pinto Beans*

| | C | F | Cb |
|---|---|---|---|
| **Chicken:** with Corn Tortillas | 1060 | 39 | 121 |
| with Flour Tortillas | 1250 | 44 | 146 |
| **Shrimp:** with Corn Tortillas | 990 | 35 | 123 |
| with Flour Tortilla | 1180 | 41 | 148 |
| **Steak:** with Corn Tortillas | 1050 | 38 | 121 |
| with Flour Tortilla | 1240 | 44 | 146 |
| **Wahoo:** with Corn Tortillas | 990 | 35 | 121 |
| with Flour Tortilla | 1180 | 40 | 146 |
| *Tacos: With Standard Toppings* | | | |
| **Americano, Soft Taco:** Carnitas | 220 | 9 | 21 |
| Chicken | 230 | 11 | 19 |
| Baja, meat varieties, average | 160 | 6 | 17 |
| Wahoo, Crispy Taco | 250 | 15 | 24 |
| *Salads: Without Dressing* | | | |
| **Baja Ensalada:** with Carnitas | 300 | 9 | 28 |
| with Chicken | 260 | 11 | 18 |
| with Shrimp | 280 | 12 | 19 |
| with Steak | 250 | 11 | 17 |
| **Tostada:** Carnitas & Pinto Beans | 1010 | 48 | 99 |
| Chicken & Black Beans | 1020 | 53 | 86 |
| Shrimp & Pinto Beans | 1000 | 51 | 90 |
| Steak & Black Beans | 1020 | 52 | 86 |
| *Sides:* Guacamole, 8 oz | 310 | 27 | 19 |
| Queso, 8 oz | 470 | 37 | 13 |
| Rice & Black Beans, 17 oz | 550 | 11 | 90 |
| Rice & Pinto Beans, 17 oz | 570 | 11 | 95 |
| Tortilla Chips, 5 oz | 710 | 28 | 99 |

*For Complete Nutritional Data ~ see CalorieKing.com*

## Baskin Robbins® (Sept '19)

*Cones:*

| | C | F | Cb |
|---|---|---|---|
| Cake | 25 | 0 | 5 |
| Fresh-Baked Waffle | 160 | 3.5 | 29 |
| Sugar | 45 | 0.5 | 9 |
| *Ice Creams: Per 4 oz Scoop* | | | |
| **Classic Flavors:** Cherries Jubilee | 230 | 11 | 28 |
| Chocolate Chip | 250 | 16 | 23 |
| Chocolate | 240 | 14 | 26 |
| Jamoca Almond Fudge | 260 | 15 | 27 |
| Mint Chocolate Chip | 250 | 16 | 23 |
| Old Fashioned Butter Pecan | 260 | 18 | 20 |
| Oreo Cookies 'n Cream | 260 | 15 | 28 |
| Peanut Butter 'n Chocolate | 300 | 20 | 25 |
| Pistachio Almond | 270 | 19 | 21 |
| Pralines 'n Cream | 270 | 14 | 31 |
| Reese's P'nut Butter Cup | 280 | 17 | 27 |
| Rocky Road | 270 | 15 | 29 |
| Rum Raisin | 240 | 11 | 29 |
| Vanilla | 240 | 16 | 21 |
| Very Berry Strawberry | 210 | 11 | 24 |
| **Wild 'n Reckless Sherbet** | 130 | 2 | 25 |

**180**

## Baskin Robbins® cont... (Sept '19)

### Ice Creams (Cont): Per 4 oz Scoop

| | C | F | Cb |
|---|---|---|---|
| **Seasonal Flavors:** Black Walnut | 260 | 18 | 20 |
| Chocolate Fudge | 240 | 15 | 27 |
| Creole Cream Cheese | 230 | 13 | 23 |
| Strawberry Cheesecake | 250 | 13 | 28 |

### Grab-N-Go: Per 1.3 oz Cookie

| | | | |
|---|---|---|---|
| Dark Chocolate Chunk Cookie | 170 | 7 | 26 |
| Double Fudge Cookie | 160 | 6 | 26 |
| Peanut Butter 'n Chocolate Cookie | 160 | 7 | 23 |
| White Chunk Macadamia Cookie | 180 | 9 | 24 |

### Ice Cream Quarts: Per ½ Cup, 2.6 oz

| | | | |
|---|---|---|---|
| Chocolate | 170 | 9 | 21 |
| Mint Chocolate Chip | 160 | 10 | 15 |
| Vanilla | 170 | 10 | 17 |

### Soft Serve:

| | | | |
|---|---|---|---|
| **Cups:** Vanilla: Kid's, 3 oz | 110 | 4.5 | 14 |
| Regular, 6 oz | 230 | 9 | 29 |
| Large, 9 oz | 340 | 14 | 43 |
| **Parfaits:** M&M's, regular | 820 | 32 | 119 |
| Oreo, regular | 710 | 28 | 104 |
| Snickers, regular | 780 | 24 | 125 |

### 31 Below' Mix-In: Per 16 oz Medium Cup

| | | | |
|---|---|---|---|
| Butterfinger | 840 | 34 | 118 |
| Choc. Chip Cookie Dough | 870 | 32 | 129 |
| Heath | 910 | 46 | 111 |
| M&M's | 1000 | 40 | 139 |
| Oreo | 720 | 29 | 99 |
| Reese's PB Cup | 910 | 45 | 109 |
| Snickers | 840 | 36 | 108 |

### Sundaes:

| | | | |
|---|---|---|---|
| Banana Royale | 680 | 33 | 90 |
| Brownie | 810 | 42 | 99 |
| Chocolate Chip Cookie Dough | 1100 | 47 | 160 |
| Made with Snickers | 1060 | 43 | 155 |
| Two Scoop | 570 | 33 | 63 |
| Warm Brownie | 810 | 42 | 99 |

### Beverages: Per Medium, 24 fl.oz

| | | | |
|---|---|---|---|
| **Blasts:** Caramel Cappuccino | 790 | 25 | 130 |
| Mocha Cappuccino | 610 | 22 | 97 |
| **Fruit Blast:** Mango | 500 | 1.5 | 123 |
| Strawberry Citrus | 350 | 0 | 89 |
| Tropical | 370 | 0.5 | 93 |
| **Milk Shakes:** Chocolate Chip | 1030 | 54 | 117 |
| Mint Chocolate Chip | 1030 | 55 | 117 |
| **Smoothie:** Mango Banana | 640 | 2 | 153 |
| Strawberry Banana | 520 | 1 | 126 |

## Big Apple Bagels® (Sept '19)

### Bagels:

| | C | F | Cb |
|---|---|---|---|
| Asiago Melt; Swiss Melt | 370 | 6 | 65 |
| Cinnamon Sugar | 370 | 2 | 78 |
| Fruit Varieties, average | 330 | 3 | 66 |
| Plain or Salt | 320 | 2 | 64 |

### Cream Cheese: Per 1.5 oz

| | | | |
|---|---|---|---|
| Chedd. & Bacon; Walnut Raisin, av | 140 | 13 | 4 |
| Plain/Scallion, average | 130 | 12 | 2 |
| Plain, Lite | 100 | 9 | 2 |
| Strawberry | 130 | 11 | 5 |
| Tomato-Basil | 140 | 13 | 3 |

### Muffins: With Whole Egg

| | | | |
|---|---|---|---|
| **Mini:** Blueberry; Lem. Poppyseed | 90 | 4.5 | 12 |
| Cinnamon Swirl Cheesecake | 90 | 5 | 9 |
| **Large:** | | | |
| Blueberry | 590 | 28 | 78 |
| Choc. Cheesecake, 6 oz | 650 | 38 | 70 |

### Breakfast Sandwiches: Per Sandwich

| | | | |
|---|---|---|---|
| French Toast w/ Egg: on BAB Bagel | 1020 | 55 | 107 |
| On MFM Bagel | 1060 | 55 | 117 |

### Salads: With Dressing

| | | | |
|---|---|---|---|
| Caesar, with Caesar Dressing | 450 | 34 | 19 |
| Chicken Club, with Ranch Dressing | 760 | 59 | 18 |
| Mediterranean Bread Salad, with Balsamic Vinaigrette | 740 | 41 | 63 |

### Beverages: Per Medium, 16 fl.oz

| | | | |
|---|---|---|---|
| Hot Chocolate | 440 | 12 | 71 |
| Mocha; White Chocolate Latte, av | 380 | 8 | 66 |
| Vanilla Creme Latte | 310 | 7 | 50 |

## Biggby Coffee® (Sept '19)

### Hot Drinks: Per Tall, 16 fl.oz, without Whipped Cream

| | C | F | Cb |
|---|---|---|---|
| **Caffe au Lait:** with 2% Milk | 100 | 4 | 9 |
| with Non-Fat Milk | 65 | 0 | 9 |
| with Soy | 90 | 3 | 11 |
| **Caffe Latte:** with 2% Milk | 175 | 7.5 | 16 |
| with Non-Fat Milk | 115 | 0 | 16 |
| with Soy | 160 | 5 | 19 |
| **Cappuccino:** with 2% Milk | 105 | 4.5 | 10 |
| with Non-Fat Milk | 70 | 0 | 10 |
| with Soy | 95 | 3 | 11 |
| **Chai Latte:** with 2% Milk | 315 | 7.5 | 51 |
| with Non-Fat Milk | 255 | 0 | 51 |
| **Dark Hot Chocolate:** w/ 2% Milk | 320 | 9 | 50 |
| with Non-Fat Milk | 260 | 1.5 | 50 |

### Frozen Creme Freeze: Per 20 fl.oz, with 2% Milk, Whipped Cream & Sugar, without Reduced Calorie

| | | | |
|---|---|---|---|
| Avalanche Latte | 640 | 19 | 108 |
| Banana Chip | 750 | 20 | 135 |
| Coconut Creme | 640 | 19 | 110 |
| Mellow Mochanut | 645 | 19 | 109 |

# Fast - Foods & *Restaurants*

## BJ's Restaurant® (Sept '19)

### Shareable Appetizers: Full Order

| | C | F | Cb |
|---|---|---|---|
| Ahi Poke | 320 | 10 | 24 |
| Chicken Lettuce Wraps | 500 | 21 | 43 |
| Mozzarella Sticks | 810 | 39 | 76 |
| Root Beer Glazed Ribs | 450 | 16 | 63 |
| Sliders | 880 | 32 | 97 |
| Wings, Bone In, 10 pieces | 750 | 57 | 6 |

### Handcrafted Burgers: With French Fries

| | C | F | Cb |
|---|---|---|---|
| Bacon Cheeseburger | 1380 | 84 | 97 |
| Bacon Guacamole Deluxe | 1590 | 98 | 103 |
| Classic Burger | 1250 | 71 | 98 |
| Crispy Jalapeno Burger | 1380 | 81 | 106 |
| Portobello Swiss Burger | 1430 | 81 | 105 |

### Brunch: Avocado Toast

| | C | F | Cb |
|---|---|---|---|
| Avocado Toast | 410 | 20 | 47 |
| Buttermilk Pancakes, short stack | 910 | 31 | 143 |
| Calif. Scramble, w/ sourdough | 1210 | 69 | 90 |
| Enlightened Veggie Omelette, with fruit | 270 | 9 | 24 |

### Enlightened Entrees: Includes Menu Set Sides

| | C | F | Cb |
|---|---|---|---|
| Cherry Chipotle Glazed Salmon | 580 | 26 | 39 |
| Lemon Thyme Chicken | 630 | 19 | 52 |
| Mediterranean Chicken Pita Tacos | 670 | 20 | 79 |
| Quinoa Bowls: Fresh Atl. Salmon | 790 | 44 | 47 |
| Roasted Chicken | 650 | 28 | 47 |
| Seared Ahi Salad | 570 | 31 | 42 |
| Vegetarian Pita Tacos | 550 | 17 | 81 |

### Pasta: Includes Garlic Knot

| | C | F | Cb |
|---|---|---|---|
| Deep Dish Ziti | 1400 | 91 | 99 |
| Gr. Chicken Alfredo | 1380 | 69 | 129 |
| Italiano Veggie Penne | 800 | 38 | 92 |
| Jumbo Spaghetti & Meatballs | 1600 | 82 | 161 |
| Shrimp & Asparagus Penne | 870 | 38 | 94 |

### Pizza, Deep Dish: Per Slice, 1/8 Med. Pizza

| | C | F | Cb |
|---|---|---|---|
| BBQ/Buffalo Chicken, average | 310 | 10 | 35 |
| California Supreme | 280 | 12 | 33 |
| Classic Combo; Pepp. Extreme, av. | 335 | 17 | 32 |
| Spicy Hawaiian Chicken | 350 | 15 | 36 |
| Sweet Pig; Vegetarian, average | 265 | 10 | 34 |

### Pizza, Tavern-Cut: Per Slice (1/12 Pizza)

| | C | F | Cb |
|---|---|---|---|
| Brewhouse; Italian Market | 110 | 6 | 9 |
| Garlic Chicken Pesto | 100 | 5 | 9 |
| Spicy Pig/Old Country Tomato, av. | 80 | 4 | 10 |

### Sandwiches: With French Fries

| | C | F | Cb |
|---|---|---|---|
| Barbeque Pulled Pork | 1600 | 82 | 172 |
| California Chicken Club | 1280 | 66 | 90 |
| Slow Roasted Turkey Club | 1660 | 111 | 104 |

### Ribs & Steaks: Without Sides

| | C | F | Cb |
|---|---|---|---|
| Baby Back Pork Ribs, half rack, with Peppered BBQ Sauce | 710 | 34 | 74 |
| Classic Rib-Eye | 1080 | 67 | 5 |
| Prime Rib Dinner | 1310 | 106 | 6 |
| Top Sirloin | 500 | 32 | 2 |

### Soups:

| | C | F | Cb |
|---|---|---|---|
| Chicken Tortilla, Bowl | 280 | 12 | 30 |
| Clam Chowder: Bowl w/ crackers | 440 | 26 | 33 |
| Sourdough Loaf, w/ crackers | 1470 | 42 | 219 |

## BJ's Restaurant® cont...(Sept '19)

### Salads: With Dressing & Toppings

| | C | F | Cb |
|---|---|---|---|
| BBQ Chicken Chopped Salad | 930 | 47 | 64 |
| Caesar Salad | 810 | 64 | 44 |
| Derby-Style Chicken Cobb Salad | 940 | 69 | 20 |
| Honey-Crisp Chicken Salad | 1370 | 103 | 77 |
| Tri-Tip Wedge Salad | 1300 | 91 | 68 |

### Sides: Broccoli

| | C | F | Cb |
|---|---|---|---|
| Broccoli | 40 | 0 | 6 |
| Classic Baked Potato | 590 | 28 | 70 |
| French Fries | 350 | 19 | 40 |
| Garlic Green Beans | 70 | 4 | 7 |
| Rice Pilaf | 230 | 6 | 39 |
| White Cheddar Mashed Potatoes | 330 | 18 | 33 |

### Desserts: Baked Beignet

| | C | F | Cb |
|---|---|---|---|
| Baked Beignet | 630 | 25 | 91 |
| Monkey Bread Pizookie | 1260 | 56 | 177 |
| Salted Caramel Pizookie | 1360 | 55 | 200 |
| Soda Floats, average all flavors | 510 | 19 | 79 |

*For Complete Nutritional Data ~ see CalorieKing.com*

## Blimpie® (Sept '19)

### Cold Deli Subs:
*Per Regular, 6" White Sub, with Standard Menu Board Toppings*

| | C | F | Cb |
|---|---|---|---|
| Blimpie Best | 470 | 17 | 54 |
| Club; Ham & Swiss | 430 | 14 | 54 |
| Roast Beef & Provolone | 460 | 14 | 53 |
| Tuna | 460 | 21 | 41 |
| Turkey & Provolone | 460 | 15 | 55 |

### Wraps: Chicken Caesar

| | C | F | Cb |
|---|---|---|---|
| Chicken Caesar | 570 | 28 | 50 |
| Southwestern; Buffalo Chicken, av. | 590 | 31 | 53 |

### Hot Deli Subs: Per Regular White Sub with Standard Menu Board Toppings Unless Indicated

| | C | F | Cb |
|---|---|---|---|
| BLT | 510 | 27 | 48 |
| Meatball Parmigiana | 740 | 38 | 59 |
| Philly Cheesesteak | 570 | 28 | 49 |

### Salads: Regular, without Dressing

| | C | F | Cb |
|---|---|---|---|
| Buffalo Chicken | 180 | 8 | 9 |
| Garden | 40 | 0 | 8 |
| Grilled Chicken Caesar | 160 | 5 | 6 |
| Ultimate Club | 310 | 16 | 11 |

### Dressings: Creamy Caesar, 1.5 oz

| | C | F | Cb |
|---|---|---|---|
| Creamy Caesar, 1.5 oz | 210 | 23 | 2 |
| Creamy Italian, 1.5 oz | 240 | 26 | 1 |
| Thousand Island | 200 | 19 | 6 |

### Soups: Per 8.6 oz

| | C | F | Cb |
|---|---|---|---|
| Chicken Noodle | 210 | 4 | 29 |
| Cream of Broccoli with Cheese | 190 | 11 | 15 |
| Cream of Potato with Bacon | 190 | 9 | 24 |
| New England Clam Chowder | 170 | 3 | 28 |
| Vegetable Beef with Barley | 100 | 3 | 14 |

### Breakfast:

| | C | F | Cb |
|---|---|---|---|
| Biscuits: Bacon, Egg & Cheese | 410 | 22 | 37 |
| Sausage, Egg & Cheese | 560 | 36 | 37 |
| Bluffin, Egg & Cheese | 240 | 8 | 29 |
| Burritos: Ham, Egg & Cheese | 570 | 27 | 51 |
| Sausage, Egg & Cheese | 710 | 43 | 50 |
| Sandwich, Grilled Bacon | 520 | 23 | 49 |

## Bob Evans® (Sept '19)

| Burgers: With Fries | C | F | Cb |
|---|---|---|---|
| **Big Farm Burgers:** | | | |
| Double Bacon Cheeseburger | 1100 | 61 | 81 |
| Double Steakhouse | 1350 | 78 | 88 |
| **Sandwiches:** With Fries | | | |
| Farmhouse Chicken | 890 | 50 | 87 |
| Handcrafted Deli Turkey | 980 | 35 | 124 |
| Shaved Ham & Swiss Melt | 1080 | 43 | 128 |
| **Slow Roasted:** | | | |
| Pot Roast | 1130 | 57 | 104 |
| Turkey Bacon Melt | 970 | 46 | 92 |
| **Dinners:** With Menu Set Sides | | | |
| Chicken 'n Noodles Deep Dish | 620 | 33 | 54 |
| Down-Home Country Fried Steak | 730 | 45 | 58 |
| Fork Tender Pot Roast | 950 | 62 | 62 |
| Heartland Chicken Pot Pie | 1430 | 87 | 106 |
| Herb Rubbed Turkey & Drssng | 820 | 40 | 81 |
| **H'style Fried Chkn:** Dark, 2 pcs | 710 | 45 | 43 |
| White, 2 pieces | 810 | 47 | 42 |
| Half Chicken | 1100 | 65 | 46 |
| **Dinners:** Without Sides | | | |
| Beef Stroganoff | 740 | 36 | 77 |
| Chicken Parm Pasta | 630 | 30 | 58 |
| Great Alaska Cod w/ Tartar Sauce | 640 | 39 | 39 |
| Potato Crusted Flounder | 260 | 13 | 13 |
| USDA Choice Sirloin w/toppings | 750 | 54 | 17 |
| **Sides:** Baked Potato | 330 | 12 | 51 |
| Loaded | 570 | 32 | 53 |
| Bread & Celery Dressing | 340 | 15 | 42 |
| Broccoli, with Butter | 110 | 10 | 5 |
| Carrots | 90 | 4.5 | 13 |
| Coleslaw | 200 | 14 | 19 |
| Corn | 170 | 10 | 20 |
| French Fries | 330 | 14 | 47 |
| Green Beans with Ham | 30 | 1.5 | 4 |
| Hash Browns | 220 | 12 | 28 |
| Home Fries | 250 | 17 | 24 |
| Mac & Cheese | 250 | 12 | 25 |
| Mashed Potatoes: w/ Chicken Gravy | 210 | 14 | 19 |
| with country gravy | 170 | 10 | 17 |
| **Sauces:** Per 1 oz Ramekin | | | |
| Bob Evans Wildfire | 50 | 0 | 13 |
| Buffalo | 60 | 6 | 1 |
| Honey Mustard | 120 | 11 | 5 |
| Ranch | 100 | 10 | 0.5 |
| **Salads:** Regular Size, with dressing | | | |
| Chicken Cobb | 1000 | 71 | 17 |
| Cranberry Pecan Chicken | 870 | 51 | 55 |

## Bob Evans® cont... (Sept '19)

| Soups: Per Bowl, with 2 Saltine Crackers | C | F | Cb |
|---|---|---|---|
| Cheddar Baked Potato | 390 | 21 | 32 |
| Chicken N Noodles | 290 | 15 | 26 |
| Hearty Beef Vegetable | 230 | 5 | 36 |
| **Kid's:** With Menu Set Items | | | |
| Chicken & Noodles | 150 | 7 | 14 |
| Cheeseburger | 760 | 36 | 84 |
| Grilled Cheese & Tomato Basil Soup | 430 | 22 | 43 |
| Grilled Chicken | 360 | 6 | 52 |
| Gr. Cheese Triangles | 330 | 15 | 40 |
| Mac & Cheese | 280 | 12 | 31 |
| Turkey Lurkey | 410 | 23 | 34 |
| **Breakfast:** With Menu Set Items, without Added Sides | | | |
| Belgian Waffle, with butter & syrup | 630 | 25 | 98 |
| Bob's Big Griddle Stacker | 1180 | 78 | 73 |
| Border Scramble | 620 | 56 | 12 |
| Brioche Fr. Toast, w/ butter & syrup | 830 | 25 | 134 |
| Cntry Fried Steak & Gravy | 540 | 33 | 38 |
| Everything Breakfast | 1130 | 73 | 63 |
| Goat Cheese Veg. Omelet | 850 | 54 | 12 |
| Ham Biscuit Benedict | 440 | 23 | 43 |
| **Hotcakes:** With Menu Set Toppings | | | |
| Buttermilk (4) | 1150 | 28 | 209 |
| Cinnamon Supreme (4) | 1070 | 26 | 190 |
| Doule Blueberry Hotcakes (4) | 1090 | 23 | 203 |
| Double Chocolate (4) | 1120 | 27 | 199 |
| Multigrain (4) | 1200 | 31 | 214 |
| Pot Roast Hash | 580 | 39 | 28 |
| Sunshine Skillet | 760 | 59 | 27 |
| Western Omelet | 650 | 50 | 11 |
| **Breakfast Sides:** | | | |
| **Eggs:** Egg White | 60 | 0 | 0.5 |
| Freshly Cracked | 200 | 16 | 0.5 |
| Scrambled | 160 | 11 | 1 |
| Homefries | 250 | 17 | 24 |
| Grits with butter | 240 | 21 | 13 |
| Hardwood Smoked Bacon | 190 | 14 | 0.5 |
| Hashbrowns | 200 | 12 | 28 |
| Hickory-Smoked Ham | 100 | 2.5 | 2 |
| Sausage Links (3) | 190 | 16 | 0 |
| Sausage Patties (2) | 320 | 26 | 2 |
| Turkey Sausage Links (2) | 140 | 7 | 2 |
| **Dessert:** Coconut Cream Pie, 1 slice | 600 | 38 | 64 |
| Chocolate Peanut Butter Pie, 1 slice | 680 | 41 | 74 |
| Double-Crust Apple Pie, 1 slice | 530 | 24 | 77 |
| Strawberry Supreme Pie, 1 slice | 590 | 38 | 6 |

## Bojangles® (Sept '19)

| Biscuit: | C | F | Cb |
|---|---|---|---|
| Plain | 340 | 17 | 40 |
| Bacon, Egg & Cheese | 480 | 28 | 42 |
| Cajun Filet | 550 | 27 | 55 |
| Country Ham | 450 | 24 | 40 |
| Gravy Biscuits | 460 | 23 | 51 |
| Sausage | 540 | 35 | 40 |
| Sausage & Egg | 580 | 38 | 40 |
| Smoked Sausage | 490 | 29 | 41 |
| Steak | 570 | 35 | 49 |
| **Biscuit Add Ons:** American Cheese | 45 | 3.5 | 1 |
| Egg | 45 | 3 | 0 |
| *Chicken:* Breast (1) | 280 | 13 | 10 |
| Leg (1) | 100 | 5 | 5 |
| Thigh (1) | 240 | 17 | 9 |
| Wing (1) | 100 | 7 | 5 |
| Homestyle Tenders, 4 pieces | 500 | 24 | 41 |
| Supremes, 4 pieces | 390 | 19 | 29 |
| *Sandwiches:* | | | |
| **Cajun Filet:** Regular | 650 | 30 | 65 |
| Club | 740 | 40 | 70 |
| **Grilled Chicken:** Regular | 470 | 22 | 41 |
| Club | 570 | 30 | 42 |
| Pulled Pork BBQ | 460 | 21 | 48 |
| *Fixins':* Per Individual Size, Unless Indicated | | | |
| Bo-Tato Rounds, medium | 370 | 19 | 45 |
| Cole Slaw | 170 | 11 | 20 |
| Green Beans | 40 | 0 | 8 |
| Macaroni & Cheese | 260 | 13 | 29 |
| Mashed Potatoes 'N Cajun Gravy | 120 | 4.5 | 17 |
| *Seasoned Fries:* Small | 250 | 16 | 37 |
| Medium | 340 | 21 | 50 |
| Picnic size | 610 | 38 | 90 |
| *Salads:* Without Dressing or Croutons | | | |
| Chicken Supreme | 450 | 24 | 31 |
| Garden | 160 | 10 | 10 |
| Grilled Chicken | 290 | 14 | 11 |
| *Sweets:* Bo-Berry Biscuit (1) | 470 | 23 | 61 |
| Cinnamon Twist (1) | 370 | 21 | 41 |
| Sweet Potato Pie | 370 | 24 | 35 |

## Boston Market® (Sept '19)

| *Sandwiches:* Per Whole Sandwich on White Sub Roll | C | F | Cb |
|---|---|---|---|
| All-White Chkn Salad, w/o Cheese | 840 | 48 | 64 |
| Meatloaf Carver | 970 | 49 | 87 |
| Pulled BBQ Rotisserie Chicken | 740 | 29 | 73 |
| Roasted Turkey Carver | 820 | 45 | 64 |
| *Individual Meals:* Without Sides or Corn Bread | | | |
| Meatloaf, regular | 470 | 33 | 17 |
| Rosemary Lemon Half Chicken | 640 | 37 | 9 |
| Rotisserie Half Chicken | 500 | 24 | 1 |
| Rotisserie Prime Rib | 630 | 47 | 0 |
| St Louis Style BBQ Ribs, half rack | 860 | 64 | 23 |

## Boston Market® cont...(Sept '19)

| *Salads:* Entree Size, with Dressing | C | F | Cb |
|---|---|---|---|
| Chicken Caesar | 430 | 28 | 15 |
| Southwest Santa Fe, 13.7 oz | 500 | 29 | 28 |
| *Sides:* Corn Bread | 160 | 3 | 31 |
| Creamed Spinach | 200 | 14 | 10 |
| Fresh Steamed Veggies | 60 | 3.5 | 7 |
| Fresh Vegetable Stuffing | 220 | 10 | 28 |
| Garlic Dill New Potatoes | 120 | 2 | 22 |
| Green Beans | 80 | 4.5 | 6 |
| Macaroni & Cheese | 260 | 9 | 34 |
| Mashed Potatoes | 240 | 10 | 32 |
| Southwest Rice | 170 | 6 | 26 |
| Sweet Corn | 130 | 6 | 17 |
| Sweet Pot. Casserole | 440 | 2 | 83 |
| *Soup,* Chicken Noodle | 240 | 9 | 20 |
| *Kid's:* Without Sides or Corn Bread | | | |
| Meatloaf | 240 | 16 | 9 |
| Turkey | 80 | 2.5 | 0 |
| White Chicken, 1 breast, 1 wing | 270 | 11 | 0 |
| *Sauce:* Beef Au Jus/Chckn Gravy | 10 | 0 | 2 |
| Horseradish | 60 | 3 | 6 |
| Tartar Sauce | 45 | 4.5 | 1 |
| Zesty BBQ | 40 | 0 | 10 |
| *Desserts:* Apple Pie, 1 slice | 430 | 21 | 59 |
| Chocolate Brownie (1) | 340 | 14 | 53 |
| Chocolate Cake, 1 slice | 570 | 33 | 66 |
| Chocolate Chunk Cookie (1) | 370 | 18 | 53 |

*For Complete Nutritional Data ~ see CalorieKing.com*

## Boston Pizza® Canada (Sept '19)

| Starters: | C | F | Cb |
|---|---|---|---|
| Medit. Hummus & Veggie Platter | 1270 | 3 | 166 |
| Oven Roasted Wings, 12.5 oz | 780 | 50 | 9 |
| Spinach & Artichoke Dip, 14.7 oz | 830 | 39 | 93 |
| *Burgers:* Dble Bacon BBQ Burger | 1110 | 78 | 60 |
| Most Valuable Burger | 1040 | 77 | 49 |
| Veggie Quinoa Burger | 800 | 46 | 71 |
| *Pastas:* Full Order, without Garlic Toast | | | |
| Boston's Lasagna | 790 | 23 | 107 |
| Montréal Smoked Meat Spagh. | 890 | 16 | 142 |
| Pesto Chicken Bowtie | 1220 | 46 | 143 |
| *Pizza:* Per 8" Individual Pizza | | | |
| **Original Crust:** Boston Royal | 790 | 27 | 97 |
| Deluxe | 720 | 24 | 92 |
| Hawaiian | 660 | 16 | 100 |
| Pepperoni | 710 | 25 | 89 |
| Vegetarian | 620 | 15 | 94 |
| **New Thin Crust Pizzas:** Per Slice of Medium Pizza | | | |
| Cherry Bomb Margherita, 2.47 oz | 150 | 6 | 17 |
| Fiesta Chicken, 2.86 oz | 200 | 11 | 18 |
| Pizza Bella, 2.3 oz | 150 | 6 | 17 |
| Potato Bianca, 3.2 oz | 170 | 5 | 24 |

## Boston Pizza® Canada cont... (Sept '19)

*Sandwiches: Without Sides*

| | C | F | Cb |
|---|---|---|---|
| Big Dipper | 1320 | 71 | 117 |
| Boston Brute | 800 | 24 | 108 |
| Chipotle Chicken Club | 950 | 40 | 86 |
| Montreal Smoked Meat | 910 | 59 | 40 |
| NY Steak Sandwich | 1000 | 49 | 104 |

*Salads: Full Order with Dressing*

| | | | |
|---|---|---|---|
| Crispy Chicken Pecan | 1090 | 83 | 49 |
| Roasted Beef & Peach | 480 | 35 | 47 |

*Desssert:*

| | | | |
|---|---|---|---|
| NY Cheesecake | 580 | 37 | 54 |
| The Panookie, with ice cream | 940 | 45 | 125 |

**For Complete Nutritional Data ~ see CalorieKing.com**

## Braum's® ~ see CalorieKing.com

## Bruegger's® (Sept '19)

*Bagels:*

| | C | F | Cb |
|---|---|---|---|
| Blueberry, 4.1 oz | 310 | 2 | 63 |
| Cinnamon Sugar, 4.1 oz | 320 | 2 | 63 |
| Everything, Whole Wheat, 4.1 oz | 280 | 2.5 | 55 |
| Jalapeno Cheddar, 5.5 oz | 440 | 9 | 75 |
| Plain, 4.1 oz | 300 | 2 | 60 |
| Rosemary Olive Oil, 4.1 oz | 330 | 6 | 59 |

*Cream Cheese: Per 1.5 oz*

| | | | |
|---|---|---|---|
| Bacon Scallion, Jalapeno, av. | 140 | 12 | 5 |
| Honey Walnut | 150 | 12 | 8 |
| Light Herb Garlic/Plain | 100 | 6 | 4 |
| Plain | 130 | 11 | 6 |
| Smoked Salmon | 150 | 13 | 3 |

*Breakfast Bagel S'wiches: With Standard Toppings*

| | | | |
|---|---|---|---|
| Egg & Cheese | 430 | 18 | 63 |
| Egg White, Cheese & Bacon | 460 | 12 | 64 |
| Plain Bagel: Smoked Salmon | 460 | 10 | 66 |
| Sriracha Egg | 650 | 30 | 70 |
| Western | 670 | 34 | 67 |

*Deli Sandwiches: With Standard Toppings*

| | | | |
|---|---|---|---|
| BLT on Wheat Bread | 610 | 44 | 38 |
| Chicken Breast on Plain Bagel | 550 | 6 | 81 |
| Garden Veggie on Plain Bagel | 360 | 2 | 72 |
| Ham On Wheat Bread | 470 | 10 | 67 |

*Deli Classics: With Standard Toppings*

| | | | |
|---|---|---|---|
| Cheese & Tomato, on Rye | 690 | 35 | 63 |
| Pastrami & Swiss Melt, on Rye | 530 | 20 | 62 |
| Tarragon Chkn Salad, on Wheatberry | 530 | 30 | 44 |
| Turkey in the Slaw, on Wheat | 520 | 23 | 49 |

*Signature & Classic Sandwiches: With Standard Toppings*

| | | | |
|---|---|---|---|
| Herby Turkey/Sesame Bagel | 570 | 15 | 75 |
| Leon. da Veggie/Asiago Parm. Bagel | 490 | 14 | 70 |
| Sm. Salmon Egg Salad/Pumpnkl Bgl | 570 | 21 | 64 |
| Turkey Chipotle Club/Evrythng Bagel | 810 | 45 | 66 |

## Bruegger's® cont... (Sept '19)

*Café Salads: Without Dressing*

| | C | F | Cb |
|---|---|---|---|
| Blue Apple, 7 oz | 360 | 18 | 30 |
| Chicken Caesar, 7.7 oz | 200 | 8 | 14 |
| Pastrami Cobb, 10.3 oz | 280 | 16 | 15 |

*Dressings: Balsamic Vinaig., 1 oz*

| | | | |
|---|---|---|---|
| Balsamic Vinaig., 1 oz | 60 | 6 | 3 |
| Caesar, 1 oz | 80 | 7 | 2 |
| Ranch | 90 | 10 | 1 |

*Dessert:*

| | | | |
|---|---|---|---|
| Chocolate Chunk Brownie, 3.3 oz | 440 | 22 | 55 |
| Marshmallow Chew, 2.7 oz | 290 | 7 | 54 |
| Oatmeal Raisin Pecan Cookie, 4 oz | 460 | 21 | 65 |

**For Complete Menu & Data ~ see CalorieKing.com**

## Burgerville® (Sept '19)

*Burgers: With Standard Ingredients*

| | C | F | Cb |
|---|---|---|---|
| American Colossal | 540 | 29 | 40 |
| American ½ lb Colossal | 790 | 47 | 40 |
| Double Cheeseburger | 490 | 28 | 31 |
| Original: Hamburger | 340 | 17 | 31 |
| Cheeseburger | 380 | 21 | 31 |
| Pepper Bacon Cheeseburger | 670 | 40 | 37 |
| Tillamook Cheeseburger | 600 | 34 | 38 |
| Chicken Tenders, (3), with Fries | 770 | 43 | 71 |

*Sandwiches: With Standard Menu Components*

| | | | |
|---|---|---|---|
| Deluxe Crispy Chkn, on Kaiser Bun | 780 | 43 | 67 |
| Deluxe Gr. Chicken, on Kaiser Bun | 550 | 25 | 42 |
| Halibut Fish, without Cheese, on Plain Bun | 460 | 27 | 40 |
| Turkey, w/out Cheese, on Sesame Seed Bun | 450 | 19 | 40 |

*French Fries: Small, 2.8 oz*

| | | | |
|---|---|---|---|
| Small, 2.8 oz | 220 | 11 | 28 |
| Regular, 5 oz | 400 | 19 | 50 |
| Large, 6.5 oz | 510 | 25 | 65 |

*Salads: Full Size, without Dressing*

| | | | |
|---|---|---|---|
| Grilled Chicken Club | 240 | 14 | 6 |
| Smoky Blue Cheese | 220 | 7 | 33 |
| Wild Smoked Salmon & Hazelnuts | 240 | 16 | 7 |

*Dressing: Balsamic Vinaigrette*

| | | | |
|---|---|---|---|
| Balsamic Vinaigrette | 180 | 18 | 5 |
| Blue Cheese | 180 | 18 | 2 |
| Honey Mustard | 200 | 19 | 8 |
| Ranch | 190 | 20 | 2 |

*Breakfast: With Standard Menu Components*

| | | | |
|---|---|---|---|
| B'fast Platter, Bacon, Engl. Muffin | 760 | 45 | 63 |
| Burger, w/ Pepp. Bacon, Chedd. Chse | 470 | 27 | 27 |
| Burrito, Ssg Patty & Chedd Cheese | 690 | 45 | 40 |

*Ice Cream Sundaes: With Whipped Cream*

| | | | |
|---|---|---|---|
| Caramel | 390 | 19 | 50 |
| Hot Fudge | 390 | 19 | 51 |
| Triple Berry | 350 | 18 | 41 |

## Burger King® (Sept '19)

### Whopper Sandwiches:

| | C | F | Cb |
|---|---|---|---|
| Whopper: Regular | 660 | 40 | 49 |
| with Cheese | 740 | 46 | 50 |
| Double Whopper | 900 | 58 | 49 |
| With Cheese | 980 | 64 | 50 |
| Bacon & Cheese | 790 | 51 | 50 |
| BBQ Bacon | 800 | 51 | 53 |
| Impossible Whopper (Vegan) | 630 | 34 | 58 |
| Whopper Jr | 310 | 18 | 27 |

### Flame Grilled Burgers:

| | C | F | Cb |
|---|---|---|---|
| Bacon Cheeseburger | 320 | 16 | 27 |
| Bacon Double Cheeseburger | 420 | 24 | 27 |
| Bacon King Sandwich | 1150 | 79 | 49 |
| Bacon King Jr. | 570 | 38 | 27 |
| Cheeseburger | 280 | 13 | 27 |
| Double Cheeseburger | 390 | 21 | 27 |
| Hamburger | 240 | 10 | 26 |
| Quarter Pound King | 580 | 29 | 49 |
| Double | 1140 | 71 | 50 |
| Rodeo King | 1250 | 100 | 69 |
| **Stacker King:** Single | 700 | 42 | 48 |
| Double | 1050 | 68 | 49 |
| Triple | 1370 | 93 | 51 |
| *Pulled Pork King* | 690 | 25 | 82 |

### Chicken Sandwiches:

| | C | F | Cb |
|---|---|---|---|
| **Chicken Jr.:** Regular | 450 | 30 | 34 |
| Spicy Chicken Jr. | 390 | 21 | 27 |
| **Crispy Chicken:** Regular | 670 | 41 | 54 |
| BBQ Bacon | 790 | 49 | 60 |
| Club | 800 | 51 | 55 |
| Rodeo | 960 | 60 | 72 |
| Spicy | 700 | 42 | 57 |
| *Crispy Taco* | 170 | 9 | 19 |
| **Chicken Nuggets:** 4 pieces | 170 | 11 | 11 |
| 6 pieces | 260 | 16 | 16 |
| *Chicken Fries,* Regular, 9 pieces | 280 | 17 | 20 |
| *Dipping Sauces:* BBQ | 40 | 0 | 11 |
| Buffalo | 80 | 8 | 2 |
| Chicken Fry | 140 | 13 | 6 |
| Ranch; Zesty Onion Ring, av. | 145 | 15 | 2 |
| *Big Fish S'wich* | 510 | 28 | 51 |
| *French Fries:* Small, 4.3 oz | 320 | 14 | 44 |
| Medium, 5.8 oz | 380 | 17 | 53 |
| Large, 7 oz | 430 | 19 | 60 |
| *Onion Rings:* Small | 320 | 16 | 41 |
| Medium | 410 | 21 | 53 |
| Large | 500 | 25 | 64 |

### Salads: *Without Dressing*

| | C | F | Cb |
|---|---|---|---|
| **Club:** with Crispy Chicken | 540 | 33 | 31 |
| with Grilled Chicken | 440 | 23 | 16 |
| **Garden:** with Crispy Chicken | 440 | 25 | 31 |
| with Grilled Chicken | 340 | 15 | 16 |
| **Garden,** Side Salad | 60 | 4 | 3 |

## Burger King® cont... (Sept '19)

### Salad Dressings:

| | C | F | Cb |
|---|---|---|---|
| Golden Italian, 1.5 oz | 160 | 17 | 4 |
| Lite Honey Balsamic Vinaigrette, 1.5 oz | 120 | 8 | 14 |
| Ranch, 1.5 oz | 260 | 28 | 2 |

### Breakfast:

| | C | F | Cb |
|---|---|---|---|
| **Biscuits:** Bacon, Egg & Cheese | 390 | 25 | 28 |
| Ham, Egg & Cheese | 370 | 22 | 29 |
| Sausage | 400 | 28 | 28 |
| Sausage, Egg & Cheese | 520 | 37 | 29 |
| **BK Ultimate Breakfast Platter** | 1170 | 65 | 122 |
| **Burrito:** Egg-Normous | 930 | 57 | 69 |
| Breakfast Burrito Jr. | 370 | 23 | 27 |
| **Croissan'wich:** | | | |
| Bacon, Egg & Cheese | 340 | 18 | 30 |
| Egg & Cheese | 300 | 15 | 30 |
| Fully Loaded | 570 | 37 | 32 |
| Ham, Egg & Cheese | 340 | 16 | 31 |
| **Double Croissan'wich:** | | | |
| with Sausage | 710 | 52 | 31 |
| with Ham & Sausage | 580 | 38 | 31 |
| with Sausage & Bacon | 580 | 40 | 31 |
| **French Toast Sandwiches:** | | | |
| Bacon, Egg & Cheese | 380 | 20 | 30 |
| Ham, Egg & Cheese | 380 | 18 | 30 |
| Sausage, Egg & Cheese | 510 | 32 | 30 |
| **French Toast Sticks,** 3 pieces | 230 | 11 | 29 |
| **Hash Browns:** Small, 3 oz | 250 | 16 | 24 |
| Medium, 6 oz | 500 | 33 | 48 |
| Large, 8 oz | 670 | 44 | 65 |
| **Oatmeal,** Orig. Maple Flavored | 170 | 3 | 32 |
| **Pancake Platter:** Regular (3) | 440 | 16 | 71 |
| Pancakes & Sausage | 610 | 31 | 72 |

### Desserts:

| | C | F | Cb |
|---|---|---|---|
| Chocolate Chip Cookie (2) | 320 | 16 | 48 |
| Cinni Minis (4) | 410 | 14 | 66 |
| **Pies:** Dutch Apple | 340 | 14 | 51 |
| Hershey's Sundae | 310 | 19 | 32 |
| **Sundaes:** Caramel | 240 | 5 | 42 |
| Chocolate Hershey's | 260 | 5 | 49 |
| **Vanilla Soft Serve,** in cone | 140 | 4 | 24 |
| *Shakes:* Chocolate w. M&M's | 840 | 22 | 144 |
| Chocolate Oreo | 610 | 19 | 99 |
| Strawberry | 640 | 15 | 113 |
| Vanilla | 580 | 15 | 98 |
| *Smoothies:* Strawb. Ban.,16 fl.oz | 310 | 1 | 71 |
| Tropical Mango, 16 fl.oz | 370 | 0 | 86 |
| *Beverages:* Frappe, av., 16 fl.oz | 405 | 16 | 62 |
| Minute Maid Orange Juice, 10 fl.oz | 140 | 0 | 33 |
| **Frozen Coke/Fanta** | 130 | 0 | 3 |
| **Icee,** Cherry, 16 oz | 140 | 0 | 38 |
| **Iced Coffee:** Medium | 150 | 8 | 19 |
| Vanilla, 16 oz | 190 | 8 | 28 |
| **Sweet Tea,** 20 oz | 120 | 0 | 35 |

Updated Nutrition Data ~ www.CalorieKing.com
Persons with Diabetes ~ See Disclaimer (Page 22)

## Captain D's Seafood® (Sept '19)

*From The Grill: Without Sides, Rice, Hushpuppies or Breadstick*

| | C | F | Cb |
|---|---|---|---|
| Blackened Tilapia | 210 | 7 | 1 |
| Grilled Wild Salmon | 230 | 10 | 2 |
| Grilled Whitefish & Shrimp Skewer | 280 | 11 | 3 |
| Lemon Pepper Whitefish Fillet | 180 | 8 | 1 |
| Shrimp Skewers (2) | 200 | 6 | 2 |

*Variety Meals:*

| | | | |
|---|---|---|---|
| Deluxe Seafood Platter | 1100 | 75 | 67 |
| Fish & Shrimp | 810 | 56 | 45 |
| Supreme Sampler | 1180 | 79 | 68 |
| White Fish, Shrimp & Crab | 940 | 64 | 52 |

*Salads: Without Dressing or Breadstick*

| | | | |
|---|---|---|---|
| Grilled Tilapia | 310 | 13 | 9 |
| Southern Style Breaded Chicken | 290 | 17 | 20 |

*Add-Ons:*

| | | | |
|---|---|---|---|
| Baked Potato, plain, (1) | 210 | 0 | 48 |
| Coleslaw, 1 order | 180 | 13 | 15 |
| French Fries, 1 serving | 330 | 22 | 28 |
| Hushpuppy (1) | 80 | 4 | 9 |
| Jalapeno Poppers | 510 | 36 | 40 |
| *Dessert,* Chocolate Cake, 1 order | 300 | 11 | 49 |

## Caribou Coffee® (Sept '19)

*With Standard Recipe Ingredients.*

| Hot Beverages: | C | F | Cb |
|---|---|---|---|
| **Chai Tea,** 20 fl.oz | 310 | 7 | 48 |
| **Chocolate,** 20 fl.oz | 450 | 22 | 49 |
| **Crafted Press Coffee:** Small, 12 fl.oz | 90 | 6 | 7 |
| Medium, 16 fl.oz | 160 | 9 | 12 |
| Large, 20 fl.oz | 190 | 11 | 17 |
| **Macchiato:** Small, 12 fl.oz | 15 | 0.5 | 1 |
| Medium, 16 fl.oz | 20 | 1 | 1 |
| Large, 20 fl.oz | 20 | 1 | 1 |

*Cold Beverages: Per Medium 20 fl.oz, without Whipped Cream*

**Blended Fruit & Yogurt Smoothies:**

| | | | |
|---|---|---|---|
| Mango Orange Key Lime | 420 | 0 | 106 |
| Strawberry Banana | 360 | 0 | 87 |

**Coolers:**

| | | | |
|---|---|---|---|
| Berry White Mocha, 20 fl.oz | 770 | 24 | 126 |
| Caramel High Rise, 20 fl.oz | 720 | 27 | 113 |
| Mint Condition, 20 fl.oz | 790 | 27 | 121 |

*For Complete Menu ~ See Calorieking.com*

## Carl's Jr.® (Sept '19)

*California menu only. Please check instore for further nutritional information.*

| Charbroiled Burgers: | C | F | Cb |
|---|---|---|---|
| Beyond Famous Star with Cheese | 710 | 40 | 61 |
| Famous Star with Cheese | 670 | 37 | 57 |
| Super Star with Cheese | 920 | 56 | 59 |
| The Big Carl | 920 | 58 | 56 |
| Western Bacon Cheeseburger | 750 | 35 | 75 |
| Double | 1010 | 55 | 76 |
| **1/2 lb Thickburgers:** Original $6 | 980 | 69 | 59 |
| Guacamole Bacon | 1200 | 89 | 51 |
| Lettuce Wrapped | 630 | 55 | 9 |

*Chicken Sandwiches:*

| | | | |
|---|---|---|---|
| Bacon Swiss Crispy Chicken Fillet | 770 | 41 | 58 |
| Big Chicken Fillet | 650 | 33 | 55 |
| **Charbroiled:** BBQ Chicken | 390 | 7 | 50 |
| Chicken Club | 580 | 28 | 46 |
| Santa Fe Chicken | 560 | 27 | 46 |
| *Chicken Tenders,* hand breaded, 5 pieces, without sauce | 440 | 21 | 21 |
| *Low Carb Options,* Chicken Club | 370 | 24 | 8 |
| *Trim It:* Charbr. BBQ Chicken S'wich | 390 | 8 | 51 |
| Famous Star | 430 | 18 | 46 |
| *Veg It,* Guacamole Thickburger | 670 | 46 | 56 |

*Breakfast:*

| | | | |
|---|---|---|---|
| Bacon & Egg Burrito | 570 | 35 | 32 |
| Breakfast Burger, Single | 730 | 43 | 47 |
| Grilled Cheese & Sausage S'wich | 660 | 43 | 43 |
| **Hash Rounds:** Small, 3.8 oz | 350 | 23 | 32 |
| Medium, 4.2 oz | 390 | 26 | 36 |
| Large, 6 oz | 560 | 37 | 52 |
| Loaded B'fast Burrito | 760 | 48 | 46 |
| Steak & Egg Burrito | 630 | 36 | 37 |
| *Fries:* CrissCut Fries, 5 oz | 450 | 29 | 42 |
| Natural Cut: Small, 3.5 oz | 300 | 15 | 39 |
| Medium, 6 oz | 430 | 21 | 55 |
| Large, 6.5 oz | 460 | 22 | 59 |
| *Fried Zucchini,* 5 oz | 330 | 18 | 36 |
| *Onion Rings,* 4.5 oz | 530 | 28 | 61 |

*Salads: W/out Dressing*

| | | | |
|---|---|---|---|
| Charbroiled Chicken | 280 | 9 | 19 |
| Garden, side | 140 | 7 | 15 |

*Dressings: Per 2 oz Package*

| | | | |
|---|---|---|---|
| House | 220 | 22 | 3 |
| Low-Fat Balsamic | 35 | 1.5 | 5 |
| *Dessert:* Choc. Chip Cookies (2) | 330 | 17 | 43 |
| Chocolate Cake, 3 oz | 290 | 11 | 46 |
| Strawberry Swirl Cheesecake, 3.5 oz | 320 | 17 | 35 |

*Shakes: With Ice Cream*

| | | | |
|---|---|---|---|
| Oreo Cookie | 710 | 39 | 79 |
| Vanilla; Chocolate; Strawberry, av. | 695 | 35 | 85 |

## Carvel® (Sept '19)

| *Carvelanche:* | C | F | Cb |
|---|---|---|---|
| **M&M'S:** Small, 12 oz | 650 | 32 | 73 |
| Regular, 16 oz | 850 | 43 | 97 |
| Large, 24 oz | 1320 | 66 | 152 |
| *Classic Sundaes: Per Small, 12 oz* | | | |
| Hot Caramel | 620 | 27 | 79 |
| Hot Fudge | 620 | 32 | 72 |
| Strawberry | 530 | 26 | 61 |
| *Sundae Dashers: Per Regular, 16 oz* | | | |
| Banana's Foster | 1050 | 33 | 171 |
| Fudge Brownie | 1250 | 62 | 166 |
| Mint Chocolate Chip | 1080 | 56 | 144 |
| Peanut Butter Cup | 1850 | 110 | 174 |
| Strawberry Shortcake | 880 | 37 | 125 |
| *Ice Cream Scoops: Per Medium* | | | |
| Butter Pecan | 750 | 51 | 57 |
| Chocolate | 520 | 27 | 59 |
| Mint Chcolate Chip | 670 | 35 | 78 |
| Peanut Butter Treasure | 680 | 41 | 73 |
| *Thick Shakes: Per 16 oz* | | | |
| Chocolate; Vanilla, av. | 650 | 27 | 90 |
| Strawberry | 590 | 27 | 73 |

## Charley's Grilled Subs® (Sept '19)

| *Philly Cheesesteaks: Per Regular* | | | |
|---|---|---|---|
| Bacon 3 Cheese Steak | 720 | 31 | 56 |
| Chicken Buffalo/Teriyaki, av. | 620 | 18 | 61 |
| Chicken California | 690 | 28 | 52 |
| Jalapeno Cheesesteak | 640 | 24 | 57 |
| Pepperoni Cheesesteak | 780 | 37 | 55 |
| Philly Cheesesteak | 640 | 24 | 58 |
| *Chicken: Per Piece* | | | |
| **Boneless:** Plain/Buffalo/Habanero | 110 | 7 | 6 |
| Garlic Parmesan | 160 | 12 | 8 |
| Nashville Hot | 180 | 14 | 9 |
| Thai Chili | 150 | 7 | 16 |
| **Classic:** Plain | 120 | 9 | 0 |
| Angry Ghost | 140 | 10 | 3 |
| Buffalo/Cajun Rub/Smokin Habanero | 130 | 9 | 1 |
| Nashville Hot | 190 | 16 | 2 |
| Thai Chili/Cajun Rub | 130 | 10 | 1 |
| **Tenders,** Plain | 190 | 13 | 11 |
| *Fries:* | | | |
| Original | 400 | 22 | 46 |
| Gourmet: Cheese & Bacon | 690 | 42 | 63 |
| Cheese | 550 | 31 | 62 |
| Ultimate | 790 | 54 | 61 |
| *Sides:* | | | |
| Baked Beans, regular | 180 | 0 | 41 |
| Celery Sticks with Ranch Dip | 210 | 21 | 3 |
| Coleslaw regular | 190 | 16 | 11 |
| Texas Toast, 1 piece | 170 | 6 | 26 |

*For Complete Menu & Data ~ see CalorieKing.com*

## Cheesecake Factory® (Sept '19)

| *Cheesecake: Per Slice* | C | F | Cb |
|---|---|---|---|
| Original | 830 | 59 | 63 |
| Godiva Chocolate | 1400 | 105 | 110 |
| Reese's P.B. Chocolate Cake | 1530 | 94 | 157 |
| White Chocolate Raspb. Truffle | 1220 | 89 | 92 |
| *Appetizers:* Avocado Egg Rolls | 930 | 48 | 111 |
| Brussels Sprouts & Kale Salad | 1330 | 118 | 43 |
| Chicken Pot Stickers | 420 | 14 | 42 |
| Fried Macaroni & Cheese | 1290 | 95 | 68 |
| Hummus | 090 | 71 | 90 |
| **Small Plates & Snacks:** *As Served* | | | |
| Beets & Avocado Salad | 290 | 12 | 40 |
| Chicken Taquitos | 390 | 22 | 31 |
| Crispy Fried Cheese | 1070 | 75 | 49 |
| Garlic Cheese Toast | 830 | 54 | 54 |
| Korean Fried Cauliflower | 1150 | 71 | 113 |
| *Flatbread Pizza:* Cheese | 980 | 50 | 83 |
| Margherita | 740 | 30 | 82 |
| Pepperpmo | 1100 | 61 | 84 |
| *Glamburgers: Without Sides* | | | |
| American Cheeseburger | 1400 | 93 | 79 |
| Bacon-Bacon Cheeseburger | 1590 | 108 | 76 |
| Classic Burger | 1340 | 87 | 69 |
| Grilled Turkey Burger | 1010 | 53 | 83 |
| Mushroom Burger | 1470 | 102 | 72 |
| Veggie Burger | 1160 | 57 | 136 |
| **Glamburger Sides:** French Fries | 530 | 23 | 76 |
| Green Salad | 130 | 12 | 6 |
| Sweet Potato Fries | 450 | 20 | 63 |
| *Fish & Seafood:* | | | |
| Fish & Chips | 1860 | 121 | 133 |
| Shrimp Scampi | 1350 | 77 | 123 |
| Seared Ahi Tuna | 1090 | 54 | 107 |
| *Pasta:* Four Cheese | 1240 | 60 | 125 |
| with Chicken | 1500 | 76 | 125 |
| Fettuccine Alfredo with Chicken | 2290 | 154 | 142 |
| Louisiana Chicken Pasta | 2120 | 125 | 168 |
| *Sandwiches:* Club | 1210 | 60 | 111 |
| Cuban | 1190 | 71 | 64 |
| Sthwst Chicken | 1040 | 57 | 80 |
| *Specialties:* Baja Chicken Tacos | 1250 | 53 | 123 |
| Cajun Chicken "Littles" | 2130 | 110 | 177 |
| Chicken Bellagio | 1670 | 86 | 135 |
| Chicken Riesling | 1430 | 84 | 88 |
| Crispy Chkn Costoletta | 1760 | 116 | 102 |
| Factory Burrito Grande | 1870 | 98 | 159 |
| Grilled Fish Tacos | 1030 | 42 | 121 |
| Grilled Steak Tacos | 1030 | 42 | 121 |
| White Chicken Chili | 590 | 6 | 33 |
| *Salads: Includes Dressing* | | | |
| Caesar | 1290 | 112 | 41 |
| Santa Fe | 1730 | 114 | 106 |
| Seared Tuna Tataki | 490 | 29 | 17 |

## Chick-fil-A® (Sept '19)

| Breakfast: | C | F | Cb |
|---|---|---|---|
| **Bagel,** Chicken, Egg & Cheese | 460 | 18 | 49 |
| **Biscuits:** Plain, buttered | 310 | 14 | 42 |
| Bacon, Egg & Cheese | 440 | 23 | 42 |
| Chicken | 440 | 20 | 48 |
| Egg White Chicken Grill | 300 | 7 | 31 |
| Sausage, Egg & Cheese | 670 | 46 | 43 |
| **Bowl,** Hash Brown Scramble | 460 | 29 | 21 |
| **Burrito,** Hash Brown Scramble | 690 | 38 | 52 |
| **Chick-n-Minis,** 4 pieces | 350 | 14 | 37 |
| **Hash Browns,** 2.7 oz | 250 | 17 | 23 |
| **Parfait,** Greek Yogurt, fruit topping | 250 | 9 | 30 |

| *Chick-fil-A Sandwiches: Without Sauce* | | | |
|---|---|---|---|
| Chicken | 440 | 19 | 40 |
| Deluxe | 500 | 23 | 42 |
| Grilled Chicken | 310 | 6 | 36 |
| Grilled Chicken Club | 440 | 16 | 36 |
| Spicy Deluxe | 540 | 25 | 43 |

| *Chicken: Without Dipping Sauce* | | | |
|---|---|---|---|
| Breaded Chick-n-Strips, 3 count | 330 | 16 | 21 |
| **Grilled Nuggets:** 6 count | 110 | 2.5 | 2 |
| 8 Count | 140 | 3.5 | 2 |

| *Salads: Without Dressing* | | | |
|---|---|---|---|
| **Cobb:** with Chick-n Strips | 620 | 33 | 41 |
| with Grilled Nuggets | 550 | 29 | 30 |
| with Spicy Grilled Filet (cold) | 410 | 20 | 22 |
| **Market:** with Nuggets | 470 | 23 | 34 |
| without Chicken | 210 | 11 | 24 |

| *Dressings:* Creamy Salsa | 290 | 31 | 2 |
|---|---|---|---|
| Fat Free Honey Mustard | 90 | 0 | 23 |
| Garlic Herb Ranch | 280 | 29 | 2 |
| Light Italian | 25 | 1 | 3 |
| *Sauces:* BBQ/Honey Roasted | 45 | 0 | 10 |
| Chick-fil-A | 140 | 13 | 6 |
| Honey Mustard Sauce | 45 | 0 | 11 |
| Sweet & Spicy Sriracha Sauce | 45 | 0 | 10 |
| *Sides:* Fruit Cup, medium | 50 | 0 | 12 |
| Chicken Noodle Soup, small bowl | 130 | 3.5 | 15 |
| Side Salad, with toppings | 160 | 10 | 13 |

| Superfood Side Salad, w/ toppings: | | | |
|---|---|---|---|
| Small | 140 | 8 | 16 |
| Large | 180 | 9 | 24 |
| Waffle Potato Fries: Med. | 360 | 18 | 43 |
| Large | 460 | 24 | 56 |
| *Dessert:* Chocolate Chunk Cookie | 350 | 16 | 49 |
| Icedream Cone, large | 250 | 6 | 43 |
| Frosted Coffee, large | 300 | 7 | 51 |
| *Milkshakes:* Chocolate, large | 740 | 26 | 114 |
| Cookies & Cream, large | 780 | 31 | 111 |
| Vanilla, large | 640 | 26 | 91 |

## Chili's® (Sept '19)

| *Appetizers: As Served* | C | F | Cb |
|---|---|---|---|
| Bottomless Tostada Chips w/ Salsa | 910 | 45 | 113 |
| **Classic Nachos:** Beef | 1610 | 105 | 56 |
| Chicken | 1390 | 88 | 59 |
| Southwestern Eggrolls | 800 | 41 | 82 |
| Texas Cheese Fries, full order | 1860 | 127 | 97 |
| **Triple Dipper:** *Serving for One* | | | |
| Big Mouth Bites | 780 | 54 | 40 |
| Original Chicken Crispers | 510 | 34 | 23 |

| *Baby Back Ribs: Full Rack, without Sides* | | | |
|---|---|---|---|
| Dry Rub | 1480 | 107 | 30 |
| Original BBQ | 1430 | 106 | 21 |
| Honey Chipotle BBQ | 1480 | 106 | 35 |
| House BBQ | 1440 | 107 | 21 |

| *Burgers: Without Side Fries* | | | |
|---|---|---|---|
| Just Bacon Beef | 1060 | 72 | 48 |
| Oldtimer, with Cheese Beef | 890 | 55 | 47 |
| Southern Smokehouse Beef | 1290 | 84 | 73 |

| *Crispers & More: As Served, with Set Sides* | | | |
|---|---|---|---|
| Cajun Pasta with Grilled Chicken | 1180 | 53 | 111 |
| Orig. Tempura, w/ Honey Mstrd | 1320 | 67 | 120 |

| *Fresh Mex: As Served* | | | |
|---|---|---|---|
| Bacon Ranch Chicken Quesadilla | 1680 | 125 | 70 |
| Chicken Enchiladas | 1140 | 53 | 104 |
| Chipotle Chicken Bowl | 1000 | 50 | 79 |
| Ranchero Chicken Tacos | 1030 | 46 | 97 |

| *Guiltless Grill: As Served* | | | |
|---|---|---|---|
| Ancho Salmon | 630 | 30 | 42 |
| Grilled Chicken Salad | 430 | 23 | 22 |
| Mango Chile Chicken | 490 | 19 | 49 |
| Margarita Grilled Chicken | 630 | 16 | 67 |
| Sirloin (6 oz), w/ Grilled Avocado | 330 | 16 | 13 |

| *Sandwiches: Without Fries* | | | |
|---|---|---|---|
| Bacon Avocado Chicken | 1140 | 60 | 74 |
| Buffalo Chicken Ranch | 880 | 48 | 69 |
| CA Turkey Club | 1100 | 65 | 87 |

| *Steaks: Without Sides* | | | |
|---|---|---|---|
| Classic Sirloin, 6 oz | 260 | 13 | 1 |
| Classic Ribeye | 630 | 40 | 0 |
| Country-Fried Steak, with gravy | 590 | 35 | 30 |

| *Sides: As Served* | | | |
|---|---|---|---|
| Awesome Blossom Petals | 820 | 56 | 70 |
| Homestyle Fries | 420 | 17 | 60 |
| Loaded Mashed Potatoes | 350 | 20 | 33 |
| Mexican Rice | 160 | 4.5 | 27 |
| Roasted Street Corn | 390 | 28 | 31 |

| *Salads: As Served* | | | |
|---|---|---|---|
| Boneless Buffalo Chicken | 970 | 67 | 44 |
| Caribbean with Seared Shrimp | 600 | 26 | 80 |
| Quesadilla Explosion | 1400 | 93 | 83 |

| *Sweet Stuff: Per Slice* | | | |
|---|---|---|---|
| Cheesecake | 720 | 43 | 74 |
| Molten Chocolate Cake | 1150 | 61 | 142 |

*For Complete Menu & Data ~ see CalorieKing.com*

**189**

## Chipotle® (Sept '19)

| Tortillas: | C | F | Cb |
|---|---|---|---|
| Burrito Size Flour Tortillas (1) | 320 | 9 | 50 |
| Taco Size: Crispy Corn Tortilla (3) | 200 | 9 | 29 |
| Soft Flour Tortillas (Taco), (3) | 250 | 8 | 40 |
| **Meal Components:** | | | |
| Barbacoa, 4 oz | 170 | 7 | 2 |
| Black/Pinto Beans, average, 4 oz | 130 | 1.5 | 22 |
| Cilantro Brown/White Rice, 4 oz | 210 | 5 | 38 |
| Carnitas, 4 oz | 210 | 12 | 0 |
| Chicken, 4 oz | 180 | 7 | 0 |
| Fajita Vegetables, 2.5 oz | 20 | 0 | 5 |
| Guacamole, 3.5 oz | 230 | 22 | 8 |
| Lettuce, 1 oz | 5 | 0 | 1 |
| Monterey Jack, 1 oz | 110 | 8 | 1 |
| Sofritas, 4 oz | 150 | 10 | 9 |
| Steak, 4 oz | 150 | 6 | 1 |
| **Condiments:** | | | |
| **Queso,** 2 oz | 120 | 8 | 4 |
| **Salsa:** Chili Corn, 3.5 oz | 80 | 1.5 | 16 |
| Green Tomatillo, 2 oz | 15 | 0 | 4 |
| Red Tomatillo, 2 oz | 15 | 0 | 4 |
| **Sour Cream,** 2 oz | 110 | 9 | 2 |
| **Extras,** Chips, 4 oz | 540 | 25 | 73 |

## Chuck E. Cheese® (Sept '19)

| Appetizers: | C | F | Cb |
|---|---|---|---|
| Cheesy Breadsticks (1) | 170 | 11 | 13 |
| French Fries, 7 oz | 380 | 12 | 59 |
| Parmesan Breadstick (1) | 240 | 10 | 30 |
| **Sandwiches & Wraps:** *Per Half Sandwich/Wrap* | | | |
| BBQ Chicken Ciabatta | 270 | 9 | 30 |
| Italian Ciabatta | 320 | 17 | 25 |
| Wraps: Chicken Caesar | 400 | 20 | 29 |
| Club | 470 | 30 | 28 |
| **Specialty Pizzas:** *Per Medium Slice* | | | |
| BBQ Chicken | 210 | 9 | 24 |
| Cali Alfredo; Meat Combo | 200 | 10 | 19 |
| Super Combo | 190 | 9 | 19 |
| Vegetarian | 160 | 6 | 19 |
| **Traditional Wings:** | | | |
| **Small:** with BBQ or Sweet Chili Sauce | 450 | 27 | 17 |
| with Lemon Pepper Sauce | 400 | 27 | 4 |
| **Desserts:** Apple Pie Pizza, whole | 440 | 7 | 89 |
| Churros (4) | 560 | 21 | 90 |

## Church's Chicken® (Sept '19)

| Chicken: *Per Serving* | C | F | Cb |
|---|---|---|---|
| **Original:** Breast, 1 piece | 250 | 14 | 9 |
| Leg, 1 piece | 150 | 8 | 6 |
| Thigh, 1 piece | 360 | 27 | 12 |
| Wing, 1 piece | 290 | 18 | 8 |
| **Spicy:** Breast, 1 piece | 280 | 17 | 12 |
| Leg, 1 piece | 160 | 9 | 9 |
| Thigh, 1 piece | 380 | 25 | 21 |
| Wing, 1 piece | 350 | 20 | 19 |
| **Tender Strips,** average, 1 piece | 110 | 5 | 6.5 |
| **Sides:** *Per Regular Serving* | | | |
| Baked Macaroni & Cheese, 4.7 oz | 210 | 12 | 19 |
| Cole Slaw, 4.2 oz | 170 | 11 | 16 |
| French Fries, 2.6 oz | 210 | 9 | 29 |
| Honey Butter Biscuits (1), 2.2 oz | 230 | 15 | 25 |
| Jalapeno Cheese Bombers (4) | 220 | 11 | 24 |
| Mashed Potatoes & Gravy, 4.5 oz | 110 | 1 | 24 |
| Okra, 3.4 oz | 260 | 15 | 30 |
| Sauces: Honey BBQ, pkt | 45 | 0 | 11 |
| Creamy Jalapeno, pkt | 120 | 13 | 2 |
| Honey Mustard/Ranch, av., pkt | 140 | 14 | 3 |
| Dessert, Apple Pie | 270 | 13 | 37 |

## Cici's Pizza® (Sept '19)

| Pizza: *Per Slice* | C | F | Cb |
|---|---|---|---|
| **Favorites:** Pepperoni | 200 | 7 | 23 |
| Alfredo; Zesty Ham & Cheddar, av. | 170 | 6 | 22 |
| **Flatbread:** Chicken Bacon | 150 | 7 | 14 |
| Honey BBQ Chkn; Spinach Alfredo, av. | 140 | 6.5 | 16 |
| **Pan,** Cheese; Meat Eater; Supreme, av. | 230 | 11 | 27 |
| **Specialty:** Meat Eater; Supreme, av. | 200 | 9 | 25 |
| Veggie | 180 | 6 | 23 |
| **Stuffed Crust,** Cheese; Pepperoni | 200 | 8 | 21 |
| **Wings:** BBQ (5) | 260 | 12 | 16 |
| Buffalo (5), average | 215 | 13 | 4 |
| Garlic Parmesan (5) | 270 | 18 | 5 |
| **Sides:** Chicken & Pasta Soup, 8 oz | 90 | 2.5 | 13 |
| Pasta Salad | 210 | 8 | 29 |
| Salad Mix | 5 | 0 | 2 |
| **Dessert:** Brownie | 140 | 6 | 21 |
| Apple/Barvarian Pizza, 1 slice | 130 | 3 | 23 |

## Cinnabon® (Sept '19)

| | C | F | Cb |
|---|---|---|---|
| Cinnabon Classic Roll (1) | 880 | 37 | 127 |
| MiniBon Roll (1), 3.4 oz | 350 | 15 | 51 |
| **Cheese Roll Paninis:** Grilled Cheese | 480 | 26 | 41 |
| Black Forest Ham | 590 | 25 | 48 |
| Smoked Turkey Club | 520 | 25 | 48 |
| **Chillata:** *Per 16 fl.oz* | | | |
| Double Chocolate Mocha | 360 | 13 | 59 |
| Oreo Cookies & Cream | 700 | 25 | 112 |
| Strawberries & Cream | 540 | 18 | 89 |

## Claim Jumper® (Sept '18)

| | C | F | Cb |
|---|---|---|---|
| ***Appetizers:*** *As Served* | | | |
| Southwest Eggrolls | 1190 | 53 | 114 |
| Three Cheese Potatocakes (3) | 1075 | 71 | 80 |
| ***Burgers & Sandwiches:*** *Without Sides* | | | |
| Grilled Cobb Sandwich | 1210 | 78 | 78 |
| Widow Maker Burger | 1370 | 87 | 84 |
| ***Calzones:*** Specialty | 1430 | 80 | 137 |
| Traditional | 1350 | 66 | 140 |
| ***Meals:*** *As Per Menu Description* | | | |
| **Favorites:** Country Fried Steak | 2030 | 107 | 189 |
| Giant Stuffed Chicken Baker | 990 | 34 | 118 |
| Meatloaf & Mashed Potatoes | 1300 | 75 | 117 |
| **Pasta:** Black Tie Pasta | 1535 | 84 | 126 |
| Parmesan Crusted Chicken | 975 | 47 | 83 |
| **Pizza:** Calif. Works, Classic Crust | 1295 | 64 | 127 |
| Steakhouse, Flatbread | 820 | 47 | 65 |
| **Specialties:** BBQ Baby Back Pork Ribs, Full Rack | 1745 | 111 | 111 |
| Roasted Tri-Tip with Demi Glaze | 800 | 47 | 19 |
| **Seafood:** Atlantic Salmon, Blcknd | 715 | 42 | 48 |
| Tilapia Bianca, with Shrimp, Artichoke Hearts & Sauce | 1165 | 80 | 56 |
| ***Entree Salads:*** *Without Dressing or Bread* | | | |
| Calif. Citrus Chkn, Charbroiled | 865 | 53 | 58 |
| Seared Ahi Spinach | 515 | 24 | 31 |
| ***Soups:*** *Per Bowl* | | | |
| New England Clam Chowder | 525 | 45 | 23 |
| Potato Cheddar | 710 | 61 | 31 |
| ***Sweets:*** Choc. Motherlode Cake | 2770 | 144 | 340 |
| Italian Lemon Cake | 1240 | 62 | 158 |

## Cold Stone Creamery® (Sept '19)

| | C | F | Cb |
|---|---|---|---|
| *Ice Cream:* | | | |
| **Amaretto:** Like it | 340 | 21 | 36 |
| Love it | 550 | 33 | 57 |
| Gotta have it | 820 | 49 | 85 |
| **Chocolate:** Like it | 330 | 20 | 34 |
| Love it | 520 | 31 | 54 |
| Gotta have it | 780 | 47 | 81 |
| *Sorbet:* | | | |
| **Strawberry Mango Banana:** | | | |
| Like it, 5 oz | 210 | 0 | 54 |
| Love it, 8 oz | 340 | 0 | 87 |
| Gotta have it, 12 oz | 510 | 0 | 130 |
| ***Shakes:*** *Per 20 oz With Whipped Topping* | | | |
| Cake Batter 'n Shake | 1440 | 76 | 176 |
| Oh Fudge | 1340 | 76 | 149 |
| Savory Strawerry | 1200 | 71 | 133 |
| Very Vanilla | 1300 | 75 | 147 |
| ***Sundaes:*** Banana Split Decision | 650 | 37 | 77 |
| Who You Callin' Shortcake | 560 | 31 | 68 |

## Costco Food Court® (Sept '19)

| | C | F | Cb |
|---|---|---|---|
| *(Approximate Figures Only)* | | | |
| ***Baked Potato,*** with Chicken Chili | 840 | 24 | 120 |
| ***French Fries,*** 11 oz | 870 | 45 | 106 |
| ***Hot Dogs:*** Hebrew National | 550 | 34 | 42 |
| KS | 570 | 33 | 46 |
| Sinai | 540 | 30 | 48 |
| ***Pizza:*** *Per Slice* | | | |
| Cheese Pizza, 9.8 oz | 700 | 28 | 70 |
| Combo Pizza, 10.7 oz | 680 | 29 | 72 |
| Pepperoni Pizza, 8.9 oz | 620 | 24 | 68 |
| ***Chicken Bake,*** 12.75 oz | 770 | 25 | 78 |
| ***Wrap,*** Turkey, 14.4 oz | 810 | 38 | 65 |
| ***Salad,*** Chicken Caesar, w/ Dressing | 650 | 40 | 34 |
| ***Sandwiches:*** Hebrew Sausage | 540 | 32 | 44 |
| Italian Sausage | 700 | 42 | 46 |
| KS Polish/Sinai Sausage, av. | 570 | 33 | 47 |
| ***Desserts:*** California Churro | 410 | 18 | 51 |
| Ice Cream Bar | 870 | 65 | 60 |
| J&J Churro | 470 | 22 | 61 |
| Yogurt, 12 oz | 390 | 0 | 82 |
| ***Smoothies:*** Fruit, 16 fl. oz | 290 | 0 | 72 |
| Strawberry Banana, 16 fl.oz | 300 | 0 | 74 |
| ***Sundae,*** Berry, 12.3 oz | 410 | 0 | 87 |
| ***Beverages:*** Hot Latte, 9.6 fl.oz | 190 | 5 | 24 |
| Hot Mocha, 11.3 fl.oz | 310 | 9 | 45 |

## Cousins Subs® (Sept '19)

| | C | F | Cb |
|---|---|---|---|
| ***Subs:*** *Per 7.5", Standard Toppings* | | | |
| **Grilled To Order:** | | | |
| Chicken Bacon Cheddar | 610 | 23 | 53 |
| Chicken Bacon Mushroom Swiss | 730 | 33 | 58 |
| Chicken Cheese Steak | 560 | 18 | 52 |
| **Classics:** | | | |
| Club, with Mayo | 670 | 32 | 53 |
| Italian Special, with Oil | 830 | 48 | 52 |
| Tuna with Mayo | 650 | 36 | 51 |
| **Deli Fresh:** | | | |
| Ham & Provolone, with Mayo | 630 | 32 | 51 |
| Roast Beef & Cheddar, with Mayo | 740 | 37 | 52 |
| Turkey Breast with Mayo | 550 | 25 | 53 |
| ***Cheese Curds:*** Regular, 4 oz | 550 | 47 | 10 |
| Large, 8 oz | 1110 | 94 | 20 |
| ***French Fries:*** Regular, 3 oz | 260 | 14 | 31 |
| Large, 5.9 oz | 520 | 27 | 62 |
| ***Soup:*** *Per Cup* | | | |
| Beef Steak with Noodles | 105 | 3.5 | 12 |
| Cheddar Cauliflower | 110 | 5 | 13 |
| Chicken Noodle | 110 | 3 | 16 |
| Cream of Potato | 170 | 8 | 21 |
| New England Clam Chowder | 150 | 2.5 | 25 |

***For Complete Nutritional Data ~ see CalorieKing.com***

# Fast - Foods & *Restaurants*

## Culver's® (Sept '19)

| ButterBurgers: | C | F | Cb |
|---|---|---|---|
| **Original:** Single | 390 | 17 | 38 |
| Double | 560 | 30 | 38 |
| Triple | 730 | 43 | 38 |
| **Cheddar:** | | | |
| Single | 470 | 24 | 38 |
| Double | 720 | 44 | 38 |
| **Culver's Bacon Deluxe:** | | | |
| Single | 610 | 38 | 40 |
| Double | 850 | 57 | 41 |
| **Culver's Deluxe:** | | | |
| Single | 570 | 35 | 41 |
| Double | 810 | 54 | 42 |
| **Mushroom & Swiss,** Single | 500 | 26 | 40 |
| **Sourdough Melt,** Single | 490 | 25 | 42 |
| *Sandwiches:* | | | |
| Beef Pot Roast | 410 | 13 | 40 |
| Crispy Chicken | 460 | 14 | 57 |
| Grilled Reuben Melt | 660 | 37 | 43 |
| North Atlantic Cod Filet | 600 | 33 | 50 |
| Pork Tenderloin | 630 | 25 | 72 |
| *Sides:* | | | |
| Chili Cheddar Fries | 690 | 32 | 80 |
| Crinkle Cut Fries, reg. | 360 | 14 | 53 |
| Green Beans, regular | 130 | 9 | 9 |
| Mashed Potatoes & Gravy, regular | 130 | 1 | 25 |
| Onion Rings | 400 | 22 | 44 |
| Wisconsin Cheese Curds, 5.3 oz | 510 | 25 | 51 |
| *Dinners:* With Fries, Cole Slaw, Dinner Roll & Butter & Accompanying Sauce | | | |
| Butterfly Jumbo Shrimp, 6 pieces | 1090 | 54 | 129 |
| North Atlantic Cod, Fried, 2 pieces | 1480 | 98 | 108 |
| *Soup:* | | | |
| Broccoli Cheese | 220 | 12 | 17 |
| Chicken Noodle | 100 | 2 | 15 |
| Potato with Bacon | 240 | 10 | 28 |
| *Salads: Without Dressing* | | | |
| Chicken Cashew w/ Gilled Chicken | 450 | 24 | 14 |
| Cranberry Bacon Bleu, with Grilled Chicken | 360 | 14 | 15 |
| Garden Fresco with Grilled Chicken | 350 | 14 | 16 |
| Side Salad | 50 | 2 | 5 |
| *Kid's Meals:* | | | |
| Corn Dog | 240 | 14 | 23 |
| Chicken Tenders, Breaded, 2 pieces | 270 | 12 | 21 |
| Grilled Cheese Sourdough Sandwich | 360 | 16 | 39 |
| *Dressings:* Chunky Bleu Chse, 1.8 oz | 310 | 33 | 2 |
| French Dressing, 1.8 oz | 190 | 13 | 19 |
| Ranch, 1.75 oz | 180 | 19 | 2 |
| Sesame Ginger, 2 oz | 70 | 0 | 16 |

## Culver's® cont... (Sept '19)

| Concrete Mixers: No Toppings | C | F | Cb |
|---|---|---|---|
| Chocolate & M&M's, reg. | 980 | 46 | 124 |
| Cookie Dough, regular | 1010 | 56 | 113 |
| *Sundaes: Per 2 Scoops* | | | |
| Banana Split | 1090 | 6 | 122 |
| Caramel Cashew | 1000 | 51 | 121 |
| Fudge Pecan | 1040 | 63 | 106 |
| Turtle | 1040 | 61 | 111 |
| *Beverages:* Chocolate Malt, reg. | 850 | 38 | 114 |
| Chocolate Shake, reg. | 820 | 38 | 108 |
| Strawberry Malt, reg. | 760 | 38 | 92 |
| Strawberry Shake, reg. | 730 | 38 | 86 |

## D'Angelo® (Sept '19)

| Burgers: | C | F | Cb |
|---|---|---|---|
| Regular, no condiments | 450 | 18 | 45 |
| Cheeseburger, no cond. | 480 | 21 | 46 |
| Steak #9 | 830 | 34 | 83 |
| Western Bacon Cheddar | 780 | 42 | 51 |
| *Deli Sandwiches: Per Medium, with Standard Toppings on Italiab Sub* | | | |
| Cranberry Pecan Chicken Salad | 980 | 58 | 78 |
| Roast Beef & Cheese | 750 | 38 | 67 |
| Tuna Salad | 950 | 68 | 61 |
| *Wraps: Per Medium, with Standard Toppings, on Tortilla Wrap* | | | |
| Buffalo Chicken | 1020 | 62 | 58 |
| Chicken Caesar | 1090 | 63 | 68 |
| Cobb BLT | 700 | 32 | 78 |
| *Fresh Entree Salads: With Dressing, without Pokket* | | | |
| **Entree:** Caesar | 630 | 53 | 26 |
| Greek | 240 | 13 | 17 |
| **Grilled Topped:** | | | |
| Chicken Cobb | 800 | 58 | 26 |
| Steak Cobb | 870 | 64 | 26 |
| Steak Greek | 780 | 62 | 20 |
| *Soup: Per Bowl* | | | |
| Beef Stew | 330 | 12 | 34 |
| Extreme Broccoli & Cheddar | 370 | 28 | 18 |
| Main Lobster Bisque | 540 | 43 | 24 |
| New England Clam Chowder | 480 | 27 | 46 |

*For Complete Menu & Data ~ see CalorieKing.com*

## Dairy Queen® (Sept '19)

| Burgers: | | | |
|---|---|---|---|
| **Cheeseburger,** Deluxe | 400 | 18 | 35 |
| **GrillBurgers:** 1/4 lb Bacon Cheese | 630 | 36 | 43 |
| 1/2 lb Cheese | 800 | 49 | 43 |
| 1/2 lb Flame Thrower | 980 | 70 | 40 |
| 1/3 Double with Cheese | 560 | 31 | 35 |

## Dairy Queen® cont... (Sept '19)

*Sandwiches:*

| | C | F | Cb |
|---|---|---|---|
| Chicken Bacon Ranch | 500 | 20 | 47 |
| Grilled Chicken | 390 | 15 | 34 |
| Turkey BLT | 580 | 28 | 45 |

*Chicken Strip Baskets: Without Beverage or Sauce*

| | | | |
|---|---|---|---|
| 4 pieces, with fries & toast | 940 | 45 | 96 |
| 6 pieces, with fries & toast | 1180 | 57 | 115 |
| *Hot Dogs:* Cheese | 390 | 24 | 26 |
| Chili Cheese | 420 | 26 | 28 |
| Classic | 340 | 20 | 28 |
| *Snack Melts:* Buffalo Chicken | 280 | 15 | 22 |
| Chicken Bacon BBQ | 280 | 11 | 28 |

*Salads: Without Dressing*

**Chicken BLT:**

| | | | |
|---|---|---|---|
| Crispy Chicken | 400 | 21 | 28 |
| Grilled Chicken | 280 | 11 | 12 |
| **Side Salad** | 25 | 0 | 5 |
| *French Fries:* regular, 4 oz | 290 | 13 | 39 |
| large | 470 | 21 | 63 |
| *Onion Rings,* 4 oz | 360 | 16 | 48 |
| *Sides:* Cheese Curds: Regular | 500 | 34 | 26 |
| Large | 1000 | 67 | 52 |
| Onion Ring: regular | 360 | 16 | 48 |
| large | 540 | 24 | 71 |
| Pretzel Sticks with Zesty Queso | 330 | 9 | 52 |

*Desserts: Per Medium*

**Blizzard Treats:** Butterfinger

| | | | |
|---|---|---|---|
| Blizzard Treats: Butterfinger | 730 | 25 | 110 |
| Choco Brownie Xtreme | 800 | 35 | 112 |
| Choc. Chip Cookie Dough | 1040 | 41 | 151 |
| Heath | 860 | 37 | 119 |
| Oreo Cookies | 780 | 29 | 117 |
| Reese's Peanut Butter Cups | 750 | 31 | 102 |
| S'mores | 1010 | 45 | 137 |
| Turtle Pecan Cluster | 900 | 48 | 105 |

**Curl On Top Treats:**

| | | | |
|---|---|---|---|
| Fudge Stuffed Cookie | 640 | 33 | 80 |
| Triple Chocolate Brownie | 540 | 24 | 75 |
| **DQ Dipped Cone,** Chocolate | 460 | 22 | 59 |
| **DQ Sundaes:** Caramel | 430 | 11 | 73 |
| Hot Fudge | 430 | 15 | 66 |
| Strawberry | 330 | 10 | 53 |
| **Shakes:** Caramel | 750 | 25 | 115 |
| Chocolate | 710 | 23 | 110 |
| Strawberry | 620 | 23 | 87 |
| Vanilla | 660 | 23 | 97 |
| **Add Malt** | 80 | 1 | 18 |

*Moo Latte: Per Medium, with Whipped Topping*

| | | | |
|---|---|---|---|
| Caramel | 570 | 17 | 96 |
| Mocha | 580 | 22 | 88 |
| Vanilla | 530 | 16 | 90 |

## Daphne's Greek Cafe® (Sept '19)

*Califonia Menu Only. Check Instore for Latest Information*

*Starters:*

| | C | F | Cb |
|---|---|---|---|
| Fire Feta & Warm Pita | 340 | 17 | 39 |
| Hummus & Warm Pita | 320 | 12 | 47 |

*Classic Pita Sandwiches: Without Tzatziki Sauce*

| | | | |
|---|---|---|---|
| with Chicken | 410 | 16 | 41 |
| with Crispy Shrimp | 410 | 17 | 48 |
| with Falafel | 640 | 17 | 96 |
| with Gyro | 680 | 45 | 49 |

*Plates: Without Pita or Tzatziki Sauce*

**Cali-Greek Bowls:**

| | | | |
|---|---|---|---|
| with Crispy Shrimp | 930 | 38 | 117 |
| with Falafel | 1160 | 39 | 165 |
| with Grilled Chicken | 930 | 37 | 109 |
| with Grilled Shrimp | 1060 | 56 | 91 |
| **Mediterranean Veggie** | 1300 | 56 | 161 |
| **Surf & Turf** | 690 | 25 | 85 |

*Classic Greek Salads: W/ Dressing, w/o Pita & Sauce*

| | | | |
|---|---|---|---|
| Crispy Shrimp | 440 | 31 | 25 |
| Falafel | 670 | 31 | 74 |
| Grilled Chicken | 440 | 30 | 18 |
| **Add,** Pita & Tzatziki | 130 | 3 | 21 |
| *Sides:* Cucumber-Tomato Salad | 120 | 11 | 5 |
| Fire Roasted Vegetables | 70 | 3 | 12 |
| French Fries | 440 | 22 | 55 |
| Greek Salad, small | 140 | 12 | 7 |
| Lemon Chicken Soup | 280 | 12 | 37 |
| Moroccan Carrot Salad | 180 | 13 | 15 |
| Pita Chips | 220 | 6 | 36 |
| Pita Bread | 190 | 3 | 36 |
| Seasoned Rice | 360 | 8 | 68 |
| Tabouli | 220 | 15 | 20 |
| *Dessert,* Traditional Baklava | 250 | 9 | 36 |

## Davanni's® (Sept '19)

*Hot Hoagies: Per Half, with 6" White Bun & Standard Toppings*

| | C | F | Cb |
|---|---|---|---|
| Assorted | 490 | 30 | 39 |
| Cheese | 500 | 31 | 39 |
| Chicken & Bacon, w/ Honey Mustard | 505 | 22 | 46 |
| Chicken Parmigiana | 445 | 16 | 40 |
| Club | 495 | 27 | 40 |
| Pastrami | 470 | 27 | 40 |
| Roast Beef | 470 | 25 | 39 |
| Southwestern Chicken | 535 | 26 | 43 |
| Tuna Melt | 645 | 44 | 42 |
| Turkey Bacon Chipotle | 565 | 33 | 39 |

*Pasta: As Served, with Garlic Toast*

| | | | |
|---|---|---|---|
| Chicken Florentine, half portion | 610 | 28 | 56 |
| Lasagna, half portion | 625 | 43 | 37 |

*continued next page...*

**193**

## Davanni's® cont... (Sept '19)

*Pizzas: Per ⅛ of Medium Pizza*

| | C | F | Cb |
|---|---|---|---|
| **Five Meat:** Thin Crust | 255 | 13 | 19 |
| Traditional Crust | 305 | 13 | 30 |
| Solo, Deep Dish | 840 | 38 | 77 |
| **Veggie:** Thin Crust | 220 | 10 | 19 |
| Traditional Crust | 275 | 10 | 30 |
| **Works:** Thin Crust | 265 | 14 | 19 |
| Traditional Crust | 315 | 15 | 30 |

## Del Taco® (Sept '19)

*Breakfast:*

| | C | F | Cb |
|---|---|---|---|
| **Burritos:** Breakfast | 430 | 21 | 38 |
| Bacon | 640 | 36 | 38 |
| Chorizo/Steak, av. | 510 | 26 | 39 |
| **Hash Brown Sticks,** 5 pieces | 230 | 17 | 18 |
| **Tacos:** Bacon | 230 | 14 | 15 |
| Chorizo | 240 | 15 | 16 |
| Carne Asada | 240 | 13 | 16 |
| Egg & Cheese | 190 | 11 | 15 |
| *Burgers: Without Fries* | | | |
| Bacon Double Del Cheeseburger | 740 | 51 | 35 |
| Del Cheeseburger | 470 | 28 | 34 |
| Double Del Chseburger | 690 | 47 | 35 |
| *Crinkle Cut Fries: Kids,* 3 oz | 160 | 10 | 17 |
| Small, 4 oz | 210 | 13 | 22 |
| Medium, 6 oz | 320 | 19 | 34 |
| Macho, 8.8 oz | 470 | 28 | 49 |
| **Chili Cheddar Fries,** 10.5 oz | 570 | 35 | 42 |
| *Burritos:* ½ lb Bean & Cheese, av. | 460 | 10 | 69 |
| Classic Gr. Chicken | 530 | 33 | 40 |
| Del Beef | 500 | 24 | 40 |
| Del Combo | 540 | 17 | 64 |
| Epic: Carne Asada | 740 | 25 | 88 |
| Cali Steak & Guacamole | 800 | 39 | 80 |
| Grilled Chicken Avocado | 830 | 36 | 88 |
| Macho Combo | 950 | 37 | 100 |
| *Loaded Nachos,* | | | |
| Queso Carne Asada/Chicken, av. | 970 | 46 | 100 |
| *Platos: Per Plate* | | | |
| Beer Battered Fish Tacos (2) | 1060 | 45 | 139 |
| **2 Street Tacos:** | | | |
| Carne Asada Steak | 950 | 34 | 124 |
| Grilled Chicken | 930 | 24 | 124 |
| Carne Asada Wet Burrito | 1290 | 47 | 147 |
| Chicken Verde, Wet Burrito | 1210 | 47 | 151 |
| *Quesadillas:* Mini Bacon | 170 | 9 | 14 |
| Cheddar | 460 | 26 | 31 |
| Chckn/ Cheddar or Spicy Jack, av. | 550 | 31 | 35 |

## Del Taco® cont... (Sept '19)

*Tacos:*

| | C | F | Cb |
|---|---|---|---|
| Beer Battered Fish | 230 | 12 | 26 |
| Chicken Street | 170 | 7 | 20 |
| **Del Taco:** Crunchy Beef | 310 | 20 | 14 |
| Soft Beef | 300 | 18 | 17 |
| Grilled Chicken | 210 | 12 | 16 |
| *Salads: Without Dressing* | | | |
| Chicken, Bacon Avocado | 590 | 46 | 23 |
| Mexican Chopped Chicken | 510 | 23 | 39 |
| Signature Taco | 550 | 29 | 38 |
| *Sides:* | | | |
| Bean & Cheese Cup, 7.8 oz | 320 | 3.5 | 52 |
| Carne Aada Fries, 12.5 oz | 810 | 59 | 46 |
| Cheddar Potato Poppers, 4 pieces | 240 | 14 | 20 |

## Denny's® (Sept '19)

*Breakfast:*

| | C | F | Cb |
|---|---|---|---|
| **Favorites:** *With Hash Browns, without Bread* | | | |
| Country Fried Steak, w/out eggs | 570 | 37 | 39 |
| T'Bone Steak without eggs, 18 oz | 660 | 42 | 16 |
| **Omelettes:** *With Hash Browns* | | | |
| Ham & Cheese, 13 oz | 780 | 54 | 20 |
| Loaded Veggie, 18 oz | 620 | 44 | 24 |
| Philly Cheesesteak | 880 | 64 | 25 |
| Ultimate | 890 | 71 | 20 |
| **Skillets:** | | | |
| Fit Fare Veggie, 18 oz | 390 | 16 | 40 |
| Santa Fe Sizzlin' w/out eggs, 10 oz | 720 | 53 | 35 |
| Supr. Sizzlin' w/out eggs, 10 oz | 590 | 44 | 32 |
| **Slams:** *Without Bread* | | | |
| All American, w/ Hash Browns, 15 oz | 930 | 74 | 19 |
| Belgian Waffle, without egg, 7 oz | 430 | 12 | 56 |
| French Toast, without egg, 11 oz | 860 | 53 | 65 |
| Lumberjack, without egg, 19 oz | 970 | 49 | 96 |
| **Pancakes (2):** *Without Hash Brown, Egg & Meat* | | | |
| Double Berry Banana | 540 | 10 | 103 |
| Dulce De Leche Crunch | 1220 | 27 | 228 |
| Salted Caramel & Banana | 1140 | 27 | 207 |
| Tres Leches | 910 | 36 | 129 |
| **Sides:** Bacon Strips (4) | 210 | 16 | 2 |
| Buttermilk Biscuit (2) | 470 | 26 | 54 |
| English Muffin, w/out Margarine | 130 | 1 | 25 |
| Grilled Ham, 3 oz slice | 90 | 3 | 1 |
| Hash Browns, 5 oz | 170 | 12 | 15 |
| Hearty Breakfast Sausage (1) | 350 | 31 | 5 |
| Oatmeal, w/ Milk & Br. Sugar, 10 oz | 240 | 2 | 45 |
| Sausage Links (40 | 320 | 31 | 3 |
| Wheat Toast, with Margarine | 230 | 11 | 29 |

## Denny's® cont... (Sept '19)

### Appetizers:

| | C | F | Cb |
|---|---|---|---|
| **Build Your Own:** *Without Sauce* | | | |
| Bacon Cheddar Tots (6) | 300 | 15 | 31 |
| Beer-Battered Onion Rings, 5 oz | 400 | 27 | 35 |
| Mozzarella Cheese Sticks (4) | 280 | 11 | 30 |
| Italian Sampler, 21 oz | 1250 | 71 | 96 |
| Loaded Nacho Tots (10) | 980 | 62 | 68 |
| Premium Chicken Tenders (5) | 680 | 40 | 38 |
| **Zesty Nachos:** Half Size, 15 oz | 870 | 55 | 70 |
| Full Size, 25 oz | 1650 | 105 | 135 |

### Lunch Burgers & Sandwiches: *Without Sides*

| | C | F | Cb |
|---|---|---|---|
| **Burgers:** American Diner, single | 790 | 47 | 50 |
| Bacon, Avocado Cheeseburger | 1000 | 66 | 53 |
| Bourbon Bacon | 920 | 53 | 60 |
| Slamburger without Egg | 840 | 48 | 56 |
| Spicy Sriracha | 920 | 55 | 55 |
| **Sandwiches:** Cali Club | 820 | 48 | 55 |
| Club | 830 | 39 | 74 |
| Grilled Tuscan Chicken | 800 | 49 | 43 |
| The Super Bird | 600 | 28 | 43 |

### Lunch Sides:

| | C | F | Cb |
|---|---|---|---|
| Bacon & Cheddar Tots (6), without Sour Cream | 300 | 15 | 31 |
| Beer Battered Onion Rings, 5 oz | 400 | 27 | 35 |
| Caesar Side Salad, 6 oz | 260 | 20 | 16 |
| Garden Salad, w/out Dressing, 7 oz | 170 | 9 | 16 |
| Seasoned Fries, 5.5 oz | 490 | 26 | 57 |
| Wavy-Cut Fries, 5 oz | 400 | 22 | 46 |

### Dinners: *Without Sides or Bread*

| | C | F | Cb |
|---|---|---|---|
| Brooklyn Spag. & M'balls, 22 oz | 920 | 46 | 85 |
| Country Fried Steak, w/ Gravy, 10 oz | 630 | 40 | 37 |
| Grilled Haddock, 6 oz | 290 | 14 | 2 |
| Homestyle Meatloaf, 12 oz | 590 | 29 | 46 |
| Medit. Grilled Chicken | 630 | 40 | 6 |
| Sirloin Steak, 8 oz | 350 | 17 | 2 |
| Slow Cooked Pot Roast | 400 | 19 | 10 |
| T-Bone Steak, 13 oz | 490 | 30 | 0 |
| Tilapia Ranchero, 9 oz | 300 | 12 | 6 |
| Wild Alaska Salmon | 310 | 19 | 2 |

### Dinner Sides:

| | C | F | Cb |
|---|---|---|---|
| Broccoli, 3 oz | 35 | 0 | 5 |
| Fresh Sauteed Zuchini & Squash, 3 oz | 70 | 6 | 3 |
| Garlic Toast/Dinner Bread, 2 pcs | 190 | 7 | 25 |
| Red-Skinned Potatoes: Plain, 4 oz | 200 | 8 | 26 |
| Mashed, without gravy | 120 | 5 | 17 |
| Southwest Creamed Corn, 4 oz | 240 | 18 | 13 |
| Whole Grain Rice, 5 oz | 240 | 2.5 | 48 |

## Denny's® cont... (Sept '19)

### Salads: *Without Bread*

| | C | F | Cb |
|---|---|---|---|
| **Caesar Salad,** with dressing, 9 oz | 440 | 0 | 9 |
| **Cobb Salad:** *Without Dressing* | | | |
| without Meat, 13 oz | 430 | 30 | 20 |
| with Chkn Tenders (3) | 840 | 54 | 43 |
| with Grilled Chicken, 18 oz | 630 | 39 | 20 |
| with Prime Rib, 15.5 oz | 560 | 38 | 23 |
| **House Salad:** *Without Dressing* | | | |
| without Meat, 10 oz | 190 | 9 | 19 |
| with Chicken Tenders (3) | 600 | 33 | 42 |
| with Grilled Chicken, 15 oz | 390 | 18 | 19 |
| with Prime Rib, 12.5 oz | 320 | 17 | 22 |
| with Wild Alaskan Salmon, 17 oz | 500 | 28 | 21 |

### Soups: *Without Bread*

| | C | F | Cb |
|---|---|---|---|
| Chicken Noodle: Cup | 260 | 10 | 28 |
| Bowl | 390 | 15 | 43 |
| Loaded Baked Potato: Cup | 360 | 24 | 25 |
| Bowl | 470 | 31 | 36 |
| Vegetable Beef: Cup | 200 | 11 | 27 |
| Bowl | 310 | 16 | 40 |
| **Condiments:** Pico de Gallo, 2 oz | 15 | 0 | 3 |
| Sour Cream, 1 oz | 45 | 4 | 1 |
| Tomato Sauce, 1.5 oz | 25 | 1 | 3 |
| Whipped Margarine, 0.5 oz | 40 | 4.5 | 0 |

### Dressings: *Per 1.5oz*

| | C | F | Cb |
|---|---|---|---|
| Blue Cheese | 160 | 16 | 2 |
| Caesar | 210 | 22 | 2 |
| French | 130 | 8 | 2 |
| Honey Mustard | 180 | 15 | 12 |
| Ranch | 200 | 21 | 1 |
| Thousand Island | 160 | 16 | 7 |

### Sauces: *Per 1.5 oz*

| | C | F | Cb |
|---|---|---|---|
| All American | 250 | 27 | 2 |
| Bourbon | 110 | 0 | 26 |
| Buffalo | 110 | 12 | 1 |

### Desserts: *As Served*

| | C | F | Cb |
|---|---|---|---|
| Caramel Apple Pie Crisp, 13 oz | 760 | 26 | 126 |
| Chocolate Lava Cake | 700 | 34 | 85 |
| New York Style Cheesecake, plain | 500 | 34 | 42 |

### Beverages:

| | C | F | Cb |
|---|---|---|---|
| Hot Chocolate, 8 oz | 190 | 3 | 37 |
| Iced Tea, sweetened, 12 oz | 160 | 0 | 40 |
| Lemonade Iced Tea, 12 oz | 80 | 0 | 21 |
| Mango Lemonade, 15 oz | 210 | 0 | 57 |
| Strawb. Lemonade, 12 oz | 210 | 0 | 55 |
| **Milk Shakes:** Chocolate, 16 oz | 870 | 43 | 111 |
| Vanilla, 16 oz | 800 | 43 | 97 |
| **Smoothie:** Groovy Mango, 15 oz | 340 | 0 | 86 |
| Strawberry Banana Bliss, 15 oz | 330 | 0.5 | 82 |

*For Complete Nutritional Data ~ see CalorieKing.com*

# Fast - Foods & *Restaurants*

## Dippin' Dots® (Sept'19)

| | C | F | Cb |
|---|---|---|---|
| ***Flavored Ices:*** *Per ½ Cup, 3 oz* | | | |
| Frozetti with Popping Candy | 110 | 0 | 28 |
| Aerage all flavors | 100 | 0 | 26 |
| ***Frozen Yogurt:*** *Per ½ Cup* | | | |
| **YoDots:** Cookies 'N Cream | 130 | 3 | 25 |
| Cookie Dough | 140 | 2.5 | 26 |
| Cotton Candy | 100 | 1.5 | 20 |
| Strawberry Cheesecake | 100 | 0 | 21 |
| ***Ice Cream:*** *Per ½ Cup* | | | |
| Banana Split | 160 | 8 | 20 |
| Choc. Chip Cookie Dough | 190 | 9 | 24 |
| Cool Mint Crunch | 190 | 9 | 24 |
| Strawberry | 160 | 8 | 18 |

## Donatos Pizza®(Sept'19)

| | C | F | Cb |
|---|---|---|---|
| ***Pizzas:*** *Per Slice* | | | |
| **Hand Tossed Signature Pizzas:** *Per Slice of 14" Pizza* | | | |
| Chicken Spinach Mozzarella | 340 | 15 | 31 |
| Founder's Favorite | 330 | 14 | 33 |
| Mariachi Beef | 310 | 12 | 34 |
| Mariachi Chicken | 230 | 6 | 33 |
| Serious Meat | 340 | 15 | 33 |
| The Works | 320 | 14 | 34 |
| **Thick Crust Signature Pizzas:** *Per Slice of 14" Pizza* | | | |
| Bourbon BBQ Bacon | 160 | 7 | 18 |
| Chicken Spinach Mozzarella | 160 | 7 | 15 |
| Double Bacon Pepperoni | 200 | 10 | 16 |
| Founders Favorite | 170 | 8 | 16 |
| Margherita | 160 | 8 | 14 |
| Serious Meat | 190 | 9 | 16 |
| The Works | 170 | 8 | 17 |
| ***Oven Baked Subs:*** | | | |
| Big Don | 600 | 25 | 62 |
| Chicken Bacon Cheddar | 770 | 37 | 62 |
| Fresh Vegy | 490 | 19 | 63 |
| Ham & Smoked Prov. | 560 | 21 | 62 |
| Hot Chicken | 840 | 42 | 73 |
| Meatball | 850 | 38 | 80 |
| ***Salad:*** *Entree Size, with Menu Set Dressing* | | | |
| Chicken Caprese | 400 | 25 | 17 |
| Chicken Harvest | 600 | 37 | 42 |
| Italian Chef | 500 | 42 | 12 |
| ***Wings:*** *Per 6 pieces, without Dipping Sauce* | | | |
| **Boneless Chkn:** Mild/Hot Sce, av. | 415 | 23 | 26 |
| BBQ Sauce | 400 | 17 | 39 |
| Sweet Thai Chili | 470 | 18 | 53 |
| ***Dessert:*** Cinnamon Bread, ¼ bread | 280 | 10 | 44 |
| Fudge Brownie (1) | 360 | 21 | 39 |
| Salty Caramel Apple Pie, 2 pieces | 330 | 10 | 53 |
| Triple Chocolate Chunk Cookie (1) | 320 | 23 | 22 |

*For Complete Nutritional Data ~ see CalorieKing.com*

## Domino's® (Sept'19)

| | C | F | Cb |
|---|---|---|---|
| *Regular Pizzas Use Regular Cheese Base* | | | |
| ***12" Hand Tossed:*** *Per Slice, ⅛ Pizza* | | | |
| Bacon, Beef, & Sausage | 290 | 14 | 27 |
| Beef, Green Pepp., On. & Mshrm | 210 | 7 | 27 |
| Black Olives, Green Peppers, Onions, Mushrooms, Tomatoes | 200 | 7 | 27 |
| Ham & Pineapple | 200 | 6 | 28 |
| Pepperoni | 220 | 9 | 26 |
| Pepperoni & Sausage | 250 | 11 | 26 |
| Sausage | 240 | 11 | 26 |
| Sausage, Beef & Pepperoni | 270 | 14 | 26 |
| ***14" Brooklyn:*** *Per Slice, ⅙ Pizza* | | | |
| Beef, Green Pepp., On. & Mshrm | 270 | 11 | 29 |
| Black Olives, Green Peppers, Onions, Mushrooms, Tomatoes | 260 | 10 | 30 |
| Ham & Pineapple | 270 | 10 | 31 |
| Pepperoni | 290 | 14 | 28 |
| Pepperoni & Sausage | 340 | 19 | 28 |
| Sausage | 330 | 18 | 28 |
| ***14" Thin Crust:*** *Per Slice, ⅛ Pizza* | | | |
| Bacon, Beef & Sausage | 300 | 19 | 19 |
| Beef, Green Pepp., On. & Mshrm | 200 | 10 | 19 |
| Black Olives, Green Peppers, Onions, Mushrooms & Tomatoes | 190 | 9 | 19 |
| Ham & Pineapple | 200 | 9 | 20 |
| Pepperoni | 210 | 12 | 18 |
| Pepperoni & Sausage | 250 | 16 | 18 |
| Sausage | 240 | 15 | 18 |
| ***12" Specialty Handmade Pan:*** *Per Slice, ⅛ Pizza* | | | |
| Cali Chicken Bacon Ranch | 370 | 21 | 30 |
| Deluxe | 310 | 16 | 30 |
| Memphis BBQ Chicken | 330 | 16 | 33 |
| Spinach & Feta | 300 | 15 | 29 |
| ***12" Specialty Hand-Tossed:*** *Per Slice, ⅛ Pizza* | | | |
| Buffalo Chicken | 260 | 12 | 26 |
| Deluxe | 230 | 10 | 27 |
| ExtravaganZZa | 280 | 13 | 28 |
| MeatZZa | 270 | 13 | 27 |
| Ultimate Pepperoni | 270 | 13 | 26 |
| ***14" Specialty Thin Crust:*** *Per Slice, ⅛ Pizza* | | | |
| Buffalo Chicken | 260 | 15 | 17 |
| Cali Chicken Bacon Ranch | 320 | 21 | 18 |
| Honolulu Hawaiian | 250 | 13 | 20 |
| Memphis BBQ Chicken | 260 | 14 | 22 |
| Wisconsin 6 Cheese | 250 | 14 | 18 |

## Domino's® cont... (Sept '19)

| | | C | F | Cb |
|---|---|---|---|---|
| **Chicken Wings:** *Without Sauce* | | | | |
| Barbecue, 4 wings | | 240 | 13 | 18 |
| Hot, 4 wings | | 200 | 13 | 8 |
| **Chicken Dipping Cups:** BBQ, 1.25 oz | | 60 | 0 | 14 |
| Blue Cheese, 1.25 oz | | 200 | 21 | 2 |
| Kicker Hot, 1.25 oz | | 45 | 3.5 | 2 |
| Ranch, 1.5 oz | | 200 | 21 | 2 |
| Sweet Mango Habanero, 1.25 oz | | 60 | 0 | 17 |
| **BreadBowl Pasta:** *Per ½ Bowl* | | | | |
| Chicken Alfredo, 10.5 oz | | 690 | 25 | 91 |
| Chicken Carbonara, 11.6 oz | | 730 | 28 | 92 |
| Italian Sausage Marinara, 11.85 oz | | 730 | 27 | 96 |
| Pasta Primavera, 11 oz | | 660 | 24 | 91 |
| **Oven Baked Sandwiches:** *Per Sandwich* | | | | |
| Buffalo Chicken with Blue Cheese | | 840 | 42 | 74 |
| Chicken Bacon Ranch | | 860 | 44 | 72 |
| Chicken Parmesan | | 760 | 30 | 74 |
| Italian | | 820 | 40 | 72 |
| Mediterranean Veggie | | 700 | 28 | 76 |
| Philly Cheese Steak | | 640 | 24 | 74 |
| Sweet & Spicy Chicken Habanero | | 800 | 32 | 84 |
| **Pasta In Dish:** Chkn Alfredo, 11.9 oz | | 620 | 30 | 60 |
| Chicken Carbonara, 13 oz | | 690 | 35 | 63 |
| Italian Sausage Marinara, 13.5 oz | | 690 | 34 | 70 |
| Pasta Primavera, 11.9 oz | | 550 | 27 | 61 |
| **Salads:** *Without Dressing* | | | | |
| Chicken Caesar | | 210 | 7 | 15 |
| Classic Garden | | 200 | 9 | 17 |
| **Salad Dressings:** *Per 1.5 oz Package* | | | | |
| Caesar Dressing | | 230 | 25 | 1 |
| Italian | | 140 | 14 | 4 |
| Light Balsamic Dressing | | 90 | 9 | 5 |
| Ranch Dressing | | 200 | 21 | 2 |
| **Bread Side Items:** | | | | |
| Garlic Bread Twists, 2 pcs | | 220 | 11 | 27 |
| Jalap. Bacon Stuffed Cheesy Bread (1) | | 170 | 8 | 17 |
| Parmesan Bread Bites, 4 pieces | | 220 | 10 | 27 |
| Spin. & Fetta Stuffed Cheesy Bread, 1 piece | | 160 | 7 | 17 |
| Stuffed Cheesy Bread, 1 piece | | 150 | 7 | 17 |
| **Bread Dipping Sauces:** *Per Container* | | | | |
| Garlic, 1 oz cup | | 250 | 28 | 0 |
| Marinara, 2 oz cup | | 30 | 0 | 6 |
| **Cinnamon Bread Twists,** 2 pcs | | 250 | 12 | 31 |
| **Sweet Icing,** Dipping Cup, 2.25 oz | | 230 | 4 | 51 |
| **Dessert:** Choc. Lava Crunch Cake, 3 oz | | 350 | 19 | 46 |
| Marbled Cookie Brownie, 1.5 oz | | 190 | 9 | 25 |

## Dunkin'® (Sept '19)

| | C | F | Cb |
|---|---|---|---|
| **Bagels:** *Per Bagel* | | | |
| Plain | 300 | 1 | 64 |
| Cinnamon Raisin | 320 | 1 | 67 |
| Everything | 340 | 3 | 67 |
| Multigrain | 380 | 8 | 63 |
| Sesame Seed | 350 | 5 | 64 |
| White Cheddar Twist | 390 | 8 | 64 |
| **Donuts:** Apple 'n Spice | 260 | 14 | 29 |
| Apple Crumb | 320 | 15 | 42 |
| Bavarian Kreme | 270 | 15 | 30 |
| Bismark | 490 | 24 | 65 |
| Boston Kreme | 300 | 16 | 37 |
| Butternut | 410 | 20 | 55 |
| Chocolate Butternut | 410 | 20 | 54 |
| Chocolate Frosted Cake | 350 | 19 | 40 |
| Chocolate Headlight | 330 | 18 | 39 |
| Coconut; Coffee Roll, average | 390 | 19 | 50 |
| Dulce de Leche | 300 | 16 | 35 |
| French Cruller | 220 | 13 | 23 |
| Glazed | 260 | 14 | 30 |
| Glazed Chocolate | 340 | 16 | 44 |
| Glazed Jelly | 310 | 14 | 42 |
| Jelly | 280 | 14 | 34 |
| Lemon | 260 | 15 | 29 |
| Maple Frosted | 280 | 15 | 32 |
| Maple Vanilla Creme | 360 | 20 | 43 |
| New Yorker | 360 | 20 | 43 |
| Old Fashioned | 290 | 19 | 28 |
| Peanut | 450 | 26 | 48 |
| Powdered | 320 | 19 | 33 |
| Sour Cream | 350 | 17 | 47 |
| Strawberry Frosted | 280 | 15 | 32 |
| Sugared | 230 | 14 | 22 |
| Vanilla Creme | 330 | 20 | 35 |
| **Muffins:** Blueberry | 460 | 15 | 76 |
| Chocolate Chip | 550 | 21 | 83 |
| Coffee Cake | 590 | 24 | 87 |
| Corn | 460 | 16 | 72 |
| **Munchkins:** Cinnamon | 60 | 3.5 | 7 |
| Glazed | 70 | 4 | 7 |
| Glazed Chocolate | 70 | 3.5 | 8 |
| Jelly | 70 | 4 | 9 |
| Old Fashioned | 60 | 3.5 | 6 |
| Powdered | 60 | 3.5 | 7 |
| **Other Bakery Items:** | | | |
| English Muffin | 180 | 2 | 34 |
| Plain Croissant | 340 | 18 | 38 |
| **Sandwiches:** | | | |
| Egg & Cheese on Plain Bagel | 460 | 13 | 66 |
| Ham, Egg & Chees on Croissant | 530 | 32 | 41 |
| Sausage, Egg & Cheese on Engl. Muffin | 550 | 34 | 37 |
| Veggie Egg White on Engl. Muffin | 310 | 10 | 38 |

*continued next page...*

## Dunkin'® cont... (Sept '19)

*Breakfast:*

| | C | F | Cb |
|---|---|---|---|
| **Hash Browns,** 6 pieces | 140 | 8 | 17 |
| **Oatmeal,** | | | |
| Brown Sugar Flavored Oatmeal, with Dried Fruit Topping | 310 | 2 | 66 |
| **Plain Bagels:** | | | |
| Bacon, Egg & Cheese | 520 | 18 | 66 |
| Egg & Cheese | 430 | 13 | 61 |
| Ham, Egg & Cheese | 460 | 14 | 61 |
| Sausage, Egg & Cheese | 670 | 33 | 67 |
| **Big N' Toasted,** with Toast | 620 | 38 | 41 |
| **Biscuit,** Chicken | 460 | 22 | 46 |
| **Croissants:** Bacon, Egg & Cheese | 560 | 35 | 41 |
| Egg & Cheese | 500 | 31 | 40 |
| Ham, Egg & Cheese | 530 | 32 | 40 |
| Sausage, Egg & Cheese | 710 | 51 | 41 |
| **English Muffins:** | | | |
| Bacon, Egg & Cheese | 390 | 19 | 37 |
| Ham, Egg & Cheese | 360 | 15 | 37 |
| Sausage, Egg & Cheese | 550 | 34 | 37 |
| **Wake-Up Wraps:** | | | |
| Bacon, Egg & Cheese | 210 | 13 | 15 |
| Egg & Cheese | 180 | 10 | 14 |
| Ham, Egg & Cheese | 190 | 11 | 15 |
| Turkey Sausage | 240 | 14 | 15 |

*Hot Beverages: Per Medium Size*

| | C | F | Cb |
|---|---|---|---|
| **Chocolate:** Original | 330 | 10 | 59 |
| Mint | 300 | 10 | 52 |
| **Dunkaccino** | 350 | 15 | 52 |

*Cold Beverages: Per Medium, 24 fl.oz*

| | C | F | Cb |
|---|---|---|---|
| **Coolatta:** | | | |
| Blue Raspberry | 360 | 0 | 92 |
| Strawberry | 360 | 0 | 92 |
| Vanilla Bean | 630 | 9 | 138 |

**Iced Latte:** *Per Medium, 24 fl.oz, with Whole Milk, without sugar*

| | C | F | Cb |
|---|---|---|---|
| Caramel Swirl | 350 | 9 | 55 |
| French Vanilla Swirl | 340 | 9 | 53 |
| Hazelnut Swirl | 340 | 9 | 54 |
| Mocha Swirl | 350 | 10 | 54 |

**Iced Macchiato:** *Per Medium, 24 fl.oz, with Whole Milk, without sugar*

| | C | F | Cb |
|---|---|---|---|
| Caramel Swirl | 290 | 6 | 49 |
| French Vanilla Swirl | 280 | 6 | 49 |
| Hazelnut Swirl | 290 | 6 | 49 |
| Mocha Swirl | 280 | 7 | 49 |

## Eat 'N Park® (Sept '19)

*Breakfast: Without Extras*

| | C | F | Cb |
|---|---|---|---|
| Bananas Foster French Toast, 2 slices | 440 | 6 | 88 |
| **Omelettes:** Ham & Cheese | 670 | 47 | 6 |
| Meat Lover's | 760 | 58 | 6 |
| **Pancakes:** | | | |
| Buttermilk (2) | 320 | 2 | 65 |
| Blueberry (2) | 330 | 3 | 68 |
| **Scramblers:** | | | |
| All-American with Sausage | 740 | 42 | 58 |

*Appetizers:*

| | C | F | Cb |
|---|---|---|---|
| Fried Cheese Sticks | 590 | 35 | 41 |
| Fried Ravioli | 870 | 61 | 64 |
| Hand-Breaded Zucchini | 830 | 57 | 60 |
| Mac 'n Cheese Bites | 940 | 74 | 54 |

*Burgers: Without Sides*

| | C | F | Cb |
|---|---|---|---|
| **Black Angus:** | | | |
| American Grill | 760 | 45 | 43 |
| Bacon Cheeseburger | 810 | 51 | 37 |
| Cheeseburger | 760 | 47 | 40 |
| Mushroom & Onion | 790 | 48 | 41 |
| **Superburgers:** Black Angus | 1100 | 71 | 39 |
| Original | 670 | 42 | 37 |

*Sandwiches: With Menu Set Ingredients*

| | C | F | Cb |
|---|---|---|---|
| Bacon Grilled Cheese | 800 | 43 | 70 |
| Crispy Buff. Chkn Wrap, with Ranch | 970 | 54 | 68 |
| Chicken Club, grilled | 810 | 49 | 39 |
| Classic Grilled Cheese | 720 | 37 | 70 |
| Hot Turkey | 500 | 8 | 73 |
| Reuben | 1020 | 72 | 45 |
| Shredded Pot Roast | 540 | 31 | 28 |
| Turkey Club | 860 | 46 | 48 |
| Whale of a Cod Fish | 930 | 35 | 96 |

*Dinners: Without Sides*

| | C | F | Cb |
|---|---|---|---|
| **Baked Chicken Parmigiana:** | | | |
| with Marinara Sauce | 920 | 41 | 84 |
| with Meat Sauce | 1030 | 50 | 75 |
| Baked Cod, 2 fillets | 410 | 24 | 6 |
| Fisherman's Platter | 1020 | 53 | 74 |
| Nantucket Cod & Stuffing, 2 pieces | 740 | 56 | 20 |
| Pasta Noodles w/ Marinara Sauce | 680 | 8 | 130 |
| Pasta Noodles with Meat Sauce | 840 | 22 | 120 |
| Smothered Ground Sirloin Steak | 450 | 27 | 8 |
| Whale of a Cod | 620 | 30 | 39 |

*Continued Next Page....*

## Eat 'N Park® cont... (Sept '19)

### Salads: *Per Menu, w/out Dressing*

| | C | F | Cb |
|---|---|---|---|
| Buffalo, with Crispy Chicken | 390 | 23 | 31 |
| Caprese with Grilled Chicken | 550 | 29 | 26 |
| Eat'n Park, with Rib Eye | 730 | 44 | 31 |
| Strawberry with Grilled Chicken | 510 | 25 | 35 |

### Sides: Baked Potato

| | C | F | Cb |
|---|---|---|---|
| Baked Potato | 190 | 0 | 44 |
| Broccoli | 40 | 0 | 8 |
| Carrots | 40 | 1 | 9 |
| Coleslaw | 120 | 8 | 12 |
| French fries | 350 | 17 | 47 |
| Gravy Fries | 370 | 17 | 50 |
| Mac'n Cheese | 450 | 22 | 44 |
| Mashed Potatoes | 110 | 6 | 13 |
| Onion Rings | 170 | 9 | 20 |
| Pasta: with Alfredo Sauce | 650 | 37 | 62 |
| with Marinara Sauce | 340 | 4 | 65 |

### Soup Bowls: Chicken Noodle

| | C | F | Cb |
|---|---|---|---|
| Chicken Noodle | 270 | 8 | 34 |
| Clam Chowder | 420 | 18 | 48 |
| Cream of Broccoli | 300 | 12 | 39 |
| Cream of Potato | 310 | 14 | 39 |

### Desserts:

| | C | F | Cb |
|---|---|---|---|
| Ice Cream, 2 scoops | 290 | 16 | 33 |
| Pies: Apple Pie, 1 sl. | 390 | 14 | 65 |
| Blueberry Pie, 1 sl. | 590 | 31 | 71 |
| Coconut Crm Pie, 1 sl. | 470 | 23 | 59 |
| Dutch Apple Pie, 1 sl. | 410 | 16 | 65 |
| Lemon Meringue Pie, 1 slice | 250 | 10 | 35 |
| Sundaes: Caramel, 2 scoops | 470 | 19 | 73 |
| Oreo | 560 | 24 | 80 |

## Edo Japan® (Sept '19)

### Bento Box: *Without Teriyaki Sauce*

| | C | F | Cb |
|---|---|---|---|
| Beef Yakisoba, 20.3 oz | 840 | 29 | 102 |
| Chicken Yakisoba, 20.5 oz | 790 | 24 | 102 |
| Sizzling Shrimp, 22 oz | 790 | 15 | 122 |
| Sukiyaki Beef, 20.3 oz | 880 | 27 | 120 |

### Teriyaki: *Without Teriyaki Sauce*

| | C | F | Cb |
|---|---|---|---|
| Beef & Shrimp, 17 oz | 660 | 18 | 82 |
| Sukiyaki Beef, 14.8 oz | 580 | 15 | 80 |

### Soup: *Per 33 oz Bowl*

| | C | F | Cb |
|---|---|---|---|
| Beef Udon | 580 | 17 | 72 |
| Chicken Udon | 550 | 13 | 72 |

### Maki Sushi: *Per 6 Pieces*

| | C | F | Cb |
|---|---|---|---|
| California Roll, 7.6 oz | 430 | 17 | 61 |
| Spicy Tuna Roll, 6.5 oz | 300 | 2.5 | 54 |

### Nigiri Sushi: *Per 1 Piece*

| | C | F | Cb |
|---|---|---|---|
| Ebi, 1.7 oz | 70 | 0.5 | 12 |
| Salmon Sashimi, 0.7 oz | 30 | 1.5 | 1 |

## Einstein Bros® (Sept '19)

### Bagels:

| | C | F | Cb |
|---|---|---|---|
| Bagels: Asiago Cheese | 300 | 4 | 54 |
| Blueberry | 290 | 1 | 59 |
| Chocolate Chip | 300 | 4 | 58 |
| Cinnamon Sugar | 320 | 6 | 59 |
| Everything | 280 | 2 | 56 |
| Garlic | 280 | 2 | 57 |
| Green Chile | 390 | 12 | 54 |
| Honey Whole Wheat | 260 | 3 | 49 |
| Onion | 270 | 2 | 55 |
| Poppyseed | 290 | 2.5 | 56 |
| Potato | 280 | 4 | 52 |
| Power Protein | 350 | 6 | 64 |
| Sesame | 290 | 3 | 56 |
| Six-Cheese | 370 | 10 | 53 |
| Spinach Florentine | 370 | 12 | 53 |

### Bagel Dogs:

| | C | F | Cb |
|---|---|---|---|
| Original | 530 | 26 | 57 |
| Asiago | 580 | 29 | 57 |

### Signature Bagel Sandwiches:

| | C | F | Cb |
|---|---|---|---|
| Albacore Tuna Salad | 590 | 28 | 57 |
| Chicken Florentine | 620 | 24 | 61 |
| Crispy Chicken & Tater | 790 | 39 | 76 |
| Green Chile Club | 680 | 33 | 59 |
| Hummus Veg Out | 450 | 16 | 64 |
| Turkey Bacon Avocado | 620 | 30 | 60 |
| Hot Sandwiches: Chse Bagel Pizza | 440 | 14 | 58 |
| Pepperoni Bagel Pizza | 530 | 23 | 59 |

### Cream Cheese: *Per 1.2 oz Schmear*

### Reduced Fat:

| | C | F | Cb |
|---|---|---|---|
| Garlic Herb/Garden Veggie | 110 | 9 | 5 |
| Honey Almond; Strawberry, av. | 120 | 8 | 10 |
| Plain | 120 | 12 | 2 |
| Onion and Chive | 120 | 10 | 4 |
| Smoked Salmon | 110 | 10 | 4 |

### Breakfast Bagel Sandwiches:

| | C | F | Cb |
|---|---|---|---|
| Avocado Toast | 400 | 12 | 61 |
| Bacon & Spinach | 700 | 42 | 57 |
| Chorizo Sunrise | 840 | 51 | 61 |
| Crispy Chicken & Tater | 800 | 38 | 76 |
| Nova Lox | 480 | 17 | 60 |
| Supernova | 510 | 18 | 60 |
| Side, Hash Brown | 170 | 11 | 11 |
| Sweets: Blueberry Muffin, 4 oz | 420 | 20 | 57 |
| Chocolate Chip Coffee Cake | 550 | 25 | 81 |
| Cinnamon Twist, 3.4 oz | 360 | 16 | 50 |

# Fast - Foods & *Restaurants*

## El Pollo Loco® (Sept '19)

| *Starters:* Per Small Serving | C | F | Cb |
|---|---|---|---|
| **Chicken Tortilla Soup:** Small | 220 | 9 | 19 |
| Large | 440 | 18 | 40 |
| Chips & Chunky Guacamole, 11.8 oz | 1010 | 65 | 100 |
| **Chips & Queso Sauce:** Small | 200 | 11 | 22 |
| Large | 760 | 42 | 86 |
| *Bowl:* | | | |
| Orig. Chicken Pollo | 530 | 7 | 80 |
| Double Chicken | 890 | 30 | 86 |
| Grand Avocado Chicken | 780 | 27 | 89 |
| *Burritos:* | | | |
| Chicken Avocado | 890 | 48 | 71 |
| Chipotle Chicken Avocado | 900 | 40 | 86 |
| Original BRC | 410 | 11 | 61 |
| *Fire-Grilled Chicken:* Skin On | | | |
| Breast; Thigh, av. | 215 | 12 | 0 |
| Leg; Wing, av. | 85 | 4.5 | 0 |
| *Stuffed Quesadilla,* | | | |
| Chicken Avocado | 940 | 59 | 60 |
| *Taco Al Carbon,* Chicken, 3.2 oz | 160 | 6 | 18 |
| *Tostada Salads:* With Shell, without Dressing | | | |
| Chicken & Avocado | 940 | 50 | 82 |
| Classic | 830 | 41 | 75 |
| Double Chicken | 1000 | 49 | 79 |
| Street Corn | 1060 | 54 | 99 |
| *Under 500 Calories:* Without Dressing | | | |
| Black Bean Bowl, Chicken, 18.7 oz | 460 | 11 | 57 |
| Chicken Avocado Tortilla Wrap | 490 | 19 | 47 |
| Double Chicken Avocado Salad | 370 | 15 | 14 |
| *Dressings:* Citrus Vinaig., 1.5 oz | 70 | 4 | 9 |
| Creamy Cilantro: 3 oz | 320 | 35 | 2 |
| Light Creamy Cilantro, 1.5 oz | 60 | 5 | 3 |
| Ranch, 1.5 oz | 220 | 24 | 2 |
| *Sides:* Black Beans: Small | 140 | 1 | 25 |
| Large | 370 | 2.5 | 65 |
| Cole Slaw, 4 oz | 130 | 10 | 9 |
| Loco Side Salad, small | 170 | 15 | 8 |
| Macaroni & Cheese: Small | 310 | 19 | 24 |
| Large | 770 | 48 | 60 |
| Mashed Potatoes & Gravy: Small | 100 | 1.5 | 21 |
| Large | 340 | 4.5 | 69 |
| Pinto Beans, small | 150 | 2.5 | 24 |
| Spanish Rice: Small | 160 | 1.5 | 32 |
| Large | 380 | 4 | 76 |
| *Condiments:* Pico de Gallo, 1.5 oz | 10 | 0 | 2 |
| **Salsa:** Avocado, 1.5 oz | 25 | 2 | 2 |
| House; Roja,1.5 oz | 10 | 0 | 2 |
| Sour Cream, 1.3 oz | 80 | 6 | 1 |
| *Dessert,* Two Cinnamon Churros | 320 | 22 | 30 |

## Fatburger® (Sept '19)

| *Burgers:* Without Extras | C | F | Cb |
|---|---|---|---|
| Burgers: Small | 400 | 21 | 37 |
| Medium | 590 | 31 | 46 |
| Large | 850 | 41 | 69 |
| Impossible Burger | 480 | 21 | 50 |
| Turkeyburger | 480 | 19 | 50 |
| Veggieburger | 560 | 31 | 55 |
| *Hot Dogs:* Without Extras | | | |
| Chili Cheese | 330 | 15 | 27 |
| Regular Hot Dog | 510 | 20 | 60 |
| *Sandwiches:* Without Extras | | | |
| Chicken: Crispy | 560 | 27 | 53 |
| Grilled | 430 | 14 | 42 |
| Fish | 740 | 39 | 47 |
| *Fries:* Fat Fries | 380 | 18 | 47 |
| with Chili & Cheese | 590 | 33 | 53 |
| Skinny Fries | 390 | 15 | 58 |
| with Chili Cheese | 600 | 30 | 64 |
| *Salad:* Buffalo Chicken | 640 | 32 | 16 |
| Cajun Chicken | 200 | 12 | 8 |
| *Wings & Tenders:* Bone In Wing (1) | 60 | 3.5 | 2 |
| Boneless Wing (1) | 50 | 2.5 | 2 |
| Chicken Tender (1) | 110 | 5 | 2 |
| Tenders (4) & Fries, 4 oz | 825 | 47 | 39 |
| Wings (6) & Tenders (4) Fries (4 oz) | 1360 | 96 | 47 |
| *Add-Ons:* American Cheese, 1 slice | 70 | 5 | 1 |
| Cheddar Cheese, 1 slice | 110 | 9 | 1 |
| Mayonnaise, 1 serving | 90 | 10 | 1 |
| Relish, 1 serving | 20 | 0 | 5 |
| *Sides:* Chili Cup | 200 | 11 | 10 |
| with Cheese & Onions | 320 | 20 | 12 |
| Onion Rings | 540 | 29 | 64 |
| *Shakes:* Chocolate | 910 | 45 | 115 |
| Cookies & Ice Cream | 1180 | 59 | 163 |
| Maui-Banana | 940 | 44 | 126 |
| Peanut Butter | 950 | 53 | 114 |
| Strawberry; Vanilla, average | 885 | 44 | 114 |

*For Complete Nutritional Data ~ see CalorieKing.com*

## Fazoli's® (Sept '19)

| *Oven-Baked Pasta:* Per Serving | C | F | Cb |
|---|---|---|---|
| Baked Ziti | 570 | 19 | 71 |
| Chicken Broccoli Penne | 800 | 35 | 74 |
| Chicken Parmigano | 840 | 25 | 114 |
| Penne with Creamy Basil Chicken | 840 | 43 | 70 |
| Spicy Sausage Penne | 770 | 38 | 76 |
| *Classic Pastas:* Chicken Fett. Alfredo | 810 | 25 | 107 |
| Fettuccine Alfredo | 690 | 22 | 104 |
| Spagh. with Marinara | 510 | 3.5 | 108 |
| Spaghetti with Meatballs | 740 | 21 | 113 |

*Continued Next Page....*

## Fazoli's® cont... (Sept '19)

*Samplers:* Per Serving

| | C | F | Cb |
|---|---|---|---|
| Classic Sampler | 820 | 25 | 120 |
| Oven Baked | 930 | 35 | 116 |
| Ultimate Sampler | 1050 | 30 | 163 |
| *Signature Pasta:* | | | |
| Chicken Carbonara | 920 | 31 | 113 |
| Three Cheese Tortellini Alfredo | 830 | 33 | 79 |
| *Submarinos:* | | | |
| Meatball da Vinci | 920 | 56 | 65 |
| Primo Italiano | 840 | 45 | 60 |
| *Salads:* With Dressing | | | |
| Buffalo Chicken | 890 | 70 | 34 |
| Chicken Bacon Caesar | 550 | 37 | 18 |
| Strawberry Spinach Bacon | 530 | 33 | 33 |

*For Complete Nutritional Data ~ see CalorieKing.com*

## Firehouse Subs® (Sept '19)

*Hot Subs:* Per Medium White Sub, Standard Toppings and Dressings

| | C | F | Cb |
|---|---|---|---|
| Ham | 760 | 38 | 69 |
| Roast Beef | 740 | 37 | 53 |
| Turkey | 680 | 35 | 58 |
| Veggie | 720 | 45 | 57 |
| **Specialty:** Club on a Sub | 770 | 40 | 63 |
| Engineer | 690 | 35 | 59 |
| Hero | 800 | 38 | 63 |
| Hook & Ladder | 720 | 36 | 62 |
| Italian | 940 | 58 | 65 |
| Meatball | 840 | 50 | 61 |
| *Sides,* Chili, Bowl | 300 | 16 | 26 |
| *Under 500 Calorie Salads:* | | | |
| **Firehouse Chopped:** Without Dressing | | | |
| with Grilled Chicken | 380 | 10 | 14 |
| with Ham | 310 | 10 | 27 |
| with Turkey | 220 | 7 | 15 |
| **Italian,** w/ Grilled Chkn, w/o drssng | 410 | 22 | 13 |

## Five Guys® (Sept '19)

*Burgers:* Without Toppings or Sauce

| | C | F | Cb |
|---|---|---|---|
| Bacon Burger | 920 | 50 | 39 |
| Bacon Cheeseburger | 1060 | 62 | 40 |
| Cheeseburger | 980 | 55 | 40 |
| Hamburger | 840 | 43 | 39 |
| **Little Burgers:** Bacon Burger | 620 | 33 | 39 |
| Bacon Cheeseburger | 690 | 39 | 40 |
| Hamburger | 540 | 26 | 39 |
| **Hot Dogs:** Bacon | 600 | 42 | 40 |
| Cheese | 590 | 41 | 41 |
| **Sandwich,** BLT | 600 | 34 | 42 |
| **Fries,** medium, 14.5 oz | 955 | 41 | 131 |

## Five Guys® cont... (Sept '19)

*Burger Sauces & Toppings:*

| | C | F | Cb |
|---|---|---|---|
| **Sauce:** A.1 | 15 | 0 | 3 |
| BBQ Sauce | 50 | 0 | 15 |
| Ketchup; Relish, average | 15 | 0 | 5 |
| Mayo | 110 | 11 | 0 |
| **Toppings:** Lettuce & Tomato | 15 | 0 | 3 |
| Grilled Onions | 10 | 0 | 2 |
| Grilled Mushrooms | 20 | 0 | 4 |
| Pickles | 4 | 0 | 1 |

## Flame Broiler® (Sept '19)

*Bowls:* With White Rice

| | C | F | Cb |
|---|---|---|---|
| Beef | 620 | 11 | 74 |
| Chicken | 600 | 14 | 68 |
| Chicken & Veggie | 510 | 14 | 49 |
| Half & Half | 610 | 13 | 71 |
| The Works | 520 | 13 | 52 |
| *Plates:* With White Rice | | | |
| Beef | 840 | 18 | 94 |
| Rib | 1100 | 44 | 95 |
| The Works | 700 | 19 | 63 |

## Freshens® (Sept '19)

*Smoothies:* 100% Juice

| | C | F | Cb |
|---|---|---|---|
| **Blended Fruit Classics:** Per 20 fl.oz | | | |
| Bangin' Berry | 330 | 0 | 80 |
| Caribbean Craze | 300 | 0 | 73 |
| Jamaican Jammer | 330 | 0 | 70 |
| Peach On The Beach | 330 | 2.5 | 75 |
| Peanut Butter Protein | 480 | 12 | 69 |
| Tropical Therapy | 530 | 4 | 81 |
| Vegan PowerUp | 320 | 0 | 71 |
| Wild Strawberry | 300 | 0 | 76 |
| *Crepes:* Buffalo Chicken | 410 | 22 | 25 |
| Chicken Caesar | 600 | 44 | 25 |
| Chipotle Ranch Turkey Melt | 520 | 31 | 25 |
| Denver, with Bacon | 520 | 29 | 27 |
| Honey Mustard Chicken | 460 | 22 | 36 |
| Pesto Chicken | 490 | 29 | 27 |
| Southwest Chicken | 580 | 33 | 36 |
| *Rice Bowls:* Buffalo Chicken | 600 | 23 | 70 |
| Florence | 550 | 11 | 73 |
| KC BBQ | 610 | 11 | 97 |
| Mexican | 710 | 29 | 83 |
| Power Protein | 700 | 28 | 75 |
| Spicy Korean | 520 | 8 | 90 |
| *Salad:* Buffalo Chicken | 480 | 27 | 29 |
| Grilled Chicken Caesar | 520 | 37 | 26 |
| Roadhouse BBQ Chicken | 420 | 17 | 42 |
| Strawberry & Kale | 490 | 15 | 56 |

**201**

# Fast - Foods & *Restaurants*

## Godfather's Pizza® (Sept '19)

| | C | F | Cb |
|---|---|---|---|
| *Golden Crust Pizza: Per Slice* | | | |
| **Cheese:** Medium, ⅛ pizza | 210 | 8 | 25 |
| Large, ⅒ pizza | 230 | 10 | 27 |
| **Combo:** Medium, ⅛ pizza | 280 | 13 | 27 |
| Large, ⅒ pizza | 310 | 15 | 29 |
| **Super Combo:** | | | |
| Medium, ⅛ pizza | 310 | 16 | 27 |
| Large, ⅒ pizza | 350 | 18 | 30 |
| *Mozza-Loaded:* | | | |
| **All Meat Combo:** Medium, ⅛ pizza | 340 | 18 | 28 |
| Large, ⅒ pizza | 380 | 20 | 30 |
| *Original Crust Pizza:* | | | |
| **BLT:** Small, ⅙ pizza | 290 | 13 | 29 |
| Medium, ⅛ pizza | 320 | 15 | 32 |
| Jumbo, ⅟₁₂ pizza | 430 | 21 | 41 |
| **Buffalo Chicken:** Small, ⅙ pizza | 250 | 8 | 29 |
| Medium, ⅛ pizza | 270 | 9 | 31 |
| Jumbo, ⅟₁₂ pizza | 370 | 14 | 41 |
| **Taco Pie:** Small, ⅙ pizza | 310 | 14 | 31 |
| Medium, ⅛ pizza | 340 | 15 | 34 |
| Jumbo, ⅟₁₂ pizza | 470 | 22 | 44 |
| *Thin Crust Pizza:* | | | |
| **BBQ Chicken:** Medium, ⅛ pizza | 190 | 8 | 19 |
| Large, ⅒ pizza | 230 | 10 | 23 |
| **Pepperoni:** Medium, ⅛ pizza | 190 | 11 | 14 |
| Large, ⅒ pizza | 270 | 16 | 18 |
| **The Don:** Medium, ⅛ pizza | 240 | 14 | 15 |
| Large, ⅒ pizza | 290 | 17 | 18 |
| *Sides:* Baked Beans, 4 oz | 120 | 1 | 25 |
| Biscuit, 1 oz | 90 | 3.5 | 13 |
| Cheesy Potatoes, 4 oz | 300 | 9 | 30 |
| Coleslaw, 4 oz | 210 | 17 | 12 |
| Gravy, 2 oz | 30 | 1 | 4 |
| Mashed Potatoes, 4 oz | 100 | 3 | 17 |
| Mixed Vegetables, 4 oz | 90 | 0 | 18 |
| Potato Wedges, 4 oz | 190 | 9 | 24 |

## Gold Star Chili® (Sept '19)

| | C | F | Cb |
|---|---|---|---|
| *Burgers:* | | | |
| Bacon Cheeseburger | 650 | 40 | 44 |
| Chili Burger | 680 | 39 | 50 |
| Hamburger | 560 | 33 | 44 |
| *Coneys:* Cheese | 300 | 18 | 21 |
| Plain | 210 | 11 | 21 |
| Mustard & Onion | 230 | 11 | 23 |
| *Ways, Origninal Chili:* | | | |
| Regular: 2-Way | 410 | 12 | 56 |
| 3-Way | 760 | 41 | 56 |
| 5-Way | 850 | 41 | 74 |
| Super, 5-Way | 1160 | 53 | 111 |
| *Chili Bowls, Original:* | | | |
| Plain, 8 oz | 200 | 11 | 12 |
| Beans & Onions, 8 oz | 290 | 12 | 30 |

## Gold Star Chili® cont...(Sept '19)

| | C | F | Cb |
|---|---|---|---|
| *Double Deckers:* With White Bread | | | |
| Ham & Bacon | 1080 | 80 | 46 |
| Ham & Turkey | 760 | 46 | 46 |
| Turkey & Bacon | 1070 | 78 | 46 |
| *Salads:* Full Salad, without Dressing | | | |
| BBQ Chicken | 490 | 24 | 36 |
| Harvest Chicken | 340 | 16 | 25 |
| *Fries:* French, regular | 460 | 19 | 67 |
| Cheese | 810 | 48 | 68 |
| Chili Cheese | 840 | 51 | 64 |
| Garlic Parmesan | 870 | 62 | 71 |
| Vegetarian Chili | 540 | 24 | 71 |

## Golden Corral® (Sept '19)

| | C | F | Cb |
|---|---|---|---|
| *Breakfast:* | | | |
| Corned Beef Hash, ½ cup | 230 | 15 | 14 |
| Hash Brown Casserole, ½ cup | 100 | 3.5 | 14 |
| Sausage & Egg Burrito | 320 | 19 | 22 |
| Scrambled Eggs, ½ cup | 180 | 14 | 2 |
| *Hot Buffet: Without Sides* | | | |
| **Beef:** Pot Roast, ¹/₂ cup | 160 | 7 | 8 |
| Roast, flat, 3 oz | 180 | 10 | 1 |
| Smoked Beef Short Ribs, 3 oz | 340 | 27 | 0 |
| Steak, Smothered Chopped, 5.9 oz | 290 | 18 | 4 |
| **Chicken:** Buffalo Chicken Sandwich | 210 | 10 | 20 |
| Fried Chicken, 3 oz | 240 | 15 | 6 |
| Orange Chicken, 6 oz | 390 | 15 | 40 |
| Smoked White Meat Chicken, 3 oz | 150 | 6 | 0 |
| **Fish:** Baked, 3 oz | 150 | 8 | 1 |
| Fried Catfish, 3 oz | 180 | 10 | 12 |
| **Pork:** Baby Back Ribs, 3 oz | 190 | 13 | 3 |
| Sweet & Sour, 6 oz | 220 | 11 | 18 |
| *Sides:* BBQ Baked Beans, ½ cup | 160 | 1 | 35 |
| Creamed Spinach, ½ cup | 170 | 12 | 10 |
| Fries, Seasoned Wedges (10) | 190 | 12 | 21 |
| Fried Okra (10) | 110 | 7 | 10 |
| Mac & Cheese, ½ c. | 180 | 10 | 19 |
| Mshd Potatoes, ½ c. | | | |
| Rice Pilaf, ½ cup | 130 | 4.5 | 18 |
| *Salad Buffet: Per ½ Cup Unless Indicated* | | | |
| Caesar, without dressing, 1 cup | 110 | 8 | 8 |
| Chicken | 250 | 22 | 3 |
| Coleslaw | 110 | 9 | 6 |
| Potato | 150 | 5 | 26 |
| Seafood | 140 | 10 | 9 |
| Spinach, 1 cup | 15 | 0 | 2 |
| Tuna | 190 | 12 | 4 |
| *Dressings:* Balsamic Vinaig., 2 Tbsp | 20 | 0 | 5 |
| Caesar, 2 Tbsp | 150 | 15 | 2 |
| Ranch, 2 Tbsp | 110 | 12 | 2 |

Updated Nutrition Data ~ www.CalorieKing.com
Persons with Diabetes ~ See Disclaimer (Page 22)

## Great American Bagel Co® (Sept '19)

| Bagels: | C | F | Cb |
|---|---|---|---|
| Asiago Cheese | 520 | 16 | 72 |
| Cheddar Herb | 390 | 8 | 66 |
| Cinnamon Raisin | 380 | 3.5 | 76 |
| Jalapeno Cheddar | 370 | 7 | 63 |
| Plain | 360 | 4 | 71 |
| Spinach Tomazzo | 640 | 20 | 86 |
| Tomazzo | 520 | 13 | 77 |
| *Paninis: On Regular Baguette* | | | |
| Chicken Pesto | 770 | 35 | 70 |
| Ham & Swiss | 600 | 26 | 58 |
| Philly Beef | 920 | 40 | 92 |
| Turkey Club | 680 | 29 | 67 |
| *Sandwiches: Asiago Omelet* | 720 | 29 | 80 |
| BLT | 550 | 17 | 72 |
| Chicken Parmigiana | 740 | 22 | 81 |
| Ham | 460 | 9 | 71 |
| Roast Beef | 465 | 9 | 71 |
| Turkey | 435 | 5 | 72 |
| *Cream Cheese Filling: Per 1 oz* | | | |
| Plain | 100 | 10 | 1 |
| Strawberry; Vegetable, average | 90 | 8 | 4 |
| *Pastries:* | | | |
| **Cookies:** Chocolate Chunk, 4 oz | 110 | 3.5 | 19 |
| Oatmeal Raisin, 4 oz | 120 | 5 | 18 |
| **Muffins:** Banana Nut, 4.25 oz | 430 | 18 | 61 |
| Blueberry, 4.25 oz | 430 | 16 | 64 |

## Green Burrito® (Sept '19)

| Burritos: | C | F | Cb |
|---|---|---|---|
| Bean, Rice & Cheese | 730 | 26 | 93 |
| **Green:** Chicken | 930 | 38 | 96 |
| Steak | 940 | 38 | 96 |
| **Grilled,** Beef; Chicken; Steak, av. | 840 | 33 | 89 |
| *Specialties:* | | | |
| **Quesadillas:** Cheese | 640 | 34 | 53 |
| Chicken | 780 | 40 | 56 |
| Steak | 790 | 39 | 56 |
| **Rice,** Bean & Chips Platter | 340 | 10 | 51 |
| **Taco Salad,** Chicken; Steak | 875 | 53 | 60 |
| **Taquitos:** Chicken, 3 pieces | 410 | 28 | 34 |
| Chicken, 5 pieces | 640 | 43 | 56 |
| *Tacos:* | | | |
| Crunchy Beef | 210 | 12 | 16 |
| Soft Chicken | 250 | 12 | 18 |
| *Sides:* Chips, 2 oz | 300 | 17 | 35 |
| Cilantro Lime Rice, 3.4 oz | 90 | 5 | 21 |
| Guacamole, 2.7 oz | 100 | 8 | 5 |
| Pinto Beans, 3.7 oz | 90 | 1.5 | 13 |

## (The) Great Steak® (Sept '19)

| Breakfast Sandwiches: | C | F | Cb |
|---|---|---|---|
| Bacon, Egg & Cheese | 550 | 31 | 38 |
| Sausage, Egg & Cheese | 660 | 42 | 38 |
| Steak, Egg & Chse | 540 | 27 | 38 |
| *Burgers:* | | | |
| Bacon Cheeseburger | 1050 | 72 | 45 |
| Cheeseburger | 840 | 54 | 45 |
| Hamburger | 730 | 46 | 44 |
| Philly Cheeseburger | 780 | 48 | 44 |
| *Sandwiches: Regular Sie* | | | |
| Bacon Cheddar Cheesesteak | 590 | 23 | 55 |
| Buffalo Chicken Philly | 750 | 38 | 61 |
| Chicagoland Cheesesteak | 610 | 24 | 59 |
| Chicken Bacon Ranch | 820 | 44 | 60 |
| Great Steak Cheesesteak | 790 | 45 | 55 |
| Ham Delight | 780 | 44 | 64 |
| Orig. Philly Cheesesteak | 510 | 17 | 55 |
| Pastrami Philly | 800 | 46 | 57 |
| Reuben Philly | 710 | 37 | 56 |
| Super Steak Cheesesteak | 800 | 45 | 57 |
| Turkey Philly | 750 | 42 | 57 |
| Ultimate Chicken Philly | 800 | 44 | 60 |
| Veggie Delight | 490 | 19 | 61 |
| Wisconsin Inside-Out | 530 | 26 | 50 |
| *Baked Potatoes:* | | | |
| Bacon & Cheese | 440 | 23 | 36 |
| Broccoli & Cheese | 250 | 6 | 45 |
| **The Great Potato:** Chicken | 460 | 19 | 49 |
| Ham | 450 | 19 | 52 |
| Steak | 470 | 20 | 46 |
| Turkey | 430 | 17 | 48 |
| The King | 540 | 32 | 38 |
| *Fries:* | | | |
| **Bacon Ranch:** Regular | 650 | 42 | 51 |
| Large | 1520 | 91 | 139 |
| **Great Fry:** Kids | 270 | 13 | 36 |
| Regular | 370 | 18 | 48 |
| Large | 930 | 40 | 132 |
| King Fry, regular | 480 | 27 | 52 |
| *Salads: Without Dressing* | | | |
| **Great Salad:** Chicken | 370 | 22 | 16 |
| Ham | 360 | 22 | 19 |
| Steak | 390 | 23 | 17 |
| Turkey | 350 | 20 | 19 |
| *Salad Dressings:* Mayo, reg., 1 oz | 200 | 22 | 0 |
| Ranch, 1 oz | 150 | 16 | 2 |
| Thousand Island, 1 oz | 130 | 12 | 4 |
| *Sauce:* BBQ, 1 oz | 50 | 0 | 12 |
| Buffalo, 1 oz | 10 | 0 | 1 |
| Honey Mustard, 1 oz | 40 | 1 | 7 |
| Teriyaki, 1 oz | 25 | 0 | 3 |

**203**

# Fast - Foods & *Restaurants*

## Haagen-Dazs® (Sept '19)

*Classic Flavors:* Per ½ Cup

| | C | F | Cb |
|---|---|---|---|
| Banana Peanut Butter Chip | 340 | 23 | 25 |
| Belgian Chocolate | 330 | 21 | 30 |
| Bourbon Praline Pecan | 380 | 21 | 42 |
| Bourbon Van. Bean Truffle | 340 | 20 | 36 |
| Butter Pecan | 300 | 22 | 20 |
| Caramel Cone | 320 | 20 | 28 |
| Cherry Van.; Choc. Chip Cookie Dough | 290 | 17 | 29 |
| Chocolate | 260 | 17 | 22 |
| Chocolate Chocolate Chip | 300 | 19 | 26 |
| Chocolate Peanut Butter | 330 | 22 | 25 |
| Coffee; Cookies & Cream, av. | 250 | 17 | 21 |
| Dulce de Leche | 270 | 16 | 28 |
| Espresso Chocolate Cookie Crumble | 310 | 21 | 25 |
| Green Tea | 250 | 17 | 20 |
| Honey Salted Caramel Almond | 290 | 18 | 26 |
| Irish Cream Brownie | 360 | 21 | 37 |
| Java Chip | 290 | 17 | 30 |
| Mango | 250 | 13 | 29 |
| Mint Chip; Peppermint Bark, av | 280 | 17 | 27 |
| PB Salted Fudge | 340 | 23 | 26 |
| Pineapple Coconut | 230 | 13 | 25 |
| Pistachio | 280 | 19 | 22 |
| Pralines & Cream; Rocky Road, av. | 280 | 17 | 28 |
| Rum Raisin; Vanilla, av | 250 | 17 | 22 |
| Rum Tres Leches | 360 | 21 | 38 |
| Sea Salt Caramel Truffle | 300 | 17 | 32 |
| Strawberry | 240 | 15 | 22 |
| Vanilla Bean | 270 | 17 | 25 |
| Vanilla Choc. Chip/Swiss Almond | 290 | 19 | 25 |
| White Chocolate Raspberry Truffle | 280 | 16 | 31 |

*Non Dairy:* Per ½ cup

| | C | F | Cb |
|---|---|---|---|
| Amaretto Black Cherry | 320 | 12 | 49 |
| Choc. Salted Fudge Truffle | 270 | 11 | 40 |
| Coconut Caramel | 240 | 11 | 34 |
| Mocha Chocolate Cookie | 240 | 9 | 38 |
| Peanut Butter Chocolate Fudge | 290 | 14 | 36 |

*Trio Crispy Layers:*

| | C | F | Cb |
|---|---|---|---|
| Coconut Caramel Chocolate | 290 | 19 | 26 |
| Coffee Vanilla Chocolate | 280 | 19 | 23 |
| Lemon Raspberry White Chocolate | 290 | 18 | 28 |
| Salted Caramel Chocolate | 300 | 20 | 26 |
| Triple Chocolate Trio | 290 | 19 | 26 |
| Van. Blackberry Chocolate | 280 | 19 | 24 |
| **Non Dairy:** Coconut Cookies & Creme | 260 | 12 | 35 |
| Crunchy Peanut Butter | 260 | 12 | 34 |

Ice Cream Bars/Cones ~ See Page 109

## Hardee's® (Sept '19)

*Burgers:*

| | C | F | Cb |
|---|---|---|---|
| **Charbroiled Slider:** Double, 5 oz | 340 | 20 | 20 |
| Single, 3.5 | 220 | 11 | 20 |
| **Cheeseburgers:** ¼ lb | 440 | 23 | 37 |
| ⅓ lb | 640 | 33 | 56 |
| Double | 380 | 19 | 33 |
| **Thickburgers:** ¼ lb | 530 | 35 | 34 |
| Original, ⅓ lb | 780 | 48 | 56 |
| Bacon Cheese, ⅓ lb | 850 | 54 | 54 |
| Frisco, ⅓ lb | 840 | 55 | 46 |
| Monster, ⅔ lb | 1300 | 90 | 53 |
| Mushroom 'N' Swiss, ⅓ lb | 680 | 38 | 53 |

*Sandwiches:*

| | C | F | Cb |
|---|---|---|---|
| **Big Hot Ham 'N' Cheese** | 530 | 20 | 51 |
| **Chicken:** Big Chicken Fillet, 11 oz | 710 | 36 | 64 |
| Charbroiled: BBQ Chkn, 7.8 oz | 350 | 6 | 46 |
| Chicken Club | 560 | 28 | 38 |
| Southern Style Tender | 530 | 23 | 58 |
| Spicy Chicken | 440 | 23 | 44 |

*Chicken Tenders: Without Sauce*

| | C | F | Cb |
|---|---|---|---|
| **Hand Breaded:** | | | |
| 3 pieces, 4.5 oz | 260 | 13 | 13 |
| 5 pieces, 7.5 oz | 440 | 21 | 21 |
| *Chili Dog,* Jumbo | 390 | 26 | 23 |

*Natural Cut Fries:*

| | C | F | Cb |
|---|---|---|---|
| Kid's, 3 oz | 240 | 12 | 31 |
| Small, 3.7 oz | 300 | 15 | 47 |
| Medium, 5.9 oz | 490 | 24 | 63 |
| Large, 6.5 oz | 530 | 26 | 69 |

*Sides:*

| | C | F | Cb |
|---|---|---|---|
| Beer Battered Onion Rings | 410 | 24 | 45 |
| **Dipping Sauce:** B'milk Ranch, 1 oz | 100 | 10 | 2 |
| Honey Mustard | 120 | 12 | 4 |
| Sweet & Bold BBQ, 0.9 oz | 50 | 0 | 13 |

*Crispy Curls:*

| | C | F | Cb |
|---|---|---|---|
| Small, 4.1 oz | 360 | 18 | 46 |
| Medium, 5.36 oz | 470 | 23 | 60 |
| Large, 6.5 oz | 570 | 28 | 72 |

*All Star Meals: Per Set Menu, without Dipping Sauce*

| | C | F | Cb |
|---|---|---|---|
| Double Cheeseburger & Hot Dog | 1160 | 64 | 111 |
| Hand Breaded Chicken Tender | 690 | 34 | 68 |

## Hardee's® cont... (Sept '19)

| Better For You Options: | C | F | Cb |
|---|---|---|---|
| **Low Carb It:** ⅓ lb Thickburger | 470 | 36 | 9 |
| Charbroiled Chicken Club S'wich | 340 | 22 | 13 |
| **Trim It:** ¼ lb Little Thickburger | 220 | 15 | 6 |
| Big Hot Ham Sandwich | 290 | 6 | 31 |
| Charbroiled BBQ Chicken Sandwich | 190 | 3.5 | 24 |
| **Veg It:** Egg & Cheese Biscuit | 410 | 23 | 38 |
| Thickburger, hold the Patty | 550 | 33 | 56 |

| *Breakfast:* | | | |
|---|---|---|---|
| **Better For You,** Frisco Sandwich | 360 | 11 | 44 |
| **Breakfast Burrito,** Loaded | 580 | 30 | 46 |

| *Made From Scratch Biscuits:* | | | |
|---|---|---|---|
| Bacon, Egg & Cheese | 610 | 38 | 46 |
| Biscuit 'N' Gravy | 620 | 39 | 57 |
| Buttermilk Biscuit, plain | 430 | 26 | 43 |
| Chicken Fillet | 650 | 41 | 53 |
| Country Ham | 500 | 30 | 44 |
| Country Fried Steak | 640 | 42 | 52 |
| Loaded Omelet | 620 | 39 | 48 |
| Monster | 880 | 61 | 48 |
| Pork Chop 'N' Gravy | 590 | 33 | 49 |
| Sausage | 620 | 43 | 44 |
| Sausage and Egg | 690 | 48 | 46 |
| Smoked Sausage, Egg & Cheese | 790 | 57 | 48 |
| **Platter,** with Bacon | 760 | 45 | 51 |
| **Sandwich,** Frisco Breakfast | 450 | 19 | 45 |
| **Sunrise Croissant** | 450 | 28 | 30 |

| *Breakfast Sides:* | | | |
|---|---|---|---|
| **Hash Rounds:** Small, 2.9 oz | 260 | 15 | 23 |
| Medium, 4.2 oz | 370 | 22 | 33 |
| Large, 5.8 oz | 510 | 30 | 45 |

| *Desserts:* | | | |
|---|---|---|---|
| Apple Turnover, w/out Cinnamon Sugar | 270 | 13 | 35 |
| Chocolate Chip Cookies (2), 2 oz | 290 | 15 | 35 |

| *Ice Cream Shakes:* Per 14 oz | | | |
|---|---|---|---|
| **Hand Scooped:** Chocolate | 710 | 33 | 87 |
| Strawberry | 710 | 33 | 87 |
| Vanilla | 710 | 33 | 87 |

## Hissho Sushi® (Sept '19)

| Natural Food Store Menu Items | C | F | Cb |
|---|---|---|---|
| *Starters:* Per Package | | | |
| Chicken Gyoza, 5.3 oz | 240 | 8 | 28 |
| Pork Gyoza, 5.3 oz | 310 | 14 | 31 |
| Spring Roll, 12.6 oz | 300 | 5 | 54 |
| Squid Salad, 4 oz | 160 | 3 | 20 |
| *Maki Sushi Rolls:* Per Package | | | |
| Blazing California, 12.24 oz | 450 | 17 | 68 |
| California, 12.24 oz | 360 | 10 | 65 |
| **Dynamite:** | | | |
| Spicy: Salmon, 12.2 oz | 460 | 17 | 64 |
| Shrimp, 12.2 oz | 430 | 15 | 63 |
| Tuna, 12.2 oz | 440 | 13 | 63 |
| Yellowtail, 12.2 oz | 510 | 22 | 63 |
| Eel, 12.45 oz | 300 | 6 | 59 |
| Philadelphia Crab, 12.2 oz | 510 | 22 | 68 |
| **Sushicado:** Salmon, 12.2 oz | 450 | 16 | 59 |
| Shrimp, 12.2 oz | 390 | 9 | 58 |
| Tuna, 12. oz | 410 | 10 | 58 |
| **Tokyo Fantasy:** Salmon, 12.17 oz | 430 | 15 | 56 |
| Shrimp, cooked, 12.17 oz | 390 | 13 | 56 |
| Yellowtail, 12.17 oz | 510 | 23 | 56 |
| **Veggie,** 12.2 oz | 330 | 9 | 63 |
| *Specialty Items:* Per Package | | | |
| Crispy Crab, 9.3 oz | 420 | 20 | 56 |
| **Living Color Roll:** | | | |
| Salmon & Eel, 10.3 oz | 300 | 10 | 47 |
| Tuna & Shrimp, 10.3 oz | 300 | 7 | 46 |
| Yellowtail & Eel, 10.3 oz | 320 | 12 | 47 |
| **Southern Charm Roll:** | | | |
| Spicy: Real Crab, 9.25 oz | 450 | 20 | 46 |
| Salmon, 9.25 oz | 430 | 22 | 49 |
| Shrimp, 9.25 oz | 420 | 20 | 46 |
| Tuna, 9.25 oz | 430 | 18 | 46 |
| Yellowtail, 9.,25 oz | 500 | 26 | 46 |

## Hot Dog on a Stick® (Sept '19)

| Menu Items: | C | F | Cb |
|---|---|---|---|
| American Cheese on a Stick | 260 | 16 | 20 |
| Beef Hot Dog on a Stick | 330 | 21 | 25 |
| Turkey Hot Dog on a Stick | 240 | 12 | 27 |
| Veggie Dog on a Stick | 200 | 6 | 26 |
| Pepperjack Cheese on a Stick | 260 | 15 | 22 |
| *French Fries:* Small, 7.2 oz | 500 | 29 | 57 |
| Regular, 14.4 oz | 1000 | 59 | 113 |
| *Beverages:* Per Regular Size, 16 fl.oz | | | |
| Lemonade: Original | 150 | 0 | 38 |
| Cherry | 210 | 0 | 52 |
| Lime | 230 | 0 | 57 |

## Hungry Howie's Pizza® (Sept '19)

*Counts may vary in Florida.*

|  | C | F | Cb |
|---|---|---|---|
| **Specialty Pizza:** *12" Pizza, Per ⅛ Slice* | | | |
| BBQ Chicken | 230 | 8 | 29 |
| Buffalo Chicken | 210 | 8 | 24 |
| Works | 250 | 11 | 26 |
| Veggie | 200 | 6 | 28 |
| **Subs:** *Per ½ of Large Sub, with Set Menu Toppings* | | | |
| Ham & Cheese | 590 | 23 | 62 |
| Italian | 620 | 27 | 62 |
| Steak & Cheese | 650 | 29 | 62 |
| Turkey Club | 840 | 46 | 60 |
| Veggie | 580 | 24 | 69 |
| **Salads:** *Regular Size, without Dressing* | | | |
| Antipasto | 400 | 26 | 14 |
| Chef | 320 | 19 | 13 |
| Garden | 90 | 2.5 | 14 |
| Greek | 230 | 11 | 18 |
| **Dressings:** *Per 1 oz* | | | |
| Caesar | 180 | 18 | 2 |
| Creamy Italian | 120 | 12 | 2 |
| Greek | 110 | 11 | 2 |
| Ranch | 140 | 14 | 1 |
| Thousand Island | 140 | 14 | 4 |

## In-N-Out Burger® (Sept '19)

|  | C | F | Cb |
|---|---|---|---|
| **Burgers:** | | | |
| **Hamburger:** with Onion | 390 | 19 | 39 |
| w/ Mstrd & Ketchup, w/o Spread | 310 | 10 | 41 |
| Protein Style w/ Lettuce Wrap, without Bun | 240 | 17 | 11 |
| **Cheeseburger:** with Onion | 480 | 27 | 39 |
| w/ Mstrd & Ketchup, w/o Spread | 400 | 18 | 41 |
| Protein Style w/ Lettuce Wrap, without Bun | 330 | 25 | 11 |
| **Double Double:** with Onion | 670 | 41 | 39 |
| w/ Mstrd & Ketchup, w/o Spread | 590 | 32 | 41 |
| Protein Style w/ Lettuce Wrap, without Bun | 520 | 39 | 11 |
| *French Fries,* 4.5 oz | 370 | 15 | 52 |
| *Drinks:* Milk, 10 fl.oz | 180 | 6 | 18 |
| Coca-Cola,16 fl.oz | 190 | 0 | 51 |
| Dr Pepper,16 fl.oz | 180 | 0 | 49 |
| Pink Lemonade, 16 fl.oz | 210 | 0 | 52 |
| Root Beer,16 fl.oz | 210 | 0 | 56 |
| *Hot Cocoa,* 8 fl.oz | 130 | 3 | 26 |
| **Shakes:** | | | |
| Chocolate, 15 fl.oz | 580 | 28 | 84 |
| Vanilla, 15 fl.oz | 580 | 30 | 65 |

## IHOP® (Sept '19)

|  | C | F | Cb |
|---|---|---|---|
| **Pancakes:** | | | |
| Cannoli (3) | 970 | 44 | 125 |
| Double Blueberry (4) | 610 | 16 | 101 |
| NY Cheesecake (4) | 920 | 37 | 124 |
| Orig. Buttermilk (3) | 430 | 17 | 56 |
| Strawberry banana (4) | 650 | 15 | 115 |
| **Toppings:** Glazed Strawb.; Peaches, av. | 55 | 0 | 12 |
| Raspberry | 80 | 0 | 20 |
| **Griddle Faves:** *With Menu Set Toppings* | | | |
| **French Toast:** Original | 740 | 36 | 84 |
| Strawberry Banana | 840 | 31 | 121 |
| Stuffed | 890 | 36 | 126 |
| **Waffles,** Belgian | 590 | 29 | 69 |
| **Crepes:** *With Set Toppings* | | | |
| Banana with Nutella | 950 | 44 | 120 |
| Chicken Florentine | 900 | 53 | 48 |
| German Crepes | 680 | 34 | 76 |
| Strawberries & Cream | 770 | 31 | 106 |
| Swedish | 660 | 30 | 81 |
| **Omelettes:** *Without Pancakes or Sides* | | | |
| Big Steak | 1080 | 74 | 39 |
| Chicken Fajita | 960 | 63 | 25 |
| Garden | 840 | 66 | 17 |
| Spicy Poblano | 1060 | 79 | 31 |
| Spinach & Mushroom | 890 | 69 | 21 |
| **Combos:** *With Two B'Milk Pancakes & Hash Browns* | | | |
| Country Fried Steak, w/ Ssg Gravy | 1470 | 96 | 112 |
| Sirloin Tips, w/ Gr. Onions & Mshrms | 960 | 51 | 78 |
| Smokehouse, with 2 Poached Eggs | 1140 | 80 | 62 |
| T-Bone Steak (12 oz), w/ 3 Fried Eggs, without Hash Browns | 970 | 46 | 58 |
| **Ultimate Steakburgers:** *Without Sides* | | | |
| Big Crunch | 1020 | 66 | 57 |
| Cowboy BBQ | 900 | 50 | 71 |
| Philly Cheeseburger | 1060 | 72 | 42 |
| **Sandwiches:** *Without Sides* | | | |
| Double BLT | 670 | 44 | 41 |
| Philly Cheese Steak Stacker | 820 | 40 | 63 |
| Roasted Turkey on Rye | 690 | 38 | 34 |
| Spicy Chicken Ranch | 730 | 38 | 62 |
| **Entrees:** *As Served, without Sides* | | | |
| Cntry Fried Steak & Country Gravy | 840 | 59 | 49 |
| Pot Roast | 370 | 20 | 15 |
| Sirloin Steak Tips | 430 | 23 | 21 |
| Tilapia Florentine | 480 | 32 | 9 |
| **55+ Lunch:** *Without Soup or Salad* | | | |
| BLT Sandwich, on White Bread | 400 | 26 | 27 |
| Grilled Cheese S'wich, on Sourdough | 680 | 34 | 61 |
| **Sides:** French Fries | 320 | 15 | 41 |
| Hash Browns | 210 | 14 | 19 |
| Onion Rings | 400 | 22 | 47 |

*For Complete Menu & Data ~ see CalorieKing.com*

## Jack in the Box® (Sept '19)

### Sandwiches & Burgers:

| | C | F | Cb |
|---|---|---|---|
| Bacon Swiss Buttery Jack | 890 | 59 | 48 |
| Bacon Ultimate Cheeseburger | 930 | 65 | 32 |
| Classic Buttery Jack | 820 | 52 | 50 |
| Double Jack | 830 | 58 | 34 |
| Jumbo Jack: with Cheese | 600 | 40 | 33 |
| without Cheese | 520 | 33 | 32 |
| Junior Bacon Cheeseburger | 480 | 31 | 32 |
| Sourdough Jack | 700 | 45 | 39 |
| Sourdough Patty Melt | 630 | 41 | 36 |
| Spicy Sriracha Burger | 680 | 45 | 38 |
| Ultimate Cheeseburger | 840 | 59 | 31 |

### Chicken & Fish Sandwiches:

| | C | F | Cb |
|---|---|---|---|
| Chkn Fajita Pita: without Salsa | 340 | 12 | 35 |
| with Salsa | 350 | 12 | 36 |
| Chicken Sandwich | 510 | 32 | 40 |
| with Bacon | 550 | 35 | 40 |
| Crispy Chicken Strips, 4 pieces | 560 | 24 | 53 |
| Homestyle Ranch Chicken Club | 710 | 33 | 66 |
| Jack's Spicy Chkn S'wich | 550 | 29 | 48 |
| with Cheese | 630 | 35 | 49 |
| Sourdough Grilled Chicken Club | 580 | 30 | 38 |

### Brunchfast: Brunch Burger

| | C | F | Cb |
|---|---|---|---|
| Brunchfast: Brunch Burger | 770 | 55 | 32 |
| Bacon & Egg Chicken Sandwich | 650 | 39 | 37 |
| Country Scrambler Plate | 770 | 54 | 37 |

### Breakfast:

| | C | F | Cb |
|---|---|---|---|
| Biscuit: Bacon, Egg & Cheese | 410 | 25 | 26 |
| Sausage, Egg & Cheese | 530 | 38 | 27 |
| Breakfast Jack: Reg. | 350 | 18 | 30 |
| with Sausage | 500 | 34 | 30 |
| Burrito: Meat Lovers, with salsa | 790 | 50 | 50 |
| Grand Sausage, with salsa | 1040 | 70 | 68 |
| Croissants: Sausage | 560 | 39 | 32 |
| Supreme | 450 | 27 | 32 |
| Hash Browns | 190 | 13 | 17 |
| Mini Pancakes (8) | 140 | 1.5 | 28 |
| Sandwiches: Extreme Sausage | 650 | 49 | 29 |
| Grilled | 620 | 29 | 53 |
| Loaded | 710 | 47 | 36 |
| Sourdough | 410 | 21 | 35 |
| Ultimate | 520 | 31 | 30 |

### Snacks & Sides:

| | C | F | Cb |
|---|---|---|---|
| Bacon Cheddar Potato Wedges | 680 | 41 | 58 |
| Chiquita Apple Bites w/ dip, 2.7 oz | 70 | 0 | 17 |
| Egg Rolls (1), 2.1 oz | 150 | 7 | 15 |
| Panko Onion Rings (8), 4.2 oz | 440 | 24 | 52 |
| Stuffed Jalapenos: 3 Pieces | 220 | 12 | 21 |
| 7 Pieces | 510 | 29 | 49 |

## Jack in the Box® cont... (Sept '19)

### Fries:

| | C | F | Cb |
|---|---|---|---|
| French Fries: Small | 300 | 14 | 40 |
| Medium | 430 | 20 | 58 |
| Large | 550 | 25 | 75 |
| Seasoned Curly Fries: Small | 280 | 16 | 30 |
| Medium | 430 | 25 | 46 |
| Large | 480 | 28 | 52 |

### Salads: Without Dressing or Croutons

| | C | F | Cb |
|---|---|---|---|
| Chicken Club: | | | |
| with Crispy Chicken | 510 | 28 | 36 |
| with Grilled Chicken | 370 | 20 | 11 |
| Grilled Chicken | 250 | 9 | 13 |
| Croutons, 0.5 oz | 70 | 3 | 9 |
| Dressing: Creamy Sthwest, 1.75 oz | 190 | 19 | 3 |
| Ranch, 1.75 oz | 250 | 25 | 5 |
| Low Fat Balsamic Vinaigrette, 1.5 oz | 25 | 1.5 | 3 |
| Dipping Sauce: Barbecue, 1 oz | 40 | 0 | 10 |
| Buttermilk, 1 oz | 110 | 11 | 2 |
| Frank's Red Hot Buffalo, 1 oz | 10 | 0 | 1 |
| Sweet & Sour, 1 oz | 40 | 0 | 10 |
| Teriyaki | 50 | 1 | 11 |

### Sandwich Sauce:

| | C | F | Cb |
|---|---|---|---|
| Creamy Bacon Mayo, 0.7 fl.oz | 120 | 13 | 1 |
| Creamy Sriracha Sauce, 0.8fl.oz | 120 | 13 | 1 |
| Mayo-Onion, 0.5 fl.oz | 90 | 10 | 0 |
| Tartar Sauce, 0.5 fl.oz | 50 | 4.5 | 2 |
| Desserts: Mini Churros (5) | 350 | 18 | 42 |
| Choc. Overload Cake | 300 | 7 | 57 |
| New York Style Cheesecake | 310 | 17 | 32 |

### Ice Cream Shakes: 16 fl.oz, with Whipped Topping

| | C | F | Cb |
|---|---|---|---|
| Chocolate | 780 | 38 | 103 |
| Oreo Cookie | 800 | 43 | 95 |
| Strawberry | 760 | 38 | 97 |
| Vanilla | 680 | 38 | 78 |

*For Complete Nutritional Data ~ see CalorieKing.com*

## Jack's® (Sept '19)

### Burgers & Sandwiches:

| | C | F | Cb |
|---|---|---|---|
| Big Bacon | 800 | 57 | 36 |
| Big Jack Burger | 720 | 47 | 43 |
| Cheeseburger | 440 | 23 | 38 |
| Double Cheeseburger | 680 | 43 | 38 |
| Grilled Chicken S'wich | 410 | 17 | 35 |
| Hamburger | 400 | 19 | 38 |
| Chicken: Fried Chicken Wing (1) | 220 | 13 | 10 |
| Fingers Dinner, 3 pce with Fries | 610 | 27 | 56 |
| Fries, regular | 260 | 16 | 27 |
| Sides: Coleslaw, 4 oz | 210 | 18 | 13 |
| Mashed Potatoes, 4 oz | 140 | 3.5 | 26 |
| Breakfast: Hash Browns | 360 | 25 | 31 |
| Special | 670 | 44 | 53 |
| Steak Biscuit | 580 | 41 | 42 |

## Jamba Juice® (Sept '19)

*Freshly Squeezed Juice: 16 fl.oz*

| | C | F | Cb |
|---|---|---|---|
| Orange Carrot Twist | 210 | 1 | 48 |
| Purely Carrot | 190 | 1 | 45 |
| Purely Orange | 220 | 1 | 52 |

*Smoothies: Per 16 fl.oz*

| | C | F | Cb |
|---|---|---|---|
| **Classic:** Caribbean Passion | 260 | 1 | 63 |
| Mango-A-Go-Go | 300 | 1 | 73 |
| Orange Dream Machine | 310 | 1.5 | 68 |
| Razzamatazz | 270 | 1 | 65 |
| Strawberry Surf Rider | 250 | 1.5 | 60 |
| Strawberries Wild | 240 | 0 | 57 |
| **Plant-Based:** Amazing Greens | 360 | 13 | 57 |
| Apple 'n Greens | 250 | 1 | 58 |
| Greens 'n ginger | 230 | 1 | 56 |
| Mega Mango | 210 | 0.5 | 50 |
| Peach Perfection | 210 | 0 | 51 |
| Strawberry Whirl | 210 | 0.5 | 51 |
| **Power:** Acai Super-Antioxidant | 340 | 4 | 69 |
| Lotta Horchata | 190 | 2.5 | 38 |
| La Vida Mocha | 270 | 2 | 58 |
| PB & Banana Protein | 540 | 22 | 51 |
| PB Chocolate Love | 400 | 14 | 64 |
| Soy Protein Berry Workout | 300 | 1 | 58 |

*Tasty Bites:*

**Artisan Flat Bread:** *Per Flatbread*

| | C | F | Cb |
|---|---|---|---|
| Four Cheese | 350 | 11 | 44 |
| Spicy 'n Sweet Chicken | 330 | 11 | 38 |

**Baked Goods:** *Per Item*

| | C | F | Cb |
|---|---|---|---|
| Apple Cinnamon Pretzel | 390 | 4.5 | 78 |
| Cheddar Tomato Twist | 250 | 5 | 41 |
| Sourdough Parmesan Pretzel | 420 | 11 | 69 |
| Sweet Belgian Waffle | 310 | 15 | 39 |

**Breakfast Sandwiches:**

| | C | F | Cb |
|---|---|---|---|
| Bacon, Rstd Tom., Spinach & Feta | 250 | 9 | 30 |
| Roasted Tomato, Spinach & Feta | 240 | 8 | 30 |

**Breakfast Wraps:** Spinach 'n Chse 240 | 7 | 30

| | C | F | Cb |
|---|---|---|---|
| Turkey Sausage 'n Cheese | 320 | 15 | 30 |

**Steel-Cut Oatmeal:** *With Soymilk*

| | C | F | Cb |
|---|---|---|---|
| Plain | 170 | 2.5 | 31 |
| Add: Banana | 50 | 0 | 13 |
| Blueberries | 10 | 0 | 2 |
| Brown Sugar Crumble | 40 | 1 | 8 |
| Clover Honey | 30 | 0 | 9 |
| Strawberries | 5 | 0 | 1 |

*Energy Bowls: Per 16 fl.oz*

| | C | F | Cb |
|---|---|---|---|
| Acai Primo | 510 | 10 | 101 |
| Chunky Strawberry | 580 | 16 | 94 |
| Island Pitaya | 480 | 8 | 102 |
| Nutty Almond Butter | 430 | 16 | 68 |

## Jersey Mike's Subs® (Sept '19)

*Cold Subs: Per Regular, on White, without Vinegar, Oil or Mayo Unless Indicated*

| | C | F | Cb |
|---|---|---|---|
| #1 BLT, with Mayo | 700 | 40 | 65 |
| #2 Jersey Shore Favorite | 570 | 16 | 68 |
| #3 Ham & Provolone | 570 | 15 | 67 |
| #5 Super Sub | 580 | 15 | 69 |
| #6 Roast Beef & Provolone | 630 | 16 | 65 |
| #7 Turkey & Provolone | 530 | 12 | 65 |
| #8 Club Sub with Mayonnaise | 850 | 44 | 67 |
| #9 Club Supreme w/ Mayonnaise | 880 | 44 | 66 |
| #10 Albacore Tuna | 780 | 42 | 67 |
| #13 Original Italian | 700 | 26 | 70 |
| #14 Veggie | 690 | 30 | 68 |

*Hot Subs: Per Reg., on White Roll, w/ Standard Menu Components*

| | C | F | Cb |
|---|---|---|---|
| #15 Meatball & Cheese | 810 | 38 | 79 |
| #17: Mike's Philly | 720 | 29 | 68 |
| #19 BBQ Beef | 670 | 9 | 87 |
| #20 Grilled Pastrami Reuben | 730 | 30 | 72 |
| #42 Chipotle Chicken Cheesesteak | 990 | 53 | 72 |
| #43 Chipotle Cheesesteak | 1000 | 59 | 68 |
| #55 Big Kahuna Chkn Cheesesteak | 720 | 27 | 72 |
| #56 Big Kahuna Cheesesteak | 770 | 33 | 70 |

*Signature Wraps: On White Wrap, w/ Standard Menu Components*

| | C | F | Cb |
|---|---|---|---|
| Baja Chicken | 660 | 26 | 65 |
| Buffalo Chicken | 760 | 38 | 66 |
| Chicken Caesar | 620 | 27 | 60 |
| Turkey | 450 | 9 | 59 |

*French Fries: 5 oz*

| | C | F | Cb |
|---|---|---|---|
| French Fries: 5 oz | 310 | 19 | 34 |
| 6 oz | 370 | 23 | 41 |

*Breakfast Subs: On White Bread, w/ Standard Menu Components, without Ketchup*

| | C | F | Cb |
|---|---|---|---|
| #2: Mini Bacon, Egg & Cheese | 490 | 25 | 41 |
| #3: Mini Sausage, Egg & Cheese | 890 | 63 | 41 |
| #4: Ham, Egg & Cheese | 510 | 22 | 43 |
| #5: Steak, Egg & Cheese | 540 | 22 | 41 |

*Kid's: On White Bun, with Standard Menu Components, without Condiments*

| | C | F | Cb |
|---|---|---|---|
| Ham Sub | 230 | 5 | 33 |
| Salami Sub | 260 | 9 | 33 |
| Turkey Sub | 230 | 4.5 | 32 |

*Desserts:*

| | C | F | Cb |
|---|---|---|---|
| Brownie, regular | 500 | 28 | 63 |
| Choc. Chip Cookie, mini | 180 | 9 | 26 |
| **Tastykake:** Butterscotch Krimpet | 320 | 9 | 58 |
| Chocolate Cupcake, regular | 340 | 10 | 59 |
| Cream Filled, regular | 390 | 14 | 62 |

*Beverages:* Coffee Frappuccino 290 | 4.5 | 53

| | C | F | Cb |
|---|---|---|---|
| Caramel | 300 | 5 | 54 |

## Jimmy John's® (Sept '19)

*Subs: (8") Figures Based on French Bread w/ Standard Menu Board Toppings*

| | C | F | Cb |
|---|---|---|---|
| #1 Pepe | 630 | 30 | 59 |
| #2 Big John | 540 | 22 | 56 |
| #3 Totally Tuna | 560 | 24 | 60 |
| #4 Turkey Tom | 510 | 20 | 57 |
| #5 Vito | 620 | 27 | 60 |
| #6 Vegetarian | 690 | 39 | 60 |
| JJBLT | 570 | 28 | 56 |

*Giant Club Sandwiches: Figures Based on French Bread w/ Standard Menu Set Toppings*

| | C | F | Cb |
|---|---|---|---|
| #7 Smoked Ham Club | 810 | 32 | 81 |
| #8 Billy Club | 830 | 33 | 79 |
| #9 Italian Night | 950 | 46 | 82 |
| #10 Hunter's Club | 850 | 35 | 77 |
| #11 Country Club | 800 | 31 | 80 |
| #12 Beach Club | 860 | 40 | 81 |
| #13 Gourmet Veggie Club | 1020 | 58 | 82 |
| #14 Bootlegger | 710 | 23 | 77 |
| #15 Club Tuna | 890 | 43 | 82 |
| #16 Club Lulu | 710 | 27 | 77 |
| #17 Ultimate Porker | 720 | 28 | 78 |

*Plain Slims: Figures Based on French Bread without Toppings, Dressing or Mayo*

| | C | F | Cb |
|---|---|---|---|
| Slim 1 Ham & Provolone Cheese | 570 | 13 | 76 |
| Slim 2 Roast Beef | 480 | 6 | 73 |
| Slim 3 Tuna Salad | 650 | 25 | 77 |
| Slim 4 Turkey Breast | 450 | 3 | 74 |
| Slim 5 Salami Capicola & Cheese | 660 | 23 | 75 |
| Slim 6 Double Provolone | 610 | 21 | 75 |

*Sides:*

| | C | F | Cb |
|---|---|---|---|
| **Jimmy Chips:** Average | 150 | 8 | 17 |
| Thinny, 1 oz | 130 | 5 | 20 |
| **Cookies:** Raisin Oatmeal, 3 oz | 370 | 13 | 57 |
| Triple Chocolate Chunk, 3 oz | 410 | 19 | 56 |
| **Jumbo Kosher Dill Pickle,** 6.9 oz | 20 | 0 | 4 |

## Johnny Rockets® (Sept '19)

*Starters:*

| | C | F | Cb |
|---|---|---|---|
| Chili Bowl | 620 | 50 | 20 |
| **Fries:** Plain | 330 | 10 | 50 |
| Bacon Cheese | 630 | 30 | 60 |
| Cheese | 540 | 30 | 60 |
| Chili Cheese | 820 | 50 | 70 |
| Sweet Potato | 390 | 20 | 60 |
| **Onion Rings:** Regular | 630 | 30 | 80 |
| Side of Onion Rings | 420 | 30 | 40 |
| **Tots:** Plain | 740 | 50 | 70 |
| Bacon Cheese | 1050 | 70 | 80 |
| Cheese | 960 | 70 | 80 |
| Chili Cheese | 1230 | 90 | 90 |

## Johnny Rockets® cont... (Sept '19)

*Burgers: Per Regular Size Bun*

| | C | F | Cb |
|---|---|---|---|
| **Bacon Cheddar/Route 66:** | | | |
| Beef Burger | 780 | 50 | 40 |
| Boca Veggie Burger | 680 | 40 | 50 |
| Gardein Burger | 730 | 40 | 60 |
| **Original:** Beef Burger | 680 | 40 | 40 |
| Gardein Burger | 640 | 40 | 70 |
| **Rocket:** Beef Burger | 690 | 40 | 40 |
| Boca Veggie Burger | 590 | 30 | 50 |
| Gardein Burger | 640 | 40 | 60 |
| **Smokehouse:** Beef Burger | 800 | 40 | 70 |
| Boca Veggie Burger | 710 | 30 | 80 |
| Gardein Burger | 760 | 40 | 90 |
| **Spicy Houston:** | | | |
| Beef Burger | 640 | 40 | 40 |
| Boca Veggie Burger | 550 | 30 | 50 |
| Gardein Burger | 600 | 30 | 60 |
| *Chicken,* Tenders, BBQ Sauce | 670 | 20 | 90 |

*Hot Dogs:*

| | C | F | Cb |
|---|---|---|---|
| Rocket Dog | 480 | 30 | 40 |
| Rocket Chili Dog | 670 | 50 | 40 |
| *Philly Cheese Steak,* Beef | 780 | 40 | 60 |

*Melts:*

| | C | F | Cb |
|---|---|---|---|
| BBQ Chicken | 940 | 30 | 100 |
| Tuna on Sourdough | 650 | 40 | 50 |

*Sandwiches: Without Substitutions*

| | C | F | Cb |
|---|---|---|---|
| BLT, on Sourdough | 690 | 50 | 50 |
| Chicken Club, on Sourdough | 800 | 40 | 50 |
| Grilled Chicken, on Wheat Bun | 550 | 30 | 40 |
| Grilled Cheese, on Sourdough | 580 | 30 | 50 |

*Salads: Without Dressing*

| | C | F | Cb |
|---|---|---|---|
| Crispy Chicken Club | 420 | 20 | 20 |
| Grilled Chicken Club | 400 | 20 | 10 |
| Garden Salad | 140 | 9 | 6 |

*Breakfast: Standard, without Subsititutions*

| | C | F | Cb |
|---|---|---|---|
| **French Toast:** 2 slices | 620 | 10 | 100 |
| with Bacon | 800 | 30 | 100 |
| with Sausage | 1120 | 60 | 100 |
| **Pancakes:** B'milk (2) w/ Sausage | 1020 | 50 | 110 |
| Buttermilk (2), with Bacon | 700 | 20 | 110 |
| **Scramblers:** Bacon Denver | 1130 | 60 | 80 |
| Biscuits, Sausage & Gravy | 2010 | 130 | 120 |
| Cheesy Bacon Lovers | 1170 | 70 | 80 |
| Philly Cheesesteak | 1270 | 70 | 80 |

*Shakes: Without Malt*

| | C | F | Cb |
|---|---|---|---|
| Banana | 830 | 40 | 90 |
| Chocolate | 910 | 40 | 110 |
| Hershey's Chocolate | 920 | 40 | 110 |
| Oreo Cookies & Cream | 1020 | 50 | 120 |
| P'nut Butter Banana | 1050 | 60 | 100 |

*For Complete Menu & Data ~ see CalorieKing.com*

## KFC® (Sept '19)

### Chicken On The Bone: *Per Piece*

| | C | F | Cb |
|---|---|---|---|
| **Original Recipe:** Breast, 6 oz | 390 | 21 | 11 |
| Drumstick, 1.87 oz | 130 | 8 | 4 |
| Thigh, 3.7 oz | 280 | 19 | 8 |
| Whole Wing, 1.5 oz | 130 | 8 | 3 |
| **Extra Crispy:** Breast, 6.3 oz | 530 | 35 | 18 |
| Drumstick, 1.9 oz | 170 | 12 | 5 |
| Thigh, 3.5 oz | 330 | 23 | 9 |
| Whole Wing, 1.7 oz | 170 | 13 | 5 |
| **Kentucky Grilled:** Breast, 4.6 oz | 210 | 7 | 0 |
| Drumstick, 1.4 oz | 80 | 4 | 0 |
| Thigh, 2.5 oz | 150 | 9 | 0 |
| Whole Wing, 1 oz | 70 | 3 | 0 |
| **Spicy Crispy:** Breast, 5.2 oz | 350 | 20 | 11 |
| Drumstick, 1.6 oz | 130 | 8 | 5 |
| Thigh, 2.8 oz | 270 | 20 | 10 |
| Whole Wing, 1.2 oz | 120 | 8 | 5 |

### Chicken, Signature Flavors:

| | C | F | Cb |
|---|---|---|---|
| **Georgia Gold:** | | | |
| **Extra Crispy:** Breast | 710 | 54 | 21 |
| Tender | 200 | 14 | 9 |
| Thigh | 460 | 36 | 11 |
| **Grilled:** Breast | 250 | 10 | 1 |
| Thigh | 170 | 11 | 0 |
| **Spicy Crispy:** Breast | 550 | 40 | 15 |
| Thigh | 360 | 29 | 12 |
| **Hot Honey:** | | | |
| **Extra Crispy:** Breast | 680 | 49 | 26 |
| Tender | 190 | 12 | 11 |
| Thigh | 440 | 32 | 15 |
| **Grilled:** Breast | 260 | 11 | 3 |
| Thigh | 180 | 12 | 2 |
| **Nashville Hot:** | | | |
| **Extra Crispy:** Breast, 7.4 oz | 770 | 60 | 21 |
| Tenders | 220 | 16 | 9 |
| Thigh, 4.72 oz | 500 | 40 | 11 |
| **Grilled:** | | | |
| Breast, 4.86 oz | 260 | 12 | 1 |
| Thigh, 2.6 oz | 180 | 12 | 0 |
| **Spicy Crispy:** | | | |
| Breast, 6 oz | 540 | 40 | 14 |
| Thigh, 3.3 oz | 390 | 32 | 12 |
| **Smoky Mountain BBQ:** | | | |
| **Extra Crispy:** Breast | 710 | 51 | 27 |
| Tender | 200 | 13 | 11 |
| Thigh | 450 | 33 | 15 |
| **Grilled:** Breast | 260 | 11 | 2 |
| Thigh | 180 | 11 | 1 |
| **Spicy Crispy:** Breast | 530 | 36 | 21 |
| Thigh | 380 | 30 | 16 |

### Popcorn Nuggets: Kids

| | C | F | Cb |
|---|---|---|---|
| Popcorn Nuggets: Kids | 290 | 19 | 19 |
| Large | 620 | 39 | 39 |

### Hot Wings: *Each, without Dipping Sauce*

| | C | F | Cb |
|---|---|---|---|
| Fiery Bufalo; Hot, av. | 70 | 4 | 4 |
| HBBQ | 90 | 4 | 9 |
| Other Flavors, av. | 90 | 7 | 4 |

## KFC® cont... (Sept '19)

### KFC Famous Bowls & Pot Pie:

| | C | F | Cb |
|---|---|---|---|
| **Chicken Pot Pie,** 14 oz | 720 | 41 | 60 |
| **Famous Bowl:** | | | |
| Snack Size | 270 | 13 | 27 |
| Large | 720 | 34 | 79 |

### Dipping Sauces & Condiments:
*Per 0.9 oz Container*

| | C | F | Cb |
|---|---|---|---|
| Buttermilk Ranch Sauce | 100 | 10 | 2 |
| Colonel's Buttery Spread | 35 | 4 | 0 |
| Creamy Buffalo Sauce | 70 | 7 | 2 |
| Finger Linkin' Good; Honey Mstrd, av. | 125 | 10 | 5 |
| Honey Sauce; Ketchup | 30 | 0 | 8 |
| Lemon Juice | 5 | 0 | 1 |
| Strawberry Jam | 35 | 0 | 9 |
| Summertime BBQ Sce | 40 | 0 | 9 |
| Sweet & Tangy Sauce | 45 | 0 | 12 |

### Sandwiches:

| | C | F | Cb |
|---|---|---|---|
| **Chicken Littles:** Regular | 300 | 15 | 27 |
| Georgia Gold; Hot Honey; Smoky Mtn | 330 | 18 | 28 |
| Nashville Hot | 340 | 19 | 27 |
| Colonel's Crispy | 480 | 25 | 37 |
| Crispy Twister | 630 | 34 | 53 |
| Georgia Gold; Nashville Hot, average | 530 | 32 | 38 |
| Hot Honey; Smoky Mtn BBQ, average | 535 | 31 | 41 |

### Salads: *W/out Dressing or Croutons*

| | C | F | Cb |
|---|---|---|---|
| Caesar, Side | 40 | 2 | 2 |
| House Side Salad | 15 | 0 | 3 |

### Dressings & Add-Ins:

| | C | F | Cb |
|---|---|---|---|
| Creamy Parmesan Caesar, 2 oz | 260 | 26 | 4 |
| Light Italian, 1 oz | 15 | 0.5 | 2 |
| Original Ranch Fat Free, 1.5 oz | 35 | 0 | 8 |
| Croutons, Parm. Garlic, 1 pouch | 60 | 3 | 8 |

### Homestyle Sides: *Per Single Portion*

| | C | F | Cb |
|---|---|---|---|
| BBQ Baked Beans, 4.5 oz | 240 | 1.5 | 43 |
| Biscuit, 2 oz | 180 | 8 | 22 |
| Coleslaw, 4.2 oz | 170 | 12 | 14 |
| Corn on the Cob, 2.5 oz | 70 | 0.5 | 17 |
| Macaroni & Cheese, 4.8 oz | 160 | 7 | 20 |
| Mashed Potatoes, with Gravy, 5 oz | 120 | 4 | 18 |
| Potato Wedges, 3.8 oz | 270 | 13 | 34 |
| Sweet Kernel Corn | 80 | 0.5 | 20 |

### Desserts:

| | C | F | Cb |
|---|---|---|---|
| Apple Turnover, 2.9 oz | 230 | 10 | 32 |
| Cafe Valley: Choc. Chip Cake, 1 slice | 300 | 15 | 39 |
| Mini Choc. Chip Cake (1) | 300 | 12 | 49 |
| Lemon Cake, 1 slice | 220 | 10 | 30 |
| Chocolate Chip Cookie (1) | 160 | 8 | 22 |
| Oatmeal Raisin Cookie (1) | 150 | 6 | 22 |
| Oreo Cookies & Creme Pie | 270 | 13 | 35 |
| Reese's Peanut Butter Pie, 2.6 oz | 300 | 17 | 33 |

## Krispy Kreme® (Sept '19)

*Doughnuts:* **C** **F** **Cb**

**Original Glazed:**

| | C | F | Cb |
|---|---|---|---|
| Regular | 190 | 11 | 22 |
| Mini size (3) | 250 | 13 | 30 |
| Apple Fritter | 350 | 19 | 42 |
| **Chocolate Iced:** Cake | 340 | 19 | 40 |
| Custard Filled | 300 | 15 | 37 |
| Glazed | 240 | 11 | 33 |
| with Sprinkles | 250 | 11 | 36 |
| Kreme Filling | 350 | 19 | 41 |
| Cinnamon Apple Filled | 270 | 15 | 31 |
| Cinnamon Bun | 270 | 16 | 29 |
| Cinnamon Sugar | 190 | 11 | 21 |
| **Cruller:** Glazed | 240 | 15 | 25 |
| Chocolate Iced Glazed | 260 | 10 | 40 |
| Double Dark Chocolate | 370 | 20 | 46 |
| Dulche De Leche | 300 | 16 | 35 |
| **Glazed:** Kreme Filling | 340 | 19 | 40 |
| Lemon Filled | 290 | 14 | 36 |
| Maple Iced | 240 | 11 | 34 |
| Sour Cream Cake | 300 | 15 | 40 |
| Strawberry Iced | 240 | 11 | 33 |
| Powdered Cake | 310 | 19 | 32 |
| Powdered Strawberry Filled | 270 | 15 | 30 |
| Powdered Lemon Kreme | 290 | 17 | 32 |

**Glazed Doughnut Holes:**

| | C | F | Cb |
|---|---|---|---|
| Blueberry Cake (4) | 180 | 7 | 28 |
| Original (5) | 210 | 12 | 25 |
| *Hot:* Chocolate, w/ 2% Milk, 12 oz | 390 | 14 | 57 |
| Mocha Latte, w/ Skim Milk, 12 oz | 260 | 4.5 | 42 |

*Frozen Coffees:* With Whipped Cream

| | C | F | Cb |
|---|---|---|---|
| Caramel, 12 fl.oz | 350 | 11 | 58 |
| Mocha, 12 fl.oz | 330 | 11 | 52 |
| Vanilla Latte, 12 fl.oz | 330 | 10 | 54 |
| *Frozen Lemonade,* 12 fl.oz | 200 | 0 | 52 |

*Iced Lattes:* Per 12 fl.oz with Skim Milk

| | C | F | Cb |
|---|---|---|---|
| Caramel Latte, with wh. cream | 310 | 8 | 52 |
| Hazelnut | 160 | 0 | 32 |
| *Iced Mocha,* skim milk, 12 fl.oz | 250 | 7 | 38 |

*Skinny Iced Lattes:*

**With Skimmed Milk:**

| | C | F | Cb |
|---|---|---|---|
| Caramel, 12 fl.oz | 160 | 1.5 | 29 |
| Vanilla, 12 fl.oz | 70 | 0 | 12 |

*For Complete Menu & Data ~ See CalorieKing.com*

## Krystal® (Sept '19)

*Krystals:* **C** **F** **Cb**

| | C | F | Cb |
|---|---|---|---|
| Original | 130 | 6 | 15 |
| with Cheese | 150 | 8 | 15 |
| Double | 190 | 11 | 16 |
| Angus Bacon & Cheese | 450 | 23 | 40 |
| Double | 680 | 42 | 41 |
| Bacon Cheese | 190 | 10 | 16 |
| Triple | 240 | 15 | 16 |
| with Cheese | 290 | 20 | 17 |
| *Chik,* regular | 280 | 16 | 23 |
| *Pups:* Chili Cheese Pup | 290 | 19 | 23 |
| Corn | 250 | 17 | 18 |
| Regular | 160 | 9 | 21 |

*Fries:*

| | C | F | Cb |
|---|---|---|---|
| **French Fries:** Small | 140 | 9 | 14 |
| Medium | 240 | 15 | 24 |
| Large | 300 | 19 | 30 |
| **Loaded:** Chili Cheese Fries | 670 | 47 | 40 |
| Junk Yard | 800 | 59 | 42 |
| *Nuggets:* 4 pieces | 240 | 19 | 8 |
| 10 pieces | 600 | 47 | 20 |
| 20 pieces | 1210 | 93 | 39 |
| **Sauce:** Honey Mustard; Ranch, av | 130 | 12 | 2 |
| Sweet & Sour/Baby Rays BBQ, av | 60 | 0 | 15 |
| *Wings,* Bone in (12) | 1170 | 90 | 36 |

*Breakfast:*

**Plates:** *With Three Eggs*

| | C | F | Cb |
|---|---|---|---|
| Bacon & Biscuit | 480 | 30 | 29 |
| Bacon & Toast | 330 | 19 | 16 |
| Sausage & Biscuit | 520 | 36 | 28 |
| Sausage & Toast | 370 | 24 | 16 |
| **Sandwiches:** Bacon on Toast | 300 | 13 | 30 |
| Krystal Sunrisers (2) | 410 | 32 | 16 |
| Sausage on Toast | 360 | 24 | 16 |
| **Sausage Gravy Biscuit** | 370 | 21 | 41 |

**Scramblers:**

| | C | F | Cb |
|---|---|---|---|
| Original: with Bacon | 300 | 19 | 17 |
| with Sausage | 340 | 24 | 16 |
| Low-Carb Scrambler, with Sausage | 360 | 34 | 2 |
| **Sides:** Grits, bowl | 210 | 5 | 36 |
| Kryspers (5) | 240 | 18 | 21 |
| *Dessert:* Apple Turnover | 290 | 18 | 31 |
| Cookies (2) | 240 | 10 | 36 |

*Hand-Spun Shakes:* Regular

| | C | F | Cb |
|---|---|---|---|
| Chocolate | 650 | 18 | 114 |
| Oreo | 650 | 22 | 101 |
| Strawberry | 560 | 17 | 92 |
| Vanilla | 510 | 17 | 80 |

*For Complete Menu & Data ~ see CalorieKing.com*

## LaRosa's Pizzeria® (Sept '19)

*Classic Pizzas:*

| | | C | F | Cb |
|---|---|---|---|---|
| **Hand Tossed:** *Per Slice, 1/8 of 12" Medium Pizza* | | | | |
| Chicken Bacon Ranch | | 325 | 16 | 27 |
| Double Pepperoni | | 290 | 12 | 29 |
| Garlic Chicken | | 260 | 11 | 27 |
| Hawaiian | | 280 | 10 | 31 |
| Zesty BBQ Chicken | | 275 | 9 | 32 |
| **Traditional:** *Per Slice, 1/12 of 14" Large Pizza* | | | | |
| Chicken Bacon Ranch | | 290 | 17 | 16 |
| Double Pepperoni | | 240 | 12 | 18 |
| Hawaiian | | 245 | 11 | 20 |
| Traditional Veggie | | 190 | 7 | 19 |
| Zesty BBQ Chicken | | 240 | 10 | 21 |

*Deluxe Pizzas:*

| | C | F | Cb |
|---|---|---|---|
| **Hand Tossed:** *Per Slice, 1/8 of 14" Large Pizza* | | | |
| Buddy Deluxe | 505 | 25 | 45 |
| Meat Deluxe | 575 | 30 | 45 |
| Original Deluxe | 500 | 24 | 45 |
| Veggie Deluxe | 350 | 10 | 48 |
| **Pan:** *Per Slice, 1/8 of 14" Large Pizza* | | | |
| Buddy Deluxe | 515 | 26 | 45 |
| Meat Deluxe | 585 | 31 | 45 |
| Original Deluxe | 510 | 25 | 47 |
| Veggie Deluxe | 360 | 11 | 48 |

*Specialty Calzones: Standard Toppings, w/out Sauce*

| | C | F | Cb |
|---|---|---|---|
| Philly Chicken with 4 cheese | 1090 | 54 | 109 |
| Philly Cheese Steak with 4 cheese | 1140 | 61 | 107 |
| Three Meat with 4 cheese | 1110 | 51 | 113 |

*Pasta Dinner: Without Bread, Soup or Salad*

| | C | F | Cb |
|---|---|---|---|
| Lasagna, with Meat Sauce | 1100 | 66 | 72 |
| **Ravioli:** Cheese, with Pasta Sauce | 750 | 29 | 89 |
| Meat, with Pasta Sauce | 730 | 26 | 89 |
| **Ziti:** Chicken Alfredo | 1180 | 57 | 121 |
| Sausage Pelucci w/ Spag. Sce | 1035 | 42 | 136 |

*Fresh Salad: Regular, w/out Dressing or Breadstick*

| | C | F | Cb |
|---|---|---|---|
| Antipasto, regular | 420 | 29 | 14 |
| Crispy Chicken | 500 | 27 | 37 |
| Grilled Chicken | 290 | 12 | 16 |
| JoJo BLT | 150 | 9 | 9 |
| Tossed Garden Salad | 145 | 9 | 9 |

*Salad Dressings: Per 2 oz Cup*

| | C | F | Cb |
|---|---|---|---|
| Blue Cheese | 280 | 30 | 2 |
| Honey French | 250 | 19 | 18 |
| Italian | 320 | 34 | 4 |

*Soup: With 2 Packets Saltine Crackers*

| | C | F | Cb |
|---|---|---|---|
| Baked Onion | 235 | 11 | 27 |
| Minestrone | 135 | 4 | 24 |

## LaRosa's Pizzeria® cont... (Sept '19)

*Appetizers:*

| | C | F | Cb |
|---|---|---|---|
| Cheesy Flatbread, w/ Pesto Sauce | 1465 | 88 | 116 |
| Fried Mozz. Chse Stick w/ Pizza Sce | 585 | 35 | 48 |
| Garlic Fries, w/ Buttery Garl. Sce | 895 | 61 | 76 |
| Onion Twists, w/ Diablo Sauce | 1110 | 72 | 107 |
| **Rondo:** | | | |
| Pepperoni, w/ Buttery & Pesto Sce | 1385 | 80 | 115 |
| Spinach, w/ Buttery & Pesto Sce | 1255 | 67 | 115 |
| *Wings, with Sauce:* BBQ (5) | 445 | 28 | 12 |
| Diablo (5) | 520 | 37 | 10 |
| Garlic-Romano (5) | 640 | 54 | 3 |

## La Salsa Fresh Mexican® (Sept '19)

*Breakfast:*

| | C | F | Cb |
|---|---|---|---|
| **Burritos:** Chicken | 660 | 30 | 56 |
| Steak | 700 | 36 | 55 |
| **Huevos Ranchero Platter:** Chicken | 500 | 14 | 59 |
| Chorizo | 610 | 27 | 61 |
| Steak | 550 | 20 | 58 |
| **Taco** | 200 | 10 | 14 |

*Burritos: Without Chips*

| | C | F | Cb |
|---|---|---|---|
| **Black Beans & Cheese:** | 720 | 37 | 62 |
| with Carnitas | 820 | 41 | 62 |
| with Grilled Chicken | 810 | 40 | 63 |
| **California Steak,** w/ Black Beans | 830 | 39 | 81 |
| **Grande, Black Beans,** | | | |
| with Carnitas/Chicken/Steak, av. | 760 | 30 | 79 |
| **Pinto Beans & Cheese:** Plain | 810 | 37 | 79 |
| with Chicken | 910 | 40 | 80 |
| with Steak | 970 | 49 | 80 |
| **Overstuffed Burrito:** | | | |
| with Carnitas | 860 | 35 | 56 |
| with Grilled Chicken | 860 | 32 | 59 |
| with Steak | 980 | 49 | 58 |

*Platters:*

| | C | F | Cb |
|---|---|---|---|
| **Enchiladas:** | | | |
| Pinto Beans: Carnitas; Chicken, av. | 985 | 53 | 59 |
| Cheese | 850 | 49 | 58 |
| Steak | 1070 | 63 | 59 |
| **Three Pepper Fajita Flour Tortilla:** | | | |
| Black Beans: Carnitas | 700 | 29 | 55 |
| Chicken | 690 | 27 | 58 |
| Steak | 820 | 44 | 57 |
| **Taquitos & Quesadillas:** | | | |
| Pinto Beans: Carnitas; Chicken, av. | 1600 | 76 | 134 |
| Cheese | 1470 | 72 | 129 |
| Steak | 1660 | 84 | 134 |

*Tacos: Without Chips*

| | C | F | Cb |
|---|---|---|---|
| Baja Grilled Fish | 260 | 12 | 23 |
| Baja Shrimp | 250 | 9 | 23 |
| Guadalajara Carnitas | 300 | 17 | 22 |

Updated Nutrition Data ~ www.CalorieKing.com
Persons with Diabetes ~ See Disclaimer (Page 22)

## La Salsa Fresh Mex® cont... (Sept '19)

*Favorites: Without Chips*

| | C | F | Cb |
|---|---|---|---|
| **Classic Quesadillas:** Carnitas | 980 | 58 | 59 |
| Cheese | 880 | 54 | 59 |
| Chicken | 980 | 57 | 60 |
| Steak | 1040 | 65 | 60 |
| **Fire Roasted Bowls:** | | | |
| Black Beans: Carnitas | 510 | 18 | 54 |
| Chicken | 500 | 16 | 55 |
| Steak | 570 | 25 | 55 |
| **Nachos:** | | | |
| Black Beans: with Carnitas | 1150 | 56 | 93 |
| with Chicken | 1150 | 54 | 95 |
| with Steak | 1210 | 63 | 94 |
| Pinto Beans: | | | |
| with Carnitas | 1190 | 56 | 101 |
| with Chicken | 1170 | 54 | 98 |
| with Steak | 1230 | 63 | 98 |
| **Stuffed Fajitas:** Carnitas | 930 | 49 | 59 |
| Cheese | 830 | 45 | 59 |
| Chicken | 930 | 48 | 60 |
| Steak | 990 | 57 | 60 |

## Little Caesars® (Sept '19)

*14" Pizza: Per Slice, 1/8 Pizza*

| | C | F | Cb |
|---|---|---|---|
| **Specialty Deep Dish:** | | | |
| 3 Meat Treat | 420 | 21 | 40 |
| Hula Hawaiian, ham/bacon, av. | 360 | 12 | 45 |
| Ultimate Supreme | 395 | 17 | 42 |
| Veggie | 340 | 12 | 42 |
| **Hot-N-Ready:** | | | |
| Classic Round Pizza: | | | |
| Cheese | 250 | 8 | 31 |
| Pepperoni | 280 | 11 | 31 |
| Deep Deep Dish: Cheese | 320 | 11 | 40 |
| Pepperoni | 350 | 14 | 40 |
| **Caesar Wings:** *Per 8 Wing* | | | |
| BBQ | 620 | 35 | 32 |
| Buffalo | 510 | 35 | 3 |
| Garlic Parmesan | 660 | 49 | 7 |
| Oven Roasted | 510 | 35 | 3 |
| **Caesar Dips:** *Per 1.5 oz Container* | | | |
| Buffalo Ranch | 230 | 24 | 3 |
| Buttery Garlic, 0.5 oz | 370 | 42 | 0 |
| Cheezy Jalapeno | 220 | 22 | 3 |
| Ranch | 240 | 24 | 4 |
| **Bread:** Crazy Bread, 1 stick | 100 | 3 | 16 |
| Italian Cheese Bread | 145 | 6 | 15 |
| **Crazy Sauce,** 1 cup | 30 | 0 | 7 |

## Long John Silver's® (Sept '19)

*Chicken Tenders,*

| | C | F | Cb |
|---|---|---|---|
| 1 piece 2.1 oz | 150 | 7 | 11 |
| *Sandwiches & Tacos:* | | | |
| Baja Fish Taco | 410 | 21 | 40 |
| Chicken | 480 | 23 | 46 |
| Crispy Fish | 400 | 16 | 44 |
| *Seafood: Without Sides* | | | |
| Baked Cod, 1 piece, 6 oz | 170 | 10 | 1 |
| **Battered:** Alaskan Pollock, | | | |
| 1 piece, 3.2 oz | 200 | 10 | 16 |
| Cod, 1 piece, 3 oz | 190 | 11 | 9 |
| Shrimp, 3 pieces, 1.5 oz | 100 | 7 | 5 |
| Crab Cake, 1 cake, 2.2 oz | 280 | 15 | 26 |
| **Snack Box:** Breaded Clam Strips | 340 | 20 | 35 |
| Popcorn Shrimp, 3 oz | 210 | 9 | 24 |
| *Sauces & Condiments:* | | | |
| **Dipping Sauces:** BBQ, 1 oz | 40 | 0 | 10 |
| Cocktail, 0.9 oz | 20 | 0 | 4 |
| Honey Mustard, 1packet | 60 | 6 | 2 |
| Ketchup, 1 pouch | 30 | 0 | 8 |
| Louisiana Hot Sauce, 1 tsp | 0 | 0 | 0 |
| Malt Vinegar, 0.5 oz | 0 | 0 | 0 |
| Marinara, 1 oz | 15 | 0 | 4 |
| Sweet Thai Chili, 1 oz | 60 | 0 | 14 |
| Tartar, 0.5 oz packet | 40 | 4 | 3 |
| *Sides:* Baked Potato, 12 oz | 300 | 0 | 67 |
| Battered Onion Rings, 4 oz | 480 | 35 | 39 |
| Breaded Mozzarella Sticks (3) | 335 | 21 | 22 |
| Broccoli, 5 oz | 40 | 0 | 7 |
| **Broccoli Cheese Bites:** 3 pieces | 185 | 15 | 11 |
| 5 pieces | 305 | 24 | 18 |
| Brocc. Cheese Soup, 1 bowl, 7.4 oz | 230 | 17 | 13 |
| Clam Chowder, 1 bowl, 8 oz | 230 | 16 | 16 |
| Cole Slaw, 4 oz | 170 | 11 | 18 |
| Corn | 160 | 8 | 9 |
| Crumblies, 1 oz | 170 | 12 | 13 |
| **Hushpuppies:** 2 pieces | 150 | 7 | 19 |
| 5 pieces | 245 | 16 | 18 |
| Jalapeno Peppers (1) | 15 | 0 | 2 |
| Macaaroni & Cheese, 4 oz | 150 | 6 | 19 |
| Rice, 5 oz | 220 | 1 | 47 |
| Seasoned Green Beans, 4 oz | 25 | 0 | 4 |
| Sweet Potato Fries, 4 oz | 240 | 15 | 27 |
| *Dessert:* Chocolate Cream Pie, 1 slice | 275 | 16 | 31 |
| Pecan Pie, 1 slice | 385 | 21 | 47 |

*For Complete Menu & Data ~ see CalorieKing.com*

**213**

# Fast - Foods & *Restaurants*

## Macaroni Grill® (Sept '19)

*Antipasti:* As Served

| | C | F | Cb |
|---|---|---|---|
| Amalfi Steamed Mussels | 560 | 23 | 25 |
| Baked Prosciutto & Mozzarella | 610 | 36 | 35 |
| Calamari Fritti | 760 | 55 | 35 |
| Crispy Brussels Sprouts | 370 | 25 | 37 |
| Crispy Fresh Mozzarella | 820 | 79 | 17 |
| Goat Cheese Peppadew Peppers | 350 | 11 | 56 |
| Spinach Artichoke Dip | 1100 | 61 | 109 |
| Stuffed Mushrooms | 510 | 38 | 20 |

*Meals:* With Menu Set Sides

| | C | F | Cb |
|---|---|---|---|
| **Carne:** Chianti Steak | 1460 | 87 | 82 |
| Grilled Lamb Chops | 790 | 63 | 19 |
| Italian Meatloaf | 1450 | 103 | 74 |
| Porterhouse Steak | 1480 | 115 | 16 |
| **Chicken:** Caprese | 560 | 22 | 40 |
| Marsala | 790 | 32 | 61 |
| San Marino Grilled | 890 | 34 | 86 |
| Scaloppine | 1240 | 76 | 83 |
| Sorrento | 1620 | 122 | 36 |
| **Pasta:** Carmela's Chicken | 1090 | 61 | 98 |
| **Eggplant:** Caponata | 1090 | 78 | 113 |
| Parmesan | 1340 | 90 | 103 |
| Fettuccine Alfredo | 1140 | 56 | 114 |
| Lasagna Bolognese | 1110 | 67 | 69 |
| Mushroom Ravioli | 930 | 66 | 53 |
| Penne Rustica | 1060 | 52 | 82 |
| Spagh. Bolognese | 730 | 51 | 96 |
| Truffle Mac & Chse | 1060 | 89 | 24 |
| **Seafood:** Grilled Salmon | 1020 | 50 | 82 |
| Lobster Ravioli | 920 | 74 | 36 |
| Parmesan-Crusted Sole | 1460 | 95 | 121 |
| Pasta Di Mare | 1030 | 43 | 101 |
| Shrimp Portofino | 1200 | 78 | 93 |
| Shrimp Scampi | 180 | 88 | 56 |

*Brick Oven Pizza:* Per Whole Meal, as Served

| | C | F | Cb |
|---|---|---|---|
| Cheese | 1170 | 41 | 146 |
| Farmhouse | 1330 | 56 | 146 |
| Margherita | 1140 | 41 | 146 |
| Pepperoni | 1280 | 76 | 143 |
| Piedmont | 1360 | 57 | 146 |
| Prosciutto & Arugula | 1310 | 53 | 140 |
| Spinach & Artichoke Chicken | 1150 | 35 | 144 |
| *Kids:* Chkn Tenders w/ Broccolini | 860 | 45 | 67 |
| Macaroni & Cheese | 540 | 31 | 44 |
| Pepperoni Pizza | 630 | 25 | 72 |
| Spaghetti, with Pomodoro Sauce | 290 | 8 | 43 |

## Macaroni Grill® cont... (Sept '19)

*Salads:* Includes Menu Set Dressing

| | C | F | Cb |
|---|---|---|---|
| Parmesan Crusted Chicken | 1080 | 48 | 100 |
| **Entree:** Bibb & Bleu with Shrimp | 590 | 43 | 18 |
| Caesar with Chicken | 630 | 41 | 15 |
| **Side Salads:** | | | |
| Bibb & Bleu | 270 | 22 | 9 |
| Florentine | 300 | 22 | 22 |
| Fresh Green | 190 | 16 | 11 |
| *Dessert:* Gelato, Vanilla | 310 | 13 | 42 |
| Decadent Choc. Cake | 1090 | 88 | 79 |
| Lemon Passion | 740 | 45 | 77 |
| New York Style Cheesecake | 690 | 41 | 70 |
| Tiramisu | 600 | 39 | 54 |

## Manhattan Bagel® (Sept '19)

*Bagels:* Per Bagel

| | C | F | Cb |
|---|---|---|---|
| Plain | 310 | 1 | 64 |
| **Californian:** Blueberry, 3.8 oz | 300 | 1 | 65 |
| Chocolate Chip, 3.8 oz | 290 | 2.5 | 58 |
| Cinnamon Raisin, 4 oz | 290 | 1 | 63 |
| Egg, 3.6 oz | 300 | 5 | 54 |
| Everything; Poppy, av., 3.7 oz | 275 | 2.5 | 56 |
| Pumpernickel, 3.6 oz | 240 | 1.5 | 53 |
| **Gourmet:** Asiago, 4.4 oz | 340 | 4 | 64 |
| Blueberry Glaze, 4.6 oz | 370 | 1 | 79 |
| Super Cinnamon, 4.6 oz | 360 | 1 | 77 |
| Garlic | 330 | 1 | 68 |
| Honey Whole Wheat | 280 | 2.5 | 59 |
| Jalapeno Cheddar | 320 | 1.5 | 67 |
| Poppy Seed | 330 | 3 | 64 |
| Salt | 310 | 1 | 64 |
| *Cream Cheese:* Plain; Lox, av. | 115 | 12 | 3 |
| Scallion, 1.3 oz | 140 | 12 | 5 |

*Breakfast:*

**Bagel Sandwich:** On Plain Bagel

| | C | F | Cb |
|---|---|---|---|
| Egg & Cheese | 530 | 19 | 64 |
| Egg Bacon & Cheese | 580 | 23 | 64 |
| Egg, Pork Roll & Chse | 770 | 37 | 66 |
| **Wrap,** Ranchero | 800 | 45 | 61 |

*Signature Lunch Sandwiches:*

| | C | F | Cb |
|---|---|---|---|
| Chelsea Chicken, on Asiago Roll | 750 | 37 | 59 |
| East Side Reuben, on Marble Rye | 580 | 27 | 54 |
| **Steak:** Bronx Bomber | 580 | 27 | 54 |
| Manhattan Chsesteak | 660 | 30 | 59 |
| SoHo Chicken Caesar Wrap | 580 | 21 | 59 |
| **Thintastic:** Avocado BLT | 440 | 23 | 48 |
| Turkey | 330 | 7 | 42 |
| *Soup:* Boston Clam Chowder | 360 | 17 | 40 |
| Chicken Noodle | 250 | 7 | 30 |
| Cream of Broccoli | 320 | 18 | 27 |
| Timberline Chili | 240 | 8 | 27 |

214

## Marie Callender's® (Sept '19)

| *Appetizers:* As Served | C | F | Cb |
|---|---|---|---|
| Crispy Chicken Tenders, 12.9 oz | 870 | 47 | 72 |
| Crispy Green Beans, 10.5 oz | 810 | 52 | 75 |
| Mozzarella Sticks, 8.6 oz | 690 | 42 | 46 |
| Onion Rings | 115 | 63 | 129 |

| *Burgers and Sandwiches:* With Fries | | | |
|---|---|---|---|
| Original Burger | 1290 | 87 | 84 |
| Albacore Tuna Melt | 1430 | 92 | 99 |
| Callender's Cheeseburger | 1450 | 99 | 85 |
| Frisco Chkn Breast On Parm Sourd. | 1290 | 81 | 95 |
| Meatloaf on Parm. Sourdough | 1250 | 78 | 96 |
| Roasted Turkey Croissant Club | 1450 | 97 | 95 |

*Main Meals:* With Menu Set Sides

| **Comfort Classics:** | | | |
|---|---|---|---|
| Chicken & Broccoli Fettuccine | 1090 | 49 | 98 |
| Crispy Fish & Shrimp Platter | 1700 | 97 | 143 |
| Home-Style Beef Stroganoff | 850 | 30 | 99 |
| Home-Style Meatloaf Dinner | 610 | 35 | 34 |
| Honey Ginger Glazed Salmon | 570 | 30 | 29 |
| Roasted Turkey Dinner | 730 | 36 | 65 |
| Shrimp & Chicken Carbonara | 1140 | 50 | 93 |
| Top Sirloin & Shrimp Dinner | 830 | 45 | 29 |
| **Pies,** Chicken Pot Pie, w/out sides | 1140 | 79 | 70 |

| **Savory Skillets:** | | | |
|---|---|---|---|
| Kickin' Chicken Bacon Broccoli | 720 | 37 | 40 |
| Spicy Beef & Chicken | 790 | 54 | 27 |
| Thai Shrimp | 730 | 43 | 52 |

| *Salads:* | | | |
|---|---|---|---|
| Cobb without Dressing | 570 | 31 | 15 |
| Combo Caesar w/ Caesar Dressing | 240 | 18 | 9 |
| Honey Mstd Chkn Crunch w/ dressing | 950 | 61 | 54 |
| Traditional Caesar w/ Caesar Dressing | 490 | 35 | 28 |

| *Sides:* Cornbread, w/ Honey Spread | 340 | 21 | 33 |
|---|---|---|---|
| French Fries, 4 oz | 380 | 20 | 45 |
| Loaded Mashed Potatoes, 6.2 oz | 340 | 23 | 23 |
| Macaroni & Cheese, 6.4 oz | 230 | 9 | 26 |
| Tater Tots, 5 oz | 330 | 20 | 33 |

| *Soups:* Per Bowl | | | |
|---|---|---|---|
| Chicken Tortilla | 230 | 10 | 26 |
| Clam Chowder | 270 | 13 | 22 |
| Hearty Vegetable | 90 | 3 | 13 |
| Potato Cheese | 590 | 40 | 49 |

| *Breakfast:* With Menu Set Items | | | |
|---|---|---|---|
| **Classics:** Croissant Sandwich | 1100 | 70 | 76 |
| Eggs Bened., California | 830 | 53 | 66 |
| Triple Egg Dare Ya | 1380 | 71 | 132 |

## Marie Callender's® cont... (Sept '19)

| *Breakfast (Cont.):* W/ Set Menu Sides | C | F | Cb |
|---|---|---|---|
| **Griddle Greats:** Belgian Waffles | 600 | 19 | 99 |
| Banana Cream Pie Pancakes | 800 | 28 | 118 |
| Buttermilk Pancakes (3) | 670 | 28 | 92 |
| Old Fashioned French Toast | 830 | 31 | 123 |
| **Omelettes:** BTA | 1210 | 66 | 103 |
| Oh My | 1340 | 74 | 98 |
| Veggie | 570 | 37 | 23 |
| **Quiche:** Bacon, 1 sl. | 990 | 79 | 45 |
| Ham, 1 slice | 1030 | 83 | 39 |
| Veggie, 1 slice | 990 | 80 | 42 |

| *Desserts:* Per Slice Unless Indicated | | | |
|---|---|---|---|
| **Pies:** Apple | 630 | 39 | 66 |
| Banana Cream, with Meringue | 510 | 24 | 66 |
| Chocolate Cream, with Meringue | 570 | 25 | 77 |
| Coconut Cream with Meringue | 590 | 29 | 75 |
| Traditional NY Style Cheesecake, slice | 740 | 52 | 58 |

## Max & Erma's® (Sept '19)

| *Shareables:* As Served | C | F | Cb |
|---|---|---|---|
| **Baja Fish Taco:** Crispy | 1120 | 43 | 134 |
| Grilled | 760 | 28 | 84 |
| Chicken Fajita Quesadilla | 820 | 54 | 51 |
| Potato Skins | 1990 | 91 | 232 |
| Spinach Dip | 710 | 46 | 57 |

| **Wings with Blue Cheese Dressing:** | | | |
|---|---|---|---|
| Cherry Cola BBQ | 2090 | 120 | 118 |
| Sweet Chili | 1840 | 120 | 54 |

| *Burgers & Sanwiches:* Without Fries | | | |
|---|---|---|---|
| BBQ Pulled Pork Sandwich | 1100 | 48 | 121 |
| Big Ol' Buffalo Chicken Sandwich | 1370 | 71 | 144 |
| Bodalicious Bacon Burger | 1240 | 82 | 59 |
| Cola BBQ Bacon Burger | 1320 | 80 | 93 |
| Garbage Burger, 6 oz | 1650 | 118 | 60 |
| Reuben Grill Sandwich | 1060 | 58 | 84 |
| Sauteed Mshroom & Swiss Burger | 1200 | 85 | 53 |
| Smokehouse Chicken Sandwich | 1040 | 58 | 76 |
| Tortilla Burger | 1260 | 84 | 61 |
| Turkey Avocado Swiss Burger | 610 | 33 | 32 |

| *Salads:* Entrée Size, w/ Dressing, w/out Breadstick | | | |
|---|---|---|---|
| 3rd Street | 1270 | 101 | 41 |
| Grilled Chicken Santa Fe | 1160 | 83 | 46 |
| Village | 430 | 37 | 14 |

| *Sides:* Baked Potato | 220 | 0 | 51 |
|---|---|---|---|
| Creamy Coleslaw | 160 | 12 | 14 |
| Fresh Fruit Salad | 90 | 0 | 23 |
| Mashed Potatoes | 290 | 11 | 43 |
| Seasoned Fries | 360 | 17 | 49 |

| *Dessert:* | | | |
|---|---|---|---|
| Banana Cream Pie | 790 | 37 | 107 |
| Chocolate Cake a la Mode | 1600 | 82 | 206 |

*For Complete Menu & Data ~ See CalorieKing.com*

## McAlister's Deli® (Sept '19)

| Sandwiches: | C | F | Cb |
|---|---|---|---|
| Black Angus Club | 850 | 42 | 74 |
| Four Cheese Griller | 670 | 31 | 62 |
| French Dip | 530 | 15 | 43 |
| Grilled Chicken Club | 830 | 35 | 78 |
| Harvest Chicken Salad | 680 | 44 | 53 |
| Horseradish Roast Beef | 660 | 25 | 68 |
| McAlister's Club | 820 | 37 | 78 |
| Reuben | 900 | 41 | 76 |
| Smoky Pepper Jack Turkey | 780 | 36 | 72 |
| Sweet Chipotle Chicken | 630 | 15 | 77 |
| The Italian | 790 | 41 | 49 |
| The Veggie | 680 | 35 | 80 |

## Mellow Mushroom® (Sept '19)

| Burger, | C | F | Cb |
|---|---|---|---|
| Ritz Burger | 1250 | 87 | 57 |
| **Calzones:** | | | |
| Chicken & Cheese | 1330 | 42 | 152 |
| Steak & Cheese | 1360 | 48 | 152 |
| **Hoagies, Whole:** Chicken & Chse | 1010 | 45 | 91 |
| Italian | 1240 | 73 | 89 |
| Meatball | 780 | 27 | 85 |
| Mushroom Club | 1280 | 73 | 94 |
| Steak & Cheese | 1090 | 59 | 89 |
| Tofu | 920 | 49 | 90 |
| **Munchies:** | | | |
| Cheese Bread | 820 | 39 | 77 |
| Magic Mushroom Soup | 350 | 24 | 15 |
| Meatball Trio | 330 | 22 | 11 |
| Rstd Red Potatoes | 150 | 3 | 27 |
| Spinach & Artichoke Dip | 790 | 47 | 67 |
| Tomato Bisque | 290 | 22 | 18 |
| **Wings:** BBQ (10) | 700 | 35 | 41 |
| Sweet Thai Chili (10) | 780 | 33 | 60 |
| *Pizzas: With Baked Crust, Per Medium Slice* | | | |
| Buffalo Chicken | 500 | 31 | 44 |
| Funky Q Chicken; House Special, av. | 445 | 22 | 47 |
| Kosmic Karma | 410 | 22 | 45 |
| **Salads:** *Per Regular Size* | | | |
| Caesar, with Caesar Dressing | 800 | 70 | 29 |
| Greek, without Dressing | 320 | 21 | 18 |
| *Dressing,* Balsamic Vinaigrette, 1 oz | 90 | 8 | 5 |
| **Desserts:** Choc Chunk Cookie | 600 | 29 | 83 |
| MJ Triple Choc Brownie | 550 | 31 | 64 |
| Peanut Butter Cookie | 580 | 32 | 65 |

*Extra Menu Items ~ See CalorieKing.com*

## McDonald's® (Sept '19)

| Beef Burgers: | C | F | Cb |
|---|---|---|---|
| Big Mac | 540 | 28 | 46 |
| Cheeseburger: Regular | 300 | 12 | 33 |
| Double | 440 | 22 | 34 |
| Hamburger | 250 | 8 | 31 |
| McDouble | 390 | 18 | 33 |
| Quarter Pounder: with Cheese | 540 | 28 | 42 |
| with Cheese Deluxe | 650 | 39 | 44 |
| with Cheese & Bacon | 640 | 34 | 44 |
| Double, with Cheese | 780 | 45 | 43 |
| *Burger Meal Combos: Includes Medium Fries + Coke* | | | |
| Big Mac Meal | 1100 | 4 | 149 |
| Cheeseburger Meal | 860 | 28 | 136 |
| Quarter Pounder | 1100 | 44 | 145 |
| *Chicken Sandwiches: On Artisan Roll Unless Indicated* | | | |
| Aritsan Grilled Chicken | 380 | 6 | 44 |
| Buttermilk Crispy Chicken | 630 | 9 | 64 |
| McChicken, regular bun | 410 | 22 | 39 |
| *Filet-O-Fish,* regular bun | 390 | 19 | 38 |
| *Chicken:* | | | |
| Buttermilk Crispy Tenders: 4 pcs | 500 | 27 | 25 |
| 6 pieces | 750 | 40 | 38 |
| McNuggets: 4 pieces | 180 | 11 | 11 |
| 6 pieces | 270 | 16 | 16 |
| 10 pieces | 440 | 27 | 26 |
| *Sauces: Per Packet* | | | |
| Creamy Ranch | 110 | 12 | 1 |
| Signature | 100 | 9 | 3 |
| Spicy Buffalo | 30 | 3 | 1 |
| Sweet 'N Sour; Tangy BBQ | 50 | 0 | 11 |
| *French Fries:* Kids, 1.3 oz | 110 | 5 | 15 |
| Small, 2.6 oz | 230 | 11 | 29 |
| Medium, 3.9 oz | 340 | 16 | 44 |
| Large, 5.9 oz | 510 | 24 | 66 |
| Ketchup, packet | 10 | 0 | 2 |
| *Breakfast:* | | | |
| Big Breakfast: with Reg. Biscuit | 750 | 49 | 53 |
| with Hotcakes | 1350 | 65 | 155 |
| **Biscuits:** *Regular* | | | |
| Bacon, Egg & Cheese | 450 | 24 | 40 |
| Sausage | 460 | 30 | 36 |
| Sausage with Egg | 530 | 34 | 38 |
| Steak, Egg & Cheese | 530 | 30 | 40 |
| **Burrito,** Sausage | 300 | 16 | 26 |
| Fruit 'N Yogurt Parfait | 210 | 3 | 40 |

## McDonald's® cont... (Sept '19)

*Breakfast (Cont):*

| | C | F | Cb |
|---|---|---|---|
| **Fruit & Maple Oatmeal:** | | | |
| with brown sugar | 310 | 4 | 62 |
| **Hash Browns,** (1), 2 oz | 150 | 9 | 16 |
| **Hotcakes:** Plain (3) | 330 | 8 | 56 |
| with Syrup and Whipped Butter | 600 | 16 | 102 |
| **McGriddle:** | | | |
| Bacon, Egg & Cheese | 420 | 18 | 45 |
| Sausage | 430 | 24 | 42 |
| Sausage, Egg & Cheese | 550 | 32 | 45 |
| **McMuffin:** Egg | 300 | 12 | 30 |
| Egg White Delight | 260 | 8 | 29 |
| Sausage | 400 | 25 | 29 |
| Sausage with Egg | 480 | 30 | 30 |

*Happy Meals:*

| | C | F | Cb |
|---|---|---|---|
| **Kids Fries:** Add to meals below | 110 | 5 | 15 |
| **Chicken McNuggets (4):** | | | |
| +Apple Slices + 1% Low Fat Milk | 295 | 13 | 27 |
| +Apple Slices + Fat Free Choc Milk | 325 | 11 | 38 |
| + Go-Gurt Strawb Yog. & Apple Jce | 310 | 12 | 30 |
| **Hamburger:** | | | |
| +Apple Slices + 1% Low Fat Milk | 365 | 11 | 47 |
| +Apple Slices +Fat Free Choc Milk | 395 | 8 | 58 |
| + Go-Gurt Strawb Yog. & Apple Jce | 380 | 9 | 60 |
| **Cheeseburger:** | | | |
| +Apple Slices + 1% Low Fat Milk | 415 | 15 | 49 |
| + Apple Slices & Fat-Free Choc Milk | 445 | 12 | 60 |
| + Go-Gurt Strawb Yog. & Apple Jce | 430 | 13 | 62 |

*Salads: Without Dressing*

| | C | F | Cb |
|---|---|---|---|
| **Bacon Ranch:** Grilled Chicken | 320 | 14 | 8 |
| Buttermilk Crispy Chicken | 480 | 28 | 27 |
| **Southwest:** Grilled Chkn, w/ glaze | 350 | 11 | 27 |
| B'milk Crispy Chicken, | | | |
| wih glaze | 520 | 25 | 46 |
| **Side Salad** | 15 | 0 | 4 |

*Salad Dressings: Per Package*

| | C | F | Cb |
|---|---|---|---|
| **Newman's Own:** Ranch, 2 fl.oz | 200 | 17 | 11 |
| Low-Fat: Balsamic Vinaig., 1.5 fl.oz | 35 | 2 | 4 |
| Family Recipe Italian, 1.5 fl.oz | 50 | 1.5 | 8 |
| *Snacks:* Apple Slices | 15 | 0 | 4 |
| Yoplait Go-Gurt, Strawberry, 1 tube | 45 | 0.5 | 87 |

*Desserts & Shakes:*

| | C | F | Cb |
|---|---|---|---|
| **Baked Apple Pie,** 2.6 oz | 240 | 11 | 35 |
| **Cookies:** Choc. Chip, (1) | 160 | 7 | 22 |
| Oatmeal Raisin (1), 1 oz | 140 | 5 | 22 |

## McDonald's® cont... (Sept '19)

*Desserts & Shakes (Cont):*

| | C | F | Cb |
|---|---|---|---|
| **McFlurry:** M&M Candies, regular | 630 | 22 | 96 |
| Oreo Cookies, regular | 510 | 17 | 80 |
| **Soft Serve:** Kiddie Cone | 45 | 1 | 8 |
| Vanilla Cone | 200 | 5 | 32 |
| **Sundaes:** | | | |
| Hot Caramel, 6.4 oz | 380 | 12 | 61 |
| Hot Fudge, 6.3 oz | 380 | 14 | 53 |
| Strawberry, 6.3 oz | 320 | 10 | 50 |
| *Juice,* Apple, box | 35 | 0 | 9 |
| *Milk:* 1% Low-Fat, 8 fl.oz | 100 | 2.5 | 12 |
| Fat-Free Chocolate Milk, 8 fl.oz | 130 | 0 | 23 |

*Shakes:*

| | C | F | Cb |
|---|---|---|---|
| **Chocolate:** 12 fl.oz cup | 530 | 15 | 87 |
| 16 fl.oz cup | 630 | 17 | 104 |
| 22 fl.oz cup | 840 | 22 | 142 |
| **Vanilla:** 12 fl.oz cup | 490 | 14 | 79 |
| 16 fl.oz cup | 590 | 17 | 96 |
| 22 fl.oz cup | 800 | 22 | 131 |

*Soda: With Ice, approximately 30%*

| | C | F | Cb |
|---|---|---|---|
| **Coca-Cola:** | | | |
| Extra Small, 12 fl.oz cup | 110 | 0 | 31 |
| Small, 16 fl.oz cup | 150 | 0 | 42 |
| Medium, 21 fl.oz cup | 220 | 0 | 59 |
| Large, 30 fl.oz cup | 290 | 0 | 80 |
| **Dr Pepper:** | | | |
| Extra Small, 12 fl.oz cup | 100 | 0 | 27 |
| Small, 16 fl.oz cup | 140 | 0 | 38 |
| Medium, 21 fl.oz cup | 200 | 0 | 54 |
| Large, 30 fl.oz cup | 280 | 0 | 75 |
| **Sprite:** Extra Small, 12 fl.oz cup | 90 | 0 | 25 |
| Small, 16 fl.oz cup | 120 | 0 | 36 |
| Medium, 21 fl.oz | 170 | 0 | 51 |
| Large, 30 fl.oz | 230 | 0 | 69 |
| **Sweet Tea,** medium | 110 | 0 | 28 |

*McCafe,*

| | C | F | Cb |
|---|---|---|---|
| **Frappes:** With Whipped Topping | | | |
| **Caramel; Mocha, average:** | | | |
| Small | 420 | 17 | 60 |
| Medium | 510 | 21 | 72 |
| Large | 670 | 27 | 98 |
| **Smoothies, av. all flavors:** | | | |
| Small, 12 fl oz cup | 195 | 0.5 | 45 |
| Medium, 16 fl oz cup | 245 | 1 | 56 |
| Large, 22 fl oz cup | 335 | 1 | 77 |

*...cont next page*

## McDonald's® cont... (Sept '19)

*McCafe:*

| | C | F | Cb |
|---|---|---|---|
| **Hot Chocolate:** *With Whipped Cream & Toppings* | | | |
| Whole Milk: Small | 370 | 14 | 51 |
| Medium | 450 | 17 | 63 |
| **Hot Mocha:** *With Whipped Cream & Toppings* | | | |
| Whole Milk: Small | 340 | 12 | 49 |
| Medium | 380 | 12 | 57 |
| **Iced Coffee:** *With Liquid Sugar & Light Cream* | | | |
| Regular: Small, 16 fl.oz | 140 | 5 | 24 |
| Medium, 22 fl.oz | 180 | 7 | 30 |
| Large, 30 fl.oz | 260 | 9 | 45 |
| Caramel: Small, 16 fl.oz | 140 | 5 | 23 |
| Medium, 22 fl.oz | 190 | 7 | 31 |
| **Iced Mocha:** *W/ Whole Milk, Whipped Cream & Toppings* | | | |
| Small | 290 | 11 | 40 |
| Medium | 350 | 13 | 50 |

## Mimi's Cafe® (Sept '19)

*Breakfast:*

| | C | F | Cb |
|---|---|---|---|
| **Benedicts:** *W/ Roasted Potatoes* | | | |
| Original | 800 | 45 | 57 |
| Smoked Salmon | 755 | 44 | 57 |
| **Omelets:** *With Roasted Potatoes* | | | |
| Bacon Avocado | 920 | 65 | 30 |
| Hickory-Smoked Ham & Cheese | 675 | 45 | 27 |
| Mushroom Bacon & Brie | 775 | 56 | 28 |
| Smoked Salmon | 555 | 35 | 24 |
| **Griddle:** *With Eggs, any Style* | | | |
| Brioche French Toast | 755 | 34 | 75 |
| Cinnamon Roll French Toast | 880 | 41 | 96 |
| Malted Berry Waffles | 585 | 28 | 61 |
| ***Lunch & Dinner:*** *Without Side Choices* | | | |
| **Burgers:** Brioche Cheeseburger | 775 | 41 | 56 |
| Hickory Bacon Cheddar | 945 | 50 | 68 |
| Mushroom & Brie | 890 | 51 | 51 |
| The French Quarter | 1285 | 90 | 48 |
| **Craft Sandwiches:** | | | |
| Chicken Cordon Bleu | 1050 | 43 | 96 |
| Roasted Turkey Club | 1045 | 60 | 76 |
| West Coast Reuben | 1335 | 72 | 99 |
| *Classic Dishes:* Beef Pot Roast | 460 | 31 | 13 |
| Chicken Pot Pie | 820 | 43 | 61 |
| French Pot Roast | 515 | 32 | 22 |
| Slow Roasted Turkey | 700 | 29 | 69 |
| *Sides:* Broccoli | 115 | 9 | 5 |
| Coleslaw | 250 | 23 | 7 |
| French Fries | 125 | 3 | 22 |
| Garlic Spinach | 70 | 4 | 4 |
| Mashed Potatoes | 130 | 4 | 21 |
| Mushroom Steak Topper | 175 | 17 | 5 |
| Roasted Potatoes | 150 | 5 | 23 |

## Mr. Goodcents® (Sept '19)

*Cold Subs:*

| | C | F | Cb |
|---|---|---|---|
| *Per 8" Wheat Bread Sub with Standard Toppings* | | | |
| Bologna | 670 | 41 | 60 |
| Centsable | 600 | 31 | 62 |
| Garden Veggie | 510 | 24 | 66 |
| Goodcents Original | 670 | 38 | 61 |
| Oven Roasted Chicken Breast | 490 | 18 | 60 |
| Penny Club | 510 | 19 | 61 |
| Pepperoni | 840 | 56 | 58 |
| Tuna Salad | 620 | 32 | 64 |
| **Toasted Sub:** *Per 8" Wheat Bread Sub with Standard Toppings* | | | |
| Chicken Bacon Ranch | 730 | 33 | 55 |
| Meatball | 720 | 29 | 69 |
| *Pasta:* *Without Garlic Bread* | | | |
| with Alfredo Sauce | 840 | 40 | 103 |
| with Marinara Sauce | 640 | 18 | 107 |
| Chicken Alfredo | 990 | 44 | 103 |
| Chicken Parmesan | 840 | 25 | 108 |
| **Garlic Bread,** 1 piece, 2 4 oz | 290 | 12 | 44 |
| **Soup:** *Per 16 oz Bowl* | | | |
| Broccoli Cheese | 360 | 28 | 16 |
| Chicken Homestyle Noodle | 140 | 4 | 20 |
| Saltine Crackers for soup bowls | 110 | 2 | 17 |

## Mr. Hero® (Sept '19)

*7" Subs & Burgers:*

| | C | F | Cb |
|---|---|---|---|
| **Burgers:** | | | |
| Cheeseburger | 720 | 49 | 44 |
| Romanburger | 805 | 56 | 46 |
| **Chicken Subs:** | | | |
| Chkn Bacon Ranch | 590 | 29 | 43 |
| Chicken Philly | 510 | 22 | 45 |
| **Deli Subs:** *Per 7" Sub with Menu Board Toppings* | | | |
| Italiano | 550 | 26 | 54 |
| Original Italian | 520 | 27 | 50 |
| Tuna 'N Cheese | 670 | 53 | 45 |
| Turkey | 330 | 2.5 | 49 |
| **Steak Subs:** Baja Fire | 625 | 36 | 44 |
| Hatta Potatta | 720 | 45 | 53 |
| Hot Buttered Cheesesteak | 580 | 31 | 42 |
| Sicilian Parm | 710 | 46 | 40 |
| Zesty Bacon & Swiss | 670 | 41 | 39 |
| *Sides:* *Per Regular Size* | | | |
| Mozzarella Sticks | 525 | 34 | 36 |
| Onion Petals | 545 | 36 | 52 |
| Potato Waffer Fries | 360 | 27 | 29 |
| *Desserts:* Brownie | 500 | 28 | 63 |
| Carrot Cake Cookies, 4 pack | 720 | 36 | 96 |
| Funnel Cake Fries w/ Crml Sce, reg. | 285 | 5.5 | 57 |

## Mrs Fields Cookies® (Sept '19)

*Brownies:* Per 2.15 oz Brownie

| | C | F | Cb |
|---|---|---|---|
| Butterscotch Blondie | 260 | 10 | 38 |
| Double Fudge; Pecan Fudge, av. | 265 | 14 | 33 |
| Special Walnut Fudge & Blondie | 260 | 13 | 35 |
| Toffee/Walnut Fudge, average | 265 | 14 | 33 |

*Brownie Bites:*

| | | | |
|---|---|---|---|
| Butterscotch Blondie (3) | 200 | 8 | 29 |
| Double/Toffee Fudge (3) | 200 | 10 | 27 |

*Coffee Cake,*

| | | | |
|---|---|---|---|
| Chocolate Chip, small, 2.35 oz | 240 | 11 | 30 |

*Bite Size Nibblers Cookies:*

| | | | |
|---|---|---|---|
| Cinnamon Sugar (3) | 180 | 8 | 25 |
| Peanut Butter (3) | 170 | 9 | 19 |
| Semi-Sweet Chocolate (3) | 170 | 8 | 23 |
| Triple Chocolate (3) | 160 | 8 | 22 |
| White Chunk Macadamia (3) | 180 | 9 | 22 |

*Cookies:* Per Cooookie

| | | | |
|---|---|---|---|
| Butter; Debra's Special, average | 200 | 8 | 28 |
| Cut Out | 280 | 11 | 44 |
| Oatmeal, Raisins & Walnuts | 200 | 9 | 27 |
| Peanut Butter | 200 | 12 | 24 |
| **Semi-Sweet:** Chocolate | 210 | 10 | 29 |
| with Walnuts | 220 | 11 | 28 |
| Triple Chocolate | 210 | 10 | 28 |
| White Chunk Macadamia | 230 | 12 | 28 |

*Muffins:* Per 1.9 oz

| | | | |
|---|---|---|---|
| Blueberry | 190 | 9 | 24 |
| Chocolate Chip | 200 | 10 | 26 |

*For Complete Nutritional Data ~ see CalorieKing.com*

## My Favorite Muffin® (Sept '19)

*Muffins:* Per Large Muffin

| | C | F | Cb |
|---|---|---|---|
| **Large:** Blueberry | 590 | 28 | 78 |
| Boston Cream Pie | 740 | 33 | 105 |
| Chocolate Chip | 790 | 39 | 100 |
| Carrot Cake | 850 | 42 | 112 |
| Deep Dish Apple Pie | 560 | 22 | 85 |
| Lemon Poppy Seed | 670 | 32 | 90 |
| Pumpkin Spice | 600 | 26 | 86 |
| Strawberry Cheesecake | 580 | 31 | 67 |

## Nathan's Famous® (Sept '19)

*Burgers:*

| | C | F | Cb |
|---|---|---|---|
| Super Cheeseburger, 5 oz | 960 | 67 | 48 |
| *Cheesesteak,* Original Philly, 10.5 oz | 680 | 33 | 52 |

*Chicken:*

| | | | |
|---|---|---|---|
| **Sandwiches:** Grilled Chicken, 8.2 oz | 470 | 21 | 43 |
| Krispy Chicken, 8.5 oz | 660 | 37 | 58 |
| **Tenders,** Krispy, 3 pieces, 6.3 oz | 520 | 31 | 32 |
| **Wings,** Original Buffalo, 10.5 oz | 690 | 49 | 34 |

## Nathan's Famous® cont... (Sept '19)

*Hot Dogs:* With Natural Casings

| | C | F | Cb |
|---|---|---|---|
| Original, 3.5 oz | 280 | 18 | 24 |
| Chili, 5.5 oz | 400 | 27 | 30 |
| Chili Cheese, 6.5 oz | 460 | 31 | 33 |
| *Hot Dog Nuggets,* 3.5 oz | 350 | 28 | 20 |
| *Corn Dog,* on a stick, 3.2 oz | 380 | 21 | 39 |

*Fries:*

| | | | |
|---|---|---|---|
| **Bacon Cheese,** regular, 10 oz | 710 | 51 | 46 |

*Crinkle Cut:*

| | | | |
|---|---|---|---|
| Cheese, regular, 9 oz | 570 | 38 | 46 |
| French, regular, 7.5 oz | 510 | 34 | 42 |
| *Onion Rings,* Beer Battered, 5.6 oz | 550 | 41 | 37 |

## New York Fries® ~ See CalorieKing.com

## Ninety Nine® (Sept '19)

*Standout Starters:* As Served

| | C | F | Cb |
|---|---|---|---|
| Boneless Wings & Skins Sampler | 1890 | 125 | 107 |
| Mozzarella Moons | 870 | 52 | 63 |
| Outrageous Pot. Skins | 1470 | 101 | 84 |

*Burgers:* Without Sides

| | | | |
|---|---|---|---|
| Bacon & Cheese | 830 | 41 | 58 |
| Black Bean | 590 | 16 | 88 |
| Cheeseburger | 750 | 34 | 58 |
| Crunchy Pickle BBQ Burger | 1340 | 83 | 96 |
| Vermont Cheddar | 970 | 54 | 61 |

*Sandwiches & Wraps:* Without Sides

| | | | |
|---|---|---|---|
| Honey BBQ Chicken Wrap | 850 | 33 | 100 |
| Triple Decker Turkey Club S'wich | 700 | 31 | 58 |

*Entrees:*

| | | | |
|---|---|---|---|
| Braised Short Rib Taco | 1100 | 55 | 13 |
| Chicken Parmigiana | 1390 | 47 | 179 |
| Cntry Fried Chkn, Mashed Pot & Bisc. | 1270 | 55 | 49 |
| Fish & Chips with Fries & Coleslaw | 1570 | 105 | 107 |
| Garlic Parm. Chicken Mac & Cheese | 1130 | 87 | 93 |
| Grilled Angus Sirloin w/ Mashed Pot. | 1330 | 87 | 93 |
| Sliced Sirloin with Mashed Potaotes | 560 | 23 | 44 |
| Stacked Apple BBQ Ribs & Biscuit | 1740 | 99 | 143 |
| S'west Fajita Bowl with Shrimp | 750 | 35 | 85 |
| Sundried Tomato Chkn Kabobs w/ Rice | 820 | 32 | 66 |

*Sides:* Baked Potato, plain

| | | | |
|---|---|---|---|
| Baked Potato, plain | 250 | 3 | 51 |
| with butter | 350 | 15 | 52 |
| Broccoli Florets | 50 | 0.5 | 9 |
| Butternut Squash | 150 | 3 | 30 |
| Coleslaw | 150 | 12 | 10 |
| Corn | 150 | 6 | 19 |
| French Fries | 1040 | 64 | 107 |
| Garden Salad, w/out dressing | 120 | 3 | 22 |
| Russet Mashed Potatoes | 260 | 11 | 36 |
| *Dessert,* Midnight Fudge Cake | 790 | 40 | 96 |

## Noodles & Company® (Sept '19)

### Noodles & Pasta: *Regular Size*

| | C | F | Cb |
|---|---|---|---|
| Alfredo MontAmore Parm Chkn | 1410 | 84 | 110 |
| BBQ Pork Mac | 1210 | 47 | 129 |
| Buffalo Chicken Mac | 1100 | 39 | 128 |
| Buttered Noodles | 760 | 35 | 98 |
| Japanese Pan Noodles | 630 | 12 | 113 |
| Pad Thai | 1040 | 42 | 143 |
| Penne Rosa, w/ Parmesan/Feta | 720 | 24 | 103 |
| Pesto Cavatappi, w/ Feta | 730 | 31 | 93 |
| Spaghetti & Meatballs | 980 | 46 | 104 |
| Spicy Korean Beef Noodles | 1000 | 32 | 138 |
| Steak Stroganoff | 1150 | 62 | 113 |
| Thai Green Curry, with Shrimp | 840 | 23 | 131 |
| Wisconsin Mac & Cheese | 980 | 38 | 119 |
| Zucchini, Aspagagus & Lmon Sce | 500 | 37 | 32 |

### Salads: *Per Regular Size*

| | | | |
|---|---|---|---|
| Grilled Chicken Caesar | 420 | 27 | 18 |
| Chicken Veracru | 650 | 47 | 30 |
| The Med, with Chicken | 390 | 16 | 33 |

### Soups: *Per Regular Size*

| | | | |
|---|---|---|---|
| Thai Chicken | 370 | 22 | 31 |
| Tomato Basil Bisque | 430 | 28 | 37 |

### Extras: Cheesy Garlic Bread, small

| | | | |
|---|---|---|---|
| Cheesy Garlic Bread, small | 350 | 15 | 44 |
| Potsticker (6), regular | 380 | 10 | 54 |
| Korean BBQ Meatballs, regular | 870 | 64 | 37 |
| Wisconsin Mac & Cheese, side | 270 | 12 | 31 |

### Dessert: Chocolate Chunk Cookie

| | | | |
|---|---|---|---|
| Chocolate Chunk Cookie | 450 | 21 | 64 |
| Rice Crispy | 540 | 19 | 87 |
| Snoodledoodle Cookie | 450 | 20 | 64 |

## O'Charley's® (Sept '19)

### Appetizers: *As Served*

| | C | F | Cb |
|---|---|---|---|
| Chicken Tenders, Chipotle | 1160 | 40 | 107 |
| Nashville Deviled Eggs | 720 | 61 | 24 |
| Spicy Jack Cheese Wedges (7) | 720 | 48 | 44 |
| Top Shelf Combo Platter | 1880 | 132 | 74 |

### Burgers: *Without Sides*

| | | | |
|---|---|---|---|
| Better Cheddar Bacon | 1000 | 68 | 49 |
| Classic Cheeseburger | 930 | 61 | 47 |

### Chicken & Pasta: *Without Sides Unless Indicated*

| | | | |
|---|---|---|---|
| Chicken Tenders & Fries | 1410 | 85 | 74 |
| Chicken Tender Dinner: Buffalo | 1070 | 64 | 31 |
| Chipotle | 1040 | 40 | 77 |
| Nashville Hot | 1260 | 87 | 44 |
| Garlic Shrimp Pasta | 950 | 43 | 104 |
| New Orleans Cajun Chicken Pasta | 1170 | 61 | 99 |
| Peach Chutney Chicken | 470 | 8 | 69 |

## O'Charley's® cont... (Sept '19)

### Classic Combos: *Without Sides*

| | C | F | Cb |
|---|---|---|---|
| Steak & Chicken Tenders, 6 oz | 1030 | 67 | 26 |
| Steak & Gr. Atlantic Salmon, 6 oz | 750 | 33 | 5 |
| Steak & Half Rack Baby Back Ribs | 890 | 49 | 48 |

### Ribs & Steak: *Without Sides*

| | | | |
|---|---|---|---|
| **Baby Back Ribs:** Regular | 1220 | 62 | 95 |
| Carolina Gold | 1220 | 62 | 96 |
| Nashville Hot | 1540 | 110 | 63 |

### Slow Roasted Prime Rib:

| | | | |
|---|---|---|---|
| 8oz | 830 | 70 | 3 |
| 12 oz | 1140 | 95 | 3 |
| 16 oz | 1460 | 120 | 4 |
| **Steak:** Bacon & Bourbon Glazed Filet | 640 | 42 | 28 |
| Filet Mignon, w/ Garlic Butter | 580 | 47 | 1 |
| Grilled Top Sirloin, 6 oz | 270 | 18 | 0 |
| Louisiana Sirloin | 600 | 43 | 3 |
| Ribeye Steak | 840 | 71 | 1 |

### Sandwiches: *Without Sides Unless Indicated*

| | | | |
|---|---|---|---|
| Carolina BBQ Chicken | 650 | 22 | 74 |
| Classic French Dip | 1020 | 55 | 79 |
| Club Sandwich | 950 | 85 | 91 |
| Nashville Hot Chicken, with Fries | 2000 | 101 | 119 |

### Seafood| Favorites: *Without Sides Unless Indicated*

| | | | |
|---|---|---|---|
| Grilled Blackened Atl. Salmon, 9 oz | 500 | 31 | 3 |
| Grilled Salmon Bowl | 990 | 70 | 44 |
| Hand Battered Fish & Chips | 1420 | 92 | 85 |
| Hand Breaded Catfish, w/ Fries & Slaw | 1720 | 124 | 103 |

### Sides: Baked Potato (1)

| | | | |
|---|---|---|---|
| Baked Potato (1) | 200 | 1 | 50 |
| Broccoli, 5 oz | 110 | 8 | 6 |
| Coleslaw | 200 | 15 | 12 |
| French Fries, 6 oz | 400 | 24 | 40 |
| Loaded Baked Potato, 1 portion | 490 | 27 | 53 |
| Mac & Cheese | 450 | 22 | 47 |
| Sweet Potato Fries, 1 portion | 280 | 19 | 27 |

### Salads: *Per Full Salad, with Dressing*

| | | | |
|---|---|---|---|
| California Chicken | 1020 | 67 | 71 |
| Classic Cobb | 1140 | 92 | 36 |
| Southern Fried Chicken | 1550 | 110 | 48 |
| Southern Pecan Chicken Tender | 1550 | 106 | 95 |

### Signature Soup: *Per Bowl*

| | | | |
|---|---|---|---|
| Chicken Harvest | 210 | 13 | 20 |
| Chicken Tortilla | 190 | 7 | 20 |

### Desserts: *Per slice*

| | | | |
|---|---|---|---|
| Country Apple Pie | 630 | 35 | 77 |
| Double-Crust Cherry Pie | 600 | 35 | 69 |
| French Silk Pie | 580 | 43 | 49 |
| Goo Goo Crunch Pie | 1450 | 93 | 155 |
| Ooey Gooey Caramel Pie | 640 | 39 | 76 |
| Southern Pecan Pie | 730 | 45 | 78 |

*For Complete Menu & Data ~ see CalorieKing.com*

Updated Nutrition Data ~ www.CalorieKing.com
Persons with Diabetes ~ See Disclaimer (Page 22)

## Old Spaghetti Factory® (Sept '19)

| | C | F | Cb |
|---|---|---|---|
| ***Appetizers:** As Served* | | | |
| Spinach & Artichoke Dip | 640 | 46 | 44 |
| Sicilian Garlic Cheese Bread | 1220 | 78 | 97 |
| with Bacon | 1450 | 95 | 97 |
| ***Entrées, Lunch/Dinner:*** | | | |
| **Founder's Favorites:** | | | |
| Baked Lasagna, 17.6 oz | 820 | 45 | 61 |
| Garlic Mizithra, 17 oz | 1360 | 85 | 102 |
| Tenderloin w/ Mizithra & Brocc. | 1260 | 87 | 59 |
| **Manager Favorites:** | | | |
| Marinara: Clam, 15 oz | 690 | 18 | 107 |
| Meat, 15 oz | 600 | 8 | 108 |
| Mushroom, 16.5 oz | 610 | 10 | 109 |
| **Signature Pasta:** | | | |
| Angel Hair Pomodoro, 16.6 oz | 570 | 8 | 98 |
| Fettuccine Alfredo, 13.3 oz | 1090 | 72 | 91 |
| Spinach & Cheese Ravioli, 11 oz | 470 | 16 | 63 |
| **Spaghetti:** w/ Clam Sauce, 15 oz | 790 | 29 | 107 |
| with Marina Sauce, 15 oz | 570 | 7 | 106 |
| with Meat Sauce, 15 oz | 650 | 11 | 108 |
| with Sicilian Meatballs, 21 oz | 1040 | 36 | 115 |
| *Soup:* Clam Chowder, 9 oz | 320 | 25 | 10 |
| Cream of Broccoli, 9 oz | 210 | 12 | 20 |
| *Dessert,* Tiramisu, 4.5 oz | 295 | 14 | 43 |

## Olive Garden® (Sept '19)

| | C | F | Cb |
|---|---|---|---|
| **Appetizers:** | | | |
| Calamari | 870 | 56 | 67 |
| Sauce: Marinara | 45 | 2.5 | 6 |
| Ranch | 210 | 21 | 3 |
| Fried Mozzarella | 860 | 59 | 48 |
| Spicy Shrimp Scampi Fritta | 560 | 37 | 34 |
| *Lunch:* Fettuccine Alfredo | 650 | 45 | 47 |
| Chicken & Cheese Piadina | 710 | 49 | 40 |
| Grilled Vegetable & Cheese Piadina | 630 | 37 | 52 |
| Lasagna Classico | 640 | 36 | 39 |
| Meatball Pizza Bowl | 950 | 56 | 64 |
| *Taste of the Mediterranean:* | | | |
| Chicken Giardino | 530 | 12 | 65 |
| Herb Grilled Salmon | 460 | 29 | 9 |
| Salmon Piccata | 570 | 39 | 11 |
| *Early Dinner Duos:* Chicken Piccata | 360 | 21 | 11 |
| Creamy Mishrom Ravioli | 830 | 57 | 61 |
| Fettuccine Alfredo | 1010 | 56 | 97 |
| *Sides:* Garlic Mashed Potatoes | 150 | 8 | 17 |
| Garlic Parmesan Fries | 260 | 13 | 32 |
| Parmesan Crusted Zuzzhini | 80 | 5 | 5 |
| Steamed Broccoli | 35 | 0 | 7 |
| *Desserts:* | | | |
| Black Tie Mousse Cake | 750 | 50 | 76 |
| Tiramisu | 470 | 27 | 54 |
| Warm Apple Crostata | 630 | 29 | 83 |
| Zeppoli, without sauce | 810 | 28 | 119 |

## On the Border® (Sept '19)

| | C | F | Cb |
|---|---|---|---|
| ***Appetizers:** As Served* | | | |
| Border Sampler | 2000 | 134 | 109 |
| Fajita Quesadillas: | | | |
| Chicken | 1190 | 82 | 58 |
| Steak | 1280 | 96 | 55 |
| Stacked Nachos | 2010 | 128 | 146 |
| ***Burritos:** Without Bean, Rice or Sauce* | | | |
| Classic Chicken Tinga | 690 | 30 | 56 |
| Classic Ground Beef | 840 | 47 | 55 |
| ***Chimichangas:** Without Beans, Rice or Sauce* | | | |
| Chicken Tinga | 810 | 43 | 57 |
| Ground Beef | 960 | 55 | 66 |
| ***Enchiladas:** Without Bean or Rice* | | | |
| Border Queso Beef | 510 | 29 | 35 |
| Ranchiladas | 1150 | 68 | 53 |
| Suizas | 800 | 43 | 57 |
| ***Salads:** W/out Dressing* | | | |
| Fajita: Chicken | 410 | 19 | 24 |
| Steak | 490 | 27 | 27 |
| **Grande Taco Salad:** Chkn Tinga | 710 | 46 | 49 |
| Ground Beef | 830 | 57 | 51 |
| ***Tacos:** W/out Beans or Rice* | | | |
| Brisket Tacos (2) | 850 | 42 | 79 |
| Gr. Fish Taco Del Mar | 370 | 20 | 30 |
| Southwest Chicken Taco (3) | 1500 | 106 | 80 |
| *Soup:* Chicken Tortilla, 1 cup | 330 | 18 | 24 |
| 1 Bowl | 540 | 27 | 46 |
| *Sides:* Black Beans | 200 | 1 | 36 |
| Cilantro Lime Rice | 180 | 2 | 37 |
| Corn Tortillas (3) | 170 | 2 | 35 |
| Mexican Rice | 220 | 6 | 37 |
| Refried Beans | 230 | 7 | 30 |
| *Dressings:* Ranch | 230 | 24 | 2 |
| Smoked Jalapeno Vinaigrette | 250 | 24 | 9 |

*For Complete Nutritional Data ~ see CalorieKing.com*

## Orange Julius® (Sept '19)

| | C | F | Cb |
|---|---|---|---|
| ***Julius Originals:** Per Medium Size* | | | |
| Berry Pomegranate | 340 | 0.5 | 84 |
| Mango Pineapple | 310 | 0 | 78 |
| OrangeBerry | 310 | 0 | 80 |
| Strawberry Banana | 460 | 7 | 100 |
| ***Premium Fruit Smoothies:** Per Medium Size* | | | |
| OrangeBerry Xtreme | 350 | 0.5 | 86 |
| Pomegranate Berry Blast | 380 | 1 | 92 |
| Strawberry | 320 | 0.5 | 80 |
| Sunshine Orange | 370 | 0.5 | 87 |
| ***Light Smoothies:** Per Medium Size* | | | |
| OrangeBerry Xtreme; Strawberry, av. | 205 | 0 | 55 |
| Strawberry Banana | 210 | 0 | 58 |
| Tripleberry | 210 | 0.5 | 55 |
| *Boost,* Banana, Small drink | 30 | 0 | 7 |

## Outback Steakhouse® (Sept '19)

*Aussie-Tizers:* Per Regular Size, with Selected Dressing/Sauce

| | C | F | Cb |
|---|---|---|---|
| Alice Springs Chicken Quesadillas | 1630 | 98 | 91 |
| Aussie Cheese Fries: Small | 1160 | 83 | 70 |
| Large | 1770 | 117 | 124 |
| Bloomin' Onion | 1950 | 155 | 123 |
| Crab Cakes | 790 | 66 | 22 |
| Kookaburra Wings (medium), reg. | 1420 | 123 | 13 |
| Seared Peppered Ahi, large | 390 | 22 | 19 |
| Steakhouse Quesadilla, regular | 1590 | 107 | 78 |
| Volcano Shrimp | 960 | 73 | 55 |

*Forkless Features:* Without Sides

| | C | F | Cb |
|---|---|---|---|
| Crispy Chicken Sandwich | 880 | 52 | 69 |
| Outback Burger, without Cheese | 710 | 43 | 42 |
| Steakhouse Philly S'wich | 1030 | 61 | 54 |
| The Bloomin' Burger | 1160 | 83 | 58 |

*Chicken & Ribs:*

| | C | F | Cb |
|---|---|---|---|
| Alice Springs Chicken & Fries, 5 oz | 930 | 52 | 69 |
| Baby Back Ribs & Fries, full order | 1280 | 75 | 78 |
| Grilled Chkn On The Barbie, 8 oz, | 360 | 7 | 16 |
| with Fresh Mixed Veggies | 520 | 16 | 34 |
| Parmesan-Herb Crusted Chicken, | 510 | 23 | 13 |
| with Mixed Veggies | 670 | 33 | 30 |
| Queensland Chicken & Shrimp Pasta | 1210 | 55 | 98 |

*Signature Steaks:* Without Sides

| | C | F | Cb |
|---|---|---|---|
| Melbourne Porterhouse, 18 oz | 910 | 64 | 4 |
| Outback Centre Cut Sirloin: 6 oz | 210 | 7 | 0 |
| 9 oz Sirloin | 320 | 10 | 0.5 |
| Ribeye, 10 oz | 540 | 35 | 0 |
| Victoria's Filet Mignon, 6 oz | 240 | 9 | 0 |

*Straight From The Sea:* Without Sides

| | C | F | Cb |
|---|---|---|---|
| Bacon Bourbon Salmon, 10 oz | 650 | 42 | 6 |
| Halibut Fish & Chips | 1030 | 43 | 104 |
| Lobster Tails (2), grilled | 650 | 45 | 2 |

*Entree Salads:*

**Aussie Cobb Salad, without dressing:**

| | C | F | Cb |
|---|---|---|---|
| with Crispy Chicken | 840 | 52 | 47 |
| with Grilled Chicken | 530 | 27 | 19 |

**Brisbane Caesar, with dressing:**

| | C | F | Cb |
|---|---|---|---|
| with Grilled Chicken | 580 | 37 | 23 |
| with Grilled Shrimp | 580 | 38 | 25 |
| **Steakhouse,** 5 oz, with dressing | 910 | 58 | 50 |

*Side Salads:* With Dressing

| | C | F | Cb |
|---|---|---|---|
| Blue Cheese Pecan Chopped | 620 | 48 | 34 |
| Blue Cheese Wedge | 510 | 40 | 27 |
| Caesar | 280 | 24 | 12 |
| House: with Blue Cheese Vinaig. | 230 | 21 | 12 |
| with Caesar Dressing | 190 | 19 | 2 |
| with Creamy Blue Cheese | 240 | 25 | 1 |
| with Honey Mustard | 230 | 21 | 12 |
| with Thousand Island | 250 | 25 | 6 |

## Outback Steakhouse® cont...(Sept '19)

*Soups:*

| | C | F | Cb |
|---|---|---|---|
| **Baked Potato:** Cup | 280 | 17 | 23 |
| Bowl | 520 | 32 | 47 |
| **Chicken Tortilla Soup:** Cup | 170 | 9 | 13 |
| Bowl | 260 | 14 | 21 |
| **Clam Chowder:** Cup | 360 | 22 | 23 |
| Bowl | 710 | 44 | 47 |
| **French Onion** | 420 | 29 | 21 |

*Sides:*

| | C | F | Cb |
|---|---|---|---|
| Aussie Fries | 410 | 17 | 57 |
| Baked Potato, with all toppings | 390 | 12 | 58 |
| Fresh Seasonal Mixed Veggies | 160 | 10 | 17 |
| Grilled Asparagus | 60 | 4 | 4 |
| Homestyle Mashed Potatoes | 240 | 15 | 20 |
| Red Rock Rice | 250 | 4.5 | 46 |
| Steamed Broccoli | 150 | 10 | 14 |
| Steamed Rice | 270 | 0 | 59 |
| Sweet Potato, with all toppings | 410 | 11 | 72 |

*Kid's Menu:* Without Sides or Drink

| | C | F | Cb |
|---|---|---|---|
| **Entrees:** Boomerang Cheeseburger | 600 | 36 | 40 |
| Chicken Fingers | 470 | 29 | 28 |
| Grilled Cheese-A-Roo | 580 | 21 | 77 |
| Grilled Chicken on the Barbie | 160 | 3.5 | 0 |
| Junior Ribs, BBQ Sauce | 300 | 21 | 2 |
| Mac-A-Roo 'N Cheese | 510 | 19 | 65 |

*Desserts:* Per Whole Dish

| | C | F | Cb |
|---|---|---|---|
| Chocolate Thunder | 1500 | 101 | 138 |
| Double Chocolate Mini Parfait | 590 | 39 | 54 |
| NY Style Cheesecake, w/ Choc. Sce | 1080 | 73 | 92 |
| Triple Layer Carrot Cake | 1290 | 68 | 174 |

*For Complete Menu & Data ~ see CalorieKing.com*

## Panda Express® (Sept '19)

*Appetizers:*

| | C | F | Cb |
|---|---|---|---|
| Chicken Egg Roll (1), 2.75 oz | 200 | 10 | 20 |
| Chicken Potsticker (3), 3.3 oz | 160 | 6 | 20 |
| Cream Cheese Rangoon (3), 2.4 oz | 190 | 8 | 24 |
| Veggie Spring Rolls (2), 3.4 oz | 190 | 8 | 27 |

*Entrées:*

| | C | F | Cb |
|---|---|---|---|
| **Beef:** Beijing Beef, 5.6 oz | 470 | 26 | 46 |
| Broccoli Beef, 5.4 oz | 150 | 7 | 13 |
| Shanghai Angus Steak, with String Beans, 6.4 oz | 310 | 19 | 17 |
| **Chicken:** | | | |
| Black Pepper, 6.3 oz | 280 | 19 | 15 |
| Breast: String Bean, 5.6 oz | 190 | 9 | 13 |
| SweetFire, 5.8 oz | 380 | 15 | 47 |
| Grilled Teriyaki, 6 oz | 300 | 13 | 8 |

## Panda Express® cont... (Sept '19)

*Entrees (Cont):*

**Chicken (Cont):**

| | C | F | Cb |
|---|---|---|---|
| Mushroom Chicken, 5.7 oz | 220 | 14 | 11 |
| Orange Chicken, 5.7 oz | 490 | 23 | 51 |
| **Shrimp:** Honey Walnut, 3.7 oz | 360 | 23 | 35 |
| Wok-Fired Shrimp, 6 oz | 190 | 5 | 19 |
| *Vegetables,* Eggplant Tofu, 6.1 oz | 340 | 24 | 23 |
| *Sides:* Chow Mein, 9.4 oz | 510 | 20 | 80 |
| Fried Rice, 9.3 oz | 520 | 16 | 85 |
| Steamed Brown Rice, 10.4 oz | 420 | 4 | 86 |
| Steamed White Rice, 8.1 oz | 380 | 0 | 87 |
| Super Greens, 7 oz | 90 | 2.5 | 10 |
| *Soup,* Hot & Sour: Cup, 12.2 oz | 120 | 5 | 14 |
| Bowl, 17.4 oz | 170 | 6 | 20 |
| *Dessert,* Choc Chip Chunk Cookie | 160 | 7 | 25 |

## Panera Bread® (Sept '19)

*Bagels:*

| | C | F | Cb |
|---|---|---|---|
| Asiago Cheese | 330 | 5 | 55 |
| Cinnamon Crunch | 420 | 6 | 82 |
| *Breakfast Sandwiches, Grilled:* | | | |
| Bacon, Egg & Cheese on Brioche | 460 | 25 | 32 |
| Sausage, Egg & Cheese on Brioche | 540 | 33 | 32 |
| Steak & Egg on Everthing Bagel | 530 | 18 | 59 |
| *Bowls,* Vegan Lentil Quinoa Broth | 270 | 7 | 43 |
| *Sandwiches: Per Full Sandwich* | | | |
| Bacon Turkey Bravo on Tomato Basil | 620 | 23 | 58 |
| Heritage Ham & Swiss, on Wh. Grain | 600 | 26 | 50 |
| Mediterranean Veggie on Tomato Basil | 440 | 13 | 66 |
| Roasted Turkey & Avocado BLT, on Country Rustic | 680 | 35 | 52 |
| Tuna Salad, on Black Pepper Foccacia | 650 | 34 | 58 |
| **Flatbread,** BBQ Chicken (1) | 400 | 18 | 37 |
| **Panini,** Frontega Chicken on Focaccia | 770 | 29 | 84 |
| *Pasta:* | | | |
| Chicken Tortellini Alfredo, 2 cups | 750 | 39 | 68 |
| **Mac & Cheese:** | | | |
| Small | 470 | 31 | 33 |
| Large | 950 | 62 | 66 |
| *Salads: Full Size, with Dressing, without Bread* | | | |
| Asian Sesame w/ Chkn | 410 | 21 | 25 |
| Chicken Caesar | 450 | 28 | 17 |
| Fuji Apple with Chicken | 570 | 35 | 36 |
| Greek | 390 | 36 | 11 |
| Strawberry Poppyseed with Chkn | 340 | 13 | 31 |

## Panera Bread® cont... (Sept '19)

*Soups: Per Cup, without Bread*

| | C | F | Cb |
|---|---|---|---|
| Baked Potato | 260 | 14 | 29 |
| Broccoli Cheddar | 190 | 8 | 20 |
| Crm of Chkn & Wild Rice | 210 | 11 | 21 |
| New England Clam Chowder | 370 | 25 | 27 |
| Vegetarian Creamy Tomato | 230 | 15 | 24 |
| *Brownie,* (1) | 390 | 13 | 69 |
| *Cookies:* Chocolate Chipper (1) | 380 | 19 | 51 |
| Oatmeal Raisin with Berries (1) | 350 | 13 | 54 |
| *Pastries & Sweets:* | | | |
| Bear Claw | 550 | 31 | 59 |
| Chocolate Croissant | 380 | 22 | 39 |
| Pecan Braid | 500 | 29 | 53 |
| *Muffin:* Choc. Chip | 640 | 28 | 91 |
| Pumpkin Muffin | 570 | 21 | 87 |
| *Muffie,* Chocolate Chip | 320 | 14 | 46 |

## Papa Gino's® (Sept '19)

*Appetizers: Per Small Serving*

| | C | F | Cb |
|---|---|---|---|
| BBQ Chicken Tenders, 5.2 oz | 360 | 18 | 33 |
| Buffalo Chicken Tenders, 5.4 oz | 390 | 25 | 22 |
| Cheese Breadsticks, 3.75 oz | 230 | 8 | 30 |
| Chicken Tenders, 8.8 oz | 350 | 20 | 24 |
| *Burgers:* Cheeseburger, 6.7 oz | 570 | 32 | 37 |
| Classic Double, 12.8 oz | 1040 | 67 | 43 |
| Hamburger, 6.3 oz | 520 | 28 | 35 |
| *French Fries:* Small, 5 oz | 470 | 24 | 66 |
| Large, 13.7 oz | 680 | 33 | 99 |
| *Pasta:* | | | |
| Mac & Cheese, 17.8 oz | 1040 | 60 | 87 |
| Ravioli, 12.4 oz | 560 | 21 | 67 |
| Spaghetti & Meatballs, 19.8 oz | 780 | 28 | 109 |
| *Pizzas:* | | | |
| **Thin Crust:** *Per Slice, ⅛ Large Pizza* | | | |
| Boss BBQ Chicken | 320 | 12 | 38 |
| Cheese | 230 | 7 | 32 |
| Crispy Buffalo, w/ Blue Cheese | 360 | 16 | 36 |
| PapaRoni | 340 | 16 | 32 |
| Pepperoni | 280 | 11 | 32 |
| Super Veggie | 250 | 8 | 35 |
| Works | 330 | 14 | 34 |
| *Subs: Per Small Sub* | | | |
| BLT | 690 | 35 | 67 |
| Italian | 590 | 24 | 64 |
| Meatball Parmesan | 790 | 38 | 79 |
| Steak & Cheese | 610 | 30 | 61 |
| Super Steak | 650 | 31 | 59 |
| Tuna | 730 | 39 | 64 |
| Turkey Club | 600 | 22 | 67 |

**223**

## Papa John's® (Sept '19)

*Pizzas:*

| | C | F | Cb |
|---|---|---|---|
| **Original Crust (14"):** *Per ⅛ of Large 14" Pizza* | | | |
| BBQ Chicken & Bacon | 340 | 11 | 45 |
| Buffalo Chicken | 380 | 17 | 40 |
| Cheese | 290 | 10 | 38 |
| Grilled Chicken & Bacon | 270 | 7 | 37 |
| Garden Fresh | 280 | 9 | 39 |
| Pepperoni | 320 | 13 | 38 |
| Sausage | 330 | 14 | 40 |
| **Thin Crust (14"):** *Per ⅛ of Large 14" Pizza* | | | |
| BBQ Chicken & Bacon | 270 | 12 | 27 |
| Buffalo Chicken | 300 | 18 | 22 |
| Cheese | 210 | 11 | 20 |
| Grilled Chicken & Bacon | 190 | 8 | 19 |
| Garden Fresh | 210 | 10 | 21 |
| Pepperoni | 250 | 14 | 20 |
| Pepperoni & Sausage | 310 | 20 | 20 |
| **Wings:** *Per 8 Wings, with Dipping Sauce* | | | |
| BBQ | 880 | 57 | 20 |
| Honey Chipotle | 900 | 57 | 27 |
| Spicy Buffalo | 840 | 58 | 8 |
| **Chicken Poppers:** 5 Poppers | 270 | 10 | 21 |
| 10 Poppers | 530 | 21 | 42 |
| 15 Poppers | 800 | 31 | 64 |
| **Sides:** | | | |
| Breadsticks, 1 X 12" | 130 | 2 | 24 |
| Garlic Parmesan, 1 X 12" | 160 | 5 | 24 |
| Cheesesticks, 1 X 10" | 90 | 4 | 10 |
| **Desserts:** Chocolate Chip Cookie | 190 | 9 | 26 |
| Double Chocolate Chip Brownie | 240 | 12 | 34 |

## Papa Murphy's® (Sept '19)

*Pizzas:*

| | C | F | Cb |
|---|---|---|---|
| **Original Crust:** *Per ½ of Family Size Pizza* | | | |
| BBQ Chicken | 340 | 13 | 37 |
| Chicken Garlic | 330 | 15 | 30 |
| Cowboy | 370 | 19 | 32 |
| Garden Veggie | 270 | 11 | 33 |
| Gourmet Vegetarian | 320 | 16 | 32 |
| Hawaiian | 270 | 10 | 33 |
| Murphy's Combo | 350 | 18 | 33 |
| Papa's Favorite | 350 | 17 | 33 |
| Pepperoni | 300 | 14 | 31 |
| Rancher | 320 | 14 | 32 |
| Thai Chicken | 340 | 12 | 40 |
| **Stuffed Pizzas:** *Per 1⁄16 of Family Size Pizza* | | | |
| 5 Meat | 460 | 18 | 52 |
| Big Murphy | 450 | 18 | 53 |
| Chicago Style | 450 | 18 | 52 |
| Chicken and Bacon | 440 | 17 | 51 |

## Papa Murphy's® cont... (Sept '19)

*Pizzas (Cont):*

| | C | F | Cb |
|---|---|---|---|
| **Salads:** *Per Whole Salad, w/out Dressing or Croutons* | | | |
| Caesar | 100 | 5 | 7 |
| Club | 270 | 16 | 12 |
| Garden | 190 | 11 | 13 |
| Italian | 270 | 19 | 11 |
| Mediterranean | 320 | 17 | 23 |
| **Desserts:** | | | |
| Choc. Chip Cookie, 1 slice | 170 | 11 | 34 |
| Cinnamon Wheel, 2 slices | 250 | 7 | 42 |
| S'mores Dessert Pizza, 2 slices | 260 | 7 | 44 |

## Pei Wei Asian Diner® (Sept '19)

*Shareables:* *Without Sauce*

| | C | F | Cb |
|---|---|---|---|
| Crab Wontons (4) | 340 | 20 | 28 |
| Chkn Lettuce Wraps | 810 | 46 | 66 |
| Trad'nl Edamame, lge | 320 | 13 | 19 |
| Vegetable Spring Rolls (4) | 480 | 24 | 60 |
| **Sauce:** Lettuce Wrap Sce, 2 oz | 60 | 3 | 3 |
| Sweet Chile Sce, 2 oz | 80 | 0 | 20 |
| Thai Peanut Dipping Sce, 2 oz | 230 | 15 | 20 |
| **House-Rolled Sushi Rolls:** *Per 4 Rolls* | | | |
| Mango California | 190 | 4 | 28 |
| Spicy Tuna Roll | 180 | 8 | 24 |
| Teriyaki Crunch | 370 | 20 | 40 |
| Wasabi Crunch | 320 | 16 | 32 |
| **Featured Items:** | | | |
| Cauli Flower Power Bowl | 750 | 37 | 44 |
| **Cauliflower Fried Rice:** Small | 510 | 30 | 27 |
| Large | 730 | 46 | 30 |
| **Wei Better Orange:** *Regular* | | | |
| Crispy Tempura Chicken | 1020 | 48 | 109 |
| Steamed Chicken | 680 | 20 | 79 |
| **Wei Veggie Orange:** *Regular* | | | |
| Crispy Tempura Chicken | 1070 | 48 | 118 |
| Steamed Chicken | 720 | 20 | 88 |
| **Noodle Bowls:** | | | |
| Dan Dan | 990 | 40 | 110 |
| Chicken Pad Thai | 1470 | 42 | 167 |
| Japanese Steak & Shrimp Chile Ramen | 1600 | 41 | 196 |
| **Salad Bowls:** *With Dressing* | | | |
| Ahi Avocado | 770 | 41 | 78 |
| Asian Chopped Chicken | 660 | 35 | 44 |
| Spicy Polynesian Poke Bowl | 760 | 33 | 90 |
| **Soup:** Hot & Sour, bowl | 180 | 6 | 15 |
| Thai Wonton, bowl | 160 | 5 | 22 |

## Pepe's Mexican® ~ *see CalorieKing.com*

Updated Nutrition Data ~ www.CalorieKing.com
Persons with Diabetes ~ See Disclaimer (Page 22)

## Perkins® (Sept '19)

### Breakfast: *Without Side Choices*

| | C | F | Cb |
|---|---|---|---|
| **Classic:** Cntry Fried Steak & Eggs | 740 | 45 | 47 |
| Eggs Benedict | 650 | 33 | 61 |
| Hearty Man's Combo | 800 | 69 | 11 |
| Steak Medallions & Eggs | 530 | 28 | 8 |
| **Omelets:** | | | |
| Everything | 550 | 40 | 14 |
| Farmer's | 660 | 54 | 8 |
| Granny's Country | 640 | 41 | 34 |
| **Platters:** Belgian Waffle | 620 | 38 | 51 |
| Brioche French Toast | 730 | 33 | 68 |
| Cinn. Roll French Toast | 810 | 45 | 73 |
| French Toast | 620 | 32 | 53 |
| Strawberry Pancake | 930 | 39 | 123 |
| **Syrups & Toppings:** | | | |
| Apricot Syrup, 2 oz | 120 | 0 | 30 |
| Glazed Blueberries, 6 oz | 200 | 0 | 51 |
| Glazed Strawberries, 6 oz | 140 | 0 | 36 |
| Pancake/Twinberry Syrup, 2 oz, av. | 130 | 0 | 33 |
| Sugar Free Pancake Syrup, 2 oz | 10 | 0 | 3 |
| **Side Choices:** Bacon, 4 slices | 140 | 12 | 0 |
| Biscuits (2), Jumbo, with butter | 650 | 36 | 68 |
| Blueberry Muffin, with butter | 650 | 33 | 81 |
| Breakfast Potatoes, 5 oz | 280 | 17 | 30 |
| Eggs (2) | 170 | 13 | 2 |
| English Muffin, with butter | 230 | 11 | 28 |
| Fresh Cut Fruit, 4 oz | 70 | 0 | 19 |
| Ham, grilled, 5.6 oz | 160 | 4.5 | 6 |
| Hash Browns, 4.3 oz | 210 | 13 | 22 |
| Homestyle Potatoes, 6.8 oz | 210 | 3 | 40 |
| Oatmeal, with butter blend, | | | |
|     2% Milk & Brown Sugar | 390 | 15 | 57 |
| Sausage Patties (2) | 380 | 38 | 1 |
| Smoked Ssg., 4.1 oz | 380 | 34 | 8 |
| Sticky Bun, with butter | 790 | 41 | 98 |
| White Toast (2), with butter | 310 | 16 | 34 |
| Whole Wheat Toast (2), w/ butter | 310 | 13 | 38 |

### Burgers: *Without Sides*

| | C | F | Cb |
|---|---|---|---|
| A-1 BBQ Bacon | 1170 | 72 | 75 |
| A-1 Tangler | 1160 | 70 | 77 |
| Classic Burger | 920 | 62 | 49 |
| Classic Cheeseburger | 1080 | 74 | 51 |

### Sandwiches: *Without Sides*

| | C | F | Cb |
|---|---|---|---|
| Chicken Strips Melt, on S'dough | 1290 | 80 | 88 |
| Country Club Melt, on S'Dough | 990 | 57 | 64 |
| Reuben Melt | 1090 | 61 | 79 |
| Roast Beef & Swiss | 730 | 50 | 33 |
| Turkey & Avocado BLT | 700 | 39 | 47 |

## Perkins® cont... (Sept '19)

### Lunch & Dinners:

**Comfort Classics:** *Without Sides*

| | C | F | Cb |
|---|---|---|---|
| Chicken Strips | 800 | 43 | 59 |
| Country Fried Steak | 570 | 32 | 45 |
| Fish 'n Chips, with Tartar Sauce | 1290 | 85 | 97 |
| Grilled Garlic Tilapia & Shrimp | 550 | 20 | 57 |
| Jumbo Shrimp, w/ Cocktail Sce | 270 | 7 | 41 |
| Steak Medallions & Mushrooms | 480 | 29 | 6 |
| Turkey & Dressing, w/- Cranb. Sce | 510 | 20 | 39 |

**Supper Skillets:** *With Menu Set Sides*

| | C | F | Cb |
|---|---|---|---|
| Bals. Glazed Salmon | 950 | 49 | 81 |
| Hibachi Fried Chicken | 860 | 33 | 107 |
| Hibachi Gr. Shrimp | 690 | 24 | 89 |
| Kickin' Chicken Tortilla | 1020 | 40 | 110 |
| Steak & Pepper | 800 | 43 | 58 |

**Sides:** Applesauce, 3 oz

| | C | F | Cb |
|---|---|---|---|
| *Sides:* Applesauce, 3 oz | 40 | 0 | 9 |
| Baked Potato,with Sour Cream | 300 | 12 | 42 |
| Buttered Corn | 150 | 8 | 17 |
| French Fries, 7 oz | 570 | 36 | 56 |
| Green Beans & Bacon, 4 oz | 45 | 2.5 | 4 |
| Herb Rice Pilaf, 6.5 oz | 270 | 6 | 50 |
| H'style Seasoned Potato, 6.8 oz | 210 | 3 | 40 |
| Macaroni & Five Cheese, 5.2 oz | 300 | 16 | 26 |
| Mashed Potatoes & Gravy, 8.6 oz | 240 | 9 | 34 |
| Sauteed Spinach, 4 oz | 70 | 3.5 | 4 |
| Tater Tots | 470 | 28 | 47 |

**Soups:** *Per Bowl, Includes Crackers*

| | C | F | Cb |
|---|---|---|---|
| Chicken Noodle | 260 | 6 | 37 |
| Loaded Potato; Tomato Basil | 460 | 26 | 46 |
| Tomato Basil | 460 | 26 | 46 |

**Salads:** *With Set Dressing Unless Indicated*

| | C | F | Cb |
|---|---|---|---|
| Honey Mstrd Chkn Crunch | 980 | 63 | 63 |
| Southwest Avocado | 820 | 50 | 61 |
| Turkey BLT w/out dressing | 380 | 19 | 11 |

### Dessert:

**Muffins:** *Includes Whipped Butter Blend*

| | C | F | Cb |
|---|---|---|---|
| Apple Cinnamon | 630 | 33 | 76 |
| Banana Nut | 790 | 46 | 85 |
| Blueberry | 650 | 33 | 81 |

**Pies:** *Per Slice*

| | C | F | Cb |
|---|---|---|---|
| Caramel Apple, 7.2 oz | 500 | 22 | 68 |
| Cherry | 580 | 27 | 75 |
| Lem. Meringue, 7 oz | 500 | 17 | 80 |
| Southern Pecan, 5.5 oz | 670 | 33 | 86 |
| Wildberry, no sugar added, 7 oz | 470 | 27 | 50 |

**225**

## Peter Piper Pizza® (Sept '19)

### Appetizers:

| | C | F | Cb |
|---|---|---|---|
| Bone In Wings (10), without sauce | 1160 | 97 | 0 |
| Boneless Wings, 10 oz, without sauce | 880 | 58 | 47 |
| Cheddar Bacon Roll (1) | 350 | 18 | 34 |
| Garlic Chse Bread, 3.25 oz | 390 | 17 | 45 |
| Handmade Breadsticks, with Marinara Sauce (6) | 1190 | 31 | 199 |

### Dipping Sauces:

| | C | F | Cb |
|---|---|---|---|
| BBQ | 240 | 0 | 60 |
| Buffalo | 120 | 9 | 6 |
| Ranch | 320 | 36 | 2 |
| Sweet Chili | 200 | 0 | 46 |
| Xtra Hot Buffalo | 90 | 6 | 5 |

### Signature Pizzas:

**Original Crust:** *Per 1/8 of Large 14" Pizza*

| | C | F | Cb |
|---|---|---|---|
| 5 Meat Supreme | 360 | 15 | 39 |
| California Veggie | 290 | 9 | 41 |
| Cheese | 320 | 11 | 39 |
| Chicago Classic | 330 | 13 | 40 |
| Hearty Hawaiian | 310 | 9 | 41 |
| New York 3 Cheese w/ Pepperoni | 390 | 18 | 39 |
| Pizza Mexicana | 390 | 18 | 39 |
| Spinach Chkn Alfredo | 350 | 15 | 37 |
| The Werx | 310 | 11 | 40 |
| Veggie Harvest | 300 | 9 | 42 |

**Original Crust:** *Per 1/12 of Extra Large 16" Pizza*

| | C | F | Cb |
|---|---|---|---|
| 5 Meat Supreme | 350 | 16 | 34 |
| California Veggie | 250 | 8 | 35 |
| Cheese | 280 | 10 | 34 |
| Chicago Classic | 300 | 12 | 35 |
| Hearty Hawaiian | 270 | 8 | 36 |
| New York 3 Cheese w/ Pepperoni | 350 | 16 | 34 |
| Pizza Mexicana | 340 | 15 | 34 |
| Spinach Chkn Alfredo | 310 | 14 | 32 |
| The Werx | 290 | 11 | 34 |
| Veggie Harvest | 260 | 8 | 36 |

### Pasta: *With Breadstick*

| | C | F | Cb |
|---|---|---|---|
| Mac & Pepperoni | 1670 | 91 | 168 |
| Spinach Alfredo | 1640 | 89 | 153 |

### Salads: *Small Size, without Dressing*

| | C | F | Cb |
|---|---|---|---|
| Caesar, with Croutons | 320 | 14 | 35 |
| Greens & Grapes | 170 | 7 | 21 |

### Dessert:

| | C | F | Cb |
|---|---|---|---|
| Cinnamon Crunch, small slice | 380 | 9 | 69 |
| Vanilla Soft Serve: Cone | 200 | 6 | 35 |
| Cup | 180 | 6 | 31 |

## P.F. Chang's® (Sept '19)

### Street Fare:

| | C | F | Cb |
|---|---|---|---|
| Cauliflower Tempura | 680 | 45 | 64 |
| Chang's BBQ Spare Ribs | 810 | 22 | 37 |
| Chang's Chicken Lettuce Wraps | 660 | 27 | 67 |
| Chang's Vegetarian Lettuce Wraps | 570 | 28 | 53 |
| Crispy Green Beans | 990 | 78 | 69 |
| Dynamite Shrimp | 640 | 48 | 36 |
| Edamame with Kosher Salt | 400 | 17 | 25 |
| Northern Style Spare Ribs | 710 | 21 | 12 |
| Tempura Calamari & Vegetables | 960 | 73 | 61 |

### Entrées:

**Beef:** *Per Whole Meal, without Rice*

| | C | F | Cb |
|---|---|---|---|
| A La Sichuan | 690 | 33 | 55 |
| Beef with Broccoli | 670 | 33 | 46 |
| Mongolian | 770 | 42 | 39 |
| Wok Fired Filet Mignon | 1140 | 72 | 72 |

**Chicken:** *Per Whole Dish, without Rice*

| | C | F | Cb |
|---|---|---|---|
| Chang's Spicy | 840 | 33 | 77 |
| Crispy Honey Chkn | 1120 | 60 | 87 |
| Ginger Chicken with Broccoli | 480 | 12 | 41 |
| Kung Pao | 960 | 58 | 46 |
| Orange Peel Chkn | 860 | 31 | 84 |
| Sesame Chicken | 870 | 36 | 75 |

**Seafood:** *Per Whole Meal, w/out Rice Unless Noted*

| | C | F | Cb |
|---|---|---|---|
| Chang's Lobster & Shrimp Rice | 1060 | 46 | 112 |
| Crispy Honey Shrimp | 1020 | 55 | 79 |
| Kung Pao Shrimp | 760 | 52 | 40 |
| Oolong Chilean Sea Bass | 560 | 35 | 30 |
| Orange Peel Shrimp | 570 | 22 | 71 |
| Salt & Pepper Prawns | 500 | 22 | 37 |
| Walnut Shrimp with Melon | 1340 | 107 | 72 |

**Vegetarian:** *Without Rice*

| | C | F | Cb |
|---|---|---|---|
| Buddha's Feast, steamed | 260 | 4 | 32 |
| Ma Po Tofu | 920 | 59 | 57 |
| Stir-Fried Eggplant | 530 | 34 | 57 |
| Thai Harvest Curry | 1070 | 74 | 74 |

### Noodles & Rice:

**Fried Rice:** Combo

| | C | F | Cb |
|---|---|---|---|
| Fried Rice: Combo | 1200 | 35 | 160 |
| with Beef | 1140 | 33 | 155 |
| with Chicken | 1100 | 26 | 159 |
| with Pork | 1190 | 37 | 161 |
| with Shrimp | 1030 | 24 | 158 |
| Hokkien Street Noodles | 1260 | 17 | 224 |
| **Lo Mein:** Beef | 980 | 31 | 127 |
| Chicken | 950 | 24 | 130 |
| Combo | 1050 | 33 | 132 |
| Pork | 1030 | 35 | 133 |
| Shrimp | 880 | 21 | 130 |
| Vegetables | 760 | 13 | 135 |
| Long Life Noodles & Prawns | 1040 | 37 | 130 |

## P.F. Chang's® cont... (Sept '19)

*Noodles & Rice (Cont):*

| | C | F | Cb |
|---|---|---|---|
| **Pad Thai:** Chicken | 1230 | 33 | 181 |
| Combo | 1210 | 32 | 181 |
| Shrimp | 1180 | 31 | 181 |

*Lunch Bowls:*

| | C | F | Cb |
|---|---|---|---|
| **Noodles:** Chiang Mai | 850 | 35 | 91 |
| Tokyo Udon with Chicken | 890 | 28 | 110 |
| **Rice:** Korean Bibimbap with Steak | 1080 | 51 | 104 |
| Mongolian Beef | 790 | 28 | 89 |
| Tempura | 1260 | 80 | 100 |

*Market Sides: Per Serving*

| | C | F | Cb |
|---|---|---|---|
| Brown Rice | 190 | 0 | 40 |
| Chili Garlic Green Beans | 530 | 40 | 39 |
| Sichuan-Style Asparagus | 450 | 34 | 31 |
| White Rice | 220 | 0 | 49 |
| Wok-Charred Brussels Sprouts | 350 | 28 | 25 |
| Wok'd Spinach w/ Garlic | 140 | 6 | 15 |
| *Sushi:* Ahi Poke Bowl | 540 | 21 | 54 |
| California Roll | 380 | 16 | 52 |
| Kung Pao Dragon Roll | 510 | 23 | 60 |
| Lobster Avocado Roll | 370 | 16 | 44 |
| Shrimp Tempura Roll | 580 | 25 | 69 |
| Spicy Tuna Roll | 300 | 6 | 43 |
| *Salad:* Asian Caesar | 410 | 30 | 21 |
| Mandarin Crunch | 730 | 46 | 71 |
| Vietnamese Noodle | 800 | 6 | 166 |
| *Dessert:* Banana Spring Rolls | 940 | 35 | 149 |
| Chocolate Dome | 610 | 43 | 61 |
| New York Style Cheese Cake | 940 | 61 | 80 |
| The Great Wall of Chocolate | 1700 | 71 | 259 |

## Pita Pit® ~ *See CalorieKing.com*

## Pizza Hut® (Sept '19)

*Hand-Tossed Style: Per 1/8 of Medium 12" Pizza*

| | C | F | Cb |
|---|---|---|---|
| Cheese | 210 | 8 | 26 |
| Chicken-Bacon Parmesan | 230 | 9 | 25 |
| Meat Lover's | 280 | 15 | 25 |
| Pepperoni | 220 | 10 | 25 |
| Pepperoni Lover's | 270 | 13 | 26 |
| Supreme | 240 | 11 | 26 |
| Ultimate Cheese Lover's | 230 | 10 | 25 |
| Veggie Lover's | 200 | 7 | 26 |

*Original Pan: Per 1/8 of Medium 12" Pizza*

| | C | F | Cb |
|---|---|---|---|
| Cheese | 260 | 12 | 28 |
| Meat Lover's | 320 | 18 | 28 |
| Pepperoni | 260 | 13 | 27 |
| Pepperoni Lover's | 320 | 17 | 28 |
| Supreme | 280 | 14 | 28 |
| Ultimate Cheese Lover's | 280 | 14 | 27 |
| Veggie Lover's | 240 | 10 | 29 |

## Pizza Hut® cont... (Sept '19)

*Personal Pan: Per 1/4 of 6" Pizza*

| | C | F | Cb |
|---|---|---|---|
| Backyard BBQ Chicken | 180 | 6 | 25 |
| Meat Lover's | 210 | 12 | 17 |
| Pepperoni | 150 | 7 | 17 |
| Pepperoni Lover's | 180 | 9 | 17 |
| Supreme | 170 | 9 | 17 |
| Ultimate Cheese Lover's | 170 | 8 | 17 |
| Veggie Lover's | 140 | 5 | 18 |

*Rectangle Slices: Per Slice, 1/8 of Pizza*

| | C | F | Cb |
|---|---|---|---|
| Backyard BBQ Chicken | 260 | 9 | 34 |
| Buffalo Chicken | 240 | 8 | 32 |
| Cheese | 240 | 10 | 29 |
| Pepperoni | 250 | 11 | 28 |
| Veggie Lovers | 220 | 8 | 29 |

*Thin 'n Crispy: Per 1/8 of Medium 12" Pizza*

| | C | F | Cb |
|---|---|---|---|
| Backyard BBQ Chicken | 210 | 7 | 27 |
| Cheese | 180 | 7 | 22 |
| Chicken-Bacon Parmesan | 220 | 10 | 21 |
| Meat Lover's | 260 | 14 | 22 |
| Pepperoni Lover's | 250 | 13 | 22 |
| Supreme | 210 | 9 | 23 |
| Ult. Cheese Lover's | 210 | 10 | 21 |
| Veggie Lover's | 170 | 6 | 24 |

*Pastas, Tuscani:*

| | C | F | Cb |
|---|---|---|---|
| Creamy Chicken Alfredo, 9.9 oz | 890 | 49 | 74 |
| Meaty Marinara, 9.6 oz | 820 | 36 | 85 |

*Soup: Per Bowl with Crackers*

| | C | F | Cb |
|---|---|---|---|
| Broccoli & Cheese | 530 | 7 | 35 |
| Creamy Tomato Basil | 390 | 23 | 37 |
| Loaded Baked Potato | 600 | 40 | 41 |
| *Sides:* Baked Bone Out Wing (1) | 60 | 2 | 4 |
| Breadstick (1), without sauce | 140 | 4.5 | 19 |
| Buffalo Chicken Nachos | 1110 | 50 | 132 |
| Cheesy Dip 'N Cheese | 660 | 36 | 78 |
| Fried Onion Rings, with Ketchup | 860 | 50 | 93 |
| Garlic Bread, 1 piece | 140 | 8 | 15 |
| Stuffed Garlic Knot | 80 | 2.5 | 10 |
| Stuffed Pizza Roller | 230 | 10 | 27 |

*Salad: Entree Size, without Dressing*

| | C | F | Cb |
|---|---|---|---|
| Asian | 330 | 15 | 24 |
| BLT | 400 | 26 | 26 |
| Chicken Caesar | 470 | 25 | 27 |
| Harvest | 470 | 19 | 48 |
| Zesty Italian | 370 | 22 | 30 |
| *Dressing:* Blue Cheese, entree size | 450 | 48 | 3 |
| Buttermilk Ranch, 1.5 oz | 200 | 22 | 2 |
| Honey French, 1.5 oz | 190 | 15 | 13 |
| *Desserts:* Fried Apple Pie | 170 | 9 | 22 |
| Hershey's: Chocolate Chip Cookie | 300 | 14 | 45 |
| Triple Choc. Brownie, 1/6 square | 380 | 16 | 56 |
| New York Style Cheesecake, slice | 840 | 57 | 69 |

## Pizza Ranch® (Sept '19)

*Pizza:*

| | C | F | Cb |
|---|---|---|---|
| **Original Crust:** *Per Slice, ⅒ of Medium Pizza* | | | |
| Bacon Cheeseburger | 180 | 7 | 20 |
| BBQ Chicken | 170 | 6 | 20 |
| Bronco | 200 | 8 | 19 |
| Buffalo Chicken | 180 | 8 | 18 |
| Chicken Bacon Ranch | 230 | 12 | 18 |
| Macaroni & Cheese | 220 | 10 | 22 |
| Prairie (Veggie) | 170 | 6 | 20 |
| Stampede | 200 | 8 | 21 |
| Sweet Swine | 170 | 6 | 21 |
| Taco Texan | 230 | 10 | 26 |
| **Thin Crust:** *Per ⅒ Slice of Medium Pizza* | | | |
| BBQ Chicken | 150 | 6 | 14 |
| Bronco | 180 | 9 | 13 |
| Cuban | 180 | 8 | 16 |
| *Wrap Meal:* Corn | 150 | 1 | 35 |
| BBQ Chicken | 1180 | 48 | 129 |
| Caesar Chicken | 1310 | 80 | 92 |
| Chicken Bacon | 1720 | 120 | 94 |
| *Sides:* Biscuit | 200 | 10 | 23 |
| Coleslaw | 180 | 16 | 11 |
| Corn | 150 | 1 | 35 |
| Mashed Potatoes & Gravy, 8 oz | 260 | 6 | 41 |
| Ranch Potato Wedges (8) | 540 | 24 | 71 |
| *Salads:* Chef | 460 | 20 | 12 |
| Chicken Fiesta | 200 | 8 | 11 |
| Strawberry Spinach | 710 | 52 | 52 |
| Taco | 600 | 36 | 50 |

*For Complete Menu & Data ~ see CalorieKing.com*

## Pollo Tropical® ~ See CalorieKing.com

## Popeye's® (Sept '19)

*Chicken Pieces: Mild & Spicy with Skin*

| | C | F | Cb |
|---|---|---|---|
| Breast | 380 | 20 | 16 |
| Leg | 160 | 9 | 5 |
| Thigh | 280 | 21 | 7 |
| Wing | 210 | 14 | 8 |
| *Nuggets:* 6 pieces | 225 | 14 | 15 |
| 9 Pieces | 340 | 20 | 23 |
| *Tenders:* Mild/Spicy, 3 pieces | 445 | 21 | 29 |
| 5 pieces | 740 | 34 | 48 |
| *Sandwiches & Wraps: Each* | | | |
| Chicken Tender Po'Boy: Blackened | 580 | 32 | 39 |
| Spicy/Mild | 600 | 33 | 55 |
| Cajun Fish Po'Boy | 750 | 52 | 75 |
| Catfish Po'Boy | 800 | 51 | 59 |
| Loaded Chicken Wrap | 310 | 12 | 35 |
| Popcorn Shrimp Po' Boy | 660 | 41 | 61 |
| *Seafood:* Catfish Fillets, 2 pieces | 460 | 29 | 27 |
| Butterfly Shrimp (8) | 420 | 25 | 34 |
| Popcorn Shrimp, 4 oz | 390 | 25 | 28 |

## Popeye's® cont... (Sept '19)

*Sides:*

| | C | F | Cb |
|---|---|---|---|
| Biscuit | 205 | 13 | 20 |
| Cajun Fries, regular | 270 | 14 | 33 |
| Cajun Rice, regular | 185 | 6 | 24 |
| Cole Slaw, regular | 140 | 10 | 12 |
| Corn on the Cob (1) | 210 | 6 | 34 |
| Mashed Potatoes, w/ Cajun Gravy | 110 | 4 | 18 |
| Onion Rings, regular | 280 | 19 | 25 |
| Red Beans & Rice, regular | 245 | 16 | 22 |
| *Breakfast:* | | | |
| **Biscuits:** Bacon | 400 | 25 | 37 |
| Chicken | 490 | 26 | 47 |
| Egg | 510 | 29 | 41 |
| Egg & Sausage | 690 | 45 | 43 |
| Sausage | 540 | 36 | 41 |
| Sausage & Gravy | 510 | 33 | 42 |
| Grits | 370 | 5 | 80 |
| Hash Rounds | 360 | 20 | 41 |
| *Desserts:* | | | |
| Hot Sweet Potato Pie 3.4 oz | 350 | 19 | 41 |
| Mardi Gras Cheesecake, 3 oz | 320 | 21 | 29 |
| Mississippi Mud Pie, 3 oz | 260 | 7 | 50 |
| Sliced Pecan Pie, 3.4 oz | 410 | 21 | 52 |

## Port of Subs® (Sept '19)

*Figures Based on West Coast Outlets*

*Classic Subs: Per 8" White Sub with Standard Menu Components*

| | C | F | Cb |
|---|---|---|---|
| #1 Ham, Salami, Capicolla, Pepperoni, Provolone | 630 | 26 | 64 |
| #2 Ham & Turkey, Provolone | 540 | 15 | 65 |
| #3 Salami & Turkey, Provolone | 580 | 20 | 65 |
| #4 Ham, Salami, Provolone | 550 | 20 | 63 |
| #5 Smoked Ham, Turkey, Cheddar | 580 | 17 | 65 |
| #6 Vegetarian, 3 Chse | 670 | 34 | 68 |
| #7 Roast Beef, Prov. | 540 | 14 | 61 |
| #8 Turkey, Provolone | 560 | 15 | 66 |
| #10 Rstd Chicken Breast, Provolone | 530 | 14 | 64 |
| #11 Ham, American Cheese | 530 | 16 | 64 |
| #12 Salami, Provolone | 590 | 25 | 63 |
| #13 Pepprd Pastrami Turkey, Swiss | 560 | 15 | 65 |
| #15 Salami, Pepperoni, Provolone | 600 | 27 | 63 |
| #16 Chkn, Pepperoni, Pepper Jack | 580 | 22 | 63 |
| #17 Tuna, Provolone | 700 | 29 | 65 |
| #18 Roast Beef, Turkey, Provolone | 550 | 14 | 64 |

## Port of Subs® cont... (Sept '19)

*Figures Based on West Coast Outlets* **C** **F** **Cb**

*Hot Subs: Per 8" White Sub with Provolone & Standard Menu Components*

| | C | F | Cb |
|---|---|---|---|
| BLT | 740 | 38 | 67 |
| **Grilled:** Buffalo Chicken | 590 | 13 | 60 |
| Chicken | 590 | 13 | 60 |
| Teriyaki Chicken | 670 | 13 | 77 |
| Hot Pastrami | 780 | 39 | 64 |
| Meatball | 940 | 48 | 78 |
| NY Steak | 650 | 28 | 59 |

*Flatbreads: With Provolone without Sauce*

| | C | F | Cb |
|---|---|---|---|
| BLT, without sauce | 470 | 26 | 38 |
| Grilled Chicken | 420 | 11 | 35 |
| Hot Pastrami | 550 | 30 | 37 |
| Meatball | 530 | 28 | 43 |
| NY Steak | 450 | 22 | 33 |

*Wraps: On Wheat Wrap with Povolone & Standard Menu Components*

| | C | F | Cb |
|---|---|---|---|
| BLT | 800 | 46 | 65 |
| Grilled Chicken Caesar | 670 | 25 | 60 |
| Hot Pastrami | 850 | 47 | 62 |

*Fresh Salads: Without Dressing*

| | C | F | Cb |
|---|---|---|---|
| Caesar | 70 | 2.5 | 10 |
| Chef | 260 | 15 | 13 |
| Garden | 70 | 2.5 | 10 |
| Grilled Chicken; Gr. Chckn Spinach | 280 | 7 | 11 |
| Gr. Chicken Caesar | 290 | 7 | 12 |
| Spinach | 60 | 2.5 | 8 |
| Tuna | 360 | 20 | 13 |

*Salad Dressings: Per 2 fl.oz*

| | C | F | Cb |
|---|---|---|---|
| Caesar | 220 | 22 | 4 |
| Honey Mustard | 260 | 26 | 10 |
| Ranch | 220 | 24 | 2 |

*Sides: Per Regular, 8 oz*

| | C | F | Cb |
|---|---|---|---|
| Macaroni Salad | 520 | 36 | 44 |
| Potato Salad | 370 | 20 | 45 |

*Soup:* Boston Clam Chowder, small

| | C | F | Cb |
|---|---|---|---|
| Boston Clam Chowder, small | 200 | 9 | 22 |
| Chicken & Wild Rice, small | 190 | 8 | 21 |
| Chicken Noodle, small | 90 | 2.5 | 12 |
| Cream of Broccoli, small | 200 | 12 | 17 |
| New England Clam Chowder, small | 180 | 7 | 22 |

*Breakfast Sub: With American Cheese & Egg*

**5" Wheat Bread:**

| | C | F | Cb |
|---|---|---|---|
| Peppered Bacon | 470 | 23 | 40 |
| Smoked Ham | 390 | 15 | 39 |
| Turkey Sausage | 480 | 22 | 38 |

**Flatbread:** Peppered Bacon

| | C | F | Cb |
|---|---|---|---|
| Peppered Bacon | 480 | 25 | 37 |
| Smoked Ham | 400 | 17 | 35 |
| Turkey Sausage | 490 | 24 | 35 |

*Desserts:*

| | C | F | Cb |
|---|---|---|---|
| Brownie | 760 | 36 | 109 |
| Chocolate Chunk Cookie, 4 oz | 500 | 23 | 71 |
| Oatmeal Raisin Cookie, 4 oz | 480 | 20 | 69 |
| White Choc.Macadamia Nut Cookie | 530 | 26 | 67 |

## Pret A Manger® (Sept '19)

*East Coast Outlets.* **C** **F** **Cb**

*Baguettes:*

| | C | F | Cb |
|---|---|---|---|
| Artichoke Caprese Artisan | 660 | 29 | 74 |
| Balsamic Chicken & Mozzarella | 590 | 21 | 65 |
| Ham & Cheese | 600 | 24 | 62 |

*Hot Food: Per Pack*

| | C | F | Cb |
|---|---|---|---|
| Chipotle Chicken Grain Bowl | 530 | 13 | 79 |
| Spinach & Tomato Mac & Cheese | 670 | 24 | 89 |

*Pots:* Banana & Honey

| | C | F | Cb |
|---|---|---|---|
| Banana & Honey | 350 | 11 | 53 |
| Blueberry & Granola | 340 | 13 | 37 |
| Little Cup of Goodness | 300 | 10 | 37 |
| Sunshine Bowl | 390 | 12 | 63 |

*Sandwiches:*

| | C | F | Cb |
|---|---|---|---|
| Balsamic Chicken & Avocado | 480 | 24 | 46 |
| California Club | 410 | 16 | 46 |
| Cheddar & Tomato | 440 | 25 | 41 |
| Chicken & Bacon | 550 | 32 | 41 |
| Egg Salad & Arugula | 430 | 25 | 37 |
| Tuna Salad | 480 | 27 | 38 |

*Soups: Per Small*

| | C | F | Cb |
|---|---|---|---|
| Chicken Pozole | 140 | 4 | 16 |
| Moroccan Lentil | 190 | 12 | 19 |
| Pumpkin Bisque | 140 | 9 | 16 |
| Tomato Feta | 130 | 7 | 13 |

*Salads: With Set Dressing*

| | C | F | Cb |
|---|---|---|---|
| Chef | 530 | 41 | 14 |
| Chicken Avocado | 680 | 51 | 32 |
| Kale Chicken Caesar | 640 | 49 | 14 |
| Salmon Cobb | 550 | 45 | 11 |
| Veggie Fiesta | 530 | 31 | 54 |

*Breakfast:*

| | C | F | Cb |
|---|---|---|---|
| Coconut Oatmeal, w/out Toppings | 230 | 11 | 30 |
| Add Almond & Dried Cranberries | 60 | 3 | 8 |
| Egg Salad & Avocado Baguette | 440 | 24 | 43 |
| Egg White & Veggie Brioche | 330 | 13 | 35 |
| Egg & Cheddar Brioche | 370 | 17 | 32 |
| Ham & Spinach Frittata | 390 | 24 | 6 |
| Southern Breakfast Wrap | 380 | 14 | 45 |

*Bakery: Per Pack*

**Croissants:** Almond

| | C | F | Cb |
|---|---|---|---|
| Almond | 370 | 21 | 39 |
| Pain au Chocolate | 300 | 15 | 34 |
| Pain au Raisin | 390 | 20 | 46 |

**Cookies:** Carrot Cake, 2.5 oz

| | C | F | Cb |
|---|---|---|---|
| Carrot Cake, 2.5 oz | 270 | 14 | 35 |
| Chocolate Chunk, 2.5 oz | 320 | 15 | 41 |
| Harvest, 2.5 oz | 280 | 12 | 40 |

| | C | F | Cb |
|---|---|---|---|
| **Muffin,** Blueberry, 4.5 oz | 420 | 16 | 63 |

## Pretzelmaker® (Sept '19)

*Pretzels: Per Small Serving*

| | C | F | Cb |
|---|---|---|---|
| **Bites:** Salted, 6 oz | 500 | 14 | 85 |
| Cinn. Sugar, 6 oz | 530 | 14 | 90 |
| **Whole:** Plain, 4 oz | 310 | 3 | 66 |
| Cinnamon Sugar, 5 oz | 450 | 12 | 79 |
| Garlic, 5 oz | 430 | 12 | 74 |
| Parmesan, 5 oz | 450 | 15 | 66 |
| Ranch, 5 oz | 440 | 12 | 72 |
| **Pretzel Dogs:** Regular | 420 | 23 | 31 |
| Mini (8) | 430 | 29 | 33 |
| Jalapeno (1), 6 oz | 450 | 24 | 34 |

*Sauces: Per 2 oz*

| | | | |
|---|---|---|---|
| Caramel | 100 | 1 | 22 |
| Cheddar/Nacho Cheese, av. | 80 | 6 | 5 |
| Cream Cheese | 200 | 20 | 2 |
| Pizza Sauce | 30 | 1 | 6 |
| Vanilla Glaze | 170 | 0 | 42 |

*Beverages: Per 20 oz Unless Indicated*

**Blended Drinks:**

| | | | |
|---|---|---|---|
| Cool Cappuccino | 430 | 22 | 58 |
| Mango Madness | 500 | 16 | 90 |
| Mocha Mania | 580 | 22 | 94 |
| Power Pomegranate | 490 | 16 | 86 |
| Strawberry Bananza | 500 | 16 | 85 |
| **Fresh Lemonade:** Original, 20 oz | 140 | 0 | 38 |
| Strawberry; Raspberry, 20 oz, av. | 210 | 0 | 53 |

## Qdoba® (Sept '19)

| | C | F | Cb |
|---|---|---|---|

*Please Note: Nutritional Information is based on a single serving of each menu ingredient listed.*

*Burritos: Each with 12.5" Flour Tortilla, Cilantro-Lime Rice, Black Beans, Salsa Verde, Lite Sour Cream, Lettuce and Shredded Cheese*

| | | | |
|---|---|---|---|
| Marinated Grilled Chkn | 1035 | 37 | 124 |
| Pulled Pork | 1005 | 33 | 129 |
| Seasoned Ground Beef | 1055 | 40 | 124 |

*Burritos: With 12.5" Flour Tortilla, 3-Cheese Queso Pinto Beans, Roasted Chili Corn Salsa, Guacamole & Lite Sour Cream*

| | | | |
|---|---|---|---|
| Marinated Grilled Chicken | 1020 | 47 | 104 |
| Marinated Gr. Steak | 1030 | 47 | 102 |
| Pulled Pork | 990 | 43 | 109 |
| Seasoned Ground Beef | 1040 | 50 | 104 |

*Grilled Quesadillas: With 12.5" Flour Tortilla, Shredded Cheese, Pico de Gallo and Fajita Vegetables*

| | | | |
|---|---|---|---|
| Grilled Chicken | 685 | 30 | 64 |
| Pulled Pork | 655 | 26 | 60 |

*3-Cheese Nachos: Per Serving, with Tortilla Chips, 3-Cheese Queso, Salsa Roja, Guacamole & Sour Cream*

| | | | |
|---|---|---|---|
| Grilled Chicken | 1120 | 64 | 98 |
| Pulled Pork | 1090 | 60 | 103 |

## Qdoba® cont... (Sept '19)

*Knock Out Tacos:*

| | C | F | Cb |
|---|---|---|---|
| Bohemian Veg | 230 | 9 | 28 |
| Drunken Yardbird | 220 | 8 | 25 |
| Mad Rancher | 230 | 10 | 21 |
| Two Timer | 290 | 13 | 28 |
| Triple Threat | 250 | 12 | 17 |
| The Gladiator | 280 | 17 | 16 |

*Taco Salads: With Crunchy Flour Tortilla Bowl, Black Beans, Lettuce, Shredded Cheese, Brown Rice, Lite Sour Cream, Guacamole & Cilantro Lime Dressing*

| | | | |
|---|---|---|---|
| Grilled Chicken | 1270 | 66 | 116 |
| Pulled Pork | 1240 | 62 | 121 |
| Seasoned Ground Beef | 1290 | 69 | 116 |

*Chips & Dip: Includes Tortilla Chips*

| | | | |
|---|---|---|---|
| 3- Cheese Queso | 750 | 41 | 81 |
| 3-Cheese Queso, Guac. & Salsa Roja | 900 | 51 | 92 |

*Breakfast Burritos: With 12" Flour Tortilla*

**Chorizo & Seasoned Potato:**

| | | | |
|---|---|---|---|
| with 3-Cheese Queso Sauce | 820 | 40 | 80 |
| with Shred. Cheese & Salsa Roja | 820 | 38 | 79 |

## Quiznos Subs® (Sept '19)

*Subs: Per 8" Regular Japaleno Cheddar Sub, with Standard Menu Toppings Unless Indicated*

**Chicken:**

| | C | F | Cb |
|---|---|---|---|
| Apple Harvest | 790 | 32 | 97 |
| Baja | 800 | 32 | 76 |
| Carbonara | 890 | 42 | 73 |
| Honey Mustard | 850 | 36 | 80 |
| Mesquite | 800 | 33 | 73 |
| Southwest Chicken | 860 | 45 | 73 |

**Steak:**

| | | | |
|---|---|---|---|
| Black Angus Steak, On Rosemary Parmesan | 780 | 27 | 88 |
| Chipotle Steak & Cheddar | 840 | 44 | 73 |
| French Dip | 760 | 30 | 79 |
| Peppercorn Steak | 840 | 42 | 76 |

**Deli Classic:**

| | | | |
|---|---|---|---|
| Classic Italian | 920 | 50 | 77 |
| Spicy Monterey | 600 | 15 | 81 |
| Tuna Melt | 660 | 22 | 76 |
| Turkey Ranch & Swiss | 670 | 25 | 73 |
| Veggie Guacamole | 810 | 44 | 81 |

*Salads: Per Full Size*

| | | | |
|---|---|---|---|
| Apple Harvest Chkn | 590 | 39 | 40 |
| Carbonara | 700 | 51 | 15 |
| Chipotle Steak & Cheddar | 670 | 56 | 13 |
| French Dip | 530 | 34 | 22 |
| Honey Mustard Chkicken | 650 | 43 | 22 |
| Peppercorn Steak | 680 | 55 | 16 |

*continued next page...*

## Quiznos Subs® cont... (Sept '19)

| Savory Soups: Per Regular | C | F | Cb |
|---|---|---|---|
| Broccoli Cheese | 220 | 14 | 18 |
| Chicken Noodle | 120 | 4 | 14 |
| Chili | 290 | 10 | 34 |
| Tomato Bisque | 290 | 21 | 21 |
| *Breakfast:* | | | |
| Biscuit: Egg & Cheddar | 460 | 31 | 31 |
| Sausage, Egg & Cheddar | 630 | 48 | 31 |
| *Subs:* | | | |
| Bacon, Egg & Cheddar | 370 | 17 | 34 |
| Ham, Egg & Cheddar | 340 | 14 | 36 |
| Sausage, Egg & Cheddar | 550 | 37 | 35 |
| *Desserts:* Choc Brownie | 350 | 18 | 46 |
| Chocolate Chunk Cookie | 390 | 19 | 54 |
| Cinnamon Sugar Cookie | 400 | 17 | 58 |
| Oatmeal Raisin Cookie | 360 | 12 | 58 |

## Rally's/Checkers® (Sept '19)

| Burgers/Sandwiches: | C | F | Cb |
|---|---|---|---|
| Bacon Roadhouse | 680 | 47 | 37 |
| Baconzilla | 910 | 62 | 43 |
| Big Buford | 660 | 39 | 39 |
| Cheese Champ | 430 | 21 | 39 |
| Cheese Double | 480 | 25 | 38 |
| *Classic Wings:* Buffalo, 5 pieces | 360 | 23 | 3 |
| Honey BBQ, 5 pieces | 430 | 23 | 19 |
| Garlic Parmesan, 5 pieces | 510 | 40 | 3 |
| *Fries:* | | | |
| Fries, medium | 500 | 24 | 63 |
| Chili Cheese | 590 | 30 | 72 |
| Fully Loaded | 870 | 56 | 72 |

## Ranch One® (Sept '19)

| Sandwiches: | C | F | Cb |
|---|---|---|---|
| Chicken & Cheese | 390 | 12 | 40 |
| Chkn Philly, 9.3 oz | 410 | 13 | 40 |
| Grilled Classic Chicken, 9.4 oz | 680 | 47 | 37 |
| Original Crispy Chicken, 11.5 oz | 640 | 31 | 60 |
| *Other Favorites:* | | | |
| Chicken Fajitas, 10 oz | 540 | 24 | 53 |
| Chicken Platter, with Rice, 11.9 oz | 270 | 6 | 28 |
| Popcorn Chicken: | | | |
| Small, 5.5 oz | 310 | 10 | 30 |
| Large, 7.5 oz | 420 | 14 | 40 |
| *Salads:* Completed | | | |
| Grilled Chicken Caesar, 13.3 oz | 430 | 30 | 14 |
| Southwest Chicken, 17.5 oz | 680 | 43 | 44 |
| *Fries:* | | | |
| Medium, 5.8 oz | 380 | 19 | 43 |
| Large, 10.9 oz | 530 | 27 | 58 |
| Cheese Fries: Medium, 7.3 oz | 490 | 27 | 46 |
| Large, 11 oz | 760 | 44 | 66 |

## Red Hot & Blue® (Sept '19)

| Starters: | C | F | Cb |
|---|---|---|---|
| Catfish Fingers | 590 | 19 | 75 |
| Nachos, with Chili | 1005 | 51 | 103 |
| Shakin' Bacon Cheese Fries | 2440 | 60 | 106 |
| *Burgers:* | | | |
| ALL IN | 915 | 52 | 46 |
| Classic Blues | 665 | 32 | 44 |
| *Ribs, Full Slab:* | | | |
| Dry | 1870 | 144 | 28 |
| Sweet | 1895 | 142 | 44 |
| *Favorite Entrees:* Delta Catfish | 835 | 42 | 57 |
| Delta Surf & Turf | 1025 | 68 | 38 |
| Southern Fried Chicken Crispers | 760 | 35 | 50 |
| Rib & Crispers Platter | 1060 | 68 | 39 |
| *BBQ Platters:* Five Meat | 935 | 63 | 15 |
| Delta Double with Memphis Chkn | 900 | 54 | 12 |
| Pulled Pork | 325 | 21 | 7 |
| Smoked Sausage | 965 | 68 | 36 |
| *Sandwiches:* | | | |
| Fried Delta Catfish | 655 | 25 | 71 |
| Grilled Chicken | 360 | 6 | 40 |
| Pulled Pork | 370 | 15 | 37 |
| Ribwich Combo | 685 | 39 | 42 |
| *Sides:* BBQ Beans | 255 | 2 | 48 |
| Collard Greens | 50 | 2 | 7 |
| Fried Ocra | 190 | 8 | 29 |
| Mashed Potatoes, with gravy | 310 | 14 | 44 |
| Memphis Fries, 6 oz | 345 | 19 | 38 |
| Potato Salad | 405 | 28 | 33 |
| Sweet Potato | 495 | 0 | 114 |
| Sweet Potato Fries | 375 | 19 | 49 |
| *Salads:* Grilled Chicken Caesar | 770 | 46 | 47 |
| Southern Fried Chicken | 710 | 31 | 60 |

## Red Lobster® (Sept '19)

| Seaside Starters: As Served | C | F | Cb |
|---|---|---|---|
| Fried Oysters | 620 | 26 | 76 |
| Lobster & Langostino Pizza | 700 | 35 | 59 |
| Mozzarella Cheesesticks | 700 | 40 | 56 |
| Oysters Half Shell (12), raw | 530 | 11 | 85 |
| Parrot Isle Jumbo Cocktail Shrimp | 610 | 39 | 52 |
| Seafood Stuffed Mushrooms | 390 | 22 | 18 |
| Signature Jumbo Shrimp Cocktail | 130 | 0 | 11 |
| Sweet Chili Shrimp | 960 | 66 | 68 |
| *Land & Sea:* With Menu Set Sides & Sauce | | | |
| Cajun Chicken Linguini, full | 1340 | 60 | 116 |
| Maple Glazed Chicken Dinner | 490 | 7 | 51 |
| Rock Lobster & NY Strip (12 oz) | 1250 | 83 | 27 |
| Steak: Grilled Filet Mignon (6 oz) | 460 | 23 | 26 |
| Grilled Sirloin (7 oz) | 480 | 22 | 26 |
| Wood-Grilled Shrimp & Sirloin | 560 | 25 | 27 |

*continued next page...*

## Red Lobster® cont... (Sept '19)

*Lunch Classics:*

*With Menu Fixed Sides & Dipping Sauce*

| | C | F | Cb |
|---|---|---|---|
| Cajun Chicken Linguini, half order | 690 | 30 | 62 |
| Crab Linguini Alfredo, half order | 610 | 28 | 57 |
| Crunchy Popcorn Shrimp | 430 | 19 | 49 |
| Farm-Raised Catfish, Blackened | 210 | 10 | 2 |
| Garlic Shrimp Scampi | 220 | 18 | 3 |
| Hand Breaded Shrimp | 240 | 11 | 23 |
| Maple Glazed Chkn | 360 | 5 | 50 |
| Sailor's Platter | 450 | 18 | 18 |

**Wild Caught Flounder:**

| | | | |
|---|---|---|---|
| Golden Fried | 710 | 50 | 38 |
| Oven Broiled | 210 | 5 | 1 |

*Savor The Sea:*

| | | | |
|---|---|---|---|
| Bar Harbour Lobster Bake | 1250 | 56 | 106 |
| Seafarer's Feast | 1140 | 73 | 69 |
| Seaside Shrimp Trio | 1100 | 58 | 94 |
| Ultimate Feast | 1120 | 69 | 68 |

*Sides:*

| | | | |
|---|---|---|---|
| Baked Potato, Plain | 210 | 2 | 45 |
| Broccoli | 40 | 0 | 8 |
| Cheddar Bay Biscuit | 160 | 10 | 16 |
| Coleslaw | 150 | 10 | 13 |
| Creamy Lobster Mashed Potatoes | 330 | 18 | 31 |
| French Fries | 290 | 12 | 42 |
| Garden Salad, without dressing | 100 | 5 | 10 |
| Mashed Potatoes | 190 | 9 | 24 |
| Rice Pilaf | 160 | 3 | 30 |
| Tomato Mozzarella Caprese | 160 | 11 | 9 |

*Salads:*

**Caesar Salad:** *With Caesar Dressing*

| | | | |
|---|---|---|---|
| with Gr. Chicken | 640 | 48 | 19 |
| with Gr. Shrimp | 610 | 50 | 18 |
| With Salmon | 830 | 65 | 18 |

*Sauces:* 100% Pure Melted Butter 300 33 0

| | | | |
|---|---|---|---|
| Blue Cheese Dressing | 230 | 24 | 2 |
| Caesar Dressing | 300 | 32 | 0 |
| Cocktail Sauce | 45 | 0 | 11 |
| Honey Mustard Dressing | 200 | 18 | 9 |
| Marinara Sauce | 35 | 2 | 4 |

*Desserts:*

| | | | |
|---|---|---|---|
| Brownie Overload | 1020 | 57 | 121 |
| Chocolate Wave | 1110 | 62 | 134 |
| Key Lime Pie | 400 | 14 | 59 |
| Warm Apple Crostada | 590 | 30 | 74 |

**For Complete Nutritional Data ~ see CalorieKing.com**

## Red Robin® (Sept '19)

*Nutritional Information varies between restaurants. Please refer to Red Robin's website for further information.*

*Appetizers:*

| | C | F | Cb |
|---|---|---|---|
| Creamy Artichoke & Spinach Dip | 820 | 44 | 71 |
| Fried Pickle Nickels | 750 | 52 | 61 |
| Guacamole, Salsa & Chips | 720 | 35 | 74 |
| NachO M.G. | 1390 | 74 | 115 |
| Pretzel Bites | 810 | 40 | 95 |
| The O-Ring Shorty | 920 | 58 | 92 |
| Towering Onion Rings | 1310 | 59 | 178 |
| Voodoo Fries, with Ranch Sauce | 1060 | 54 | 121 |

*Jump Starters:* *Without Dressing*

| | | | |
|---|---|---|---|
| Cheese Sticks | 550 | 30 | 43 |
| Fresh Fried Mshrms | 420 | 23 | 53 |
| Fried Jalapeono Coins | 560 | 41 | 38 |
| Sweet Potato Fries | 380 | 15 | 59 |

**Wings:** Bone In Bar with Buzz Sauce 1240 85 26

| | | | |
|---|---|---|---|
| with Banzai Sauce | 1180 | 67 | 50 |
| with Whisky River Sauce | 1240 | 73 | 53 |

*Entrées:* *With Menu Set Sides*

| | | | |
|---|---|---|---|
| Arctic Cod Fish & Steak Fries | 1520 | 89 | 136 |
| Clucks & Fries | 1340 | 82 | 104 |
| Ensenada Chicken Platter | 490 | 20 | 27 |
| Prime Rib Dip | 860 | 43 | 59 |
| Sear-ious Salmon | 470 | 37 | 9 |
| Shrimp & Cod Duo | 1110 | 67 | 94 |

*Burgers:* *Without Fries or other Options*

**Finest:** Black & Bleu 970 61 53

| | | | |
|---|---|---|---|
| Citrus Harissa Salmon | 940 | 67 | 50 |
| The MadLove | 1140 | 63 | 72 |
| The Southern Charm | 1220 | 72 | 80 |

**Fire Grilled Burgers:** Bleu Ribbon 1140 5 67

| | | | |
|---|---|---|---|
| Burnin' Love | 910 | 59 | 56 |
| Chili Chili Chseburger | 860 | 47 | 56 |
| Guacamole Bacon | 930 | 58 | 51 |
| Keep It Simple, Beef | 530 | 24 | 44 |
| Prime Chophouse | 1040 | 57 | 82 |
| Red Robin Gourmet Cheeseburger | 770 | 47 | 47 |
| Royal Red Robin | 1110 | 78 | 48 |
| Sauteed 'Shroom | 770 | 40 | 53 |
| Whiskey River BBQ | 1130 | 74 | 71 |

**Tavern Menu Burgers:** Big Ghost 700 35 53

| | | | |
|---|---|---|---|
| Big Pig Out | 1080 | 70 | 62 |
| Four Cheese Melt | 720 | 42 | 51 |
| Haystack Double | 680 | 43 | 37 |
| The Big Cowboy Ranch | 810 | 4 | 57 |

## Red Robin® cont... (June'19)

### S'wiches & Wraps: W/out Sides

| | C | F | Cb |
|---|---|---|---|
| BLTA Croissant | 680 | 41 | 50 |
| Caesars Chkn Wrap | 820 | 50 | 59 |
| Nacho Chicken Bacon Wrap | 1160 | 70 | 82 |
| Whiskey River BBQ Chicken Wrap | 1020 | 58 | 79 |
| Wrappin' California Club | 1000 | 64 | 64 |

### Soups:

| | C | F | Cb |
|---|---|---|---|
| Baked Potato: 1 cup | 260 | 15 | 23 |
| 1 Bowl | 460 | 29 | 39 |
| Clam Chowder: With Slice Garlic Toast | | | |
| 1 Cup | 230 | 13 | 19 |
| 1 Bowl | 420 | 26 | 32 |
| French Onion: With Slice Garlic Toast | | | |
| 1 Cup | 210 | 11 | 15 |
| 1 Bowl | 380 | 22 | 23 |

### Salads: Without Dressing Unless Indicated

| | C | F | Cb |
|---|---|---|---|
| Avo-Cobb-O | 560 | 28 | 34 |
| Crispy Chicken Tender | 910 | 50 | 66 |
| Mighty Caesar, with Caesar Drssng | 670 | 51 | 24 |
| Simply Grilled Chicken | 320 | 9 | 29 |
| Southwest | 940 | 64 | 50 |

### Sides: Chili Chili Cheese Fries

| | C | F | Cb |
|---|---|---|---|
| | 900 | 60 | 64 |
| Coleslaw | 210 | 15 | 17 |
| Mac 'n' Cheese | 290 | 16 | 25 |
| Onion Rings | 280 | 1 | 61 |
| Steamed Broccoli | 30 | 0 | 6 |
| Steak Fries | 210 | 9 | 29 |

### Desserts:

| | C | F | Cb |
|---|---|---|---|
| Gooey Chocolate Brownie Cake | 950 | 37 | 150 |
| Mountain High Mudd Pie | 1360 | 59 | 193 |

## Roly Poly® (Sept '19)

### Wraps:
*Per 6" White Tortilla Unless Indicated*

| | C | F | Cb |
|---|---|---|---|
| Chicken: Basil Cashew Chicken | 300 | 10 | 30 |
| Chicken Caesar | 310 | 11 | 30 |
| Chicken Fajita | 315 | 9 | 28 |
| Santa Fe Chicken | 305 | 11 | 28 |
| Beef/Ham: Philly Melt | 280 | 11 | 25 |
| Ranch Roast | 320 | 15 | 28 |
| Tuna: Classic Tuna Melt | 340 | 17 | 26 |
| Popeyes Tuna on Wheat | 305 | 10 | 31 |
| Texas/Thai Hot Tuna, average | 300 | 11 | 30 |
| Turkey: Applejack | 320 | 12 | 30 |
| California | 330 | 12 | 30 |
| Veggie & Cheese: | | | |
| California Humer | 305 | 13 | 32 |
| Nutty Avocado on Wheat Tortilla | 265 | 12 | 35 |

### Salads: Without Dressing

| | C | F | Cb |
|---|---|---|---|
| Alpine Chef | 315 | 15 | 13 |
| Chipotle Caesar | 520 | 25 | 21 |
| Just Veggies | 95 | 0 | 19 |
| Walnut Spinach | 420 | 33 | 14 |

## Round Table Pizza® (Sept '19)

### Appetizers:

| | C | F | Cb |
|---|---|---|---|
| Boneless Wings, Oven Roasted: | | | |
| with BBQ Sauce (1) | 100 | 2 | 13 |
| with Buffalo Sauce (1) | 90 | 3.5 | 8 |
| Garlic Bread: 1 piece | 70 | 3.5 | 9 |
| with Cheese, 1 piece | 110 | 6 | 9 |
| Garlic Parmesan Twists, 1 twist | 170 | 5 | 25 |

### Pizzas: Per ½ of Large 14" Pizza

| | C | F | Cb |
|---|---|---|---|
| Original Crust: Cheese | 230 | 10 | 24 |
| Gourmet Veggie | 230 | 10 | 25 |
| Guinevere's Garden Delight | 220 | 8 | 26 |
| Hawaiian | 220 | 8 | 27 |
| Italian Garlic Supreme | 270 | 14 | 24 |
| King Arthur Supreme | 270 | 13 | 26 |
| Maui Zaui, with Polynesian Sce | 260 | 10 | 29 |
| Montague's All Meat Marvel | 290 | 15 | 24 |
| Smokehouse Combo, Pepperoni | 290 | 14 | 27 |
| Triple Play Pepperoni | 250 | 12 | 24 |
| Pan Crust: Cheese | 280 | 10 | 35 |
| Gourmet: Chkn & Garlic | 290 | 10 | 35 |
| Veggie | 280 | 10 | 35 |
| Guinevere's Garden Delight | 270 | 9 | 36 |
| Hawaiian | 280 | 8 | 37 |
| Italian Garlic Supreme | 320 | 14 | 35 |
| King Arthur Supreme | 320 | 13 | 35 |
| Maui Zaui w/ Polynesian Sauce | 340 | 12 | 41 |
| Montague's All Meat Marvel | 340 | 16 | 35 |
| Smokehouse Combo, Chicken | 350 | 12 | 37 |
| Triple Play Pepperoni | 330 | 14 | 36 |
| Skinny Crust: Cheese | 210 | 10 | 19 |
| Gourmet: Chkn & Garlic | 220 | 11 | 19 |
| Gourmet Veggie | 210 | 10 | 20 |
| Guinevere's Garden Delight | 200 | 9 | 21 |
| Hawaiian | 210 | 8 | 22 |
| Italian Garlic Supreme | 260 | 15 | 19 |
| King Arthur Supreme | 260 | 14 | 21 |
| Maui Zaui w/ Polynesian Sauce | 240 | 11 | 23 |
| Montague's All Meat Marvel | 290 | 17 | 20 |
| Smokehouse Combo, Chicken | 260 | 12 | 22 |
| Triple Play Pepperoni | 240 | 13 | 19 |

### Sandwiches: Chicken Club

| | C | F | Cb |
|---|---|---|---|
| | 670 | 27 | 58 |
| Ham Club | 670 | 30 | 59 |
| Italian Meats | 840 | 49 | 59 |
| Meatball | 750 | 37 | 70 |
| RT Pizza Veggie | 550 | 21 | 62 |
| Turkey Club | 650 | 27 | 59 |
| Tukey Pesto | 710 | 37 | 56 |
| Turkey Sante-Fe | 730 | 40 | 51 |

*For Complete Nutritional Data ~ see CalorieKing.com*

**233**

## Rubio's Coastal Grill® (Sept '19)

*Burritos:* Flour Tortilla, w/o Chips

| | C | F | Cb |
|---|---|---|---|
| **Beef:** California, with Steak | 1120 | 63 | 88 |
| Especial, with Steak | 930 | 39 | 103 |
| **Chicken:** Especial, with Chicken | 880 | 34 | 105 |
| **Seafood:** Ancho Shrimp | 830 | 34 | 103 |
| Beer Battered Fish | 890 | 55 | 75 |
| Classic Grilled Shrimp | 720 | 34 | 73 |
| Grilled Wild Mahi Mahi | 740 | 34 | 75 |
| Shrimp & Bacon | 920 | 51 | 75 |
| Wild Alaska Coho Salmon | 740 | 35 | 78 |

*Tacos:* With Corn Tortilla Unless Indicated

| | C | F | Cb |
|---|---|---|---|
| **Chicken, Grilled:** Classic | 250 | 12 | 21 |
| Gourmet | 350 | 19 | 22 |
| Street | 100 | 3 | 10 |
| **Seafood, Grilled:** Cocktail Trio | 840 | 46 | 72 |
| House Blackened: Mahi Mahi | 240 | 10 | 24 |
| Wild Gropher | 280 | 14 | 25 |
| Mango Wild Mahi Mahi, Flour Tortilla | 280 | 15 | 24 |
| Salsa Verde Shrimp, Flour Tortilla | 290 | 17 | 23 |
| Wild Alask. Salmon | 230 | 10 | 23 |
| Wild Mahi Mahi | 230 | 9 | 22 |
| **Steak, Grilled:** Classic | 270 | 14 | 20 |
| Gourmet | 370 | 21 | 22 |
| Street | 120 | 5 | 9 |

*Sides:*

| | C | F | Cb |
|---|---|---|---|
| **Black Beans:** Reg., 4 oz | 100 | 2 | 15 |
| Large, 9.4 oz | 280 | 3 | 46 |
| **Citrus Rice:** Reg., 2.3 oz | 100 | 2 | 21 |
| Large, 6 oz | 270 | 4 | 55 |
| **Mexican Rice:** Regular, 2.3 oz | 100 | 2 | 20 |
| Large, 6 oz | 270 | 4 | 53 |
| **No Fried Pinto Beans:** Reg., 4 oz | 110 | 1 | 17 |
| Large, 10.9 oz | 300 | 2 | 51 |
| **Tortilla Chips:** Regular, 1.8 oz | 210 | 3 | 43 |
| Large, 4 oz | 460 | 5 | 96 |
| **Salsas,** average all types | 10 | 0 | 2 |

*Salad & Bowls:* Entrée Size, Includes Dressing

| | C | F | Cb |
|---|---|---|---|
| California Bowl, Chkn Salsa Verde | 670 | 23 | 83 |
| Chipotle Orange Shrimp Salad | 430 | 26 | 38 |
| **Chopped Salad with:** | | | |
| Blackened Coho Salmon | 520 | 34 | 25 |
| Grilled Chicken | 490 | 32 | 21 |
| Grilled Mahi Mahi | 490 | 33 | 19 |
| Grilled Veggies | 450 | 33 | 30 |
| Pan Seared Shrimp | 440 | 34 | 19 |

## Ruby Tuesday® (Sept '19)

*Shareables:* As Served

| | C | F | Cb |
|---|---|---|---|
| Crispy B'milk Chicken Bites, classic | 705 | 38 | 37 |
| Shrimp Fondu, with Chips | 1170 | 66 | 100 |
| Spinach Artichoke Dip, with Chips | 900 | 57 | 72 |
| Tater Totchos | 1450 | 94 | 94 |

*Burgers:* With Fries Unless Indicated

| | C | F | Cb |
|---|---|---|---|
| Bacon Cheeseburger, w/o fries | 815 | 47 | 36 |
| Classic | 665 | 35 | 36 |
| Classic Cheeseburger, w/o fries | 720 | 39 | 36 |
| Hickory Bourbon Bacon | 945 | 53 | 45 |
| Mushroom & Swiss | 870 | 50 | 40 |
| Smokehouse | 975 | 52 | 61 |

*Lunch/Dinner Entrees:* Without Sides

| | C | F | Cb |
|---|---|---|---|
| **Chicken:** Asiago Bacon | 480 | 27 | 9 |
| Parmesan | 1525 | 69 | 135 |
| Fresco | 370 | 22 | 2 |
| Hickory Bourbon | 250 | 5 | 18 |
| **Pasta:** | | | |
| Cajun Chicken & Shrimp | 600 | 21 | 40 |
| Chicken & Broccoli | 1395 | 81 | 101 |
| Parmesan Shrimp Pasta | 505 | 20 | 48 |
| **Ribs & Chops:** | | | |
| Hickory Boubon Pork Chop | 570 | 22 | 23 |
| Classic BBQ Ribs: Half Rack | 470 | 22 | 21 |
| Full Rack | 940 | 47 | 42 |
| Texas Dusted Ribs: Half Rack | 590 | 33 | 24 |
| Full Rack | 1100 | 68 | 30 |
| **Seafood:** | | | |
| Grilled Salmon | 490 | 30 | 0 |
| Blackened Tilapia | 205 | 6 | 2 |
| Hickory Bourbon Salmon | 575 | 30 | 18 |
| New Orleans Seafood | 345 | 14 | 4 |
| **Steak:** New York Strip, 10 oz | 565 | 40 | 0 |
| Hickory B'rbon Bacon Sirloin, 6 oz | 285 | 7 | 12 |
| Ribeye, 12 oz | 760 | 55 | 1 |
| Top Sirloin, 8 oz | 420 | 22 | 2 |

*Lunch Combos:*

| | C | F | Cb |
|---|---|---|---|
| Chicken Quesadilla | 850 | 41 | 46 |
| **Sandwiches:** | | | |
| Crispy Chicken & Pimento | 1095 | 64 | 75 |
| Spicy Crispy Chicken & Pimento | 1445 | 100 | 80 |
| **Sliders:** | | | |
| Classic Cheese: with Fries | 790 | 41 | 70 |
| with Tater Tots | 745 | 38 | 65 |
| Crispy Chicken Club: with Fries | 845 | 42 | 78 |
| with Tater Tots | 800 | 39 | 73 |
| **Salads:** Caesar w/ drssng | 590 | 52 | 17 |
| Garden without dressing | 265 | 18 | 13 |
| **Soup:** Broccoli Cheese | 260 | 18 | 17 |
| Garden Vegetable | 85 | 1 | 16 |
| Roasted Tomato | 270 | 14 | 24 |
| Turkey Burger | 650 | 35 | 36 |

Updated Nutrition Data ~ www.CalorieKing.com
Persons with Diabetes ~ See Disclaimer (Page 22)

## Ruby Tuesday® cont... (Sept '19)

*Sandwiches: Without French Fries*

| | C | F | Cb |
|---|---|---|---|
| Avocado Grilled Chicken | 710 | 35 | 38 |
| Avocado Turkey Burger | 825 | 49 | 38 |
| Cajun Chicken | 810 | 41 | 49 |
| **Crispy Chicken:** Original | 1715 | 31 | 67 |
| with Pimentos | 1095 | 64 | 75 |
| Spicy | 1060 | 67 | 72 |
| with Pimentos | 1445 | 100 | 80 |

*Sides:*

| | C | F | Cb |
|---|---|---|---|
| Braised Green Beans | 50 | 2 | 6 |
| Caesar Salad, with Caesar Dressing | 590 | 52 | 17 |
| Coleslaw | 125 | 8 | 9 |
| Dirty Rice | 240 | 7 | 28 |
| French Fries | 505 | 24 | 63 |
| Fresh: Baked Potato | 250 | 3 | 51 |
| Grilled Zucchini | 20 | 0 | 2 |
| Steamed Broccoli | 45 | 1 | 4 |
| Garden Salad, without Dressing | 265 | 18 | 13 |
| Hush Puppies with BBQ Ranch | 290 | 11 | 38 |
| Loaded Baked Potato | 560 | 27 | 51 |
| Mac 'N Cheese | 560 | 29 | 46 |
| Mashed Potatoes | 295 | 16 | 32 |
| Onion Rings | 340 | 19 | 37 |
| Rice Pilaf | 190 | 1 | 40 |
| Southern Green Beans | 130 | 6 | 10 |
| Sweet Potato Fries | 445 | 23 | 55 |
| Tater Tots | 365 | 16 | 45 |

*Salads: With Dressing*

| | C | F | Cb |
|---|---|---|---|
| BBQ Chicken Cobb | 625 | 31 | 25 |
| Crispy Chkn Ranch | 1030 | 67 | 56 |
| Grilled Chkn Caesar | 855 | 53 | 33 |

*Soups:* Broccoli & Cheese

| | C | F | Cb |
|---|---|---|---|
| Broccoli & Cheese | 260 | 18 | 17 |
| Garden Vegetable | 85 | 1 | 16 |
| Roasted Tomato | 270 | 14 | 24 |

*Desserts: As Served*

| | C | F | Cb |
|---|---|---|---|
| Apple Crumble Skillet | 875 | 46 | 103 |
| Cake: Caramel Crunch | 760 | 37 | 99 |
| Chocolate Fall | 1375 | 59 | 180 |
| Key Lime | 765 | 44 | 86 |
| Molten Chocolate Lava | 620 | 31 | 76 |
| Oreo Cookies & Cream | 725 | 32 | 95 |
| New York Cheesecake | 975 | 61 | 90 |
| New York Choc. Chip Cookie Skillet | 1350 | 69 | 172 |

*For Complete Menu ~ see CalorieKing.com*

## Runza® (Sept '19)

*Burgers:*

| | C | F | Cb |
|---|---|---|---|
| ¼ LB: BBQ Bacon & Swiss | 530 | 32 | 26 |
| Bacon Cheeseburger | 490 | 28 | 23 |
| Cheeseburger | 410 | 22 | 23 |
| French Onion | 490 | 29 | 26 |
| Hamburger | 350 | 18 | 21 |
| Spicy Jack | 570 | 38 | 23 |
| Swiss Cheese M'shrm | 480 | 29 | 24 |

*Chicken Sandwiches:*

| | C | F | Cb |
|---|---|---|---|
| BBQ Grilled | 400 | 11 | 40 |
| Buffalo Grilled | 360 | 11 | 37 |
| Spicy Jack Grilled | 530 | 28 | 26 |
| **Wraps:** Buffalo Jr. | 330 | 17 | 32 |
| Ranch Jr. | 330 | 17 | 31 |
| *Chicken Strips,* 2 pieces | 220 | 12 | 14 |

*Runza Sandwiches:* Original

| | C | F | Cb |
|---|---|---|---|
| Original | 530 | 20 | 67 |
| Cheese Runza | 590 | 25 | 69 |
| Original Vegetarian | 530 | 9 | 94 |
| Spicy Jack Runza | 750 | 41 | 69 |
| SW Black Bean Vegetarian | 470 | 12 | 76 |
| Swiss Cheese Mushroom Runza | 620 | 28 | 68 |

*Sides:* Chili

| | C | F | Cb |
|---|---|---|---|
| Chili | 290 | 11 | 26 |
| French Fries: Small | 210 | 9 | 28 |
| Medium | 300 | 13 | 40 |
| Large | 440 | 19 | 59 |
| French Onion Dip | 70 | 5 | 3 |
| Frings, Medium | 320 | 17 | 39 |
| Onion Rings: Medium | 320 | 19 | 35 |
| Large | 550 | 31 | 58 |
| Side Salad | 20 | 0 | 4 |

*Salads: Without Dressing*

| | C | F | Cb |
|---|---|---|---|
| Southwest Chicken Salad, w/ Salsa | 360 | 18 | 32 |
| Sweet Berry Chicken | 400 | 20 | 20 |
| *Dressings:* Honey Mustard | 200 | 18 | 9 |
| SW Ranch | 220 | 24 | 4 |

*Soups: Per Bowl*

| | C | F | Cb |
|---|---|---|---|
| Boston Clam Chowder | 280 | 15 | 29 |
| Broccoli Cheese | 240 | 16 | 20 |
| Chicken Tortilla | 150 | 6 | 16 |
| Potato Bacon | 260 | 14 | 30 |
| *Kids:* Chkn Strip Meal, w/o drink | 430 | 21 | 42 |
| **Junior:** Cheeseburger, plain | 260 | 13 | 18 |
| Hamburger, plain | 200 | 9 | 16 |
| Swiss Cheese Mushroom Burger | 300 | 17 | 17 |

*Desserts:*

| | C | F | Cb |
|---|---|---|---|
| Choc. Chip Cookie | 370 | 18 | 53 |
| Ice Cream Cones, all flavors | 210 | 6 | 32 |
| Shake, Cappuccino, regular | 490 | 12 | 82 |
| **Sundaes:** Caramel; Chocolate | 300 | 7 | 51 |
| Turtle | 360 | 13 | 53 |

## 7-Eleven® (Sept '18)

*Breakfast Sandwiches:*

| | C | F | Cb |
|---|---|---|---|
| **Biscuits:** | | | |
| Sausage, 3.3 oz | 330 | 22 | 28 |
| Spicy Chicken, 4.5 oz | 270 | 14 | 30 |
| **Croissants:** | | | |
| Sausage, Egg & Cheese, 4.7 oz | 450 | 32 | 23 |
| **English Muffin:** | | | |
| Egg, Bacon & Chse, 4.5 oz | 300 | 14 | 28 |
| Egg, Cheese & Sausage, 5 oz | 390 | 25 | 24 |
| *Salads:* Per Container | | | |
| Balsamic Garden Salad, | | | |
| with Chicken, 6.5 oz | 170 | 9 | 18 |
| BLT, 8 oz | 270 | 18 | 12 |
| Caprese Salad, 4.5 oz | 150 | 11 | 7 |
| Chicken Caesar, 7.5 oz | 390 | 28 | 17 |
| Chicken Caesar Pasta Salad, 9 oz | 540 | 24 | 61 |
| Kale & Quinoa Salad, 6 oz | 300 | 18 | 30 |
| Mediterranean Pasta Salad, 8.5 oz | 490 | 29 | 49 |
| Side, 5 oz | 30 | 0 | 7 |
| *Sandwiches/Melts:* | | | |
| Chicken, Bacon Ranch Melt, 7.4 oz | 560 | 22 | 56 |
| Chicken Salad Sandwich, 6.6 oz | 470 | 21 | 49 |
| Double Cheeseburger, | | | |
| with American Cheese, 9.6 oz | 800 | 54 | 35 |
| Egg Salad Sandwich, 6.8 oz | 480 | 24 | 50 |
| Go!Smart Turkey Sandwich, 8.8 oz | 300 | 2.5 | 48 |
| Grilled Chicken Sandwich, | | | |
| with Honey Mustard BBQ Sauce, 6 oz | 340 | 10 | 39 |
| Italian Melt, 7.8 oz | 610 | 39 | 38 |
| Southwest Turkey Sandwich, 8 oz | 560 | 28 | 48 |
| Steak & Cheese Melt, 7.8 oz | 680 | 35 | 57 |
| *Sides:* Hash Brown (1), 2 oz | 100 | 5 | 12 |
| Potato Wedges (6), 0.7 oz | 240 | 4.5 | 27 |
| *Taquitos,* | | | |
| Chicken & Monterey Jack, (2), 5.3 oz | 330 | 12 | 44 |
| *Drinks:* Cappuccino, 8 fl.oz | 180 | 4 | 36 |
| Caramel Macchiato, 8 fl.oz | 190 | 5 | 34 |
| Cuban Coffee, with milk, 8 fl.oz | 200 | 7 | 34 |
| French Vanilla Cappuccino, 8 fl.oz | 190 | 6 | 34 |
| Skinny, 8 fl.oz | 140 | 4.5 | 30 |
| Hot Chocolate, 8 fl.oz | 170 | 2.5 | 37 |
| Peppermint Mocha, 8 fl.oz | 180 | 4 | 36 |
| Pumpkin Spice Late, 8 fl.oz | 190 | 6 | 35 |
| *Slurpees,* average all flavors: | | | |
| 12 oz cup | 95 | 0 | 26 |
| 22 oz cup | 175 | 0 | 44 |
| 28 oz cup | 220 | 0 | 56 |
| Sugar Free, 12 oz cup | 30 | 0 | 9 |

## Saladworks® (Sept '19)

*Salads:* W/out Dressing or Bread

| | C | F | Cb |
|---|---|---|---|
| Bently | 290 | 15 | 11 |
| Buffalo Bleu | 350 | 12 | 29 |
| Chicken Caesar | 370 | 15 | 29 |
| Cobb | 370 | 23 | 19 |
| Farmhouse | 270 | 12 | 28 |
| Fire Roasted Cabo | 350 | 17 | 25 |
| Greek | 200 | 11 | 17 |
| Mandarin Chicken | 230 | 4 | 25 |
| Mediterranean | 330 | 23 | 16 |
| Sophie's Salad | 310 | 13 | 35 |
| Thai Chicken | 200 | 6 | 20 |
| Tivoli | 470 | 21 | 41 |
| Turkey Club | 290 | 7 | 38 |
| *Paninis:* Buffalo Chicken | 870 | 36 | 85 |
| Caprese | 940 | 47 | 94 |
| Chicken Parmesan | 870 | 32 | 93 |
| Turkey Melt | 1020 | 49 | 90 |
| *Sandwiches:* Avocado BLT | 830 | 55 | 60 |
| Loaded Chicken Salad | 370 | 9 | 28 |
| Tuna Salad | 410 | 8 | 57 |
| West Coast Turkey | 580 | 30 | 51 |
| *Wraps:* Bentley | 550 | 21 | 63 |
| Buffalo Bleu | 660 | 20 | 82 |
| Chicken Caesar | 610 | 20 | 81 |
| Cobb | 690 | 33 | 71 |
| Farmhouse | 590 | 20 | 82 |
| Fire Roasted Cabo | 670 | 25 | 78 |
| Madarin Chicken | 530 | 12 | 83 |
| Mediterranean | 650 | 34 | 92 |
| Sophie's Salad | 550 | 17 | 81 |
| Thai Chicken | 410 | 9 | 70 |
| Tivoli | 610 | 27 | 63 |
| Turkey Club | 460 | 14 | 61 |
| *Soups:* Per Medium Serve, without Bread Roll | | | |
| Baked Potato | 345 | 23 | 28 |
| Broccoli Cheddar | 275 | 19 | 18 |
| Chicken Dumpling | 180 | 5.5 | 21 |
| Chicken Noodle | 180 | 5 | 18 |
| Chicken Tortilla | 260 | 14 | 19 |
| Homestyle Tomato | 300 | 21 | 25 |
| Lasagna, with Turkey Sausage | 235 | 11 | 21 |
| Maine Lobster Bisque | 470 | 39 | 21 |
| New England Clam Chowder | 370 | 26 | 22 |

**236**

## Sandella's® (Sept '19)

### Grilled Flatbread:

| | C | F | Cb |
|---|---|---|---|
| BBQ Cheese | 430 | 9 | 67 |
| Bacon & Cheddar | 630 | 34 | 54 |
| Chicken Fajita | 500 | 18 | 52 |
| Chicken Parmesan | 560 | 20 | 55 |
| El Paso | 710 | 19 | 97 |
| Ham & Cheddar | 570 | 25 | 51 |
| Meatball | 630 | 29 | 56 |
| Olympian | 480 | 26 | 53 |
| Pesto & Peppers | 530 | 27 | 52 |
| Spinach & Artichoke | 610 | 33 | 54 |
| Thai Chicken | 630 | 24 | 66 |
| Tomato Bacon | 580 | 26 | 58 |

### Paninis: With Standard Toppings

| | C | F | Cb |
|---|---|---|---|
| Americana | 580 | 25 | 54 |
| Arizona Chicken | 660 | 23 | 78 |
| BBQ Chicken | 490 | 2.5 | 92 |
| Beef Fajita | 630 | 27 | 58 |
| Bistro Ham & Brie | 560 | 19 | 70 |
| Brazilian Beef, without cheese | 500 | 6 | 86 |
| Holiday Ham | 770 | 21 | 110 |
| Napoli Chicken | 440 | 17 | 49 |
| Pastrami Melt | 670 | 33 | 55 |
| Philly Cheese | 590 | 25 | 55 |
| Spinach & Bacon | 610 | 29 | 65 |
| Toasted Caprese | 380 | 14 | 50 |

### Quesadillas: With Standard Toppings

| | C | F | Cb |
|---|---|---|---|
| Barbecue | 570 | 18 | 66 |
| Beef Fajita | 570 | 22 | 55 |
| Buffalo Chicken | 510 | 20 | 49 |
| Thai Veggie | 570 | 27 | 60 |

### Salads: With ½ Flatbread, without Dressing

| | C | F | Cb |
|---|---|---|---|
| Apple Walnut | 370 | 13 | 60 |
| Napa Valley | 770 | 60 | 54 |
| Panzanella | 190 | 3 | 36 |
| Siesta | 310 | 15 | 44 |
| Thai Chicken | 330 | 13 | 35 |

### Rice Bowls: Includes Flatbread & Standard Toppings

| | C | F | Cb |
|---|---|---|---|
| Asian Chicken & Broccoli | 680 | 3 | 138 |
| Mesquite BBQ | 930 | 21 | 140 |
| Southwest Veggie | 810 | 20 | 126 |
| Thai Peanut Saute | 680 | 16 | 116 |

### Wraps: With Standard Toppings

| | C | F | Cb |
|---|---|---|---|
| California Turkey | 410 | 10 | 55 |
| Greek Salad | 370 | 13 | 55 |
| Nut & Honey | 800 | 32 | 116 |
| Seven Layer | 570 | 23 | 66 |
| Swiss Salad | 500 | 20 | 62 |
| Texas Beef | 420 | 10 | 58 |
| The Russian | 400 | 7 | 60 |
| Veggie & Cheese | 450 | 19 | 52 |

## Sarku Japan® (Sept '19)

### Bento Box:

| | C | F | Cb |
|---|---|---|---|
| Fried Rice: Beef | 830 | 32 | 98 |
| Chicken | 820 | 35 | 95 |
| Shrimp | 750 | 27 | 96 |

### D'Lite Meals, Vegetarian:

| | C | F | Cb |
|---|---|---|---|
| Fried Rice | 430 | 10 | 79 |
| Noodles | 640 | 14 | 109 |
| Steamed Rice | 410 | 6 | 83 |

### Teriyaki Meals: With Steamed Rice

| | C | F | Cb |
|---|---|---|---|
| Beef | 580 | 16 | 80 |
| Beef & Shrimp | 690 | 21 | 85 |
| Chicken | 640 | 24 | 79 |
| Chicken & Shrimp | 750 | 29 | 85 |
| Shrimp | 530 | 12 | 80 |

### Sushi Rolls: California

| | C | F | Cb |
|---|---|---|---|
| California | 330 | 8 | 57 |
| Chicken Teriyaki | 360 | 11 | 53 |
| Green Dragon | 650 | 35 | 71 |
| Hand Rolls: Salmon Skin | 210 | 7 | 27 |
| Seafood | 170 | 1.5 | 29 |
| Spicy Tuna | 180 | 3.5 | 27 |
| Philadelphia | 430 | 18 | 49 |
| Salmon | 220 | 5 | 33 |
| Tuna | 190 | 0 | 33 |
| Sauce, Teriyaki, 1.5 oz | 45 | 0 | 9 |
| Sides: Chicken Egg Roll | 160 | 6 | 21 |
| Dumplings (6) | 260 | 12 | 29 |
| Edamame | 170 | 7 | 11 |
| Miso Soup | 50 | 2 | 6 |
| Seaweed Salad | 70 | 2 | 13 |
| Shrimp Tempura (3) | 390 | 30 | 23 |
| Vegetable Spring Roll | 190 | 9 | 15 |

## Schlotzsky's® (Sept '19)

### Sandwiches: Per Medium

| | C | F | Cb |
|---|---|---|---|
| Angus Beef & Cheese | 780 | 30 | 81 |
| Bacon Grilled Cheese | 660 | 36 | 60 |
| Chicken Bacon Smokecheesy | 860 | 31 | 80 |
| Chipotle Chicken | 530 | 9 | 78 |
| Cuban Brisket | 770 | 30 | 75 |
| Deluxe Original | 980 | 47 | 81 |
| Fiesta Chicken | 810 | 31 | 78 |
| Fresh Veggie | 500 | 14 | 74 |
| Ham & Cheese, Orig. | 730 | 25 | 81 |
| Smoked Turkey Breast | 500 | 6 | 80 |
| The Original | 780 | 34 | 78 |
| The Sicilian | 730 | 43 | 42 |
| The Tuscan | 700 | 35 | 49 |
| Turkey Bacon Club | 770 | 30 | 81 |
| Turkey Original | 820 | 33 | 81 |
| Turkey & Guacamole | 520 | 11 | 78 |

*continued next page...*

**237**

## Schlotzsky's® cont... (Sept '19)

### Pizzas: Per 10" Pizza

| | C | F | Cb |
|---|---|---|---|
| BBQ Chkn & Jalapeno | 920 | 21 | 148 |
| Double Cheese | 840 | 27 | 115 |
| Fresh Veggie | 920 | 35 | 118 |
| Grilled Chicken & Pesto | 910 | 29 | 114 |
| Pepperoni & Double Cheese | 980 | 42 | 115 |

### Mac: Brisketeer

| | C | F | Cb |
|---|---|---|---|
| Brisketeer | 1090 | 49 | 69 |
| Double Cheese | 830 | 43 | 69 |
| Poultry In Motion | 1130 | 47 | 70 |
| Shrimpy The Best | 1070 | 45 | 71 |
| Smokey Brisketeer | 1120 | 50 | 74 |

### Salads: Without Dressing or Breadsticks

| | C | F | Cb |
|---|---|---|---|
| Chicken Caesar | 680 | 17 | 29 |
| Cranberry, Apple, Pecan & Chicken | 640 | 27 | 68 |
| Southwest Chicken | 600 | 29 | 44 |
| Turkey Avocado Cobb | 610 | 33 | 42 |

### Dressing: Blue Cheese, 3 oz

| | C | F | Cb |
|---|---|---|---|
| Blue Cheese, 3 oz | 460 | 49 | 3 |
| Caesar, 3 oz | 430 | 45 | 2 |
| Italian, 3 oz | 280 | 28 | 3 |
| Thousand Island, 3 oz | 360 | 12 | 5 |

### Soup: Per 10 oz Bowl

| | C | F | Cb |
|---|---|---|---|
| Broccoli Cheese | 185 | 12 | 14 |
| Chicken & Wild Rice | 280 | 14 | 25 |
| Chicken Tortilla | 315 | 16 | 27 |
| Loaded Potato | 385 | 31 | 29 |
| Timberline Chili | 380 | 21 | 27 |
| Tomato Basil | 320 | 26 | 21 |

### Chips:

| | C | F | Cb |
|---|---|---|---|
| Baked: Regular; BBQ | 130 | 3 | 25 |
| Other varieties, average | 230 | 14 | 24 |

### Kidz Meals: Without Cookie or Drink

| | C | F | Cb |
|---|---|---|---|
| Cheese Pizza | 540 | 17 | 78 |
| Ham Sandwich | 220 | 2 | 40 |
| Pepperoni Pizza | 590 | 22 | 78 |
| Turkey Sandwich | 220 | 2 | 40 |

### Desserts:

| | C | F | Cb |
|---|---|---|---|
| Brownie (1) | 420 | 23 | 46 |
| Cookies: Chocolate Chip (1) | 160 | 7 | 24 |
| Oatmeal Raisin; Sugar, (1), av. | 155 | 5 | 24 |

### Breakfast: Per Whole Burrito/Sandwich

| | C | F | Cb |
|---|---|---|---|
| Burritos: Bacon | 460 | 22 | 41 |
| Ham | 490 | 21 | 44 |
| Sausage | 570 | 31 | 41 |
| Veggie | 430 | 19 | 44 |
| Sandwiches: Bacon; Veggie | 500 | 21 | 51 |
| Ham | 530 | 22 | 50 |
| Sausage | 650 | 32 | 49 |
| Tacos: Bacon; Sausage, average | 250 | 14 | 18 |
| Ham | 290 | 17 | 18 |
| Veggie | 220 | 10 | 21 |
| Sides: Hash Brown, 1 piece | 60 | 5 | 8 |
| Mixed Fruit, 1 scoop | 20 | 0 | 5 |

## Second Cup® ~ *see CalorieKing.com*

## Shake Shack® (Sept '19)

### Burgers: Per Single Burger

| | C | F | Cb |
|---|---|---|---|
| Bacon Cheeseburger | 540 | 33 | 25 |
| Cheeseburger | 470 | 28 | 25 |
| Crackle Shack | 580 | 37 | 25 |
| Green Chile CheddarShack | | | |
| Hamburger | 400 | 22 | 24 |
| Lockhart Link | 810 | 60 | 27 |
| Shack Stack | 800 | 49 | 50 |
| Shroom Burger | 550 | 31 | 49 |
| SmokeShack | 610 | 39 | 28 |
| Veggie Shack | 530 | 27 | 56 |

### Chicken: Bites (6)

| | C | F | Cb |
|---|---|---|---|
| Bites (6) | 300 | 15 | 18 |
| Hot Chick'N Sandwich | 560 | 31 | 38 |

### Flat-Top Dogs: Chicken Dog

| | C | F | Cb |
|---|---|---|---|
| Chicken Dog | 310 | 13 | 27 |
| Garden Dog | 220 | 10 | 28 |
| Hot Dog | 390 | 26 | 25 |
| Shack-Cago Dog | 410 | 26 | 29 |

### Fries:

| | C | F | Cb |
|---|---|---|---|
| Bacon Cheese | 840 | 52 | 65 |
| Cheese | 710 | 44 | 64 |
| Regular | 470 | 22 | 63 |
| Floats, Creamsicle; Purple Cow, av. | 450 | 15 | 77 |

### Shakes:

| | C | F | Cb |
|---|---|---|---|
| Chocolate | 750 | 45 | 76 |
| Salted Caramel | 840 | 42 | 99 |
| Vanilla | 680 | 36 | 72 |

### Breakfast: Bacon Sandwich

| | C | F | Cb |
|---|---|---|---|
| Bacon Sandwich | 440 | 27 | 25 |
| Egg & Cheese Sandwich | 370 | 23 | 25 |
| Sausage Sandwich | 460 | 25 | 26 |

## Shakey's® (Sept '19)

### Pizzas: Per Slice, ¹⁄₁₀ Medium Size ¹²" Pizza

| | C | F | Cb |
|---|---|---|---|
| **Big Island:** Pan Crust | 210 | 6 | 30 |
| Thin Crust | 160 | 6 | 19 |
| **California Pizzarito:** Pan Crust | 265 | 12 | 30 |
| Thin Crust | 215 | 11 | 19 |
| **Cheese:** Pan Crust | 190 | 5 | 30 |
| Thin Crust | 135 | 5 | 17 |
| **Firehouse:** Pan Crust | 280 | 13 | 30 |
| Thin Crust | 230 | 12 | 20 |
| **Garden Veggie:** Pan Crust | 205 | 6 | 30 |
| Thin Crust | 150 | 6 | 19 |
| **Rustic Garlic Chicken:** Pan Crust | 215 | 6 | 30 |
| Thin Crust | 160 | 6 | 19 |
| **Shakey's Special:** Pan Crust | 255 | 11 | 30 |
| Thin Crust | 200 | 10 | 18 |
| **Texas BBQ Chicken:** Pan Crust | 220 | 6 | 32 |
| Thin Crust | 165 | 5 | 20 |
| **Ultimate Meat:** Pan Crust | 310 | 15 | 30 |
| Thin Crust | 260 | 14 | 20 |

## Shakey's® cont... (Sept '19)

### Golden Fried Chicken: Per Piece

| | C | F | Cb |
|---|---|---|---|
| Breast | 360 | 11 | 16 |
| Leg | 175 | 10 | 6 |
| Thigh | 350 | 24 | 9 |
| Wing | 130 | 9 | 4 |

### Rice: Per ½ Cup

| | C | F | Cb |
|---|---|---|---|
| Mexican Fiesta | 100 | 0 | 22 |
| Pilaf | 120 | 3 | 22 |

### Sides & Extras:

| | C | F | Cb |
|---|---|---|---|
| Enchilada (1) | 80 | 2 | 37 |
| Boneless Chicken Strip (1) | 125 | 7 | 10 |
| Garlic Bread, 1 piece | 180 | 4 | 30 |
| Macaroni & Cheese, 1 cup | 350 | 17 | 33 |
| Macaroni Salad, ½ cup | 220 | 14 | 19 |
| Mashed Potatoes, ½ cup | 65 | 1 | 13 |
| Mojo Potatoes, medium | 430 | 23 | 51 |

## Shari's® (Sept '19)

### Breakfast: As Served

| | C | F | Cb |
|---|---|---|---|
| Bacon & Eggs without extras | 290 | 22 | 1 |
| Buttermilk Pancakes | 800 | 27 | 123 |
| Country Sausage Benedictq | 1470 | 102 | 90 |
| Double Smoked Sausage & Egg | 450 | 32 | 6 |
| French Toast | 960 | 62 | 82 |
| Meat Lover's Skillet | 1100 | 86 | 38 |
| Sausage & Eggs without extras | 630 | 57 | 1 |
| Shari's Sampler | 1610 | 105 | 116 |
| Ultimate Country Fried Steak | 1060 | 72 | 67 |
| Waffle | 340 | 14 | 48 |

### Lunch: Without Side Choices

| | C | F | Cb |
|---|---|---|---|
| Chicken Strips | 340 | 18 | 23 |

### Salads: Entrée Size, with Dressing

| | C | F | Cb |
|---|---|---|---|
| Caesar | 460 | 40 | 15 |
| Northwest Steak | 890 | 50 | 65 |
| Rustic Tuscan Chicken | 510 | 32 | 21 |

### Sandwiches: Per Whole Sandwich

| | C | F | Cb |
|---|---|---|---|
| BLT on Texas Toast | 540 | 26 | 51 |
| Cajun Chicken Avocado Club | 1360 | 74 | 115 |
| Cuban on Ciabatta Roll | 680 | 30 | 60 |
| Grilled Ham & Four Cheese Melt, on Sourdough | 1140 | 68 | 78 |
| Hot Turkey on Whole Wheat | 1040 | 31 | 126 |
| Prime Rib Dip on French Roll | 680 | 33 | 63 |
| Traditional Club | 1310 | 72 | 114 |

### Dinner: With Menu Set Sides & Bread

| | C | F | Cb |
|---|---|---|---|
| Beer Battered Fish & Chips | 1600 | 119 | 104 |
| Chopped Steak | 930 | 50 | 50 |
| Country Fried Steak | 1010 | 63 | 83 |
| Grilled Lemon Chicken | 450 | 17 | 17 |
| Slow Roasted Turkey | 980 | 50 | 50 |

## Shari's® cont... (Sept '19)

### Sides, Add-Ons:

| | C | F | Cb |
|---|---|---|---|
| Baked Potato, Plain | 160 | 0 | 37 |
| French Fries | 370 | 24 | 36 |
| Loaded Mashed Potatoes | 410 | 21 | 42 |
| Onion Rings (6) | 390 | 24 | 39 |
| Red Skin Mshd Potato | 260 | 8 | 40 |
| Rice Pilaf | 90 | 5 | 10 |
| Sauteed Button Mushrooms | 220 | 23 | 1 |
| Shrimp Scampi | 360 | 30 | 2 |
| Stuffed Hashbrowns | 420 | 28 | 32 |
| Shrimp Skewers (2) | 190 | 11 | 1 |
| Steakhouse Mac 'n Cheese | 510 | 27 | 45 |
| Tater Tots: Plain | 370 | 26 | 33 |
| with Chipotle Mayo | 650 | 56 | 36 |

### Desserts:

| | C | F | Cb |
|---|---|---|---|
| Chocolate Lava Cake | 660 | 27 | 100 |

### Classic Pies:

| | C | F | Cb |
|---|---|---|---|
| Banana Cream Dream | 460 | 24 | 53 |
| Chocolate Cream Supreme | 540 | 30 | 62 |

### Gourmet Pies:

| | C | F | Cb |
|---|---|---|---|
| Creamy Caramel Pecan Crunch | 770 | 49 | 76 |
| Peanut Butter Chocolate Silk | 660 | 45 | 60 |
| Velvet Chocolate Silk | 580 | 38 | 56 |

## Sheetz® (Sept '19)

### Breakfast Sandwiches:

| | C | F | Cb |
|---|---|---|---|
| Dreamy Bacon Croissant | 400 | 25 | 28 |
| Twisted BLT | 710 | 42 | 53 |
| Walker Breakfast Ranger | 550 | 23 | 58 |

### Burgerz: Big Mozz

| | C | F | Cb |
|---|---|---|---|
| Big Mozz | 600 | 27 | 48 |
| Boss Bacon | 710 | 50 | 26 |
| Cowboy | 650 | 33 | 46 |
| Twisted Swiss | 730 | 40 | 50 |

### Hot Dogs: With Standard Hot Dog

| | C | F | Cb |
|---|---|---|---|
| BLT | 450 | 28 | 33 |
| Junkyard | 340 | 16 | 38 |
| Philly | 330 | 17 | 35 |
| Shmokehouse | 370 | 18 | 37 |

### Mac & Cheese Platter: Boom Chicka

| | C | F | Cb |
|---|---|---|---|
| Boom Chicka | 510 | 27 | 40 |
| Meatball | 610 | 37 | 35 |
| Morning | 480 | 28 | 35 |

### Sandwichez:

#### Deli: Boom Boom BLT

| | C | F | Cb |
|---|---|---|---|
| Boom Boom BLT | 820 | 46 | 52 |
| Ciabatta Bing | 620 | 34 | 53 |
| Garden of Eatin | 440 | 16 | 54 |

#### Grilled Chicken: Big Mozz

| | C | F | Cb |
|---|---|---|---|
| Big Mozz | 560 | 18 | 51 |
| Carolina Slaw | 440 | 16 | 37 |
| Twisted Brunch | 770 | 40 | 50 |

### Subz: Per Half

| | C | F | Cb |
|---|---|---|---|
| Big Philly Sub, on Pretzel Sub | 640 | 25 | 66 |
| Cali Turkey Flatbread Sub | 820 | 43 | 65 |
| Southwest Veggie, on White Sub | 440 | 18 | 56 |

*continued next page...*

## Sheetz® cont... (Sept '19)

### Sidez:

| | C | F | Cb |
|---|---|---|---|
| Coleslaw | 250 | 11 | 35 |
| Crispy Chicken Stripz, w/out sauce: | | | |
| 3 pieces | 330 | 11 | 39 |
| 5 pieces | 550 | 18 | 65 |
| Fryz, w/out sauce, 1 cup | 390 | 13 | 64 |
| Hard Cooked Egg (1) | 70 | 4.5 | 0 |
| Jalapeno Poppers, w/out Sce | 330 | 18 | 35 |
| Loaded Fryz, w/out toppings | 600 | 20 | 97 |
| Mac & Cheese, w/out toppings | 190 | 7 | 25 |
| Onion Rings, w/out sauce, 1 cup | 470 | 27 | 52 |
| Popcorn Chicken, without Sauce: | | | |
| Regular | 300 | 14 | 28 |
| Large | 610 | 28 | 55 |

## Sizzler® (Sept '19)

### Burgers & Sandwiches:

| | C | F | Cb |
|---|---|---|---|
| ⅓ lb Burgers: Bacon Chseburger | 950 | 67 | 44 |
| Classic: Burger | 830 | 57 | 44 |
| Cheese Burger | 920 | 64 | 45 |
| Turkey Patty | 510 | 30 | 39 |
| Double Mega Bacon | 1250 | 91 | 44 |
| Malibu Melt | 1840 | 155 | 69 |
| Sandwiches: Grilled Chicken Club | 580 | 19 | 39 |
| Grilled Chicken | 390 | 4.5 | 37 |
| Malibu Chicken | 870 | 63 | 52 |

***Entrees:*** *Without Sides, Condiments, Dipping Sauce or Optional Accompaniments*

| | C | F | Cb |
|---|---|---|---|
| **Chicken:** *Small Plate* | | | |
| Grilled Hibachi Chicken | 220 | 2 | 7 |
| Grilled Italian-Herb Chicken, 7 oz | 230 | 6 | 1 |
| **Pasta:** Fettuccine Alfredo | 960 | 51 | 85 |
| Cajun Penne | 1030 | 71 | 108 |
| **Ribs:** | | | |
| BBQ: 6 bones | 1870 | 145 | 32 |
| 9 Bones | 2820 | 213 | 61 |
| **Seafood:** Fish & Chips, 2 pieces | 1410 | 102 | 93 |
| Grilled Salmon, 6 oz | 370 | 23 | 3 |
| Ultimate Shrimp Trio | 1230 | 62 | 85 |
| **Steaks:** | | | |
| Burgundy Mushroom Sirloin Tips | 480 | 16 | 38 |
| Combos: Steak & Hibachi Chicken | 550 | 14 | 20 |
| Steak & Lobster Tail | 720 | 51 | 2 |
| Steak & Malibu Chicken | 920 | 73 | 14 |
| Porterhouse, 20 oz | 1430 | 108 | 2 |
| Tri Tip: Slow Roast BBQ, 5 oz | 680 | 39 | 52 |
| 6 oz | 790 | 44 | 54 |
| Tri Tip Sirloin: 8 oz | 340 | 16 | 0.5 |
| 10 oz | 440 | 20 | 3 |
| 12 oz | 530 | 24 | 3 |

## Sizzler® cont... (Sept '19)

### Sides:

| | C | F | Cb |
|---|---|---|---|
| **Baked Potato:** Foil | 350 | 13 | 54 |
| Loaded Foil | 530 | 32 | 54 |
| Salted | 510 | 30 | 55 |
| Loaded | 760 | 57 | 55 |
| Baked Yam with Maple Topping | 410 | 11 | 75 |
| Balsamic Brussels Sprouts | 150 | 7 | 20 |
| Broccoli, steamed | 40 | 0 | 7 |
| with Butter | 70 | 4.5 | 7 |
| Button Mushroom Saute | 180 | 17 | 5 |
| Cilantro Lime Rice | 150 | 0 | 31 |
| Garlic Mashed Potatoes | 150 | 2.5 | 29 |
| Green Beans | 80 | 5 | 8 |
| Grilled Onions | 80 | 6 | 7 |
| Roasted Corn with Herb Butter | 80 | 2.5 | 13 |
| Roasted Red Potatoes | 130 | 0 | 28 |
| Spinach Saute | 70 | 5 | 5 |
| Street Fries, 5 oz | 350 | 22 | 37 |
| Sweet Potato Fries | 610 | 48 | 39 |
| Vegetable Medley | 80 | 4.5 | 8 |
| Zucchini Planks | 20 | 0 | 3 |

*For Complete Menu & Data ~ see CalorieKing.com*

## Skyline Chili® (Sept '19)

### Burritos:

| | C | F | Cb |
|---|---|---|---|
| Chili Deluxe | 610 | 33 | 38 |
| Original | 610 | 31 | 54 |
| ***Coneys/Sandwiches:*** | | | |
| **Coneys:** Cheese, w/ onions & mstrd | 350 | 23 | 25 |
| Coney, plain | 220 | 13 | 22 |
| **Sandwiches:** Chili Cheese, | | | |
| with onions & mustard | 290 | 17 | 24 |
| Chili, with onions & mustard | 180 | 8 | 23 |
| ***Ways:*** *Per Regular Serving* | | | |
| Chili Spaghetti with Bean & Onion: | | | |
| Small | 250 | 10 | 34 |
| Regular | 490 | 19 | 68 |
| Large | 670 | 26 | 94 |
| **Bowls:** Chili | 200 | 12 | 0 |
| Loaded Chili | 480 | 28 | 20 |
| Vegetarian Black Beans & Rice | 400 | 14 | 48 |
| ***Steamed Potatoes:*** | | | |
| 3-Way Potato | 620 | 26 | 65 |
| Cheddar Potato | 630 | 33 | 65 |
| Sour Cream Potato | 460 | 19 | 65 |
| ***Salads:*** *Without Dressing* | | | |
| Buffalo Chicken | 220 | 11 | 12 |
| Greek | 210 | 12 | 17 |
| **Fries:** Chili Cheese | 840 | 53 | 61 |
| Regular | 430 | 24 | 51 |

Updated Nutrition Data ~ www.CalorieKing.com
Persons with Diabetes ~ See Disclaimer (Page 22)

## Smoothie King® (Sept '19)

*Fruit Smoothies: Per 20 oz Cup* **C F Cb**

**Fitness Blends:** *Without Turbinado*

| | C | F | Cb |
|---|---|---|---|
| Orig. High Prot.: Banana | 330 | 12 | 32 |
| Chocolate | 390 | 12 | 41 |
| Pineapple | 310 | 12 | 26 |
| Peanut Power Plus: Choc. | 600 | 24 | 77 |
| Strawberry | 590 | 23 | 87 |
| The Activator: Chocolate | 190 | 2 | 21 |
| Blueberry Strawberry | 310 | 1.5 | 54 |
| Strawberry Banana | 270 | 2 | 42 |
| The Hulk: With Turbinado | | | |
| Chocolate; Vanilla | 700 | 23 | 101 |
| Strawberry | 840 | 24 | 136 |

**Slim Blends:** *With Stevia*

| | C | F | Cb |
|---|---|---|---|
| Slim-N-Trim: Chocolate | 210 | 2.5 | 36 |
| Strawberry | 220 | 2 | 47 |
| Vanilla | 180 | 2.5 | 34 |

**Take A Break Blends:** *With Turbinado*

| | C | F | Cb |
|---|---|---|---|
| Banana Boat | 450 | 6 | 93 |
| Caribbean Way | 390 | 0 | 98 |
| Passion Passport | 410 | 0 | 102 |
| Pineapple Surf | 410 | 1.5 | 96 |

**Wellness Blends:** *Without Turbinado*

| | C | F | Cb |
|---|---|---|---|
| Blueberry Heaven | 260 | 1.5 | 58 |
| Vegan Mango Kale/Nutty Super Grain | 330 | 6 | 66 |
| Vegan Dark Chocolate Banana | 350 | 1.5 | 81 |
| Vegan Pineapple Spinach | 360 | 6 | 75 |

## Snappy Tomato® (Sept '19)

*Snappetizers:* **C F Cb**

| | C | F | Cb |
|---|---|---|---|
| Bone In Wings (6) | 460 | 34 | 4 |
| Flatbread, medium, ⅙ flatbread | 270 | 12 | 33 |
| Wedge Fries, plain | 220 | 10 | 28 |

**Hoagies:**

| | C | F | Cb |
|---|---|---|---|
| Italian Combo | 650 | 23 | 69 |
| Steak & Cheese | 760 | 35 | 73 |
| Veggie Melt | 490 | 11 | 74 |
| *Pasta:* Plain Spaghetti/Rigatoni, av. | 340 | 1.5 | 68 |

*Toppings:* Bacon | 120 | 8 | 1 |

| | C | F | Cb |
|---|---|---|---|
| Black or Green Olives | 50 | 4.5 | 2 |
| Cheese | 90 | 7 | 1 |
| Chicken | 120 | 2.5 | 1 |
| Pepperoni | 140 | 10 | 0 |
| Tomatoes | 5 | 0 | 1 |
| *Sauce:* Ranch | 570 | 60 | 8 |
| Snappy | 80 | 2 | 8 |
| *Salads:* Crispy Chkn, w/o dressing | 280 | 9 | 24 |
| Garden, without dressing | 90 | 4.5 | 11 |
| Grilled Chicken, w/out dressing | 160 | 2.5 | 10 |
| *Dessert:* Cinnabread, med., ⅙ slice | 350 | 13 | 57 |
| Raspberry Cinnabread, ⅙ slice | 370 | 13 | 62 |

## Sonic Drive-In® (Sept '19)

*Burgers:* **C F Cb**

| | C | F | Cb |
|---|---|---|---|
| Bacon Cheeseburger, with Mayo | 770 | 46 | 53 |
| Bacon Dble Cheeseburger, with Mayo | 1030 | 65 | 54 |
| Cheeseburger: w/ Mayo | 680 | 39 | 54 |
| with Ketchup | 600 | 28 | 56 |
| ¼ lb Double Chseburger w/ Mayo | 960 | 59 | 55 |
| Jalap. Dble Chseburger, w/ Mstrd | 850 | 48 | 54 |
| Jr. Burger | 330 | 16 | 32 |
| Jr. Deluxe Cheeseburger | 440 | 27 | 32 |
| Veggie Burger, w/ Mayo | 530 | 22 | 69 |

*Chicken:*

| | C | F | Cb |
|---|---|---|---|
| **Sandwiches:** Classic Crispy Chicken | 570 | 31 | 51 |
| Classic Grilled Chkn | 490 | 22 | 42 |
| Crispy Tender Chicken | 460 | 24 | 41 |

**Boneless Wings:** *6 Pieces*

| | C | F | Cb |
|---|---|---|---|
| Asian Sweet Chili | 470 | 24 | 32 |
| Honey BBQ | 470 | 24 | 33 |
| Buffalo | 440 | 28 | 17 |
| **Tenders:** Crispy 3 piece Dinner | 980 | 50 | 102 |
| 5 piece Dinner | 1170 | 60 | 113 |

*Coneys & 6" Hot Dogs:*

| | C | F | Cb |
|---|---|---|---|
| All American Dog | 410 | 21 | 41 |
| Chicago Dog | 400 | 20 | 41 |
| Chili Cheese Coney | 470 | 29 | 34 |
| New York Dog | 400 | 23 | 35 |
| Original Pretzel Dog | 320 | 20 | 23 |
| *Wraps:* Crispy Chicken | 570 | 22 | 56 |
| Grilled Chicken | 480 | 14 | 39 |
| *Natural Cut Fries:* Small | 250 | 12 | 33 |
| Medium | 290 | 13 | 38 |
| Large | 470 | 22 | 63 |

*Sides: Per Medium Serving*

| | C | F | Cb |
|---|---|---|---|
| Ched 'R' Bites | 410 | 46 | 35 |
| Chili Cheese Fries | 450 | 26 | 42 |
| Handmade Onion Rings | 580 | 29 | 74 |
| Mozzarella Sticks | 560 | 29 | 61 |
| Tots with Cheese | 450 | 28 | 43 |

*Breakfast:*

| | C | F | Cb |
|---|---|---|---|
| Breakfast Bacon Toaster | 610 | 31 | 52 |
| Breakfast Burrito: Bacon | 470 | 25 | 35 |
| Ham | 440 | 20 | 38 |
| Sausage | 500 | 30 | 35 |
| **CroiSonic Sandwich:** with Bacon | 560 | 37 | 31 |
| with Ham | 490 | 29 | 33 |
| with Sausage | 670 | 49 | 31 |
| Cinnasnacks (3), without Frosting | 340 | 15 | 44 |
| French Toast Sticks, (4) w/out Syrup | 480 | 25 | 54 |

*continued next page...*

## Sonic Drive-In® cont... (Sept '19)

| Ice Cream Cone, | C | F | Cb |
|---|---|---|---|
| Vanilla | 250 | 12 | 30 |
| **Ice Cream Sundaes:** | | | |
| Caramel | 490 | 22 | 61 |
| Chocolate | 430 | 22 | 51 |
| Hot Fudge | 520 | 26 | 65 |
| Strawberry | 440 | 21 | 55 |
| **Add Ons,** Pecans | 60 | 6 | 1 |
| **Classic Shakes:** Per Medium | | | |
| Caramel | 830 | 41 | 97 |
| Chocolate | 810 | 43 | 95 |
| Fresh Banana | 850 | 41 | 108 |
| Hot Fudge | 940 | 48 | 113 |
| Peanut Butter | 940 | 58 | 89 |
| Strawberry | 790 | 41 | 92 |
| Vanilla | 820 | 45 | 89 |
| **Master Shakes:** Per Medium | | | |
| Cheesecake | 840 | 43 | 101 |
| Oreo Cheesecake | 1030 | 51 | 131 |
| Oreo Chocolate | 1000 | 51 | 125 |
| Oreo Peanut Butter | 1300 | 80 | 125 |
| Strawberry Cheesecake | 890 | 43 | 113 |
| **Sonic Blast:** Per Medium | | | |
| Butterfingers Pieces | 960 | 48 | 121 |
| Choc. Chip Cookie Dough | 920 | 45 | 118 |
| M&M's Minis Choc. Candy | 1060 | 54 | 127 |
| Oreo Pieces | 860 | 44 | 103 |
| Reese's Peanut Butter Cups | 990 | 55 | 110 |
| Snickers Bars | 890 | 46 | 103 |
| **All Natural Lemonade:** Small | 160 | 0 | 42 |
| Medium | 270 | 0 | 69 |
| Large | 400 | 0 | 105 |
| **Frozen Limeade:** Small | 190 | 0 | 52 |
| Medium | 280 | 0 | 74 |
| Large | 430 | 0 | 116 |
| **Iced Coffee:** Per Medium | | | |
| **Original:** No add ins | 100 | 6 | 11 |
| w/- French Vanilla add in | 140 | 6 | 20 |
| w/- Praline Pecan add in | 140 | 6 | 20 |

*For Complete Nutritional Data ~ see CalorieKing.com*

## Souplantation® (Sept '19)

| Soups: Per 3 fl.oz Cup | C | F | Cb |
|---|---|---|---|
| Asian Ginger Broth | 10 | 0.5 | 2 |
| Big Chunk Chicken Noodle | 30 | 1 | 3 |
| Deep Kettle Chili | 90 | 3 | 11 |
| Yankee Clipper Clam Chowder | 100 | 7 | 7 |

## Souplantation® cont... (Sept '19)

| Hot Bar: Per Cup | C | F | Cb |
|---|---|---|---|
| Classic Macaroni & Cheese | 340 | 13 | 44 |
| Four Cheese Alfredo with Fettuccine | 320 | 11 | 44 |
| Garden Veggie Marinara w/ Spag. | 250 | 5 | 41 |
| **Prepared /Tossed Salads:** Per 1 Cup | | | |
| Bok Choy Citrus Slaw | 70 | 3 | 10 |
| Caesar Asiago | 130 | 11 | 6 |
| Fresh Berry | 110 | 9 | 7 |
| Joan's Broccoli Madness | 320 | 24 | 20 |
| Tuna Tarragon | 420 | 22 | 42 |
| Wonton Happiness | 100 | 6 | 12 |
| **Bakery:** | | | |
| **Bread:** Buttermilk Cornbread, | | | |
| 1 piece | 140 | 5 | 21 |
| Multigrain, East Coast | 80 | 2 | 12 |
| Sourdough: California | 70 | 0 | 13 |
| West Coast | 110 | 0 | 22 |
| **Focaccia:** Cheesy Garlic, | 60 | 2 | 9 |
| Quattro Formaggio | 70 | 2 | 9 |
| **Muffins:** Chocolate | 380 | 22 | 46 |
| Wild Blueberry | 160 | 7 | 22 |
| **Desserts:** | | | |
| Fresh Sliced Strawberries, 2 tbsp | 5 | 0 | 2 |
| Individual Shortcake | 190 | 7 | 30 |
| Red Raspberry Gelatin, ½ cup | 110 | 0 | 26 |
| Sugar Free Chocolate Mousse, ⅓ cup | 40 | 3 | 4 |
| Tapioca Pudding, ½ cup | 140 | 2.5 | 25 |

*For Complete Nutritional Data ~ see CalorieKing.com*

## Southern Tsunami® (Sept '19)

| Rolls: With White Rice | C | F | Cb |
|---|---|---|---|
| **Classic Rolls:** California, 10.5oz | 440 | 10 | 80 |
| Crab, 10.5 oz | 460 | 13 | 73 |
| Cream Cheese: Baby Shrimp, 10.5 oz | 490 | 15 | 70 |
| Eel, 10.5 oz | 570 | 22 | 75 |
| Imit. Crab, 10.5 oz | 530 | 17 | 78 |
| Salmon, 10.5 oz | 550 | 21 | 70 |
| Smoked Salmon, 10.5 oz | 550 | 21 | 71 |
| Tuna, 10.5 oz | 500 | 15 | 71 |
| **Crunchy,** Shrimp, 10.5 oz | 580 | 20 | 84 |
| **Hybrid:** | | | |
| Berry: Eel, 8 oz | 380 | 13 | 59 |
| Immitation Crab, 8 oz | 370 | 13 | 60 |
| Blueberry: Salmon, 10 oz | 530 | 26 | 55 |
| Smoked Steelhead, 10 oz | 530 | 25 | 55 |
| Tuna, 10 oz | 450 | 16 | 55 |
| Deluxe Roll: Salmon, 8.5 oz | 470 | 20 | 58 |
| Steelhead, 8.5 oz | 460 | 19 | 58 |

## Southern Tsunami® cont... (Sept '19)

*Rolls (Cont):* With White Rice  **C** **F** **Cb**

**Plus Rolls:**

| | C | F | Cb |
|---|---|---|---|
| California, 14 oz | 590 | 13 | 107 |
| Cream Cheese Plus: Eel. 14 oz | 760 | 30 | 100 |
| Salmon/Smoked, 14 oz | 730 | 28 | 94 |
| Seaside Plus: Eel, 13.5oz | 740 | 16 | 128 |
| Salmon/Smoked, 13.5 oz | 690 | 14 | 119 |
| Spicy Plus: Salmon/Smoked, 14 oz | 680 | 24 | 95 |
| Tuna, 14 oz | 580 | 11 | 96 |
| Vegetable Plus, 14 oz | 520 | 10 | 102 |
| *Wraps:* Berry Salmon, 7 oz | 160 | 9 | 15 |
| California, 8 oz | 260 | 16 | 23 |
| Cream Cheese & Tuna, 8 oz | 240 | 14 | 16 |
| Mango, 8 oz | 130 | 4.5 | 22 |
| Spicy Cream Chse & Salmon, 8 oz | 320 | 23 | 16 |
| *Salads:* Without Dressing | | | |
| Edamame, 8 oz | 320 | 12 | 27 |
| Hawaiian Poke, w/ Steelhead, 13.8 oz | 690 | 22 | 100 |
| Sea Breeze, 4 oz | 90 | 2.5 | 17 |
| Tropical Mango, 8.5 oz | 400 | 33 | 25 |
| *Dressings/Sauces:* | | | |
| Hot Garlic Sauce, 1 oz | 50 | 1.5 | 9 |
| Spicy Sauce, 1 oz | 150 | 15 | 4 |
| Sweet Chili Sauce, 1.4 oz | 100 | 0 | 25 |
| Wasabe Sauce, 1 oz | 150 | 15 | 2 |

## Starbucks® (Sept '19)

*Brewed Coffee:* Per16 fl.oz Grande without Whipped Cream  **C** **F** **Cb**

**Caffe Misto (Au Lait):**

| | C | F | Cb |
|---|---|---|---|
| with Almond Milk | 50 | 3.5 | 4 |
| with Coconut Milk | 70 | 4.5 | 7 |
| with Nonfat Milk | 70 | 0 | 10 |
| with Soy Milk | 100 | 3 | 13 |
| with Whole Milk | 130 | 7 | 10 |

*Chocolate:* Per 16 fl.oz Grande without Whipped Cream

**Hot Chocolate:**

| | C | F | Cb |
|---|---|---|---|
| with 2% Milk | 320 | 9 | 47 |
| with Almond Milk | 240 | 8 | 38 |
| with Coconut Milk | 270 | 10 | 42 |
| with Soy Milk | 320 | 8 | 51 |
| with Whole Milk | 360 | 13 | 47 |

## Starbucks® cont... (Sept '19)

*Vanilla Creme (Hot):*  **C** **F** **Cb**
Per 16 fl.oz Grande w/out Whipped Cream

| | C | F | Cb |
|---|---|---|---|
| with 2% Milk | 270 | 7 | 37 |
| with Coconut Milk, 16 fl.oz | 210 | 9 | 33 |
| with Nonfat Milk, 16 fl.oz | 210 | 0 | 38 |
| with Soy Milk | 260 | 6 | 42 |
| with Whole Milk | 310 | 12 | 37 |

*Hot Espresso Beverages:*
Per 16 fl.oz Grande without Whipped Cream

| | C | F | Cb |
|---|---|---|---|
| **Caffe Latte:** with Almond Milk | 100 | 6 | 9 |
| with Coconut Milk | 140 | 8 | 14 |
| with Nonfat Milk | 130 | 0 | 20 |
| with Soy Milk | 190 | 6 | 24 |
| with Whole Milk | 230 | 12 | 19 |
| **Caffe Mocha:** with Almond Milk | 220 | 7 | 34 |
| with Coconut Milk | 250 | 9 | 39 |
| with Nonfat Milk | 250 | 2.5 | 42 |
| with Soy Milk | 290 | 7 | 46 |
| with Whole Milk | 330 | 12 | 42 |
| **Cappuccino:** with Almond Milk | 100 | 6 | 9 |
| with Coconut Milk | 140 | 8 | 14 |
| with Nonfat Milk | 80 | 0 | 12 |
| with Soy Milk | 120 | 3.5 | 16 |
| with Whole Milk | 140 | 7 | 12 |
| **Caramel Macchiato:** w/ Alm. Milk | 170 | 6 | 27 |
| with Coconut Milk | 200 | 8 | 32 |
| with Nonfat Milk | 200 | 1.5 | 36 |
| with Soy Milk | 250 | 6 | 39 |
| with Whole Milk | 280 | 11 | 35 |
| **Cinn. Dolce Latte:** w/ Alm. Milk | 190 | 6 | 32 |
| with Coconut Milk | 220 | 7 | 37 |
| with Nonfat Milk | 220 | 0 | 42 |
| with Whole Milk | 310 | 11 | 41 |
| **Espresso:** 1 Doppio, 2 fl.oz | 10 | 0 | 2 |
| 1 Solo, 1 fl.oz | 5 | 0 | 1 |
| Espresso Con Panna, 1 Solo, 1 fl.oz | 30 | 2.5 | 2 |
| **Latte Macchiato:** with 2% Milk | 190 | 7 | 19 |
| with Soy Milk | 180 | 5 | 23 |
| with Whole Milk | 220 | 11 | 19 |

*Iced Espresso:* Per 16 fl.oz Grande w/out Whipped Cream

| | C | F | Cb |
|---|---|---|---|
| **Caffe Latte:** with Coconut Milk | 90 | 5 | 10 |
| with Nonfat Milk | 90 | 0 | 13 |
| with Soy Milk | 130 | 3.5 | 17 |
| with Whole Milk | 150 | 7 | 13 |
| **Vanilla Latte:** with 2% Milk | 190 | 4 | 30 |
| with Coconut Milk | 160 | 4.5 | 28 |
| with Nonfat Milk | 160 | 0 | 31 |
| with Whole Milk | 210 | 6 | 30 |

*continued next page...*

## Starbucks® cont... (Sept '19)

**Frappuccino Blended Coffee:** | C | F | Cb
*Per 16 fl.oz Grande w/ Whole Milk, w/out Whipped Cream*

| | C | F | Cb |
|---|---|---|---|
| Caffe Vanilla | 320 | 3 | 69 |
| Caramel | 280 | 3.5 | 60 |
| Coffee | 240 | 3 | 50 |
| Java Chip | 350 | 7 | 68 |
| Mocha | 300 | 4 | 51 |
| White Chocolate Mocha | 300 | 5 | 61 |

**Frappuccino Blended Creme:** *Per 16 fl.oz Grande, with Whole Milk and Whipped Cream*

| | C | F | Cb |
|---|---|---|---|
| Chai Creme | 360 | 15 | 52 |
| Double Chocolaty Chip Creme | 420 | 20 | 57 |
| Vanilla Bean Creme | 400 | 16 | 60 |

**Refreshers:** *Per 16 oz Grande*

| | C | F | Cb |
|---|---|---|---|
| Mango Dragonfruit Lemonade | 140 | 0 | 33 |
| Pink Drink | 140 | 2.5 | 27 |
| Very Berry Hibiscus Lemonade | 120 | 0 | 30 |
| Violet Drink | 110 | 3 | 22 |

**Teas:** *Per 16 fl.oz Grande, with Whole Milk*

| | C | F | Cb |
|---|---|---|---|
| **Hot Tea Latte:** Chai Latte | 270 | 7 | 45 |
| Matcha Green Tea, swtnd | 280 | 11 | 34 |
| **Iced Tea Latte:** Chai | 260 | 7 | 44 |
| Matcha Green Tea, sweetend | 230 | 8 | 29 |

**Drink Extras:**

| | C | F | Cb |
|---|---|---|---|
| **Caramel Drizzle,** 1 teaspoon | 15 | 0.5 | 2 |
| **Flavored Syrup:** 1 pump | 20 | 0 | 5 |
| Sugar-Free, 1 pump | 0 | 0 | 0 |
| **Mocha Syrup,** 1 pump | 25 | 0.5 | 6 |

**Sweetened Whipped Cream:**

| | C | F | Cb |
|---|---|---|---|
| Grande/Venti, cold drinks, av. | 115 | 11 | 3 |
| Grande/Venti, hot drinks | 70 | 7 | 2 |

**Breakfast:**

| | C | F | Cb |
|---|---|---|---|
| Ham & Egg Croissant | 320 | 17 | 38 |
| Bacon & Gyuyere Sous Vide Egg Bites | 310 | 22 | 9 |
| Chicken Sausage & Bacon Biscuit | 450 | 22 | 35 |
| Hearty Blueberry Oatmeal | 220 | 2.5 | 43 |

**Mercato:**

| | C | F | Cb |
|---|---|---|---|
| Chipotle Chicken Wrap | 470 | 19 | 55 |
| Gr. Chicken & Caulif. Tabbouleh | 390 | 18 | 30 |
| Smoked Port Cubano | 450 | 25 | 66 |
| Turkey Pastrami Reuben | 500 | 21 | 50 |

**Sandwiches:**

| | C | F | Cb |
|---|---|---|---|
| Bacon, Gouda & Egg | 370 | 18 | 33 |
| Sausage, Cheddar & Egg | 500 | 28 | 41 |
| Slow Rsoasted Ham, Swiss & Egg | 460 | 23 | 43 |
| Spicy Chorizo, Monterey Jack & Egg | 500 | 30 | 35 |
| Spinach, Feta & Egg White Wrap | 290 | 10 | 33 |

**Paninis:**

| | C | F | Cb |
|---|---|---|---|
| Chicken Caprese | 500 | 18 | 58 |
| Chicken & Double Smoked Bacon | 620 | 26 | 65 |
| Roasted Tomato & Mozzarella | 350 | 13 | 42 |
| Turkey Pesto | 540 | 21 | 55 |

**Protein Boxes:**

| | C | F | Cb |
|---|---|---|---|
| Chicken BLT | 580 | 23 | 58 |
| Cheese & Fruit | 450 | 27 | 34 |
| PB & J | 520 | 26 | 53 |
| Smoked Turkey | 570 | 23 | 54 |

## Starbucks® cont... (Sept '19)

**Greek Yogurt Parfait,** | C | F | Cb

| | C | F | Cb |
|---|---|---|---|
| with Blueberries, Honey & Granola | 240 | 2.5 | 42 |

**Bakery:** *Each*

| | C | F | Cb |
|---|---|---|---|
| 8-Grain Roll | 340 | 5 | 68 |
| Almond Croissant, 3.5 oz | 420 | 22 | 45 |
| Banana Nut Bread, 4.4 oz | 420 | 22 | 52 |
| Blueberry Muffin, 3.9 oz | 360 | 15 | 52 |
| Blueberry Scone, 3.5 oz | 380 | 17 | 54 |
| Butter Croissant, 2.2 oz | 260 | 15 | 27 |
| Cheese Danish, 2.8 oz | 290 | 14 | 33 |
| Chocolate Chip Cookie, 2.8 oz | 360 | 18 | 47 |
| Classic Coffee Cake, 3.5 oz | 330 | 15 | 43 |
| Dble Choc. Chunk Brownie | 480 | 28 | 55 |
| Iced Lemon Loaf Cake, 4.4 oz | 470 | 20 | 68 |
| Old-Fashioned Glazed Donut, 4 oz | 480 | 27 | 56 |

**Bottled Drinks ~ See Page 37**

## Steak Escape® (Sept '19)

**Cheesesteaks:** *Per Medium* | C | F | Cb

| | C | F | Cb |
|---|---|---|---|
| Bourbon & Bacon | 1100 | 64 | 89 |
| Grand Escape | 690 | 28 | 66 |
| Original Philly | 710 | 30 | 68 |
| Sriracha | 790 | 34 | 73 |
| Steakhouse Sirloin | 1040 | 64 | 74 |

**Sandwiches:**

| | C | F | Cb |
|---|---|---|---|
| Chicken Bacon Club | 980 | 58 | 62 |
| Crispy Buffalo Chicken | 1020 | 48 | 90 |
| Grandest Chicken | 660 | 19 | 68 |
| Ragin' Cajun | 700 | 27 | 63 |
| Simply Chicken | 550 | 13 | 60 |

**Wraps:**

| | C | F | Cb |
|---|---|---|---|
| Crispy Buffalo Chicken | 930 | 47 | 81 |
| Cubano | 820 | 46 | 57 |
| Grandest Chicken | 590 | 21 | 56 |
| Grand Escape | 600 | 27 | 57 |
| Italian Hottie | 770 | 43 | 57 |
| Ragin' Cajun Chicken | 610 | 26 | 54 |

**Fries:**

| | C | F | Cb |
|---|---|---|---|
| Buffalo Chicken; Cajun Bleu | 950 | 60 | 83 |
| Loaded Cheese & Bacon, small | 920 | 63 | 79 |
| Naked, regular | 650 | 34 | 78 |
| Sriracha Steak | 900 | 53 | 87 |

**Salads:**

| | C | F | Cb |
|---|---|---|---|
| Bourbon & Bacon | 720 | 54 | 33 |
| Cubano | 530 | 38 | 10 |
| Hangover | 630 | 29 | 50 |

**Potatoes:**

| | C | F | Cb |
|---|---|---|---|
| Bourbon & Bacon | 1010 | 63 | 80 |
| Delerious Dagwood | 1090 | 75 | 53 |
| Hangover | 800 | 37 | 67 |
| Simply Chicken | 460 | 12 | 51 |
| Triple Cheesesteak | 900 | 54 | 57 |

**For Complete Nutritional Data ~ see CalorieKing.com**

## Steak 'n Shake® (Sept '19)

| *Steakburgers:* Without Fries | C | F | Cb |
|---|---|---|---|
| Bacon Lovers | 880 | 59 | 34 |
| **Bacon 'n Cheese:** Single | 450 | 26 | 29 |
| Double | 590 | 38 | 29 |
| Cajun Double | 740 | 53 | 30 |
| **Guacamole:** Single | 540 | 37 | 36 |
| Double | 700 | 50 | 37 |
| Jalapeno Crunch | 790 | 53 | 42 |
| Portobello & Swiss | 740 | 50 | 36 |
| Royale | 800 | 56 | 32 |
| Single Burger with Cheese | 660 | 42 | 33 |
| **The Original:** Double | 460 | 26 | 33 |
| with Cheese | 530 | 33 | 33 |
| Western BBQ 'N Bacon | 810 | 48 | 52 |
| *Chili:* 3-way | 710 | 21 | 98 |
| 5-way | 1160 | 57 | 103 |
| **Chili Deluxe:** Bowl | 1000 | 56 | 71 |
| Cup | 500 | 28 | 36 |
| **Chili Mac:** Regular | 1200 | 61 | 112 |
| Supreme | 1410 | 78 | 114 |
| *Melts:* Frisco | 980 | 67 | 52 |
| Veggie, with Portobellos | 620 | 45 | 44 |
| *Steak Franks:* | | | |
| Chili Cheese Frank | 710 | 44 | 46 |
| Steak Frank, footlong, with mustard | 390 | 23 | 32 |
| *Salads:* Without Dressing | | | |
| Beef Taco | 950 | 73 | 43 |
| Fried Chicken | 600 | 36 | 34 |
| *Fries:* Per Regular | | | |
| Reg.; Cajun; Parm. & Garlic Herb, av. | 450 | 24 | 55 |
| Cheese Fries | 590 | 35 | 63 |
| Chili Cheese Fries | 760 | 41 | 83 |
| *Sides:* Baked Beans | 310 | 0 | 64 |
| Coleslaw | 160 | 11 | 13 |
| Onion Rings, regular | 330 | 17 | 39 |
| *Breakfast:* | | | |
| **Breakfast Bowl** with Hash Browns | 460 | 42 | 11 |
| **Bagel Sandwich:** with Bacon | 460 | 17 | 53 |
| with Sausage | 700 | 38 | 53 |
| Banana Pancakes | 950 | 16 | 187 |
| **Biscuits:** Bacon | 380 | 25 | 33 |
| Bacon, Egg & Cheese | 530 | 36 | 34 |
| Sausage, Egg & Cheese | 770 | 57 | 34 |
| **Hash Browns,** Shredded | 300 | 28 | 15 |
| *Milk Shakes:* Per Regular | | | |
| Banana | 680 | 18 | 125 |
| Birthday Cake | 820 | 27 | 135 |
| Reese's Choc. Peanut Butter | 920 | 43 | 119 |
| White Chocolate | 620 | 19 | 105 |

## Subway® (Sept '19)

| *Fresh Fit Sandwiches:* | C | F | Cb |
|---|---|---|---|
| *Includes 9 Grain Wheat Sub, cucumbers, green peppers lettuce, red onions, spinach & tomatoes. Without any condiments* | | | |
| Black Forest Ham | 260 | 4 | 41 |
| Oven Roasted Chicken | 270 | 3.5 | 40 |
| Roast Beef | 290 | 4.5 | 40 |
| Subway Club | 290 | 4 | 41 |
| Sweet Onion Chicken Teriyaki | 330 | 4 | 53 |
| Turkey Breast | 250 | 3 | 40 |
| Veggie Delite | 230 | 2.5 | 44 |
| *Sandwiches on 6" 9-Grain Wheat Sub:* Includes cucumbers, green peppers, lettuce, red onions, spinach & tomatoes. Without any condiments | | | |
| Chicken & Bacon Ranch Melt | 530 | 26 | 42 |
| Cold Cut Combo | 320 | 11 | 42 |
| Oven Roasted Chkn | 270 | 3.5 | 40 |
| Roast Beef | 290 | 4.5 | 40 |
| Rotisserie Style Chicken | 310 | 6 | 40 |
| Subway Club | 290 | 4 | 41 |
| Turkey Breast | 250 | 3 | 40 |
| Veggie Delite | 200 | 2 | 39 |
| *Sandwiches on Italian Sub:* Includes cucumbers, green peppers, lettuce, red onions & tomatoes. Without any condiments | | | |
| Classic Tuna | 450 | 25 | 38 |
| Italian B.M.T. | 380 | 17 | 40 |
| Spicy Italian | 450 | 24 | 40 |
| *Sandwiches on Tomato Basil Wraps:* Includes cucumbers, green peppers, lettuce, red onions, spinach & tomatoes. Without any condiments | | | |
| Black Forest Ham, w/ Monterey Jack Cheese | 490 | 16 | 56 |
| Cold Cut Combo | 570 | 27 | 57 |
| Italian BMT | 490 | 22 | 55 |
| Oven Rstd Chicken | 380 | 10 | 53 |
| Roast Beef | 400 | 10 | 53 |
| Rotisserie Style Chicken | 430 | 12 | 53 |
| Spicy Italian | 560 | 30 | 55 |
| Subway Sub | 400 | 10 | 54 |
| Sweet Teriyaki | 440 | 10 | 65 |
| Turkey Breast | 370 | 9 | 54 |
| Veggie Delite | 310 | 8 | 53 |
| *Other Sandwiches:* On Italian Sub | | | |
| Meatball Marinara, w/ Parm Chse | 430 | 18 | 48 |
| Steak & American Cheese, with green peppers & red onions | 340 | 10 | 39 |

*continued next page....*

## Subway® cont... (Sept '19)

### Sandwich Condiments & Extras:

*For 6" Sandwiches*

| | C | F | Cb |
|---|---|---|---|
| Bacon Strips, 0.5 oz | 70 | 6 | 1 |
| **Cheese:** American, 0.4 oz | 40 | 3.5 | 1 |
| Cheddar; Swiss, 0.5 oz, av. | 55 | 4.5 | 0 |
| Chipotle Southwest Sauce, 0.5 oz | 80 | 7 | 1 |
| Honey Mustard Sce, Fat-Free, 0.5 oz | 20 | 0 | 4 |
| **Mayonnaise:** 1 Tbsp, 0.5 oz | 100 | 11 | 0 |
| Light, 1 Tbsp, 0.5 oz | 50 | 5 | 1 |
| Yellow Mustard, 0.5 oz | 10 | 0 | 1 |
| Olive Oil Blend, 0.2 oz | 45 | 5 | 0 |
| Ranch Dressing, 0.5 oz | 70 | 8 | 1 |
| Sweet Onion, Fat-Free, 0.63 oz | 30 | 0 | 8 |

*Chopped Salads (6g Fat or Less): Figures based on lettuce, tomatoes, spinach, onions, green peppers, olives & cucumbers. Dressing or croutons not included.*

| | C | F | Cb |
|---|---|---|---|
| Black Forest Ham | 120 | 3 | 12 |
| Oven Roasted Chicken | 130 | 2.5 | 12 |
| Roast Beef; Subway Club, average | 140 | 3.5 | 12 |
| Rotisserie Style Chicken | 170 | 5 | 11 |
| Turkey Breast | 110 | 2 | 12 |
| Veggie Delite | 60 | 1 | 11 |

### Soup: *Per 8 oz Bowl*

| | C | F | Cb |
|---|---|---|---|
| Beef Chili, with Beans | 360 | 22 | 20 |
| Black Bean | 210 | 1 | 39 |
| Broccoli Cheddar | 170 | 9 | 18 |
| Creamy Chicken & Wild Rice | 190 | 11 | 16 |
| Homestyle Chicken Noodle | 110 | 3 | 14 |
| Loaded Baked Potato, with Bacon | 210 | 13 | 15 |
| Mediterranean Vegetable | 110 | 3 | 14 |
| Spicy Chicken Tortilla | 110 | 4.5 | 12 |

### Breakfast:

**Omelet Sandwiches on 6" 9 Grain Bread:** *With Regular Egg & American Cheese*

| | C | F | Cb |
|---|---|---|---|
| Bacon, Egg & Cheese | 410 | 18 | 40 |
| Black Forest Ham, Egg & Chse | 370 | 13 | 40 |
| Egg & Cheese | 340 | 12 | 39 |
| Steak, Egg & Chse | 400 | 15 | 41 |

**Omelet Sandwich on 6" Flatbread:** *With Regular Egg & American Cheese*

| | C | F | Cb |
|---|---|---|---|
| Bacon, Egg & Cheese | 450 | 20 | 45 |
| Black Forest Ham, Egg & Chse | 410 | 16 | 45 |
| Egg & Cheese | 380 | 15 | 44 |
| Steak, Egg & Cheese | 450 | 18 | 46 |

## Subway® cont... (Sept '19)

### Breakfast (Cont):

**Egg White Omelet on 6" Flatbread:** *With Egg White & American Cheese*

| | C | F | Cb |
|---|---|---|---|
| Bacon, Egg & Cheese | 410 | 15 | 45 |
| Black Forest Ham, Egg & Cheese | 370 | 11 | 45 |
| Egg & Cheese | 340 | 10 | 44 |
| Steak, Egg & Cheese | 410 | 12 | 46 |

## Sweet Tomatoes® *Same Menu & Data as Souplantation ~ See Page 242*

## Swiss Chalet® (Sept '19)

*Canadian Outlets*

| | C | F | Cb |
|---|---|---|---|
| **Starters:** Chicken Spring Rolls (4) | 340 | 16 | 31 |
| Caesar Salad, without Dressing | 90 | 3 | 13 |
| Chalet Wings (10), w/out Sce | 560 | 34 | 13 |
| Cheese Perogies (7) | 470 | 15 | 71 |
| Stuffed Garlic Cheese Loaf | 860 | 57 | 63 |

**Burgers:** *Without Sides or Accompanying Sauce*

| | C | F | Cb |
|---|---|---|---|
| Classic Hamburger, with Mayo | 520 | 25 | 44 |
| Ultimate Bacon Cheeseburger | 730 | 42 | 46 |
| Veggie Burger with Mayo | 440 | 15 | 50 |

**Ribs:** *Without Add On Sauce or Sides*

| | C | F | Cb |
|---|---|---|---|
| **BBQ Side Ribs:** ⅓ Rack | 480 | 33 | 1 |
| ½ Rack | 720 | 50 | 1 |
| Full Rack | 1440 | 100 | 2 |
| **BBQ Back Ribs:** ½ Rack | 460 | 30 | 0 |
| Full Rack | 920 | 61 | 1 |

**Rotisserie Beef/Chicken:** *Without Sides, Sauces or Bread*

| | C | F | Cb |
|---|---|---|---|
| ½ Rack Back Ribs & Rot. Beef Combo | 980 | 50 | 51 |
| Beef & Shrimp Combo | 550 | 23 | 40 |
| Chicken Pot Pie, 1 pie | 670 | 36 | 54 |
| **Double Leg:** with skin | 490 | 31 | 0 |
| without skin | 320 | 16 | 0 |
| **Half Chicken:** with skin | 530 | 27 | 0 |
| without skin | 380 | 14 | 0 |
| **Quarter Chicken:** | | | |
| Dark Meat: with skin | 240 | 16 | 0 |
| without skin | 160 | 8 | 0 |
| White Meat: with skin | 290 | 11 | 0 |
| without skin | 220 | 6 | 0 |

**Sandwiches:** *Without Sides or Accompanying Sauce*

| | C | F | Cb |
|---|---|---|---|
| **Chicken Kaiser:** Dark Meat | 540 | 19 | 40 |
| White Meat | 450 | 8 | 40 |
| **Classic Hot Chicken:** | | | |
| Dark Meat | 610 | 21 | 51 |
| White Meat | 520 | 11 | 51 |

**Entree Salads:** *Without Dressing*

| | C | F | Cb |
|---|---|---|---|
| Rotisserie Chicken Caesar | 420 | 11 | 38 |
| Sweet Heat Chicken | 340 | 9 | 30 |

## Swiss Chalet® cont... (Sept '19)

*Sides: Per Serving*

| | C | F | Cb |
|---|---|---|---|
| Caesar Salad without Dressing | 50 | 1.5 | 8 |
| Creamy Coleslaw | 200 | 14 | 15 |
| Fresh Cut Fries | 720 | 37 | 86 |
| Fresh Vegetable Medley | 50 | 0.5 | 11 |
| Gravy | 45 | 1.5 | 7 |
| Jasmine Rice | 380 | 1 | 85 |
| Mashed Potatoes | 170 | 5 | 27 |
| Multigrain Roll | 110 | 1 | 22 |
| Poutine | 910 | 50 | 94 |
| Seasoned Rice Pilaf | 270 | 4 | 53 |
| Sweet Potato Fries | 410 | 23 | 48 |
| White Roll | 110 | 0 | 22 |

*Dressings:* Caesar, 1 oz

| | C | F | Cb |
|---|---|---|---|
| Caesar, 1 oz | 180 | 18 | 2 |
| Ranch, 1 oz | 140 | 14 | 2 |
| Swiss Signat. Chalet House, 1.5 oz | 220 | 19 | 10 |

*Sauce:* Chalet Dipping, 1 oz

| | C | F | Cb |
|---|---|---|---|
| Chalet Dipping, 1 oz | 25 | 0.5 | 5 |
| Plum, 2 oz | 140 | 0 | 35 |
| Smoky BBQ, 1 oz | 50 | 0 | 12 |

*Desserts/Pies: Slice*

| | C | F | Cb |
|---|---|---|---|
| Apple Pie, 6 oz | 440 | 20 | 63 |
| Classic Vanilla Cheesecake, 4.1 oz | 380 | 25 | 32 |
| Coconut Cream Pie, 6.1 oz | 490 | 28 | 55 |
| Lemon Meringue Pie, 6.5 oz | 410 | 15 | 65 |
| Pecan Pie w/ Caramel Sauce, 6 oz | 680 | 31 | 95 |

## Taco Bell® (Sept '19)

*Burritos: W/ Standard Components*

| | C | F | Cb |
|---|---|---|---|
| 7-Layer, no meat | 440 | 16 | 59 |
| Bean | 380 | 11 | 55 |
| Beefy 5-Layer | 500 | 19 | 64 |
| Beefy Fritos | 440 | 18 | 57 |
| Beefy Nacho Loaded Griller | 370 | 15 | 48 |
| Black Bean | 390 | 11 | 60 |
| Burrito Supreme | 400 | 15 | 52 |
| Cheesy Bean & Rice | 430 | 17 | 57 |
| Cheesy Potato Griller | 340 | 13 | 50 |
| Chili Cheese, no meat | 370 | 17 | 40 |
| Chipotle Chicken Loaded Griller | 340 | 16 | 36 |
| Quesarito | 650 | 33 | 68 |
| Shredded Chicken | 420 | 20 | 47 |
| XXL Grilled Stuft | 870 | 40 | 97 |
| *Nachos,* Triple Layer | 320 | 15 | 41 |

*Power Menu: With Standard Menu Component*

| | C | F | Cb |
|---|---|---|---|
| **Power Bowls:** Fire Grilled Chicken | 500 | 20 | 54 |
| Seasoned Beef | 550 | 26 | 58 |
| Veggie | 480 | 19 | 65 |
| **Power Burritos:** Fire Grilled Chkn | 450 | 20 | 41 |
| Seasoned Beef | 490 | 26 | 46 |
| Veggie | 430 | 19 | 52 |

## Taco Bell® cont... (Sept '19)

*Specialties: W/Standard Components*

| | C | F | Cb |
|---|---|---|---|
| **Chalupa Supreme:** Grilled Steak | 330 | 16 | 32 |
| Fire Grilled Chicken | 330 | 16 | 31 |
| Seasoned Beef | 350 | 18 | 33 |
| Shredded Chicken | 340 | 18 | 32 |
| **Cheesy Gordita Crunch,** | | | |
| Shredded Chicken | 480 | 27 | 39 |
| **Gordita Supreme:** Grilled Steak | 270 | 9 | 30 |
| Fire Grilled Chicken | 260 | 9 | 29 |
| Seasoned Beef | 280 | 12 | 31 |
| Shredded Chicken | 270 | 11 | 30 |
| **MexiMelt,** Seasoned Beef | 250 | 13 | 19 |
| **Nachos BellGrande,** Seas'nd Beef | 750 | 38 | 85 |
| **Quesadillas:** Cheese | 460 | 26 | 37 |
| Seasoned Beef | 530 | 30 | 40 |
| Shredded Chicken | 520 | 30 | 38 |
| **Taco Salads:** Fiesta, Seasoned Beef | 760 | 39 | 78 |
| Expr. Fiesta, Shredded Chicken | 560 | 24 | 62 |

*Tacos: With Standard Menu Components*

| | C | F | Cb |
|---|---|---|---|
| **Crunchy:** Seasoned Beef | 170 | 9 | 13 |
| Supreme, S'nd Beef | 190 | 11 | 15 |
| **Double Decker:** | | | |
| Seasoned Beef: Regular | 320 | 13 | 36 |
| Supreme | 340 | 15 | 39 |
| **Soft:** Grilled Steak | 200 | 10 | 17 |
| Shredded Chicken: Regular | 170 | 8 | 16 |
| Supreme | 200 | 9 | 18 |
| Spicy Potato, no meat | 230 | 12 | 27 |

*Sides: Regular Size*

| | C | F | Cb |
|---|---|---|---|
| Black Beans & Rice | 190 | 4 | 35 |
| Cheesy Fiesta Potatoes | 230 | 12 | 28 |
| Chips & Guacamole | 230 | 14 | 23 |
| Chips & Nach Cheese | 220 | 12 | 24 |
| Pintos 'n Cheese | 190 | 7 | 22 |
| Seasoned Rice | 120 | 2 | 23 |

*Breakfast: With Standard Menu Components*

| | C | F | Cb |
|---|---|---|---|
| **Crunchwrap:** Bacon & Egg | 660 | 42 | 51 |
| Ssg Patty & Egg | 700 | 46 | 51 |
| **Grilled Fiesta Potato Burrito:** | | | |
| Bacon & Egg | 400 | 19 | 44 |
| Grilled Steak & Egg | 390 | 16 | 44 |
| **Quesadillas:** Bacon & Egg | 510 | 28 | 37 |
| Sausage Crumbles & Egg | 500 | 29 | 37 |
| Steak & Egg | 500 | 26 | 38 |
| **Sweets:** Caramel Apple Empanada | 280 | 13 | 38 |
| **Cinnabon Delights:** | | | |
| 4 Pack | 310 | 18 | 35 |
| 12 Pack (serves 4) | 930 | 53 | 104 |
| **Cinnamon Twist** | 170 | 6 | 27 |

*Note: Nutritional data in New York outlets may vary slightly. Please check Taco Bell website*

## Taco Cabana® (Sept '19)

**Burritos:** C F Cb

*Includes Flour Tortilla, Rice, Refried Beans, Romaine, Meat, Shredded Cheese, Pico de Gallo & Sour Cream*

| | C | F | Cb |
|---|---|---|---|
| Beef Cabana | 720 | 29 | 79 |
| Brisket Canana | 790 | 40 | 76 |
| Chicken Cabana | 770 | 30 | 81 |
| Flame Grilled Chicken Fajita | 730 | 26 | 79 |
| Steak Fajita | 990 | 44 | 107 |

**Cabana Bowls:** *Includes Shell, Rice, Lettuce, Meat, Shredded Cheese, Pico de Gallo & Sour Cream*

| | C | F | Cb |
|---|---|---|---|
| Beef | 710 | 36 | 64 |
| Brisket | 780 | 48 | 60 |
| Chkn/Chkn Breast, av. | 740 | 35 | 65 |
| Steak Fajita | 740 | 39 | 63 |

**Enchiladas:**

| | C | F | Cb |
|---|---|---|---|
| Beef (1) | 200 | 11 | 14 |
| Cheese (1) | 320 | 23 | 13 |
| Chicken (1) | 280 | 13 | 21 |

**Quesadillas:** *Small, with Lettuce, Guac. & Sour Cream*

| | C | F | Cb |
|---|---|---|---|
| Brisket | 920 | 63 | 51 |
| Cheese | 770 | 50 | 51 |
| Flame-Gr. Chkn Fajita | 840 | 52 | 52 |
| Steak | 850 | 55 | 52 |

**Tacos:**

| | C | F | Cb |
|---|---|---|---|
| **Crispy:** Beef | 180 | 8 | 15 |
| Shredded Chicken | 200 | 9 | 16 |
| **Soft:** Bean & Cheese | 300 | 14 | 31 |
| Beef, ground | 210 | 9 | 21 |
| Black Bean | 220 | 5 | 38 |
| Brisket | 280 | 13 | 31 |
| Carne Guisada | 210 | 8 | 20 |
| Chkn Breast Fajita, flame grilled | 210 | 6 | 21 |
| Shredded Chicken | 240 | 9 | 23 |
| Steak | 220 | 9 | 21 |
| **Street,** Beef (3) | 460 | 25 | 40 |

**Salads:** *Includes Shell, Lettuce Meat, Shredded Cheese, Pico de Gallo & Sour Cream*

| | C | F | Cb |
|---|---|---|---|
| Beef, ground | 570 | 34 | 37 |
| Chicken, shredded | 610 | 35 | 39 |
| Chicken Fajita, flame grilled | 570 | 31 | 36 |
| Steak | 600 | 36 | 36 |

**Sides & Add-Ons:**

| | C | F | Cb |
|---|---|---|---|
| Borracho Beans, 8 oz | 290 | 6 | 40 |
| Combo Chips & Queso/Guacamole | 490 | 29 | 50 |
| Guacamole, 3 oz | 110 | 9 | 7 |
| Queso, 3 oz | 110 | 8 | 5 |
| Refried Beans with Cheese, 8 oz | 530 | 29 | 49 |
| Rice, 8 oz | 310 | 6 | 58 |
| Salsa, all flavors, 1 oz | 5 | 0 | 1 |
| Sour Cream, 3 oz | 160 | 15 | 3 |

## Taco Del Mar® (Sept '19)

**Burritos:** *Includes Flour Tortilla,* C F Cb *Rice, Refr. Beans, Protein, Cheese, Pico de Gallo & Sour Crm*

| | C | F | Cb |
|---|---|---|---|
| **Regular:** Chicken | 910 | 31 | 115 |
| Ground Beef | 950 | 37 | 116 |
| Pork | 900 | 31 | 115 |
| Shredded Beef | 910 | 31 | 116 |
| Steak | 870 | 27 | 117 |
| Vegan | 390 | 9 | 68 |
| Veggie | 470 | 16 | 69 |

**Burrito Bowls:** *Per Regular Bowl, with Rice, Refried Beans, Protein, Cheese, Pico de Gallo & Sour Cream*

| | C | F | Cb |
|---|---|---|---|
| Beef, shredded | 600 | 24 | 64 |
| Chicken | 600 | 24 | 63 |
| Pork | 590 | 24 | 63 |
| Steak | 560 | 20 | 65 |
| Vegan | 370 | 8 | 63 |
| Veggie | 530 | 22 | 67 |

**Nachos:** *Includes Chips, Refried Beans, Protein, Cheese, Pico de Gallo, Guacamole & Sour Cream*

| | C | F | Cb |
|---|---|---|---|
| **Beef:** Ground | 1210 | 78 | 90 |
| Shredded | 1160 | 71 | 90 |
| Cheese | 1040 | 66 | 88 |
| Chicken | 1170 | 72 | 89 |
| Fish | 1200 | 74 | 100 |
| Pork | 1150 | 71 | 89 |
| Steak | 1130 | 68 | 91 |

**Enchilada Platters:** *Includes Protein, Cheese, Rice, Refried Beans, Lettuce, Pico, Guacamole, Sour Crm & Sauce*

| | C | F | Cb |
|---|---|---|---|
| Beef, ground (2) | 890 | 37 | 106 |
| Cheese (2) | 810 | 32 | 105 |
| Chicken (2) | 850 | 31 | 105 |
| Fish (2) | 880 | 33 | 116 |
| Pork (2) | 830 | 30 | 104 |
| Steak (2) | 810 | 27 | 107 |

**Quesadillas:** *Includes Flour Tortilla, Meat, Cheese & Pico*

| | C | F | Cb |
|---|---|---|---|
| Beef: shredded | 710 | 34 | 59 |
| Cheese | 590 | 29 | 57 |
| Chicken | 720 | 35 | 58 |
| Fish | 750 | 37 | 69 |
| Pork | 700 | 34 | 58 |
| Steak | 680 | 31 | 60 |

**Taco Salads:** *Includes Shell, Cheese, Refried Beans, Lettuce, Meat & Pico de Gallo*

| | C | F | Cb |
|---|---|---|---|
| Beef, ground | 750 | 45 | 60 |
| Chicken | 710 | 38 | 59 |
| Fish | 730 | 41 | 70 |
| Pork | 690 | 38 | 58 |
| Shrimp | 650 | 33 | 60 |
| Steak | 670 | 35 | 61 |

*Note: Nutritional Information varies from state to state. Please refer to Taco Del Mar Website*

## Taco John's® (Sept '19)

| *Burritos:* | C | F | Cb |
|---|---|---|---|
| Bean, 6.6 oz | 360 | 10 | 54 |
| Combination, 6.6 oz | 400 | 15 | 48 |
| Grilled Beef, 8.7 oz | 590 | 31 | 54 |
| Grilled Chicken, 8.7 oz | 580 | 28 | 53 |
| **Meat & Potato:** Beef, 8.35 oz | 510 | 24 | 59 |
| Chicken, 8.35 oz | 480 | 19 | 58 |
| Crunchy Chkn, 8.85 oz | 580 | 25 | 68 |
| **Super,** 8.85 oz | 440 | 18 | 51 |
| *Mexi Rolls: Without Nacho Cheese* | | | |
| 4 Pieces, 8 oz | 370 | 21 | 30 |
| 6 Pieces, 10 oz | 550 | 32 | 45 |
| *Super Nachos:* | | | |
| Beef, 12.62 oz | 800 | 43 | 82 |
| Sirloin Steak,13.1 oz | 810 | 42 | 81 |
| *Quesadillas:* | | | |
| Cheesy, 5.5 oz | 450 | 24 | 40 |
| Chicken, 8.6 oz | 530 | 25 | 48 |
| *Super Potato Oles,* reg., 16.86 oz | 1090 | 67 | 98 |
| *Tacos:* Crispy Taco, 3.25 oz | 170 | 10 | 11 |
| **Softshell Taco:** | | | |
| Beef, 4 oz | 210 | 10 | 21 |
| Chicken, 4 oz | 180 | 5 | 20 |
| **Single Street:** Chkn, 3.25 | 170 | 6 | 7 |
| Sirloin Steak, 3.25 | 180 | 5 | 20 |
| Stuffed Grilled Taco, 7.4 oz | 540 | 25 | 58 |
| **Taco Bravo,** 6.5 oz | 320 | 13 | 36 |
| *Salads: Without Dressing* | | | |
| Beef Taco Salad | 540 | 33 | 45 |
| Chicken Taco Salad | 500 | 27 | 44 |
| Crunch Chicken | 630 | 36 | 58 |
| *Sides:* | | | |
| **Chips:** with Nachos | 380 | 20 | 45 |
| with Queso | 430 | 22 | 50 |
| **Potato Oles:** Small | 480 | 27 | 52 |
| Medium | 670 | 38 | 73 |
| Large | 860 | 49 | 94 |
| Refried Beans, 9.5 oz | 320 | 17 | 46 |
| Side Salad, without dressing 3.2 oz | 40 | 2.5 | 3 |
| *Condiments:* | | | |
| Bacon Ranch Dressing, 1.5 oz | 120 | 9 | 10 |
| House Dressing, 1.5 oz | 70 | 7 | 2 |
| Nacho Cheese Sce, 3 oz | 110 | 9 | 5 |
| Salsa, 2 oz | 10 | 0 | 2 |
| Sour Cream, 2.5 oz | 140 | 13 | 4 |
| *Breakfast:* | | | |
| **Burritos:** Bacon & Potato, 7.7 oz | 540 | 25 | 57 |
| Bacon Scrambler, 8.7 oz | 550 | 25 | 59 |
| Sausage Scrambler, 8.7 oz | 650 | 33 | 60 |
| **Potato Ole Scrambler,** sausage | 1080 | 68 | 86 |
| *Desserts:* Churro, 2 oz | 200 | 9 | 29 |
| Mexican Donut Bites, 3.2 oz | 290 | 12 | 47 |

## Taco Mayo® (Sept '19)

| *Burritos:* | C | F | Cb |
|---|---|---|---|
| Bean | 450 | 14 | 63 |
| Chicken Burrito Supreme | 420 | 19 | 40 |
| **Double Smothered Dble Queso:** | | | |
| Beef | 930 | 43 | 88 |
| Chicken | 850 | 39 | 83 |
| **Mexicali Gr. Chicken** | 635 | 38 | 48 |
| **Super:** Regular | 525 | 21 | 56 |
| Beef | 525 | 21 | 56 |
| *Mexicali Bowls:* Chipotle Chicken | 1225 | 71 | 91 |
| Insalata Little Big | 275 | 16 | 14 |
| Little Big | 450 | 18 | 41 |
| Queso Chicken | 1035 | 48 | 92 |
| *Nachos:* | | | |
| **Classic:** Beef Supreme | 790 | 38 | 81 |
| Cheese | 370 | 20 | 44 |
| Chicken Supreme | 710 | 34 | 77 |
| Ultimate Grande | 990 | 51 | 93 |
| *Quesadillas:* Chicken Platter | 690 | 40 | 45 |
| Beef Melt | 655 | 35 | 45 |
| Chicken Melt | 575 | 30 | 41 |
| *Tacos:* Crispy Beef | 160 | 9 | 10 |
| Fish | 280 | 13 | 27 |
| Soft Taco: Beef | 230 | 10 | 19 |
| Chicken | 185 | 8 | 16 |
| Taco Burger | 360 | 15 | 32 |
| *Tamale Ole* | 415 | 38 | 64 |
| *Tostadas* | 235 | 0 | 28 |
| *Salads: As Per Menu Description* | | | |
| Beef | 665 | 33 | 55 |
| Chicken | 445 | 26 | 31 |
| *Sides:* Cheddar & Chips | 555 | 31 | 62 |
| Guacmole & Chips | 575 | 35 | 63 |
| Mexicali Rice | 180 | 10 | 17 |
| Queso & Chips | 575 | 30 | 62 |
| Potato Locos, small | 400 | 25 | 37 |
| Queso-N-Chips | 575 | 35 | 62 |
| Refried Beans | 225 | 4 | 34 |
| *Kids Meals:* | | | |
| **Burritos:** with Fruit Cup | 505 | 14 | 78 |
| with Potato Loco | 845 | 39 | 99 |
| **Quesadillas:** with Fruit Cup | 270 | 12 | 31 |
| with Potato Loco | 605 | 37 | 52 |
| **Tacos:** | | | |
| Crispy: Beef with Fruit Cup | 220 | 7.5 | 29 |
| with Potato Loco | 560 | 33 | 50 |
| Soft: Beef with Fruit Cup | 290 | 10 | 35 |
| with Potato Loco | 630 | 36 | 56 |

## Taco Time® (Sept '19)

| | C | F | Cb |
|---|---|---|---|
| **Burritos:** | | | |
| 5 Alarm | 420 | 15 | 58 |
| Chicken B.L.T. | 600 | 31 | 46 |
| Sweet Pork | 550 | 18 | 72 |
| **Big Juan:** Chicken | 590 | 16 | 79 |
| Seasoned Beef | 650 | 22 | 83 |
| **Casita:** Chicken | 450 | 16 | 44 |
| Seasoned Beef | 510 | 22 | 48 |
| **Crisp Burrito:** | | | |
| Chicken | 380 | 17 | 39 |
| Meat | 390 | 17 | 43 |
| Pinto Bean | 380 | 13 | 53 |
| **Soft Burrito:** Pinto Bean | 380 | 10 | 56 |
| Seasoned Beef | 420 | 16 | 46 |
| **Veggie** | 440 | 17 | 60 |
| *Nachos:* Original | 900 | 39 | 91 |
| Chicken | 970 | 39 | 92 |
| Seasoned Beef | 1020 | 45 | 96 |
| **Optionals:** | | | |
| **Green Chili Pork:** Burrito | 460 | 18 | 43 |
| Chimichanga | 590 | 21 | 65 |
| Enchiladas | 340 | 12 | 26 |
| **Soup,** Enchilada, 8 oz | 130 | 0.5 | 20 |
| *Quesadillas:* Cheese | 450 | 23 | 39 |
| Chicken | 520 | 24 | 42 |
| **Tacos:** | | | |
| **Soft Tacos:** Chicken | 360 | 10 | 42 |
| Junior | 300 | 13 | 29 |
| Pork; Seasoned Beef, av. | 425 | 16 | 44 |
| **Super Soft Tacos:** Chicken | 500 | 16 | 61 |
| Pork | 590 | 21 | 62 |
| Seasoned Beef | 560 | 21 | 65 |
| **Fries:** | | | |
| **Mexi:** Small, 3.2 oz | 190 | 12 | 19 |
| Regular, 4.7 oz | 300 | 19 | 29 |
| **Stuffed:** Small, 4.5 oz | 320 | 20 | 29 |
| Regular, 6.6 oz | 460 | 28 | 42 |
| **Salads:** | | | |
| **Fiesta,** Chicken,12.3 oz | 340 | 11 | 37 |
| **Taco:** Chicken, 8 oz | 310 | 14 | 26 |
| Seasn'd Beef , 7.5 oz | 360 | 19 | 28 |
| **Breakfast:** | | | |
| **Burritos:** *Regular Size* | | | |
| Bacon & Egg | 450 | 20 | 48 |
| Egg & Cheese | 370 | 16 | 40 |
| Enchilada | 450 | 20 | 46 |
| Sausage & Egg | 560 | 30 | 48 |
| Ultimate | 760 | 48 | 50 |
| **Quesadilla** | 300 | 17 | 18 |
| **Taters & Gravy,** regular | 410 | 27 | 36 |
| *Churros:* Plain | 210 | 16 | 15 |
| Bavarian Cream | 320 | 8 | 54 |
| Cinnamon Crustos | 320 | 5 | 64 |

## TCBY® (Sept '19)

| | C | F | Cb |
|---|---|---|---|
| **Soft Serve Frozen Yogurt:** | | | |
| *Per ½ Cup, 4 fl.oz* | | | |
| **Dairy Free/Sorbet:** | | | |
| Chocolate Almond | 100 | 1 | 28 |
| Coconut | 125 | 5 | 18 |
| Kiwi Strawberry Sorbet | 90 | 0 | 22 |
| Mango Sorbet | 95 | 0 | 24 |
| Orange Sorbet | 90 | 0 | 23 |
| Watermelon Sorbet | 100 | 0 | 25 |
| **No Sugar Added:** Chocolate; Strawb. | 65 | 0 | 18 |
| Mountain Blackberry | 65 | 0 | 18 |
| Salted Caramel | 70 | 0 | 18 |
| **Super Fro Yo:** Bananas Foster | 90 | 0 | 23 |
| Cake Batter; Golden Vanilla | 105 | 2 | 22 |
| Chocolate | 100 | 1.5 | 22 |
| Dutch Chocolate | 95 | 0 | 23 |
| Graham Cracker | 105 | 2 | 25 |
| Greek Honey Vanilla | 100 | 0 | 20 |
| New York Cheesecake | 115 | 2 | 23 |
| Old Fashioned Vanilla | 90 | 0 | 23 |
| Peppermint | 105 | 2 | 22 |
| White Chocolate Mousse | 120 | 1.5 | 24 |
| **Hand-Scooped Frozen Yogurt:** *Gluten Free* | | | |
| **Butter Pecan:** Kid's, 4 fl.oz | 220 | 10 | 27 |
| Small, 6.4 fl.oz | 350 | 16 | 43 |
| Regular, 12.8 fl.oz | 705 | 32 | 86 |
| **Chocolate Chocolate:** | | | |
| Kid's, 4 fl.oz | 120 | 2.5 | 20 |
| Small, 6.4 fl.oz | 190 | 4 | 38 |
| Regular,12.8 fl.oz | 385 | 8 | 76 |
| **Cookies & Cream:** | | | |
| Kid's, 4 fl.oz | 200 | 6 | 32 |
| Small, 6.4 fl.oz | 320 | 10 | 51 |
| Regular, 12.8 fl.oz | 640 | 19 | 102 |
| **Peanut Butter Delight:** | | | |
| Kid's, 4 fl.oz | 250 | 13 | 30 |
| Small, 6.4 fl.oz | 400 | 21 | 48 |
| Regular, 12.8 fl.oz | 800 | 42 | 96 |
| **Pralines & Cream:** Kid's 4 fl.oz | 210 | 6 | 27 |
| Small, 6.4 fl.oz | 335 | 10 | 43 |
| Regular, 12.8 fl oz | 670 | 19 | 86 |
| **Vanilla Bean:** | | | |
| Kid's,4 fl.oz | 170 | 4.5 | 27 |
| Small, 6.4 fl.oz | 270 | 7 | 43 |
| Regular, 12.8 fl.oz | 545 | 14 | 86 |

## TGI Friday's® (Sept '19)

| Appetizers/Snacks: | C | F | Cb |
|---|---|---|---|
| BBQ Chicken & Bacon Flatbread | 620 | 32 | 50 |
| Bucket of Bones | 1570 | 82 | 120 |
| Cheeseburger Sliders (2) | 620 | 37 | 45 |
| Chips & Salsa | 290 | 13 | 51 |
| Chicken Quesadilla | 1190 | 82 | 56 |
| Giant Onion Rings | 1190 | 55 | 155 |
| Loaded Potato Skins, with Ranch Sour Cream | 1510 | 73 | 179 |
| Mozzarella Sticks, w/ Marinara | 840 | 52 | 54 |
| Pan Seared Potstickers, w/ Szechuan Sauce | 590 | 25 | 72 |
| Spinach Artichoke Dip | 720 | 50 | 63 |
| Wings Roulette Platter, w/o drssng | 2170 | 120 | 148 |

| Burgers: *Without Sides* | | | |
|---|---|---|---|
| Bacon Cheeseburger | 840 | 54 | 47 |
| Beyond Meat Cheeseburger | 890 | 57 | 55 |
| Buffalo Wingman's | 920 | 60 | 45 |
| Cheeseburger | 820 | 53 | 46 |
| Philly Cheesesteak | 1000 | 65 | 58 |
| Signature Whiskey-Glazed | 1110 | 55 | 110 |

| Chicken & Seafood: | | | |
|---|---|---|---|
| Crispy Checken Tenders, with Fries & Honey Mustard | 1030 | 59 | 87 |
| Fish & Chips, Coleslaw & Tartar Sce | 890 | 55 | 73 |
| Fried Shrimp, with Coleslaw & Cocktail Sce | 880 | 52 | 81 |
| Gr. Salmon, Jasmine Rice & Veggies | 830 | 38 | 86 |
| Parmesan Crusted Chicken, with Mashed Potatoes & Broccoli | 700 | 38 | 43 |
| Pasta: Cajun Shrimp & Chicken | 1510 | 83 | 114 |
| Chicken Parmesan, full order | 1800 | 106 | 137 |
| Lemon & Garlic Shrimp | 1390 | 77 | 117 |

| Ribs: *With Coleslaw & Seasoned Fries* | | | |
|---|---|---|---|
| **BBQ:** Half Rack | 910 | 50 | 80 |
| Full Rack | 1290 | 74 | 93 |
| **Whiskey Glazed:** Half Rack | 1110 | 51 | 129 |
| Full Rack | 1630 | 75 | 178 |

| Sandwiches: *W/out Sides* | | | |
|---|---|---|---|
| Bacon Ranch Chicken | 690 | 36 | 42 |
| French Dip | 950 | 49 | 74 |
| Southern Fried Chicken | 930 | 57 | 67 |
| Whiskey Glazed Chicken | 1110 | 57 | 100 |

*Steaks: With Mashed Potatoes & Lemon Butter Broccoli*

| Centre Cut Sirloin: | | | |
|---|---|---|---|
| w/ Parm. Butter | 640 | 41 | 34 |
| w/ Whiskey Glaze | 710 | 31 | 76 |
| **New York Strip:** with Parm Butter | 985 | 56 | 37 |
| with Whiskey Glaze | 1100 | 46 | 91 |

## TGI Friday's® cont... (Sept '19)

| Salads: | C | F | Cb |
|---|---|---|---|
| House, without dressing | 220 | 8 | 29 |
| Caesar, with Breadstick & dressing | 440 | 31 | 33 |
| Soups: French Onion | 590 | 18 | 84 |
| New England Clam Chowder | 500 | 30 | 45 |
| Tomato Basil | 300 | 24 | 20 |
| White Cheddar Broccoli Cheese | 280 | 20 | 18 |

| Salad Dressing: *Per 1.25 oz* | | | |
|---|---|---|---|
| Balsamic Vinaigrette | 50 | 2 | 9 |
| Bleu Cheese | 200 | 21 | 1 |
| Caesar | 190 | 20 | 1 |
| Honey Mustard | 200 | 18 | 8 |
| Ranch | 130 | 14 | 1 |

| Signature Sides: Coleslaw | 130 | 10 | 10 |
|---|---|---|---|
| Giant Onion Rings | 510 | 26 | 61 |
| Jasmine Rice | 420 | 11 | 72 |
| Lemon Butter Broccoli | 150 | 11 | 11 |
| Loaded Fries | 600 | 40 | 50 |
| Mashed Potatoes | 220 | 11 | 21 |
| Seasoned Fries | 320 | 16 | 40 |
| Sweet Potato Fries | 390 | 20 | 50 |

| Desserts: *Per Whole Dish* | | | |
|---|---|---|---|
| Brownie Obsession | 1200 | 60 | 153 |
| Oreo Madness | 500 | 21 | 76 |
| Tennessee Whiskey Cake | 1110 | 52 | 151 |

| Signature Slushes: | | | |
|---|---|---|---|
| Blue Raspberry | 170 | 0 | 42 |
| Mango Peach Lemonade | 170 | 0 | 44 |
| Red Bull Passion, regular | 210 | 0 | 54 |
| Strawberry Lemonade | 150 | 0 | 38 |

## Thundercloud Subs® (Sept '19)

| Subs: *Small, with Standard Toppings* | C | F | Cb |
|---|---|---|---|
| **Classic:** BLT | 365 | 17 | 35 |
| Genoa Salami | 265 | 6 | 35 |
| Roast Beef | 290 | 4 | 35 |
| Smoked Chicken | 270 | 4 | 35 |
| Turkey | 255 | 4 | 36 |
| **Signature Subs:** | | | |
| Club | 445 | 19 | 38 |
| California Club | 475 | 23 | 40 |
| NY Italian | 540 | 30 | 37 |
| Office Favorite | 790 | 39 | 71 |
| Texas Tuna | 675 | 44 | 39 |
| Veggie Delite, with Hummus | 385 | 19 | 52 |

## T.J. Cinnamons® (Sept '19)

| Bakery: | C | F | Cb |
|---|---|---|---|
| Orig. Gourmet Cinn. Roll, 7.8 oz | 840 | 42 | 106 |
| Pecan Stick Bun, 8.3 oz | 940 | 49 | 111 |

## Tim Hortons® (Sept '19)

*Breakfast:*

| | C | F | Cb |
|---|---|---|---|
| **Biscuit Sandwich:** | | | |
| Sausage, Egg & Cheese | 530 | 34 | 33 |
| Turkey, Egg & Cheese | 425 | 23 | 34 |
| **English Muffin Sandwich:** | | | |
| Sausage, Egg & Cheese | 450 | 27 | 30 |
| Turkey, Egg & Cheese | 350 | 16 | 31 |
| **Grilled B'Fast Wraps:** | | | |
| Farmer's Breakfast Grilled Wrap | 450 | 38 | 54 |
| Steak & Cheddar Grilled Wrap | 440 | 21 | 40 |
| **Oatmeal,** with Mixed Berries, reg. | 210 | 3 | 44 |
| *Hash Brown,* 1.9 oz | 130 | 7 | 16 |
| *Hot Bowls: Per Regular Size* | | | |
| Cream of Broccoli Soup | 150 | 7 | 16 |
| Chili | 330 | 18 | 18 |
| Chicken Noodle Soup | 120 | 1.5 | 21 |
| Clam Chowder | 190 | 7 | 23 |
| Harvest Vegetable Soup | 80 | 0.5 | 14 |
| Spicy Thai Chicken Soup | 210 | 12 | 21 |
| Mac & Cheese | 490 | 27 | 48 |
| Potato Bacon Cheddar Soup | 260 | 15 | 22 |
| *Sandwiches:* | | | |
| BLT | 430 | 16 | 59 |
| Chicken Salad Croissant | 410 | 22 | 34 |
| Ham & Cheddar | 470 | 15 | 58 |
| *Wraps:* Chicken Bacon Ranch | 380 | 14 | 39 |
| Chicken Salad | 350 | 13 | 38 |
| Chipotle Cheddar Chicken | 430 | 19 | 40 |
| Ham & Chedar | 380 | 16 | 40 |
| Turkey Bacon Club | 420 | 17 | 37 |
| *Potato Wedges,* 6 oz | 250 | 10 | 37 |
| *Donuts:* Apple Fritter | 310 | 8 | 53 |
| Chocolate Dip | 200 | 6 | 34 |
| Double Chocolate | 260 | 14 | 32 |
| Honey Cruller | 280 | 18 | 27 |
| Sour Cream Glazed | 320 | 16 | 40 |
| *Timbits:* Choc. Glazed; Sour Crm (1), av. | 90 | 4 | 24 |
| Honey Dip (1) | 60 | 1 | 12 |
| Old Fashioned/Filled (1), av. | 50 | 1.5 | 7 |
| *Cinnamon Roll,* glazed | 320 | 12 | 47 |
| *Cookies:* Chocolate Chunk | 240 | 10 | 34 |
| Oatmeal Raisin Spice | 210 | 8 | 32 |
| Peanut Butter | 280 | 17 | 27 |
| *Muffins:* Wild Blueberry, 4 oz | 340 | 11 | 57 |
| Wh. Grain Pecan Banana Bread | 350 | 11 | 60 |

## Tim Hortons® cont... (Sept '19)

*Beverages:*

| | C | F | Cb |
|---|---|---|---|
| **Hot:** Cappuccino, 14 fl.oz | 120 | 4.5 | 11 |
| Mocha Latte, 14 fl.oz | 240 | 6 | 37 |
| **Iced:** Caramel Latte, 17.4 fl.oz | 220 | 5 | 37 |
| Coffee, 12.8 fl.oz | 120 | 7 | 12 |
| **Yogurt Smoothies:** | | | |
| Strawb. Banana, 12.8 fl.oz | 140 | 1 | 30 |
| Tropical Fruit, 12.8 fl.oz | 150 | 1 | 32 |

## Togo's® (Sept '19)

*California Outlet ~ Please check local outlet for menu items and nutritional information*

*Cold Sandwiches: Per Regular 6", with Menu Set Components on White Bread*

| | C | F | Cb |
|---|---|---|---|
| #1: Chicken | 580 | 19 | 69 |
| #2: Ham & Swiss | 690 | 28 | 70 |
| #3: Turkey & Cheddar | 800 | 39 | 68 |
| #4: Turkey, Salami & Cheddar | 980 | 56 | 68 |
| #5: Turkey & Cranberry | 650 | 18 | 86 |
| #7: Roast Beef | 710 | 21 | 67 |
| #8: Roast Beef & Turkey | 880 | 40 | 69 |
| #16: The Italian | 880 | 47 | 70 |
| #20: Albacore Tuna | 670 | 27 | 72 |
| #23: Salami & Provolone | 1020 | 61 | 68 |

*Hot Sandwiches: Per Regular 6", with Menu Set Components on White Bread*

| | C | F | Cb |
|---|---|---|---|
| Meatball | 890 | 40 | 81 |
| Pastrami | 740 | 34 | 73 |
| Pepperjack Melt | 1010 | 59 | 73 |

*Wraps: Per Whole 12" Spinach Tortilla Wrap, with Menu Set Components*

| | C | F | Cb |
|---|---|---|---|
| Asian Chicken | 650 | 28 | 70 |
| Bacon Ranch Chicken | 680 | 33 | 55 |
| Cali Veggie | 810 | 49 | 63 |
| Chicken Caesar | 570 | 21 | 62 |
| Greek Veggie | 760 | 45 | 78 |
| Santa Fe Chicken | 710 | 34 | 69 |

*Salads: Per Full Salad, with Dressing*

| | C | F | Cb |
|---|---|---|---|
| Asian chicken | 670 | 43 | 44 |
| Chicken Caesar | 450 | 26 | 22 |
| Farmer's Market | 480 | 39 | 26 |
| Santa Fe Chicken | 780 | 55 | 37 |

*Soups: Per Regular, 10 fl.oz*

| | C | F | Cb |
|---|---|---|---|
| Broccoli Cheddar | 350 | 25 | 18 |
| Chicken Noodle | 110 | 3.5 | 16 |
| Chicken Tortilla | 120 | 3 | 15 |
| Hearty Vegetable | 100 | 0.5 | 9 |
| *Brownie,* Choc. Chunk, 3 oz | 440 | 23 | 56 |
| *Cookies:* Choc. Chunk, 3 oz | 410 | 21 | 54 |
| Oatmeal Raisin, 3 oz | 370 | 13 | 58 |

## Tropical Smoothie Cafe® (Sept '19)

*Menu & Nutrition Differ from Outlets to* **C** **F** **Cb**
*Outlet. Please Check Instore. Figures below Based On Irvine, CA*

**Breakfast:**

| | C | F | Cb |
|---|---|---|---|
| All American Omelet Wrap | 430 | 20 | 37 |
| Peanut Butter Crunch Flatbread | 590 | 24 | 77 |
| Southwest Omelet Wrap | 580 | 36 | 38 |
| **Bowls:** Baja Chicken | 470 | 21 | 37 |
| Buffalo Chicken | 420 | 25 | 16 |
| Caribbean Jerk Chicken | 440 | 12 | 52 |
| Hummus Veggie | 620 | 42 | 48 |
| **Pressed Sandwiches:** Chicken Caprese | 730 | 30 | 64 |
| with Bacon | 790 | 35 | 64 |
| Cuban | 790 | 42 | 64 |
| **Quesadillas:** | | | |
| Island Chicken | 570 | 27 | 51 |
| Santa Fe Chicken | 600 | 28 | 50 |
| Three Cheese Chicken | 550 | 27 | 41 |
| **Toasted Sandwiches:** *Per Whole Ciabatta Sandwich* | | | |
| Turkey Apple Dijon | 640 | 31 | 52 |
| Turkey Bacon Ranch | 560 | 20 | 59 |
| Tropical Chicken Salad | 610 | 33 | 52 |
| **Toasted Wraps:** *In Flour Tortilla* | | | |
| Baja Chicken | 640 | 24 | 67 |
| Buffalo Chicken | 510 | 21 | 44 |
| Caribbean Jerk Chkn | 590 | 17 | 74 |
| Hummus Veggie | 740 | 38 | 83 |
| Supergreen Caesar Chicken | 610 | 31 | 42 |
| Thai Chicken | 500 | 15 | 62 |
| **Classic Smoothies:** *Per 24 oz with Turbinado* | | | |
| Bahama Mama | 500 | 4.5 | 117 |
| Beach Bum | 550 | 5 | 129 |
| Blimey Limey | 440 | 0 | 111 |
| Blueberry Bliss | 340 | 5 | 86 |
| Health Nut, with Soy | 530 | 4.5 | 101 |
| Lean Machine | 490 | 0 | 124 |
| Mocha Madness | 660 | 5 | 152 |
| Muscle Blaster, with Pea | 520 | 2 | 98 |
| Peanut Paradise, with Pea | 740 | 17 | 107 |
| Peanut Butter Cup | 710 | 20 | 127 |
| Sunrise | 390 | 0 | 98 |
| Sunrise Sunset | 360 | 0 | 89 |

## Tubby's® (Sept '19)

**Subs:** *Per Regular 8" Sub, w/ Standard Ingredients, w/out Added Sauce or Dressing* **C** **F** **Cb**

| | C | F | Cb |
|---|---|---|---|
| **Deli-Subs:** | | | |
| Ham & Cheese | 540 | 11 | 78 |
| Turkey Breast & Cheese | 550 | 11 | 77 |
| **Grilled Burger Subs:** Big Tub | 790 | 35 | 78 |
| Cheeseburger Italiano | 790 | 35 | 78 |
| Loaded Burger | 820 | 36 | 83 |
| Pizza Burger | 810 | 36 | 81 |

## Tubby's® cont... (Sept '19)

**Subs (Cont):** *Per Reg. 8" Sub, with* **C** **F** **Cb**
*Standard Ingredients, w/out Added Sauce or Dressing*

| | C | F | Cb |
|---|---|---|---|
| **Grilled Chicken Subs:** Gr. Chicken | 450 | 4.5 | 75 |
| Chicken & Broccoli | 550 | 11 | 78 |
| Chicken & Cheddar | 540 | 11 | 75 |
| Chicken Fajita | 550 | 11 | 79 |
| **Grilled Steak Subs:** | | | |
| Loaded Steak | 650 | 18 | 81 |
| Pepper Steak & Cheese | 630 | 17 | 77 |
| Portabella Mushroom Steak | 630 | 17 | 78 |
| Steak & Cheese | 620 | 17 | 76 |
| **Specialty Subs:** BLT | 570 | 21 | 72 |
| Cold Veggie | 490 | 10 | 86 |
| Italian Sausage | 600 | 22 | 78 |
| Meatball | 790 | 33 | 83 |
| Tuna | 570 | 11 | 76 |

## Uno Pizzeria & Grill® (Sept '19)

| | C | F | Cb |
|---|---|---|---|
| **Appetizers:** *Per Whole Dish* | | | |
| Mozzarella Sticks | 1100 | 57 | 108 |
| Muchos Nachos | 1700 | 71 | 199 |
| Shrimp & Crab Dip | 1120 | 81 | 64 |
| **Burgers:** *With Fries* | | | |
| Bacon Cheddar | 1800 | 132 | 70 |
| Bacon Me Happy | 2060 | 144 | 107 |
| Uno | 1450 | 105 | 70 |
| Whole Hog | 3510 | 252 | 146 |
| **Entrees:** | | | |
| **Chicken:** *Without Breadstick* | | | |
| Baked Stuffed Spinoccoli | 330 | 15 | 6 |
| Herb Rubbed Chicken | 310 | 20 | 1 |
| Romano Crusted Chicken Parm. | 1120 | 42 | 128 |
| **Pasta:** *With Housemade Bread* | | | |
| Chicken Spinoccoli | 1260 | 62 | 105 |
| Deep Dish Mac & Cheese | 1740 | 103 | 140 |
| Shrimp Scampi | 1190 | 54 | 128 |
| **Steak & Seafood:** *Without Sides or Breadstick* | | | |
| Grilled Shrimp & Sirloin | 690 | 45 | 1 |
| Shrimp Skewer | 130 | 8 | 1 |
| Sirloin, 10 oz | 560 | 37 | 0 |
| Sirloin Steak Tips | 470 | 20 | 4 |
| **Deep Dish Individual Pizza:** *Per Slice, ¼ Pizza* | | | |
| Chicago Classic | 560 | 39 | 28 |
| Numero Uno | 460 | 31 | 30 |
| Prima Pepperoni | 430 | 30 | 28 |
| **Sides:** French Fries, 7.5 oz | 450 | 33 | 35 |
| House Made Bread | 120 | 1 | 18 |
| Jumbo Onion Rings, 7.5 oz | 370 | 7 | 68 |
| Loaded Mashed Potatoes | 420 | 26 | 37 |
| Red Bliss Mashed Potatoes | 280 | 14 | 36 |
| Roasted Seasonal Veggies, 7.2 oz | 70 | 4 | 8 |
| **Dessert:** All American | 640 | 28 | 90 |
| Uno Deep Dish Sundae | 1520 | 74 | 206 |

# Fast - Foods & *Restaurants*

## Villa Fresh Italian® (Sept '19)

*Pizzas: Per Slice*

| | C | F | Cb |
|---|---|---|---|
| **Neapolitan:** Buffalo | 770 | 46 | 52 |
| Deluxe | 530 | 22 | 55 |
| Sausage & Pepperoni | 550 | 25 | 53 |
| **Stuffed:** Baked Ziti | 845 | 33 | 97 |
| Spinach & Mushroom | 735 | 33 | 79 |

*Entrees:*

| | C | F | Cb |
|---|---|---|---|
| Chicken Pasta Primavera, 16 oz | 505 | 20 | 58 |
| Fettuccini Alfredo, 14 oz | 765 | 38 | 85 |
| Mac & Cheese, 14 oz | 725 | 54 | 39 |
| Pasta Primavera, 18 oz | 495 | 21 | 66 |
| Spaghetti & Meatballs, 18 oz | 840 | 28 | 112 |

*Sides:* Caesar Salad, 4 oz | 90 | 5 | 9

| | C | F | Cb |
|---|---|---|---|
| Caesar Salad, 4 oz | 90 | 5 | 9 |
| Garlic Roll | 260 | 10 | 34 |
| Garden Salad, 3 oz | 15 | 1 | 3 |
| Greek Salad, 6 oz | 125 | 10 | 7 |
| Roasted Potatoes, 6 oz | 210 | 12 | 24 |
| Sauteed Vegetables, 6oz | 85 | 6 | 6 |

## Vocelli Pizza® (Sept '19)

*Pizzas:*

**Artisan:** *Per 1/8 of Medium Pizza, with Menu Set Components*

| | C | F | Cb |
|---|---|---|---|
| BBQ Chicken | 290 | 10 | 35 |
| Chicken Carbonara | 270 | 11 | 27 |
| Chicken Pesto | 260 | 10 | 27 |
| Deluxe | 260 | 11 | 29 |
| Hawaiian | 280 | 11 | 29 |
| Meat Magnifico | 290 | 13 | 28 |
| Philly Steak | 270 | 12 | 28 |
| Quattro Cheese | 260 | 10 | 27 |
| Spring Veggie | 220 | 7 | 29 |

**Pasta:** *Single Serving*

| | C | F | Cb |
|---|---|---|---|
| Chicken Alfredo | 1200 | 54 | 129 |
| Chicken Parmesan | 960 | 26 | 144 |
| Chicken Pesto | 1230 | 57 | 128 |

*House Baked Subs: On Italian Bread*

| | C | F | Cb |
|---|---|---|---|
| Buffalo Chicken | 950 | 39 | 86 |
| Chkn Parmesan | 990 | 39 | 105 |
| Meatball | 1170 | 55 | 103 |

*Salads: Per Regular Size, without Dressing*

| | C | F | Cb |
|---|---|---|---|
| Chicken Caesar | 180 | 4 | 14 |
| Mediterranean | 230 | 11 | 22 |
| Tuscan Grilled Chicken | 320 | 13 | 22 |

*Stromboli: With Marinara Sauce*

| | C | F | Cb |
|---|---|---|---|
| Pepperoni, w/o veggie toppings | 1410 | 62 | 149 |
| Spicy Italian | 1430 | 56 | 156 |
| Steak | 1350 | 48 | 156 |

## Wahoo's Fish Taco® (Sept '19)

*Bowls: W/ White Rice & Black Beans*

| | C | F | Cb |
|---|---|---|---|
| Blackened: Chicken | 920 | 23 | 133 |
| Fish | 875 | 18 | 133 |
| Carne Asada | 995 | 32 | 132 |
| Carnitas | 1090 | 34 | 134 |
| Salmon | 905 | 22 | 132 |

*Banzai Burritos: With Brown Rice & White Beans*

| | C | F | Cb |
|---|---|---|---|
| Blackened/Charbroiled Chicken, av. | 585 | 19 | 75 |
| Blackened/Charbroiled Fish, av. | 540 | 14 | 75 |
| Carne Asada | 650 | 27 | 75 |
| Carnitas | 735 | 29 | 77 |
| Shrimp | 530 | 15 | 77 |
| Tofu | 535 | 17 | 78 |
| Vegetarian | 485 | 14 | 82 |
| *Side Kicks,* Corn Tortillas, each | 145 | 2 | 29 |

*Shredder Sandwiches:*

**Blackened or Charbroiled:**

| | C | F | Cb |
|---|---|---|---|
| Chicken, average | 360 | 17 | 29 |
| Fish | 385 | 21 | 29 |
| Carne Asada | 350 | 18 | 30 |

*Wahoo Salads:*

| | C | F | Cb |
|---|---|---|---|
| Banzai Veggie | 295 | 18 | 24 |

**Blackened or Charbroiled:**

| | C | F | Cb |
|---|---|---|---|
| Chicken, average | 415 | 22 | 14 |
| Fish, average | 470 | 28 | 14 |
| Carne Asada | 400 | 23 | 16 |
| *Soup,* Chicken Tortilla | 55 | 1 | 5 |

*For Complete Nutritional Data ~ see CalorieKing.com*

## WAWA® (Sept '19)

*Breakfast Sizzlis:*

| | C | F | Cb |
|---|---|---|---|
| **Bagels:** Bacon, Egg & Cheese | 410 | 18 | 42 |
| Pork Roll, Egg & Cheese | 420 | 19 | 42 |
| Sausage, Egg & Cheese | 510 | 29 | 42 |
| Turkey Ssg, Egg & Cheese | 430 | 27 | 28 |
| **Biscuit,** Sausage, Egg & Cheese | 670 | 45 | 48 |

**Croissants:**

| | C | F | Cb |
|---|---|---|---|
| Bacon, Egg & Cheese | 420 | 28 | 27 |
| Chorizo | 500 | 36 | 28 |
| Sausage, Egg & Cheese | 520 | 39 | 27 |
| **Muffin,** Sausage, Egg & Cheese | 450 | 30 | 28 |

*Sourdough Melts: With Egg Omelet & Cheddar Cheese*

| | C | F | Cb |
|---|---|---|---|
| Fully Loaded; Bacon, Turkey & Egg, av. | 870 | 38 | 78 |
| Spicy Sausage & Egg | 980 | 54 | 77 |
| Western | 670 | 22 | 78 |

*Cold Hoagies: On Shorti Roll w/out Any Toppings/Spread*

| | C | F | Cb |
|---|---|---|---|
| Egg Salad | 560 | 34 | 48 |
| Italian | 400 | 14 | 44 |
| Roast Beef | 380 | 4 | 42 |
| Tuna Salad | 600 | 36 | 50 |
| Veggie | 220 | 2 | 42 |

## WAWA® cont... (Sept '19)

| Hot Hoagies: On Classic Roll, without Toppings or Spread | C | F | Cb |
|---|---|---|---|
| Beefsteak | 600 | 21 | 64 |
| Chicken Steak | 510 | 11 | 64 |
| Meatball Parmesan | 1190 | 65 | 94 |

**Quesadillas:** *Without Toppings*

| | C | F | Cb |
|---|---|---|---|
| BBQ Pork & Provolone | 630 | 22 | 66 |
| Beef & Cheddar Cheese | 560 | 28 | 44 |
| Chicken & Cheddar Cheese | 500 | 21 | 44 |

**Soups:** *Per Medium Serving without Toppings*

| | | | |
|---|---|---|---|
| Baked Potato w/ Cheddar & Bacon | 400 | 27 | 26 |
| Broccoli Cheddar Soup | 300 | 22 | 15 |
| Chicken Noodle | 190 | 6 | 20 |
| New Eng. Clam Chowder | 310 | 20 | 23 |
| Tomato Soup | 330 | 22 | 28 |

**Sides:** *Per Medium*

| | | | |
|---|---|---|---|
| Chili | 340 | 15 | 33 |
| Macaroni & Cheese | 490 | 24 | 48 |
| Mashed Potatoes | 470 | 27 | 47 |
| Meatballs in a Cup | 320 | 21 | 18 |
| Rice | 210 | 0 | 45 |

**Bakery:** Apple Fritter

| | | | |
|---|---|---|---|
| Apple Fritter | 510 | 19 | 79 |
| Brownie | 490 | 22 | 72 |
| Muffins: Banana Walnut | 610 | 33 | 74 |
| Blueberry | 570 | 28 | 72 |
| Chocolate Chip | 680 | 34 | 86 |

**Hot Beverages:** *Per 16 oz, without Extras*

| | | | |
|---|---|---|---|
| Hot Cappuccino, with 2% milk | 130 | 5 | 13 |
| Mocha Latte, with 2% milk | 330 | 7 | 59 |
| Milkshake, Chocolate, w/ Cream, 16 oz | 970 | 50 | 117 |

## Wendy's® (Sept '19)

**Hamburgers:**

| Bacon Jalapeno Cheeseburger: | C | F | Cb |
|---|---|---|---|
| Single | 750 | 49 | 44 |
| Double | 990 | 66 | 45 |
| Triple | 1280 | 87 | 47 |
| **Baconator** | 950 | 62 | 40 |
| **Daves:** Single | 570 | 34 | 40 |
| Double | 810 | 51 | 41 |
| Triple | 1090 | 72 | 43 |
| **Double Stack** | 390 | 21 | 26 |
| **Jr.:** Bacon Cheeseburger | 380 | 22 | 25 |
| Cheeseburger | 280 | 13 | 26 |
| Cheeseburger Deluxe | 340 | 19 | 27 |
| **Son of Baconator** | 630 | 39 | 37 |

## Wendy's® cont... (Sept '19)

| Sandwiches: | C | F | Cb |
|---|---|---|---|
| **Crispy:** Chicken | 330 | 16 | 33 |
| Chicken BLT | 420 | 23 | 35 |
| **Grilled:** Avocado BLT Chicken | 600 | 31 | 36 |
| Barbecue Chicken | 520 | 18 | 49 |
| Chicken | 380 | 10 | 38 |
| S'Awesome Bacon Chicken | 530 | 24 | 36 |
| **Homestyle:** Avocado BLT Chicken | 740 | 42 | 53 |
| Barbecue Chicken | 650 | 28 | 66 |
| Chicken | 510 | 22 | 51 |
| S'Awesome Bacon Chicken | 670 | 34 | 52 |
| **Spicy:** Avocado BLT Chicken | 730 | 39 | 55 |
| Barbecue Chicken | 650 | 26 | 67 |
| Chicken | 510 | 19 | 53 |
| S'Awesome Bacon Chicken | 660 | 32 | 54 |
| **Wraps:** Gr. Chicken | 300 | 13 | 26 |
| Spicy Chicken | 370 | 20 | 31 |

**Chicken:** *Nuggets:*

| | | | |
|---|---|---|---|
| **Nuggets:** 4 pieces | 170 | 11 | 10 |
| 6 pieces | 250 | 16 | 14 |
| 10 pieces | 420 | 27 | 24 |
| **Tenders:** 3 piece | 330 | 16 | 22 |
| 4 piece | 430 | 21 | 29 |

**Dipping Sauces:** *Per 1 oz*

| | | | |
|---|---|---|---|
| Barbecue | 45 | 0 | 11 |
| Buttermilk Ranch | 120 | 12 | 2 |
| Creamy Sriracha | 120 | 12 | 3 |
| Honey Mustard | 90 | 7 | 7 |
| Sweet & Sour | 45 | 0 | 12 |

**Fresh-Made Salads:** *Full Size w/ Menu Set Dressing*

| | | | |
|---|---|---|---|
| Apple Pecan Grilled Chicken | 560 | 24 | 52 |
| Harvest Chicken | 570 | 23 | 47 |
| Spicy Chkn Caesar | 720 | 42 | 44 |

**Sides:**

| | | | |
|---|---|---|---|
| Baconator Fries | 500 | 29 | 46 |
| **Baked Potatoes:** | | | |
| Bacon Cheese | 440 | 14 | 64 |
| Cheese | 460 | 15 | 66 |
| Sour Cream & Chives | 320 | 2.5 | 63 |
| Chili Cheese Fries | 510 | 25 | 55 |
| **Crispy Chicken Nuggets:** 4 pieces | 170 | 11 | 10 |
| 6 pieces | 250 | 16 | 14 |
| **French Fries:** Jr. | 230 | 10 | 30 |
| Small, 4 oz | 320 | 15 | 43 |
| Medium, 5 oz | 420 | 19 | 56 |
| Large, 6.5 oz | 530 | 24 | 70 |
| **Garden Fresh Salad,** w/ dressing | 260 | 18 | 19 |
| **Rich Meaty Chili:** Small | 160 | 4 | 19 |
| Large | 250 | 6 | 29 |

**Frosty:**

| Chocolate; Vanilla, average: | | | |
|---|---|---|---|
| Small | 345 | 9 | 57 |
| Medium | 460 | 12 | 77 |
| Large | 580 | 15 | 96 |

*For Complete Nutritional Data ~ see CalorieKing.com*

**255**

## Whataburger® (Sept '19)

### Burgers & Sandwiches:

| | C | F | Cb |
|---|---|---|---|
| **Whataburger:** | | | |
| #1 Original | 590 | 25 | 62 |
| #2 Double Meat | 830 | 44 | 62 |
| #3 Triple Meat | 1080 | 63 | 62 |
| #4 Jalapeno & Cheese | 680 | 32 | 63 |
| #5 Bacon & Cheese | 750 | 37 | 62 |
| #6 Double Meat Jr. | 420 | 20 | 37 |
| #7 Whataburger Jr. | 310 | 11 | 37 |
| ***Other Burgers & Sandwiches:*** | | | |
| Avocado Bacon Burger | 820 | 52 | 51 |
| Chop House Cheddar Burger | 1080 | 67 | 60 |
| Green Chili Double | 980 | 58 | 59 |
| Monterey Melt | 1110 | 71 | 62 |
| Sweet & Spicy Bacon Burger | 1080 | 62 | 69 |
| ***Whatachick'n:*** | | | |
| **Bites:** 6 pieces, w/out sce | 450 | 22 | 33 |
| 9 pieces w/o sce | 640 | 31 | 45 |
| Sandwich | 600 | 26 | 57 |
| Strips, 3 pieces, w/out sce | 530 | 28 | 42 |
| ***French Fries:*** Small, 3 oz | 280 | 14 | 35 |
| Medium, 4.5 oz | 420 | 21 | 52 |
| Large, 6 oz | 560 | 28 | 70 |
| ***Hash Brown Sticks,*** 2 oz | 190 | 11 | 21 |
| **Onion Rings:** Medium, 3.2 oz | 300 | 17 | 32 |
| Large, 4.8 oz | 450 | 25 | 49 |
| ***Salad:*** *Without Dressing* | | | |
| Apple & Cranberry Chicken | 390 | 13 | 38 |
| Garden, | | | |
| w/ Grilled Chicken | 290 | 12 | 12 |
| ***Breakfast:*** | | | |
| **Biscuits:** Plain | 290 | 16 | 32 |
| with Bacon | 360 | 22 | 32 |
| with Gravy | 470 | 29 | 46 |
| with Sausage | 520 | 38 | 32 |
| Honey Butter Chicken | 560 | 33 | 51 |
| Biscuit Sandwich with Bacon | 470 | 29 | 32 |
| **Cinnamon Roll** | 570 | 17 | 94 |
| **Taquitos:** *Without Cheese* | | | |
| with Bacon | 350 | 19 | 28 |
| with Potato | 400 | 21 | 38 |
| with Sausage | 380 | 23 | 28 |
| ***Desserts:*** | | | |
| Chocolate Chunk Cookie | 230 | 11 | 31 |
| Hot Apple Pie, 3 oz | 270 | 14 | 34 |
| ***Malts:*** Chocolate, 20 oz | 570 | 11 | 109 |
| Vanilla, 20 oz | 520 | 12 | 93 |
| ***Shake,*** Chocolate, 20 oz | 550 | 12 | 101 |

## White Castle® (Sept '19)

***Note:*** *Nutritional Information varies* C F Cb
*from state to state. Please check instore*

| | C | F | Cb |
|---|---|---|---|
| ***Sliders:*** | | | |
| The Original | 140 | 7 | 16 |
| Double Original | 250 | 13 | 24 |
| Bacon Cheese | 220 | 14 | 15 |
| Cheese | 170 | 9 | 16 |
| **Chicken Breast:** | | | |
| Crispy with Cheese | 230 | 10 | 22 |
| Savory Grilled | 190 | 7 | 15 |
| **Chicken & Waffles:** Crispy | 350 | 18 | 36 |
| Savory Grilled | 340 | 18 | 30 |
| Fish with Cheese | 320 | 22 | 22 |
| Impossible | 210 | 11 | 17 |
| Jalapeno Cheese | 170 | 9 | 16 |
| Surf & Turf with Cheese | 520 | 36 | 31 |
| **Veggie:** with Ranch | 320 | 23 | 23 |
| with Honey Mustard | 170 | 5 | 25 |
| ***Sides:*** Clam Strips, medium | 410 | 34 | 9 |
| Chicken Rings: 3 piece | 160 | 10 | 6 |
| 6 piece | 320 | 20 | 12 |
| Fish Nibblers: Small | 320 | 16 | 28 |
| Medium | 590 | 29 | 51 |
| Mozzarella Cheese Sticks (3) | 460 | 33 | 26 |
| Onion Chips, medium | 930 | 65 | 73 |
| Onion Rings, small, 5 oz | 480 | 33 | 40 |
| ***French Fries:*** Kids, 4 oz | 250 | 16 | 24 |
| Small, 5.2 oz | 350 | 21 | 34 |
| Medium, 9.4 oz | 630 | 39 | 60 |
| **Cheese Fries**, 7 oz | 400 | 27 | 35 |
| **Loaded Fries**, 5.7 oz | 460 | 38 | 20 |
| ***Breakfast:*** *With Cheddar Cheese* | | | |
| **Sliders:** Bacon, Egg & Cheese | 260 | 18 | 15 |
| Bologna, Egg & Cheese | 360 | 25 | 17 |
| Egg & Cheese | 200 | 12 | 15 |
| Orig., w/ Egg & Chse | 280 | 18 | 17 |
| Saus., Egg & Chse | 350 | 26 | 15 |
| **Waffle Sliders:** | | | |
| with Bacon, Egg & Cheese | 390 | 27 | 27 |
| with Sausage, Egg & Cheese | 490 | 36 | 28 |
| **Toasted Sandwiches:** | | | |
| Bacon, Egg & Chse | 380 | 23 | 29 |
| Egg & Cheese | 280 | 14 | 29 |
| Sausage, Egg & Chse | 430 | 28 | 30 |
| **Hash Round Nibblers:** | | | |
| Small | 360 | 28 | 25 |
| Medium | 600 | 46 | 42 |
| ***Dessert:*** | | | |
| **On A Stick:** Fudge Dipped Brownie | 250 | 12 | 33 |
| Fudge Dipped Cheesecake | 180 | 10 | 21 |

Updated Nutrition Data ~ www.CalorieKing.com
Persons with Diabetes ~ See Disclaimer (Page 22)

## Wienerschnitzel® (Sept '19)

*Hot Dogs: On Hot Dog Bun*

| | C | F | Cb |
|---|---|---|---|
| **Original:** Chicago Dog | 330 | 15 | 37 |
| Chili Dog | 300 | 15 | 30 |
| Chili Cheese Dog | 350 | 20 | 30 |
| Deluxe Dog | 290 | 14 | 30 |
| Junkyard Dog | 430 | 24 | 42 |
| Kraut Dog | 280 | 14 | 29 |
| Mustard Dog | 280 | 14 | 28 |
| Street Dog | 350 | 20 | 30 |
| **Hot Dog Substitute,** add: | | | |
| All Beef Dog | 100 | 10 | 1 |
| Polish Sausage | 140 | 12 | 2 |
| **Pretzel Bun Substitute,** add | 80 | 1 | 15 |
| *Burgers:* | | | |
| BBQ Bacon Chseburger | 640 | 34 | 52 |
| Chili Cheeseburger | 450 | 24 | 27 |
| Classic w/ Thousand Island Drssng | 460 | 25 | 30 |
| *Sandwiches:* | | | |
| BBQ Bacon Chicken | 640 | 34 | 52 |
| Classic Ranch Chicken | 490 | 28 | 44 |
| *Specialties:* | | | |
| Corn Dog | 230 | 13 | 21 |
| Polish Sausage S'wich | 500 | 34 | 36 |
| *Sides: Per Regular* | | | |
| **Chili Cheese Fries** | 530 | 29 | 53 |
| Bacon Ranch | 630 | 39 | 54 |
| Tapatio | 530 | 29 | 54 |
| Thousand Island | 710 | 45 | 60 |
| **French Fries:** Small | 310 | 16 | 38 |
| Medium | 440 | 23 | 54 |
| Large | 750 | 39 | 92 |
| *Breakfast:* | | | |
| **Biscuits:** Egg, Bacon, Cheese | 490 | 30 | 36 |
| Egg, Sausage, Cheese | 580 | 39 | 40 |
| **Burritos:** | | | |
| Egg, Bacon, Cheese | 420 | 20 | 38 |
| Egg, Sausage, Cheese | 510 | 29 | 42 |
| *Desserts:* | | | |
| **Classic Banana Split** | 760 | 24 | 131 |
| **Cones:** Regular, Plain, 5 oz | 250 | 9 | 41 |
| Chocolate Dipped, 5 oz | 450 | 27 | 50 |
| **Freezee,** | | | |
| Oreo; M&M, Reese's, av. | 630 | 24 | 99 |
| **Shakes,** Chocolate with Oreo | 950 | 35 | 155 |
| **Sundaes:** | | | |
| Caramel; Choc; Hot Fudge, av. | 400 | 15 | 64 |
| Strawberry | 370 | 14 | 59 |

## Winchell's® (Sept '19)

*Donuts: Per Donut*

| | C | F | Cb |
|---|---|---|---|
| Buttermillk Bars, Choc Iced/Glazed | 420 | 19 | 61 |
| Jelly Filled: | | | |
| Apple with Cinnamon Crumb | 370 | 15 | 53 |
| Raspberry with Glaze | 390 | 13 | 61 |
| Strawberry with Sugar | 380 | 13 | 60 |
| Old Fashioned, Glazed; Maple Iced | 410 | 17 | 60 |
| Raised Ring: Chocolate Iced | 270 | 10 | 41 |
| Coconut | 240 | 12 | 30 |

## WingStreet (Sept '19)

*Chicken: Without Dipping Sauce*

**Bone Out Wings:** *Per Wing*

| | C | F | Cb |
|---|---|---|---|
| Buffalo, Mild | 90 | 4 | 10 |
| Garlic Parmesan | 130 | 9 | 6 |
| Honey BBQ | 100 | 4 | 11 |
| Ranch Rub | 80 | 4 | 6 |
| **Traditional Bone In Wings:** *Per Wing* | | | |
| Buffalo, Medium/Hot | 100 | 4.5 | 5 |
| Garlic Parmesan | 140 | 11 | 1 |
| Spicy Garlic | 120 | 8 | 3 |
| *Sides:* Bacon Cheesesticks | 1420 | 99 | 104 |
| Bacon Chedd. Fries w/ Ranch Sce | 140 | 4.5 | 19 |
| Straight Cut Fries, with Ketchup | 510 | 24 | 69 |
| Stuffed Garlic Knot | 80 | 2.5 | 10 |

## Woody's Bar-B-Q® (Sept '19)

*Starters:*

| | C | F | Cb |
|---|---|---|---|
| Breaded Wings (10) | 700 | 47 | 13 |
| Beef Chili Cheese Fries | 805 | 38 | 63 |
| *Dinner Entrees: Without Sides* | | | |
| ½ Chicken | 840 | 56 | 0 |
| Baby Back Combo | 680 | 48 | 1 |
| Baby Back Ribs | 520 | 40 | 2 |
| Beef Prime Rib | 760 | 62 | 1 |
| New York Strip | 490 | 36 | 2 |
| Pork Sampler | 1010 | 62 | 4 |
| Ribeye Steak | 735 | 54 | 2 |
| *Sandwiches: Per Regular, without Sides* | | | |
| Beef | 390 | 14 | 28 |
| Pork | 490 | 26 | 29 |
| *Wraps: Without Sides* | | | |
| Beef BBQ | 380 | 13 | 31 |
| Pork BBQ | 440 | 21 | 31 |
| *Extras:* BBQ Beans | 170 | 8 | 20 |
| Cobettes | 80 | 1 | 18 |
| French Fries | 185 | 7 | 28 |
| Garlic Toast | 120 | 6 | 14 |
| Green Beans | 50 | 2.5 | 6 |
| Okra | 95 | 1 | 21 |
| Squash | 140 | 1 | 28 |

# Fast - Foods & *Restaurants*

## Yard House® (Sept '19)

| | C | F | Cb |
|---|---|---|---|
| **Appetizers:** *With Sides & Sauce* | | | |
| California Roll | 1000 | 56 | 97 |
| Chicken Nachos | 2380 | 148 | 155 |
| Chicken Lettuce Wraps | 730 | 28 | 84 |
| Poke Nachos | 870 | 59 | 51 |
| Spinach Cheese Dip | 1280 | 98 | 73 |
| **Snacks:** Asado Taco (1) | 250 | 14 | 16 |
| Guacamole & Chips | 760 | 49 | 75 |
| Hot Spicy Edamame | 500 | 41 | 19 |
| Sweet Potato Fries | 660 | 35 | 78 |
| **Grilled Burgers:** *Without Fries* | | | |
| BBQ Bacon Cheddar Burger | 1170 | 78 | 51 |
| Black Truffle Cheeseburger | 930 | 57 | 46 |
| Kurobuta Pork Burger | 930 | 52 | 63 |
| **Fries,** 1 Serving | 360 | 14 | 52 |
| **House Favorites:** *With Sides & Sauce* | | | |
| Fish & Chips | 1360 | 95 | 85 |
| Mac & Cheese, w/ Chicken, full | 1860 | 124 | 113 |
| Parmesan Crusted Pork Loin | 1130 | 45 | 81 |
| Spicy Jambalaya Pasta, full | 1310 | 67 | 103 |
| **Pizza:** Margherita | 840 | 28 | 110 |
| The Carnivore | 1400 | 75 | 101 |
| **Seafood:** *With Sides & Sauce* | | | |
| Ginger Crusted Salmon | 1060 | 62 | 65 |
| Lobster Garlic Noodles | 1030 | 57 | 76 |
| **Soups:** | | | |
| Chicken Tortilla, bowl | 980 | 75 | 45 |
| Clam Chowder, bowl | 480 | 35 | 29 |
| **Salads:** *Full Entree Size, with Dressing* | | | |
| Cobb Chicken | 1020 | 71 | 29 |
| Kale, Grilled Shrimp Caesar | 710 | 46 | 34 |
| **Dessert:** Mini Trio Sampler | 1230 | 66 | 153 |
| Brownies: Caramel | 960 | 40 | 139 |
| S'mores | 1360 | 52 | 213 |

*For Complete Nutritional Data ~ see CalorieKing.com*

## Yoshinoya® (Sept '19)

| | C | F | Cb |
|---|---|---|---|
| **Entrees:** *As Served* | | | |
| **Grilled Steak Bowl:** Regular | 570 | 11 | 97 |
| Large | 850 | 17 | 144 |
| **Beef Bowl:** Regular | 730 | 27 | 91 |
| Large | 1040 | 38 | 131 |
| With Vegetables: Regular | 650 | 20 | 95 |
| Large | 960 | 29 | 141 |
| **Teriyaki Chicken Bowl:** | | | |
| Regular, without Skin | 740 | 15 | 110 |
| Large, without Skin | 1090 | 21 | 166 |
| **Grilled Tilapia:** | | | |
| with Rice & Slaw | 570 | 13 | 91 |
| with Rice, Veggies & Teriyaki Sce | 590 | 12 | 100 |
| **Sides,** Clam Chowder Soup | 210 | 7 | 34 |
| **Kid's Meals:** Beef | 350 | 11 | 48 |
| Teriyaki Chicken without skin | 340 | 6 | 53 |

*For Complete Nutritional Data ~ see CalorieKing.com*

## Zaxby's® (Sept '19)

| | C | F | Cb |
|---|---|---|---|
| **Zappertizers:** *With Menu Set Sauce* | | | |
| Buffalo Dip & Tater Chips | 1020 | 70 | 77 |
| Cheddar Bites, with Marinara Sauce | 690 | 42 | 58 |
| Fried Mushrooms, with Zestable Sce | 590 | 46 | 39 |
| Tater Chips, with Ranch Sauce | 880 | 64 | 70 |
| **Zalads:** *With Texas Toast, Without Dressing* | | | |
| Blackened Blue | 540 | 27 | 32 |
| Buffalo Blue | 690 | 37 | 43 |
| Fried Cobb Zalad | 820 | 46 | 42 |
| Fried House Zalad | 700 | 38 | 41 |
| Garden House Zalad | 400 | 24 | 31 |
| Grilled Cobb Zalad | 680 | 35 | 34 |
| Grilled Caesar Zalad | 440 | 16 | 25 |
| **Dressings:** *Per 1.2 oz Serving* | | | |
| Blue Cheese | 180 | 19 | 2 |
| Caesar | 90 | 8 | 2 |
| Honey French | 150 | 12 | 9 |
| Mediterranean | 140 | 14 | 4 |
| Ranch | 160 | 16 | 2 |
| **Most Popular:** | | | |
| Boneless Wings & Things | 1560 | 93 | 114 |
| Buffalo Boneless Wings & Things | 1580 | 95 | 114 |
| Buffalo Chicken Finger Plate (4) | 1270 | 72 | 104 |
| Chicken Finger Plate (4) | 1240 | 70 | 101 |
| Traditional Wings & Things | 1490 | 94 | 87 |
| **Sandwich Meals:** *With Menu Set Components* | | | |
| Cajun Club | 1040 | 49 | 92 |
| Chicken Finger | 1190 | 64 | 106 |
| Chicken Salad | 990 | 58 | 90 |
| Grilled Chicken | 900 | 38 | 97 |
| Kickin' Chicken | 1130 | 57 | 102 |
| Nibblerz | 1340 | 69 | 131 |
| Zaxby's Club | 1300 | 75 | 101 |
| **Wings & Fingers:** *With Sweet & Spicy Sauce* | | | |
| **Boneless:** 5 Wings | 410 | 19 | 37 |
| 10 Wings | 810 | 37 | 73 |
| **Traditional:** 5 Wings | 340 | 20 | 10 |
| 10 Wings | 670 | 39 | 20 |
| **Chicken Finger:** 1 Finger | 120 | 5 | 8 |
| 5 Fingers | 600 | 23 | 42 |
| **Sides:** | | | |
| **Crinkle Fries:** | | | |
| Regular, 5 oz | 370 | 16 | 50 |
| Large, 8 oz | 590 | 36 | 86 |
| **Texas Toast:** | | | |
| 1 Slice, 1.5 oz | 150 | 7 | 19 |
| Basket, 4.5 oz | 460 | 22 | 56 |
| **Kidz Meals:** | | | |
| Kiddie Finger, 8.5 oz | 720 | 41 | 63 |
| Kidz Nibbler, 7.5 oz | 670 | 31 | 78 |
| Kiddie Cheese, 8.5 oz | 840 | 46 | 91 |

## Zero Sub's® ~ *see CalorieKing.com*

## Notes on Cholesterol

- **Cholesterol** is a white waxy substance produced mainly by our liver. It is also found in animal food products. Plant foods have no cholesterol.

- **Cholesterol is essential to life.** It is a structural part of every body cell wall and is the building block for vitamin D, sex hormones, and bile acids which help in the digestion of dietary fats. **Cholesterol is also vital for a healthy brain** (which contains some 20% of total body cholesterol).

- **The body makes sufficient cholesterol** for its needs and does not rely on cholesterol in the diet. Dietary fats have a major influence on blood cholesterol levels. (See next page)

- **A high blood cholesterol level increases** the risk of atherosclerosis - the thickening of arteries that can reduce or block blood flow to the heart, brain, eyes, kidneys, sex organs and other body parts.

  **This in turn increases the risk of heart attack,** stroke, blindness, kidney failure, impotence and other blood circulatory problems.

  **Other risk factors which increase the risk of atherosclerosis include high blood pressure, smoking, obesity and uncontrolled diabetes.**

### HEART ATTACK WARNING SIGNALS

Many victims die before reaching the hospital by ignoring warning signals and delaying medical help. Symptoms vary and commonly include:

- **Chest pain,** vice-like squeezing or burning sensation in center of the chest or between the shoulder blades, or in the mid-back. Pain may even feel like severe indigestion.
- **Pain** may be felt in the arms, shoulders, neck or jaw.
- **Shortness of breath** often occurs with or before chest discomfort.
- **Other signs,** with or without pain, include a cold sweat, nausea or light-headedness.

*If you experience any of the above symptoms call IMMEDIATELY for medical help. Every minute counts.*

***Call 9-1-1*** *or your emergency number*

---

### BLOOD CHOLESTEROL

#### CHECK YOUR RISK!

| Total Cholesterol Level (mg/dl) ▼ | | Risk of Heart Attack ▼ |
|---|---|---|
| 240 and above | ~ | **High Risk** |
| 200 - 239 | ~ | **Borderline/High** |
| Below 200 | ~ | **Desirable** |

- ♥ **Know your cholesterol level, particularly if there is a family history of heart disease or stroke. If your level is high, see your doctor.**

- ♥ **All adults should have their cholesterol, HDL and triglycerides tested at least every 5 years.**

▲ **Atherosclerosis can clog arteries and impede blood flow to the heart or other body organs.**

▼ **A thrombus (blood clot) can form on unstable, festering athero-sclerotic plaque and rapidly block blood flow. A heart attack or stroke can result.**

# Fats & Cholesterol Guide

The amount and type of dietary fat has the greatest influence on blood cholesterol levels.

**Fats in food are a mixture of 3 basic types:** saturated, monounsaturated, and polyunsaturated. Animal fats are mainly saturated while plant oils and fish oils are mainly mono- and polyunsaturated.

**Saturated fats** have subgroups known as long-chain, medium-chain, and short-chain fats. Most of the long chain fats raise blood cholesterol, and increase the risk of blood clots and thrombosis leading to artery blockage.

**Long-chain saturated fats** are found mainly in full-cream milk, cheese, butter, cream, fatty meats and sausages, and processed foods.

**Medium-chain fats (MCT)** have little effect on LDL-cholesterol but may raise "good" HDL. *Note: Coconut oil has some MCT but is mainly saturated fat – so limit use.*

**Monounsaturated fats** tend to more selectively lower 'bad' LDL cholesterol and maintain the protective 'good' HDL cholesterol in the bloodstream – but only if they replace saturated fats in the diet. Foods rich in monounsaturates include canola and olive oils, canola margarine, peanuts, and avocados.

**Polyunsaturated fats** consist of two main classes. **Omega-6** polyunsaturates tend to lower blood cholesterol. Rich sources include safflower, sunflower and corn oils.

**Omega-3** polyunsaturated fats can lower blood cholesterol; significantly lower blood triglycerides; and reduce the rise of thrombosis, heart arrythmmia, and artery spasm.

**Best practical omega-3 sources** include canola oil and margarine, soybean oil and fish.

**A balanced intake** of the two omega classes is important for optimal health. For most Americans, slightly increasing omega-3 intake would help attain a more ideal balance.

**Trans fats** from hydrogenated vegetable oils and shortenings should also be avoided. They are common in commercial baked and fried food products such as cakes, muffins, pastries, doughnuts, fried snacks and french fries.

## DIETARY FATS COMPARISON

■ Saturated Fat　　■ Monounsaturated Fat
**Polyunsaturated Fats:**
□ Linoleic (Omega-6)　■ Alpha-Linolenic (Omega-3)

### OILS — PERCENTAGE CONTENT

| OIL | Saturated | Monounsaturated | Linoleic | Alpha-Linolenic |
|---|---|---|---|---|
| CANOLA OIL | 7 | 63 | 20 | 10 |
| LINSEED/FLAX OIL | 9 | 19 | 17 | 55 |
| SAFFLOWER OIL | 9 | 14 | 77 | |
| GRAPESEED OIL | 10 | 22 | 68 | |
| SUNFLOWER OIL | 11 | 23 | 66 | |
| CORN OIL | 14 | 32 | 52 | 2 |
| OLIVE OIL | 14 | 76 | | 10 |
| SOYBEAN OIL | 15 | 23 | 54 | 8 |
| PEANUT OIL | 19 | 45 | 34 | 2 |
| COTTONSEED OIL | 26 | 16 | 58 | |
| PALM OIL | 51 | 39 | | 10 |

### SPREADS & FATS
Saturated Fat includes 'Trans Fats'　□ WATER CONTENT

| SPREAD | Saturated | | Mono | Poly | | Water |
|---|---|---|---|---|---|---|
| LIGHT MARGARINE | 14 | 14 | 21 | 51 | | |
| CANOLA MARGARINE | 18 | | 45 | 12 | 6 | 19 |
| POLYUNSATURATED MARG | 24 | 20 | 36 | | 20 | |
| BUTTER | 57 | | 18 | 2 | 24 | |
| LARD | 41 | | 47 | | 12 | |
| BEEF FAT | 44 | | 37 | 4 | 15 | |

## GOOD SOURCES OF OMEGA-3 FATS

**Plant Sources**　　**Omega-3 Fats (Grams)**

| | |
|---|---|
| Canola Oil, 1 Tbsp, ½ fl.oz | **1.5g** |
| Flaxseed Oil, 1 Tbsp | **8g** |
| Soybean Oil, 1 Tbsp | **1.2g** |
| Canola Margarine, 1 Tbsp, ½ oz | **1g** |
| Soybeans, cooked, ½ cup, 4 oz | **0.5g** |
| Walnuts, ½ oz | **0.5g** |

**FISH** - *Per 4 oz Serving*

**High Content:** Salmon (Chinook), Tuna, **3g**
Trout (Lake), Sardines, Herring, Mackerel **3g**
**Medium Content:**
　　Salmon, (Pink/Red/Coho), 4 oz **2g**
**Fair Content:** *Per 4 oz Serving*
Bass, Catfish, Cod, Grouper, Hake,
Halibut, Kingfish, Perch, Pollock, Shark, **0.5-1g**
Trout (Rainbow), Tuna, Crab,
Oysters, Blue Mussels, Shrimp, Squid

## How Much Is Needed?

**As little as 1-2 grams daily of omega-3 fats** may benefit general health. High doses of fish-oil supplements should only be taken as directed by your Healthcare provider.

## Dietary Cholesterol

Cholesterol in food varies in its effect on blood cholesterol level (BCL) from person to person. Much depends on the amount and type of fat and fiber eaten at the same meal.

Any elevating effect of dietary cholesterol on BCL is more likely to occur when the diet is high in saturated fat. Little elevation, if any, generally occurs when dietary fats are balanced in favor of mono- and poly-unsaturated fats (including omega-3 fats).

**Example:** While fish does contain cholesterol, the omega-3 fats can prevent any increase in BCL. Conversely, a meal containing no cholesterol but rich in saturated fat may result in a significant increase in BCL - as well as impairing artery wall functions.

**Consequently, the need to be overly concerned about dietary cholesterol is being de-emphasized in favor of simply limiting total fat, saturated fat, and trans fat in particular – and substituting unsaturated fats (including omega-3 fats).**

**Note:** Persons with familial (genetic) hyper-cholesterolemia should limit cholesterol; and ideally follow a plant-based diet.

**The liver usually cuts back its own cholesterol production** in response to cholesterol in the diet. Many people can consume high-cholesterol foods without concern.

However, it is difficult to identify just who is at risk - the so-called 'hyper-responders'. Because over 50% of Americans have a BCL above ideal levels, it may be prudent to limit cholesterol intake to less than 300mg daily, as well as to adopt a heart-healthy diet.

This limitation still allows the inclusion of most foods that are regularly eaten – even the overly maligned egg.

*Avocados (like all plant foods) contain no cholesterol. Their fats are mainly monounsaturated and can lower blood cholesterol.*

## CHOLESTEROL COUNTER

**Cholesterol is found only in foods of animal origin. Plant foods contain no cholesterol.**

| | Cholesterol mg |
|---|---|
| **Meat** - Average all types: | |
| Lean Meat, cooked, 120g | 100 |
| Fatty Meat, cooked, 120g | 100 |
| Fat, thick strip, 60g | 40 |

*Note: While lean meat and fat have similar amounts of cholesterol, choose lean meat to limit fat intake.*

| | Cholesterol mg |
|---|---|
| **Chicken/Turkey,** average, 120g | 100 |
| **Organ Meats:** Liver, fried, 4 oz | 500 |
| Brains, beef, pan fried, 3 oz | 1700 |
| **Sausages:** Frankfurter, 40g | 25 |
| Salami, 2 slices, 55g | 40 |
| **Bacon:** 3 slices, cooked, 30g | 20 |
| **Fish:** Fish fillets, average, ckd, 120g | 70 |
| Tuna/Salmon, canned, 100g | 50 |
| Scallops, 9 medium, 3 oz | 30 |
| Prawns, raw, 100g | 110 |
| Oysters, raw, 6 medium, 85g | 45 |
| Crayfish, Crab, cooked, 100g | 70 |
| **Eggs** (Chicken), 1 large | 210 |
| 1 medium | 180 |
| Egg White, *Scramblers* | 0 |
| **Milk/Yoghurt:** Whole, 1 cup, 250ml | 30 |
| Light/low-fat Milk (1%), 1 cup | 10 |
| Skim/Non-fat, 1 cup | 10 |
| **Soy Milk, Tofu, Tempeh** | 0 |
| **Cheese:** Natural/Hard/Cream, 30g | 30 |
| Cottage, low-fat, 2 Tbsp, 40g | 5 |
| Cream Cheese, 30g | 25 |
| **Fats:** Butter, 1 Tbsp, 20g | 45 |
| Margarine, Oils (vegetable) | 0 |
| Mayonnaise, 1 Tbsp | 10 |
| **Cream:** Heavy, whipping, 2 Tbsp, 40g | 40 |
| Light/Sour, 2 Tbsp | 10 |
| **Ice Cream:** Full-fat (10-11%), 100ml/50g | 20 |
| Low-fat (less than 4%), 50g | 5 |
| **Fruit, Vegetables,** Avocados | 0 |
| **Nuts, Seeds, Grains** | 0 |
| **Coffee, Tea, Beer, Wine** | 0 |

*For Comprehensive Food Listings ~ see www.CalorieKing.com*

# Blood Cholesterol ~ Diet Hints

## DIETARY HINTS TO LOWER BLOOD CHOLESTEROL

1. **Maintain a healthy weight.**
   If overweight, lose weight with a sensible, low-fat meal plan and daily exercise.

2. **Reduce saturated fat intake by:**

   **(a) eating less dairy fat.** Choose low-fat or fat-reduced varieties of milk, yogurt, soy drinks, cheese, and ice cream.

   **(b) replacing saturated fats** with fats and oils rich in monounsaturated and polyunsaturated fats. Choose vegetable oils such as extra-virgin olive, canola and soybean. Avoid solid frying fats.

   Note: *Promise Active* and *Benecol* spreads contain plant stanol esters which can lower total and LDL cholesterol.

   **(c) eating less fat from meat and poultry.** Choose lean cuts of meat and skinless chicken. Go easy on lunch meats, salami and fatty sausages. Enjoy fish.

   **(d) eating less saturated and trans fats** from baked and fried fast-foods. Avoid deep-fried foods. Avoid donuts, cakes, pastries and cookies unless made with healthier fats and oils.

3. **Increase your soluble fiber intake.**
   Foods rich in soluble fiber include beans, lentils, chickpeas, hummus, nuts, seeds, psyllium-seed husks and psyllium-fiber supplements. Oat bran, rice bran and barley are also good sources, as are fruit, vegetables and avocados.
   *(See Fiber Guide - Page 264-269).*

4. **Eat more soy bean products such as:**
   soy drinks, tofu, tempeh (cultured soy beans), soy flour, soy vegetarian foods and edamame (fresh green soybeans).

   Soy protein in place of animal protein can significantly decrease high blood cholesterol levels as well as 'bad' LDL cholesterol and blood triglycerides while 'good' HDL cholesterol is maintained. For best results, eat at least 25g of soy protein per day (from 3-4 servings).

5. **Eat more fruit, vegetables, and whole grains** in place of high-fat foods. Aim for 2 fruits and 5 servings of vegetables per day. They also contain valuable antioxidants. The fat of avocados (and most nuts) is mainly unsaturated and can lower blood cholesterol levels.

6. **Limit cholesterol to 300mg per day.**
   (Extra Notes ~ See Previous Page)

7. **Avoid brewed unfiltered coffee** (espresso; plunger-style). Several cups per day may raise blood cholesterol. Filtered coffee is fine.

8. **Spread your food intake over the day.**
   Have 5-6 small meals per day rather than just 2-3 large meals. Nibbling, versus gorging, favors lower blood cholesterol.

## ALCOHOL – WINE

Alcohol is a mixed bag. Moderate amounts of 1-2 drinks daily appear to reduce the risk of heart attack and ischemic stroke in older persons.

However, larger amounts increase the risk of high blood pressure, obesity, heart failure and hemorrhagic stroke, and can aggravate hypertriglyceridemia: as well as many other health hazards. (See Alcohol Guide – Page 23)

The speculative benefits of moderate alcohol intake have been overstated in the media. The overriding harmful effects of excess alcohol do not allow its recommendation for any aspects of health promotion.

*Fruit, Vegetables & Tea Also Protect:*

**Red wine and red grapes (more so than white) contain antioxidants which may help protect cholesterol in the blood from becoming oxidized.**

**Many fruits, vegetables, grains, nuts and tea also contain protective antioxidants.**

**Fats in the diet affect more than blood cholesterol levels.** They can also strongly influence blood clot formation and thrombosis, as well as blood flow and ultimate oxygen delivery to body parts and organs.

While advanced atherosclerosis can impede blood flow to the heart and other organs, it is thrombosis (complete blockage by blood clots) or arterial spasm which commonly results in a heart attack or stroke.

**Plant and fish oils rich in omega-3 fats** lessen the risk of blood clots, thrombus formation, and artery spasm by reducing platelet stickiness and adhesion to artery walls. This also reduces inflammation of the artery wall lining. This in turn reduces the risk of atherosclerotic plaque becoming unstable and reactive.

**Omega-3 fats also improve blood flow** by reducing blood viscosity and increasing the flexibility of red blood cells that need to flex and twist on themselves in order to squeeze through tiny narrow capillaries often half their diameter.

**A diet high in saturated fats** (longer chain) has the opposite effect by stiffening red blood cell membranes and increasing blood viscosity, thereby hindering blood flow.

Stiff red blood cells may also form aggregates that resemble coin stacks. In narrow blood vessels, this further impedes blood flow and impairs oxygen release through the much-lessened surface area of red blood cell membranes exposed to blood.

**Note:** Smoking, lack of exercise, and stress can have similar adverse effects on thrombosis, red blood cell flexibility, and blood flow.

▲ *Picture of Healthy Blood Flow*

*Flexible red blood cells twist and slide through tiny capillaries - often half the diameter of red blood cells.*

▲ *A Not-So-Healthy Picture!*

*Red blood cells have lost their flexibility and ability to twist and slip through capillaries. They are stacked up, thereby impeding blood flow.*

*A diet high in saturated fats can contribute to this picture - as can smoking, lack of exercise, and stress.*

# Fiber Guide

## Introduction `Fiber`

Fiber is the general term for those parts of plant food that we cannot digest (although bacteria in the large bowel partly digests fiber through fermentation). It is not found in foods of animal origin (meats, dairy products).

**Fiber promotes intestinal health,** bowel regularity, can benefit diabetes and blood cholesterol levels, and may help prevent colon cancer. High-fiber foods also assist weight control.

**Most Americans don't eat enough fiber – less than 20 grams/day – instead of a healthier 25 to 35 grams/day.**

## Types of Fiber

Plant foods contain a mixture of different fibers in varying proportions. Insoluble and soluble fiber categories are based on their solubility in water. All types of fiber are beneficial to the body.

♦ Insoluble fibers (cellulose, hemi-celluloses, lignin) make up the structural parts of plant cell walls.

   **Best food sources** are wheat bran, corn bran, rice bran, wholegrain cereals and breads, beans and peas, nuts, seeds, and the skins of fruits and vegetables.

These fibers absorb many times their own weight in water. They create a soft bulk and hasten the passage of waste products through the intestines.

**They promote bowel regularity,** and aid in the prevention and treatment of uncomplicated forms of **constipation, diverticulosis and hemorrhoids.**

**The risk of colon cancer** may also be reduced by fiber's diluting effect on potentially harmful substances.

♦ Soluble fibers **(pectin, gums, mucilages)** are found mainly within plant cells, soy milk (whole bean) and products.

*A fiber-rich diet assists the growth of friendly gut microbes that can benefit our metabolism, weight and blood glucose levels – as well as hunger, mood and our immune system.*

**Best Sources of Soluble Fiber:**

Fruits and vegetables, oat bran, barley, beans and peas, prunes, psyllium and flax seed.

These fibers form a gel which slows both stomach emptying and the absorption of sugars from the intestines. **This helps to control blood sugar levels.**

**Weight control** is also aided by the slower emptying of the stomach and the feeling of **fullness provided by soluble fiber.**

**Soluble fiber can also lower blood cholesterol** by binding bile acids and excreting them. More body cholesterol must then be broken down to supply bile acids for emulsification of dietary fats. **Rice bran, while not high in soluble fiber, can also lower blood cholesterol.**

♦ **Resistant starch** is that part of starchy foods (approx. 10%) which is tightly bound by fiber and resists normal digestion. Friendly bacteria in the large bowel ferment and change the resistant starch into short-chain fatty acids, which are important to bowel health and may protect against colon cancer.

**Starchy foods include** bread, cereals, rice, pasta, potatoes and legumes.

# Fiber Guide

## Fiber & Weight Control

**Fiber can assist weight control** in several ways. Fiber-rich foods such as fresh fruit and vegetables, potatoes and wholegrain bread contain few calories for their large volume (due to their low-fat, high-water content).

**Their bulk fills the stomach** and satisfies the appetite much sooner than fiber-depleted foods. The extra chewing time also contributes to satiety, and gives the stomach time to register a feeling of fullness. Excessive calories are less likely to be consumed.

**Fiber-depleted foods and drinks** are more concentrated in calories; e.g. fats, sugar, candy, soft drinks, fruit juices, alcohol. They require little or no chewing. Large amounts with excessive calories can be consumed before the appetite is satisfied.

**Example:** Whereas one fresh apple might satisfy the appetite, an apple juice drink with the equivalent sugars and calories of 2-3 apples only minimally satisfies the appetite. (See illustration below.)

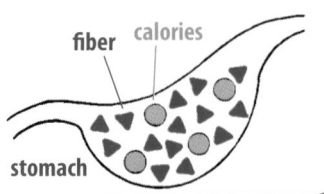

*High-fiber foods fill the stomach. Fewer calories are consumed.*

*Low-fiber foods are more concentrated in calories. More food must be eaten to fill the stomach.*

## EFFECTS OF REMOVING FIBER FROM FOOD

*2-3 pieces of fresh fruit produces 1 glass of fruit juice. The removal of fiber concentrates the sugars and calories.*

FIBER REMOVED

| FRESH FRUIT | (Comparison) | FRUIT JUICE |
|---|---|---|
| Higher Fiber | ← | Negligible Fiber |
| Low Calorie Density | ← | High Calorie Density |
| Long Eating Time | ← | No Eating Time (Drink) |
| Satisfies Hunger | ← | Does Not Satisfy Hunger |
| Sugars Slowly Absorbed | ← | Sugars More Quickly Absorbed |
| Less Insulin Required | ← | More Insulin Required |
| Supports Gut Microbes | ← | Fewer Benefits to Microbes |

# Fiber Guide ~ Constipation

## Constipation

**Constipation** can reasonably be defined as a failure to have a bowel movement at least every second day – and just as importantly, without straining or pain.

Typically, constipated stools are too hard, too narrow and too small.

The **main cause** is simply a lack of dietary fiber. Other contributing factors include insufficient fluids, too little exercise, emotional stress, gastrointestinal disease, lack of proper dentition to chew high-fiber foods, and some medications (e.g. some antacids, antidepressants, pain medications).

**Note:** Check with your doctor to rule out any underlying medical problem – especially if you have a change in bowel habits in middle-age or later years.

### DESIRABLE FIBER INTAKE

Adults: **25-35gm per day**
Children (under 18): **Age + 5gm**
**Example: 6-year old (6 + 5)= 11gm**

### SAMPLE FOOD QUANTITIES
**For 35 Grams of Fiber/Day**

| | Fiber |
|---|---|
| Breakfast Cereal (higher-fiber) | 5g |
| **plus** 4 slices wholegrain Bread | 6g |
| **plus** 3 servings fresh Fruit | 9g |
| **plus** 1 medium Potato (w. skin) | } 4g |
| **or** 1 cup Brown Rice | |
| **or** ½ cup wholegrain Pasta | |
| **plus** 3-4 servings Veggies/Salad | 6g |
| **plus** 1 cup Bean Soup | |
| **or** ¼ cup Baked/Soy Beans | |
| **or** ½ cup Corn/Peas/Lentils | } 5g |
| **or** 1¼ oz Almonds (natural) | |
| **or** 3 medium Figs | |

## HINTS TO INCREASE FIBER AND AVOID CONSTIPATION

**❶ Breakfast is an important** contributor to daily fiber intake. Eat high-fiber breakfast cereals (bran-based cereals, oatmeal etc.). Add 1-2 tablespoons of unprocessed bran.

Dried fruits, chopped nuts, soy grits, and seeds are also excellent additions to cereals.

*Note:* A gradual increase in fiber will prevent bloating, gas or pain. People intolerant to bran may benefit from psyllium-based fiber supplements and cereals.

**❷ Drink adequate water daily.** Fiber works by absorbing many times its own weight in water.

**❸ Eat wholegrain breads,** or fiber-enriched breads. They have over double the fiber of regular white bread.

**❹ Enjoy fruit as fresh fruit** with skin rather than as fruit juice. Enjoy wholegrain pasta, barley, brown rice, nuts and seeds.

**❺ Eat more vegetables,** salads and legumes – especially cooked beans, lentils, potatoes with skins, avocado, broccoli, brussels sprouts, cabbage, carrots, celery, and peas.

**❻ Add bran** (barley/rice/wheat) or soy grits to soups, casseroles, yogurt, desserts, cookies, cakes. Also use whole-meal flour or soy flour in place of white flour. Use nuts, seeds, and ground linseed.

**❼ Snack** on fresh or dried fruits, carrot or celery sticks, popcorn, nuts or seeds, wholegrain crackers, high-fiber bars (low-fat). Limit amounts if overweight.

**❽ Exercise regularly** to strengthen abdominal muscles and stimulate the gut. Keep up water intake, especially in warm weather.

**❾ Avoid** indiscriminate and regular use of harsh laxatives. They can overstimulate the intestinal muscles and may make normal bowel activity impossible. It may take several weeks to restore normal bowel function.

## Breakfast Cereals · Fiber

**General Mills:**

| | Fiber |
|---|---|
| Basic 4, 1 cup, 2 oz | 3 |
| Cheerios (Honey Nut; Multigrain), 1 cup, 1 oz | 2 |
| Fiber One, 1/2 cup, 1.1 oz | 14 |
| Multi-Bran Chex, 1 cup, 2 oz | 7 |
| Oatmeal Crisp Almond, 1 cup, 2 oz | 4 |
| Raisin Nut Bran, 1 1/4 cup, 2 oz | 6 |
| Total, average all types, 3/4 cup, 1 oz | 3 |
| Wheat Chex, 1 cup, 2 oz | 6 |
| Wheaties 3/4 cup, 1 oz | 3 |

**Health Valley:**

| | |
|---|---|
| Amaranth Flakes, 3/4 cup, 1 oz | 3 |
| Crunches & Flakes, 3/4 cup, 1.9 oz | 4 |
| Fiber 7 Flakes, 3/4 cup, 1 oz | 7 |
| Golden Flax, 3/4 cup, 1.9 oz | 6 |
| Granola (Low-Fat), 3/4 cup, 2 oz | 6 |
| Healthy Fiber Flakes, 3/4 cup, 1.1 oz | 4 |
| Oat Bran Flakes, all types, 3/4 cup, 1 oz | 2 |
| Oat Bran O's, 3/4 cup, 1 oz | 3 |
| Real Oat Bran, 1/2 cup, 1.7 oz | 5 |

**Kellogg's:**

| | |
|---|---|
| All-Bran, 1/2 cup, 1.1 oz | 10 |
| All-Bran w. Extra Fiber, 1/2 cup, 1 oz | 13 |
| All-Bran Bran Buds, 1/3 cup, 1.1 oz | 13 |
| Corn Flakes, Fruit Loops, Smacks 1 cup, 1 oz | 1 |
| Cocoa/Rice Krispies Treats, 1 1/4 cup, 1 oz | 0 |
| Complete: Wheat Flakes, 3/4 c., 1 oz | 5 |
| Oat Bran Flakes, 3/4 cup, 1.1 oz | 4 |
| Corn Pops, 1 cup, 1.1 oz | 0 |
| Cracklin' Oat Bran, 3/4 cup, 1.7oz | 6 |
| FiberPlus Antioxidants: | |
| Berry Yogurt Crunch, 1 c., 1.9 oz | 10 |
| Cinnamon Oat Crunch 3/4 c., 1.1 oz | 9 |
| Frosted Mini Wheats, 24 bisc., 2 oz | 5 |
| Granola w. Raisins, 2/3 cup, 2.1 oz | 3 |
| Raisin Bran, 1 cup, 2.1 oz | 7 |
| Smart Start, Strong Heart, Cinnamon Raisin, 1 cup, 1.8 oz | 4 |
| Special K, 1 cup, 1.1 oz | 0.5 |

**Fiber** ~ Fiber (grams)

### Breakfast Cereals (Cont) · Fiber

**Kashi:**

| | |
|---|---|
| GoLEAN Cereal, 1 cup, 1.8 oz | 10 |
| GoLEAN Crunch!, 1 cup, 1.9 oz | 8 |
| GoLEAN Bars, avg. (1) | 6 |
| Good Friends: Original, 1 cup, 1.9 oz | 12 |
| Cinna-Raisin Crunch, 1 cup, 1.8 oz | 8 |
| Heart to Heart, 3/4 cup, 1.2 oz | 5 |
| 7 Whole Grain Pilaf, 1/2 cup, cooked, 5 oz | 7 |
| 7 Whole Grain Puffs, 1 cup, 0.7 oz | 1 |

**Quaker:**

| | |
|---|---|
| Cap'n Crunch, 3/4 cup, 1 oz | 1 |
| 100% Natural Granola, avg., 1/2 cup, 1.8 oz | 3 |
| Crunchy Corn Bran, 1 cup, 1 oz | 5 |
| Life Cereal, 3/4 cup, 1.1 oz | 2 |
| Oat Bran, 1/2 cup, 1.4 oz | 6 |
| Oatmeal, average, 1 packet | 3 |

**Post:**

| | |
|---|---|
| 100% Bran, 1/3 cup, 1 oz | 9 |
| Alpha Bits, 1 cup, 1 oz | 2 |
| Blueberry Morning, 1 cup, 1.9 oz | 5 |
| Cranberry Almond Crunch, 1 cup, 1.8 oz | 3 |
| Fruit & Bran, 1 cup, 1.9 oz | 6 |
| Grape-Nuts, 1/2 cup, 2 oz | 7 |
| Great Grains, 2/3 cup, 1.9 oz | 5 |
| Honey Bunches of Oats, 3/4 cup, 1.1 oz | 2 |
| Shredded Wheat & Bran, 1/2 cup, 2 oz | 8 |

### Brans & Supplements, Metamucil

| | |
|---|---|
| **Oat Bran:** 1 Tbsp (level) | 1 |
| 1/3 cup, (5 1/3 Tbsp), 1 oz | 5 |
| **Rice Bran,** raw. 1/3 cup, 1 oz | 6 |
| **Wheat Bran,** Unprocessed: | |
| Raw, 1 Tbsp | 1.5 |
| 2 Tbsp (level), 1/4 oz | 3 |
| 1/4 cup, (4 Tbsp), 1/2 oz | 6 |
| **Wheat Germ,** Raw, 1/4 cup, 1 oz | 4 |
| **Psyllium Seed Husks,** 2 Tbsp | 8 |
| **Fibersure,** 1 heaping tsp | 5 |
| **Metamucil:** Orange, 1 rnd Tbsp, 11g | 3 |
| Fiber Wafers (2) | 6 |

### Hot Cereals, Oatmeal

| | |
|---|---|
| Bulgur (cracked Wheat), ckd, 1 cup | 8 |
| Corn/Hominy Grits, dry, 3 Tbsp, 1 oz | 0.5 |
| Cream of Wheat, cooked, 3/4 cup | 1 |
| Oatmeal (uncooked 1/3 cup), ckd, 2/3 cup | 3 |

# Fiber Counter

## Breads & Crackers | Fiber
**Bread:** White, 1 slice, 1 oz — 0.6
Whole-wheat, 1 slice, 1 oz — 1.5
Wholegrain, 1 slice, 1 oz — 2
Rye, Pumpernickel, 1 oz — 1.5
Bagel/Roll/Bun, 1 medium, 2 oz — 1.5
Pita, whole wheat, 6.5" pocket — 4.5
**Crackers:** Graham, average, 2 — 0.4
Saltine, 4 crackers — 0.4
**Crispbreads,** average, 2 — 4
**Matzo,** 1 board, 1 oz — 1
**Rice Cakes,** average, 1 cake — 0.3
**Tortilla:** Regular, 6" — 0.5
Whole-wheat, 6" — 1.3

## Barley, Pasta, Rice & Flours
**Barley,** pearled, raw, 1/4 cup, 1.7 oz — 8
**Rice:**
White, cooked, 1 cup — 0.6
Brown, cooked, 1 cup — 3.5
*Rice-A-Roni,* average, 1 cup, prepared — 1.5
**Spaghetti/Noodles:** Cooked, 1 cup — 2
Whole-Wheat, cooked, 1 cup — 4
**Flour:** Wheat, All-purpose, 1 cup, 4.5 oz — 3.5
Whole-Wheat, 1 cup, 4.5 oz — 15
Cornmeal, stone ground, 1 cup, 4.5 oz — 13
Carob Flour, 1 cup, 3.5 oz — 41
Hemp Wholemeal Flour, 1 cup, 3.5 oz — 41
Rye Flour, 1 cup, 3.5 oz — 15
Soy Flour: Defatted, 1 cup, 3.5 oz — 17
Full-fat, raw, 1 cup, 3 oz — 8
Soy Meal, defatted, 1 cup, 4.5 oz — 14

## Frozen Entrees & Dinners
*Average All Brands*: Per Serving
Beans/Chili base, average — 6-10
Potato/Pasta base, average — 4-6
Vegetable base, average — 3
Meat/Chicken base, average — 2-3
**Pizzas,** 1/4 large, average — 3
**Vegetarian Soy Burgers,** 1 pattie — 4

## Soups
Chicken Noodle, 1 cup — 0.5
Tomato Soup, average, 1 cup — 0.5
Vegetable Soup, average, 1 cup — 3
*Health Valley: Per 1 Cup*
Black Bean; Minestrone — 8
Tomato — 1
5 Bean Vegetable; Lentil & Carrots — 10
Mushroom Barley; Vegetable — 4
Split Pea — 8
*Progresso,* High Fiber, all flavors, 1 cup — 7

## Fast Foods & Restaurants | Fiber
**Hamburgers:** Small, average — 1.5
Large/Whopper, average — 2.5
**Hot Dog,** Regular — 1.5
**French Fries:** Small serving, 2.5 oz — 2.5
Regular/Medium, 3.5 oz — 3.5
**Chicken Nuggets,** 6 pack — 0.5
**Chicken Sandwich,** average — 2
**Taco,** average — 4
**Sundaes,** Shakes, Soft Drinks — 0
*Arby's,* Classic Roast Beef Sandwich — 1
*Burger King:* Whopper — 2
Impossible Whopper — 4
*Denny's:* Grilled Chicken Salad, no bread — 4
Classic Burger, no fries — 4
Club Sandwich, no fries — 2
Grilled Chicken Sandwich, no fries — 4
*Domino's:* 12", Classic/Thin, 1 slice — 1
Deep Dish, 1 slice — 3
Feast Pizza, Classic/Thin, 1 slice — 2
*McDonald's:* Big Mac — 3
Hamburger — 1
Egg McMuffin — 2
Grilled Chicken Caesar Salad — 4
Quarter Pounder — 3
*Pizza Hut: Per 1 Slice, Medium*
Pan Pizza: Cheese, Pepperoni — 1
Supreme — 2
Thin 'n Crispy, Supreme — 2
Hand-Tossed, average all varieties — 2
*Subway:* Sandwich, white roll, av. — 4
With Honey Wheat Roll, average — 3
Salads, average — 4

## Cakes, Cookies, Snack Bars
**Apple/Fruit Pie,** 1 serving, 4 oz — 2
**Cake:** With plain flour, 1 serving, 3.4 oz — 1.5
With whole-wheat flour, 1 serving — 3
**Carrot Cake,** 4 oz — 4
**Cookies,** oatmeal, (3 small/1 large) — 1
**Donuts,** medium, 1.7 oz — 0.7
**Fruit Cake,** 1 serving, 1.5 oz — 2
**Fig Bars,** 1 cookie, 0.5 oz — 0.7
**Muffins,** Oat Bran (2 small, 1 large), 4 oz — 5
**Granola Bars,** average, 1 bar — 2
*Atkins Advantage Bars,* av. — 7
*Clif Bars,* 2.5 oz — 5
*Fi-Bar Chewy & Nutty,* 1 bar — 1
*Fiber One (Gen. Mills),* 1.4 oz bar — 9
*FiberPlus,* all bars, 1.2 oz — 9
*Health Valley:* Fruit/Granola Bars — 3
Cereal Bars — 1
*Luna Bars,* avg., 1.7 oz — 3
*Special K,* Protein Meal Bar, 1.6 oz — 5

# Fiber Counter

## Chocolate, Chips, Popcorn | Fiber

| | Fiber |
|---|---|
| **Cheese Balls/Curls/Twists** | 1 |
| **Chocolate,** Hard Candy, 1 oz | 0 |
| **Chocolate with nuts/fruit,** 2 oz bar | 1.5 |
| *Mars Bar,* 1.8 oz | 1 |
| **Potato Chips; corn chips,** 1 oz | 1 |
| **Popcorn,** 3 cups | 3 |
| **Pretzels,** Twists (6) | 1 |

## Nuts, Seeds

| | Fiber |
|---|---|
| **Almonds:** Natural, 25 nuts, 1 oz | 3.5 |
| Blanched (skins removed), 1 oz | 3 |
| **Cashews,** Filberts, Pecans, 1 oz | 1.7 |
| **Hepm Seeds,** 3 Tbsp, 1 oz | 9 |
| **Peanuts,** Mixed Nuts, Coconut, 1 oz | 2.5 |
| **Peanut Butter,** 2 Tbsp, 1 oz | 2 |
| **Pistachio Nuts,** dried, shelled, 1 oz | 3 |
| **Walnuts,** Black/English, dried, 1 oz | 2 |
| **Seeds:** Amaranth, 2$^1$/$_2$ Tbsp, 1 oz | 3.5 |
| Flax Seeds, 3 Tbsp, 1 oz | 7 |
| Psyllium Seed Husks, 5 Tbsp, 1 oz | 20 |
| Quinoa Seeds, 3 Tbsp, 1 oz | 1.7 |
| Sesame Seeds, whole, 1 oz | 3.4 |
| Sesame Butter/Tahini, 2 Tbsp, 1.1 oz | 1.4 |
| Sunflower Kernels,$^1$/$_4$ cup, 1 oz | 3.8 |

## Fruit – Fresh

| | Fiber |
|---|---|
| **Apples:** 1 medium, 5$^1$/$_2$ oz (whole) | |
| with skin + core | 3.7 |
| with skin, no core | 3.2 |
| without skin, no core | 1.7 |
| **Apricots,** 2 medium, 4 oz | 1.5 |
| **Avocado,** average, $^1$/$_2$ medium | 6 |
| **Banana,** 1 medium, 6 oz (w. skin) | 3 |
| **Blueberries,** raw, $^1$/$_2$ cup, 2.5 oz | 1.7 |
| **Cherries,** sweet, raw, 8 fruits, 1.6 oz | 1 |
| **Grapefruit,** average, $^1$/$_2$ fruit, 10 oz | 1.4 |
| **Grapes,** 1 medium bunch, seedless, 7 oz | 2 |
| **Kiwifruit,** 1 medium, 2.7 oz | 2.3 |
| **Mango,** 1 medium, 11 oz (whole) | 1.6 |
| **Melons,** Cantaloupe, 4 oz (edible) | 1 |
| **Nectarine,** 1 medium, 4 oz | 1.9 |
| **Olives,** average all types, 7 jumbo, 2 oz | 1.5 |
| **Oranges,** 1 medium (7-8 oz w. skin) | |
| 5$^1$/$_2$ oz (peeled) | 3.8 |
| **Passionfruit,** 2 medium, 2.5 oz | 5 |
| **Peaches,** 1 large, 6 oz | 2 |
| **Pears,** raw, 1 medium, 6 oz | 4.5 |
| **Pineapple,** 1 slice, 3 oz | 1.2 |
| **Plums,** 2 medium, 6 oz | 1.8 |
| **Strawberries,** 6 medium/3 large, 2 oz | 1 |
| **Watermelon,** 4 oz (edible) | 0.5 |

## Fruit – Dried, Juice | Fiber

| | Fiber |
|---|---|
| **Dried** Fruit: Apricots, 8 halves, 1 oz | 2.2 |
| Dates (3 med); Raisins (2 Tbsp), 1 oz | 1.5 |
| Figs, 3 medium,1$^1$/$_2$ oz | 5 |
| Prunes, 4 medium, 1 oz | 2 |
| **Fruit Juice:** Orange/Apple etc, 1 glass | <0.5 |
| Prune Juice, 5 oz | 1.4 |
| Carrot Juice, 8 oz | 1.8 |

## Vegetables

| | Fiber |
|---|---|
| **Asparagus,** 4 medium spears | 1.3 |
| **Bean Sprouts,** $^1$/$_2$ cup, 2 oz | 1 |
| **Beans:** Snap/Green, $^1$/$_2$ cup, 2 oz | 2 |
| Baked Beans in Tom Sce, $^1$/$_2$ c, 4.5 oz | 5 |
| Dried Beans, ckd, average, $^1$/$_2$ cup | 7 |
| **Beets,** ckd, slices, $^1$/$_2$ cup, 3 oz | 1.7 |
| **Broccoli,** cooked, $^1$/$_2$ cup, 3 oz | 2.4 |
| **Brussels Sprouts,** ckd, $^1$/$_2$ cup, 3 oz | 3.5 |
| **Cabbage:** White, ckd, $^1$/$_2$ cup, 2.5 oz | 1 |
| Red, ckd, $^1$/$_2$ cup,2.5 oz | 2 |
| **Carrots,** 1 medium (7$^1$/$_2$"), $^1$/$_2$ cup, 3 oz | 2.5 |
| **Cauliflower,** cooked, 3 flowerets, 2 oz | 1.5 |
| **Celery,** raw, diced, 1 cup, 3.5 oz | 1.6 |
| **Chickpeas (Garbanzos),** ckd, $^1$/$_2$ c., 3 oz | 6.5 |
| **Corn:** Kernels, cooked, $^1$/$_2$ cup, 2$^1$/$_2$ oz | 2.5 |
| Corn on the Cob, 1 ear, 5 oz | 4 |
| **Cucumber/Lettuce/Mushrooms,** 2 oz | 0.5 |
| **Eggplant,** raw, sliced, $^1$/$_2$ cup , 1.5 oz | 2 |
| **Lentils,** cooked, $^1$/$_2$ cup, 3.5 oz | 8 |
| **Mixed Vegetables,** frozen, cooked, $^1$/$_2$ cup | 3 |
| **Onions:** Raw, 1 medium, 4 oz | 1.5 |
| Spring Onions, chop., $^1$/$_4$ cup, 1 oz | 0.7 |
| **Peas:** Green, raw, $^1$/$_2$ cup, 2.5 oz | 3.7 |
| Cowpeas (Black-eyed), ckd, $^1$/$_2$ cup | 10 |
| Split Peas, cooked, $^1$/$_2$ cup | 8 |
| **Peppers,** sweet, raw, 1 large, 6 oz | 3 |
| **Potatoes:** 1 medium, with skin, 5 oz | 4 |
| 1 medium, without skin | 2.5 |
| $^1$/$_2$ cup mashed, 3.5 oz | 1.5 |
| French Fries, small, 2.6 oz | 3 |
| **Spinach,** cooked, $^1$/$_2$ cup, 3 oz | 2.2 |
| **Squash:** Summer, cooked, $^1$/$_2$ cup, 3 oz | 2.5 |
| Winter, cooked, $^1$/$_2$ cup, 3.5 oz | 2.4 |
| **Tomatoes:** 1 medium, 4.5 oz | 1.5 |
| Tomato Sauce, 1 cup | 0.3 |
| **Soybean Products:** Miso, $^1$/$_2$ c., 5 oz | 7.4 |
| Tempeh, cooked, 1 piece, 3 oz | 2 |
| Tofu, $^1$/$_2$ cup, 4.4 oz | 0.4 |

## Salads:

| | Fiber |
|---|---|
| **Side Salad,** average | 1 |
| **Bean Salad,** $^1$/$_2$ cup | 5 |
| **Coleslaw,** $^1$/$_2$ cup | 1 |
| **Potato Salad,** $^1$/$_2$ cup | 2 |

# Protein Guide

## General Notes

- **Protein has many important body functions.** It builds and repairs muscle, and is the basis of our body's organs, hormones, enzymes, and antibodies to fight infection.

- **Protein is also an emergency fuel** in the absence of sufficient carbohydrate and fats. For this reason, weight loss should be gradual so as to preserve protein levels in muscle, the heart and other body organs.

- **It is easy to obtain sufficient protein,** even if vegetarian. **Plant proteins are not inferior to animal proteins.** In fact, eating more soy and other plant proteins, and less animal protein, may help to build stronger bones and prevent osteoporosis, and may help to control blood cholesterol levels.

- **When changing to a vegetarian diet,** include legume beans (soy, chickpeas etc.), lentils, nuts, seeds, tofu, tempeh; as well as wholegrain cereals and flours. Also try nutritional yeast flakes, and plant-based meat substitutes (*Beyond Meat; Impossible* burgers). Dairy products (lower fat) and eggs can enhance nutrient intake.

## Protein & Muscle

- Although muscles are built of protein, protein is not a special fuel for working muscle cells – carbohydrates and fats are.

- In fact, a diet high in protein (and fat) and low in carbohydrate can significantly reduce the performance of endurance sports athletes. **Carbohydrates** are the best fuel for muscles exercised for long periods.

- Any **extra protein** required by athletes and body-builders can easily be obtained from the extra food eaten to satisfy hunger and energy needs.

- Remember, **excessive protein** intake will not build bigger muscles. Any excess is converted and stored as fat. Excess protein can also strain the kidneys, which excrete the waste products of protein metabolism.

Elderly people (and dieters) must eat sufficient food to ensure adequate protein intake.

Inadequate protein leads to a drop in immune response with greater susceptibility to illness and infections. Muscle strength and muscle mass also drop.

Protein needs are easily met with sensible eating. Athletes who eat enough food for their energy needs can obtain sufficient protein.

### RECOMMENDED DAILY PROTEIN INTAKE ~ HEALTHY RANGE ~
**(Lower figure is RDA)**

| | | PROTEIN |
|---|---|---|
| Children: | 1-3 yrs | 13g-26g |
| | 4-8 yrs | 19g-38g |
| | 9-13 yrs | 34g-64g |
| Males: | 14-18 yrs | 52g-120g |
| | 19+ | 56g-120g |
| Females: | 14+ | 46g-110g |
| Pregnancy: | | 71g-120g |
| Breastfeeding: | | 71g-120g |

**Note:** On lower-calorie diets, aim for higher amounts of protein within the Healthy Range.

# Protein Counter

**Pro** ~ Protein (grams)

## Meats, Sausages | Pro

| | |
|---|---|
| **Bacon,** 3 medium slices | 6 |
| **Ground Beef Patty,** lean, cooked, 3 oz | 21 |
| **Ham:** Luncheon, 2 slices, 1 1/2 oz | 7 |
| Roasted, 2 pieces, 3 oz | 18 |
| **Lamb chop,** broiled, 3 oz | 22 |
| **Liver,** cooked, 3 oz | 23 |
| **Pastrami,** 3 slices, 1 3/4 oz | 10 |
| **Pork,** cooked, lean, 3 oz | 24 |
| **Roast Beef,** lean, 2 slices, 3 oz | 24 |
| **Sausages:** Bologna, 2 sl., 2 oz | 7 |
| Braunschweiger, 2 sl., 2 oz | 8 |
| Pork link, thick, 2 oz | 6 |
| Frankfurter, 1 1/3 oz | 5 |
| Salami, hard, 3 slices, 1 oz | 7 |
| **Steak:** Average all cuts, lean (no fat) | |
| Small (4 oz raw/3 oz cooked) | 23 |
| Medium (6 oz raw/4 1/4 oz cooked) | 34 |
| Large (10 oz raw/7 1/4 oz cooked) | 57 |

## Meat Substitutes (Vegan)

| | |
|---|---|
| **Beyond Meat:** Beef/Burger, 4 oz | 20 |
| Sausages, 1 link | 16 |
| **Impossible,** 4 oz Patty | 19 |
| **Vegetarian Patties,** av., 4 oz | 13 |

## Chicken/Turkey: *Without Skin*

| | |
|---|---|
| **Chicken,** cooked: Breast, Roasted, 4 oz | 36 |
| Leg/Thigh,Roasted, 2 oz | 14 |
| 1/2 Whole Chicken | 60 |
| Drumstick, Rstd, 1 med., 3 oz | 13 |
| **Turkey:** Light meat, cooked, 3 oz | 28 |
| Dark meat, lean, 3 oz | 24 |

## Fish

| | |
|---|---|
| **Fresh Fish:** *Per 4 oz, cooked* | |
| Cod, Flounder/Sole, Pollock | 28 |
| Catfish, Haddock, Halibut, M/Mahi | 28 |
| Ocean Perch, Swordfish, Orange Roughy | 28 |
| **Canned Fish:** Tuna, av., 3 oz | 25 |
| Salmon, pink, 3 oz | 17 |
| Salmon, red, 3 oz | 17 |
| Sardines, 3 whole (3"), 1 1/4 oz | 9 |
| **Shellfish:** Crabmeat, 3 oz | 17.5 |
| Clams, raw, 4 large/9 sml, 3 oz | 11 |
| Crayfish, cooked, 3 oz | 20 |
| Lobster, cooked, 3 oz | 17 |
| Oysters, raw, 6 medium, 3 oz | 7 |
| Scallops, 2 lge/5 small, 1 oz | 5 |
| Shrimp, raw, 6 large, 1 1/2 oz | 8.5 |
| **Fish Products:** Fish Sticks, 4 sticks | 10 |
| Fish Portions, in batter, 4 oz | 13 |
| Gefilte Fish, 1 medium ball, 2 oz | 8 |

## Eggs | Pro

| | |
|---|---|
| **1 Large Egg,** whole | 6 |
| Egg Yolk | 3 |
| Egg White | 3 |
| **Omelet:** Plain, 2 eggs | 13 |
| Ham & cheese | 17 |
| **Egg Substitutes,** (liquid): | |
| *Egg Beaters,* 1/4 cup, 2 oz | 4.5 |
| *Better 'n Eggs/Scramblers,* 1/4 cup, 2 oz | 6 |

## Milk, Yogurt, Ice Cream

| | |
|---|---|
| **Milk:** Whole: 2%, 1 cup | 8 |
| Low-Fat (1%); Fat-Free, 1 cup | 8.5 |
| **Chocolate Milk,** 1 cup | 8 |
| **Thick Shake:** Chocolate, 10 oz | 9 |
| Vanilla, 10 oz | 11 |
| **Soymilk,** (fortified), average, 1 cup | 7 |
| *Soy Dream,* Enriched, shelf-stable, 1 cup | 7 |
| **Yogurt,** average all brands: | |
| Plain, 6 oz | 8 |
| Fruit flavors, 6 oz | 7 |
| *Chobani,* Greek, Plain, 6 oz | 14 |
| Soy, fruit flavors, 6 oz | 7 |
| **Ice Cream:** Rich, 1/2 cup | 2 |
| Regular, Vanilla, 1/2 cup | 2.5 |
| **Sherbet,** 1/2 cup | 1 |
| **Custard,** baked, 1/2 cup | 7 |

## Cheese

| | |
|---|---|
| **Hard Cheeses,** average, 1 oz | 7 |
| **Cottage Cheese,** 1/2 cup | 13 |
| **Cream Cheese,** avg., 1 oz | 2 |
| **Ricotta,** part skim, 1/2 cup | 14 |

## Bread, Bagels, Biscuits

| | |
|---|---|
| **Bread:** *With enriched flour* | |
| 1 slice, 1 oz | 2 |
| 4 thin slices, 4 oz | 8 |
| 4 thick slices, 6 oz | 12 |
| **Bagel,** plain 2 oz | 6 |
| **Biscuits,** 1 oz | 2 |
| **Pita Bread,** 1 pita, 1 1/2 oz | 4 |
| **Pumpernickel,** 1 slice, 1 oz | 3 |

## Infant/Baby Foods | Pro

| | |
|---|---|
| **Infant Formula Milk:** | |
| *Enfamil/Gerber/Similac,* Regular/Low Iron , 5 fl.oz | 2.2 |
| *Isomil/Nursoy/ProSobee,* | 3 |
| **Baby Cereals:** *Average all brands* | |
| Dry, 4 Tbsp, 1/2 oz | 1 |
| Jars, with fruit, 4 1/2 oz | 1 |

# Protein Counter

## Breakfast Cereals **Pro**

**Hot Cereals** ~ *Cooked:*
**Bulgur,** cooked, 1 cup, 5 oz — 9
**Oatmeal:** Reg., non-fortified, 1 cup — 6
   Instant, fortified, avg., 1 pkt — 4
   *Quaker,* all flavors, 1/2 cup — 5
**Corn/Hominy Grits:** 1 cup — 3
   *Quaker: Reg.,* 3 Tbsp, 1 oz — 2
   Instant White, 1 packet — 2
**Cream of Wheat,** 1 cup — 4

**Brands** ~ *Ready-To-Eat*
**General Mills:**
   Cheerios, Original, 1 cup, 1 oz — 3
   Chex, Corn, 1 cup, 1.1 oz — 2
   Kix, Original, 1 1/4 cups, 1 oz — 2
   Lucky Charms, Original, 3/4 cup, 1 oz — 2
   Total, Raisin Bran, 1 cup, 1.8 oz — 3
   Wheaties, 3/4 cup, 1 oz — 2
**Health Valley:**
   Amaranth Flakes, 1 1/4 cups, 2 oz — 6
   Bran Flakes, w/ Raisins, 1 cup, 1.8 oz — 5
   Corn Crunch-Ems, 1 cup, 1 oz — 2
   Oat Bran Flakes, w/ Raisins, 1 cup, 1.9 oz — 5
   Rice Crunch-Ems, 1 1/4 cups, 1 oz — 2
**Kashi:**
   Good Friends, 1 cup, 1.9 oz — 5
   GoLean Crunch!, 1 cup, 1.9 oz — 9
   7 Whole Grain Flakes, 1 cup, 1.75 oz — 6
**Kellogg's:**
   All-Bran, Original, 1/2 cup, 1 oz — 4
   Apple Jacks, 1 cup, 1 oz — 1
   Corn Flakes, 1 cup, 1 oz — 2
   Low-fat Granola
     with Raisins 2/3 cup, 2.1 oz — 5
   Product 19, 1 cup, 1 oz — 3
   Rice Krispies, 1 1/4 cup, 1.2 oz — 2
   Smart-Start Strong Heart, 1 c., 1.75 oz — 4
   Special K: All flavors, 1 c., 1.1 oz — 2
     Protein, 3/4 cup, 1.1 oz — 10
**Post:**
   Grape Nuts, Original, 1/2 cup, 2 oz — 8
   Raisin Bran, 1 cup, 2 oz — 5
**Quaker:**
   Corn Bran Crunch, 3/4 cup, 1 oz — 2
   Granola, 1/2 cup, 1.7 oz — 5
   Honey Graham Oh's, 3/4 cup, 1 oz — 1
   Life, Original, 3/4 cup, 1.1 oz — 3

## Brans & Wheatgerm **Pro**

**Oat Bran,** raw, 1 Tbsp — 2
**Rice Bran,** raw, 2 Tbsp — 1
**Wheat Bran,** unprocessed, 2 T. — 1
**Wheat Germ,** 2 Tbsp, 1/2 oz — 4

## Grains & Flours, Yeast

**Amaranth grain,** cooked, 1/2 cup, 4.5 oz — 5
**Barley,** 1/2 cup, 3.2 oz — 12
**Buckwheat Flour,** Whole-groat, 1 cup — 15
**Carob Flour,** 1 cup, 3.6 oz — 5
**Corn Flour,** 1 cup, 4 oz — 11
**Corn Meal,** 1 cup, 4 1/2 oz — 8
**Flour:** White, 1 cup, 5.6 oz — 9
   Wholegrain, 1 cup, 4 1/4 oz — 16
**Hemp Wholemeal Flour,** 1 cup, 3.5 oz — 30
**Millet,** wholegrain, 1 cup, 3 1/2 oz — 12
**Quinoa,** raw, 1/3 cup, 1.5 oz — 6
**Rye Flour:** Dark, 1 cup, 4 1/2 oz — 18
   Light, 1 cup, 3 1/2 oz — 9
**Soy Flour,** full fat, 1 cup, 3 oz — 29
**Yeast:** Brewers, 2 Tbsp, 1/2 oz — 8
   Nutritional Yeast Flakes *(Red Star),*
     1 heaping Tbsp, 1/2 oz — 8

## Rice, Spaghetti, Macaroni

**Rice:** Brown/White, average
   1 cup cooked, 6 1/2 oz — 5
**Spaghetti/Macaroni/Noodles (enriched):**
   Cooked, 1 cup, 4 1/2 oz — 7
   Canned: in Tomato Sce, 1/2 cup — 2
     with Meatballs, 1 cup, 8 oz — 10
   Macaroni & Cheese, 1 cup, 9 oz — 8

## Soups

With Noodles/Vegetables, 1 cup — 3
With Meat/Beans/Peas, 1 cup — 8

## Fruit

**Fresh/Canned:**
   Average, all types,
     1 medium/2 small fruit — 1
**Avocado,** 1/2 medium — 2
**Dried Fruit:** Apricots, 8 halves, 1 oz — 1
   Dates, 6 dates, 2 oz — 1.5
   Figs, 4 medium figs, 2 oz — 2
   Prunes, 5 medium, 1 1/2 oz — 1
   Raisins, 1 oz — 1
**Fruit Juice:** Average, 1 cup — 0.5
   Prune Juice, 6 fl.oz — 1
   Tomato Juice, 1 cup, 8 fl.oz — 1.5

## Vegetables   **Pro**

**Beans:** Snap/green, $^1/_2$ cup, 2 oz — 1
  Dried: Average all types,
  cooked, $^1/_2$ cup — 7
  Baked Beans, $^1/_2$ cup 4$^1/_2$ oz — 5
**Bean Sprouts,** mung, 1 c., 4 oz — 3
**Broccoli,** raw, $^1/_2$ cup, 1$^1/_2$ oz — 1.5
**Cabbage; Cauliflower,** raw, 1 c. 3 oz — 1.5
**Chickpeas,** cooked, ½ cup, 3 oz — 8
**Corn:** Raw, $^1/_2$ cup kernels, 3 oz — 2.5
  1 ear trimmed to 3$^1/_2$" — 2
**Lentils,** cooked, $^1/_2$ cup 3$^1/_2$ oz — 9
**Mushrooms,** raw, $^1/_2$ c., sliced — 1
**Peas:** Green, raw, $^1/_2$ c., 2$^1/_2$ oz — 4
  Split Peas, cooked, 1 cup, 7 oz — 16
**Potatoes:** *Cooked:*
  1 medium, with skin, 5 oz — 3.3
  without skin, 4 oz — 2.3
  French Fries, small, 2.6 oz — 2
**Potato Salad,** $^1/_2$ cup, 4 oz — 3.5
**Pumpkin,** $^1/_2$ cup mashed, 4.3 oz — 1
**Seaweed,** kelp, 1 oz — <1
**Spinach,** cooked, $^1/_2$ cup, 3 oz — 2.7
**Squash,** ckd, all types, $^1/_2$ cup — 1
**Tomatoes,** 1 medium, 4$^1/_2$ oz — 1
**Vegetables,** mixed, ckd, 1 cup — 2.5
**Soybeans,** cooked, $^1/_2$ cup, 3 oz — 14

## Tofu, Tempeh, Miso

Tofu, raw, firm, $^1/_2$ cup, 4$^1/_2$ oz — 10
Tempeh, $^1/_2$ cup, 3 oz — 16
Miso, $^1/_2$ cup, 5 oz — 16
Miso Soup, 1 cup — 3
**Soybean Protein** *(TVP)*, 1 oz — 18

## Cakes, Pastries, Pies

Banana Nut Bread, 4 oz — 6
Carrot w. cream cheese frosting, 4 oz — 4
Cheesecake, 1 piece, 4 oz — 6
Chocolate, 1 piece, 2 oz — 2
Fruitcake, 1 piece, 3 oz — 4
Croissant, plain, small, 2 oz — 5
Danish Pastry, 1 pastry, 2$^1/_4$ oz — 4
Donuts, average, 2 oz — 4
Muffins, average, 1 med., 1$^1/_2$ oz — 3
Pancakes, 4" diam., two, 2 oz — 4
Pies: Fruit, 1 piece, 5$^1/_2$ oz — 4
  Pecan, 1 piece, 5 oz — 7
Puddings, average, $^1/_2$ cup, 4$^1/_2$ oz — 4
Waffles, 1 large, 2$^1/_2$ oz — 7

## Peanut Butter   **Pro**

**Regular:** 2 Tbsp, 1.1 oz — 8
  *Peter Pan Plus,* 2 Tbsp, 1.1 oz — 8

## Sugar, Honey, Jam

**Sugar:** White — 0
  Brown, 1 Tbsp — 0
**Molasses:** Light/Med., 1 Tbsp — 0
  Blackstrap, 1 Tbsp, $^3/_4$ oz — 0
**Corn Syrup,** 1 Tbsp, $^3/_4$ oz — 0
**Honey, Jams, Jelly** — 0

## Candy, Chocolate, Carob

**Candy**, sugar-based — 0
**Chocolate:** Plain, 2 oz bar — 4
  with nuts, 2 oz bar — 6
**Carob,** plain, 2 oz — 6

## Cookies, Crackers, Chips

**Cookies**, average, 4 cookies — 2
**Crackers**, Graham, 2$^1/_2$" sq., (2) — 1
**Rice Cakes**, average, one — 1
**Corn/Potato Chips**, 1 oz — 2

## Nuts:

Almonds, shelled, 20-25 nuts — 6
Brazil Nuts, 7-8 medium nuts, 1 oz — 4
Cashews, 12-16 nuts, 1 oz — 5
Hemp Seeds, 3 tbsp, 1 oz — 9
Macadamias, 1 oz — 2
Peanuts, dry rsted, 40 nuts, 1 oz — 6
Pecans, 24 halves, 1 oz — 2
Walnuts, 15 halves, 1 oz — 4

## Seeds:

Chia Seeds, raw, 2 Tbsp, 1.1 oz — 5
Flax Seeds, 3 Tbsp, 1 oz — 6
Sesame Seeds, dry, 1 Tbsp — 2
Pumpkin Kernels, dry, hulled, 1 oz — 7
Sunflower Seeds, dried, hulled, 1 oz — 6

## Granola & Food/Protein Bars

**Granola Bars**, average, 1 bar, 2 oz — 2
*Balance* Bars, Original, average all, 1.76 oz — 14
*Bariatrix,* Proti-Bars (1), 1.4 oz — 15
*Cliff,* Builder's Protein, av., 1 bar — 20
*GeniSoy,* Protein Bar, 1.6 oz — 15
*Jenny Craig,* Bars, av., 1.8 oz — 5
*Luna Protein,* av., 1 bar — 12
*Met-Rx,* "Big 100", av., 3.5 oz — 27
*Myoplex 30,* all flavors, 3 oz — 30
*Optifast 800,* all flavors, 2 oz — 14
*PowerBar:* Energize, 2 oz — 6
  Plant Protein, 1.76 oz — 10
*Slim-Fast:* Protein Meal Bars, 1.7 oz — 10
  Keto Meal Bar, 1.48 oz — 7
*Special K:* Protein Meal, 1.6 oz — 10
  Protein Snack, 0.9 oz — 4

# Protein Counter

## High Protein Drinks & Powders `Pro`

| | |
|---|---|
| **Atkins,** Shakes, 11 fl.oz | 18 |
| **Bob's Red Mill,** Protein Powders: | |
| Chai Protein, 2 scoops, 1.5 oz | 20 |
| Pea Protein, ¼ cup, 1oz | 21 |
| Hemp Protein, ¼ cup, 1 oz | 14 |
| Soy Protein, ¼ cup, 0.75 oz | 17 |
| **Boost,** High Protein, 8 fl.oz bottle | 15 |
| Max 30g Protein Shake, 11 fl oz | 30 |
| **Carnation,** B'fast Essentials, 11 fl.oz | 10 |
| **Ensure,** Plus, 8 fl.oz bottle | 13 |
| **Gatorade,** Protein Recovery Shake, 11 oz | 20 |
| **GNC,** Lean Shake, 14 fl oz | 25 |
| **Hemp Protein Powder,** 1/4 cup, 1 oz | 14 |
| **Met-Rx,** Meal Replacement, RTD | 40 |
| 51 Shake, 15 fl.oz | 51 |
| **Myoplex,** Original Nutrition Shake, 1 pkt | 42 |
| **Optifast 800,** prepared, 8 fl oz | 14 |
| **Premiere Protein,** Clear, 16.9 fl.oz | 20 |
| **Pure Protein Shake,** 11 fl.oz | 35 |
| **Slim-Fast Shakes:** Meal, 10 oz can | 10 |
| High Protein Meal, 10 fl.oz bottle | 20 |
| **Special K,** Protein Shakes, 10 fl.oz | 15 |
| **Weider,** Mass 1000, 4 scoops, 7 oz | 34 |
| **Pumpkin Protein Powder,** 2 Tbsp, ½ oz | 9 |
| **Whey Protein Powder:** 100%, plain, 1 oz | 24 |
| Choc Flavor, 1 scoop, 0.8 oz | 18 |

## Coffee, Tea, Soda

| | |
|---|---|
| Coffee, Coffee Substitutes, 1 cup, 8 fl.oz | 0 |
| Coffee, with 2 oz milk, 1 cup, 8 fl.oz | 2 |
| Caffe latte, large, 16 fl.oz | 12 |
| Cappuccino, large, 16 fl.oz | 8 |
| Frappuccino, average, 16 fl.oz | 6 |
| Hot Chocolate, with milk, 1 cup, 8 fl.oz | 8 |
| Soft Drinks/Soda | 0 |
| Tea, all types | 0 |

## Beer, Wine, Spirits

| | |
|---|---|
| Beer, 12 fl.oz | 1 |
| Wines, red/white, 1 glass | 0 |
| Spirits/Liquor | 0 |

## Fast-Foods/Burgers

| | |
|---|---|
| **Pancakes,** average all outlets, 3 | 8 |
| **Shakes,** Chocolate, 16 fl.oz | 12 |
| **Sundaes,** Average all outlets | 7 |
| **Arby's:** | |
| Buffalo Chicken Slider | 12 |
| Buttermilk Crispy Chicken S'wich | 24 |
| Roast Beef Sandwich: Classic | 23 |
| Double | 38 |
| **Burger King:** Cheeseburger | 15 |
| Double Bacon Cheeseburger | 25 |
| Impossible Whopper | 25 |
| Triple Stacker King | 85 |
| Whopper Sandwich | 28 |

## Fast Foods/Burgers (Cont) `Pro`

| | |
|---|---|
| **Carl's Jr:** Beyond Famous Star with Cheese | 30 |
| Charbroiled Chicken Club Sandwich | 42 |
| Famous Star Burger with Cheese | 28 |
| Super Star Burger with Cheese | 48 |
| **Domino's Pizza:** Hand Tossed (12") | |
| Buffalo Chicken, 1 slice | 13 |
| Honolulu Hawaiian, 1 slice | 11 |
| Ultimate Pepperoni, 1 slice | 12 |
| **KFC:** Original Breast | 39 |
| Extra Crispy Chicken Tenders | 10 |
| Grilled, Breast | 38 |
| **McDonald's:** Big Mac | 25 |
| Buttermilk Crispy Chicken S'wch | 28 |
| Cheeseburger | 15 |
| Chicken McNuggets (4) | 10 |
| Filet-O-Fish | 18 |
| Hamburger | 13 |
| Quarter Pounder with Cheese | 31 |
| French Fries: Small, 2.5 oz | 3 |
| Large, 5.4 oz | |
| Salad, Bacon Ranch | 33 |
| Shakes, medium | 14 |
| Breakfast: Egg McMuffin | 18 |
| Bacon, Egg & Cheese McGriddles | 18 |
| Sausage Burrito | 12 |
| Sausage McMuffin with Egg | 21 |
| **Pizza Hut:** Per Medium, 1 slice, ⅛ Pizza | |
| Thin 'n Crispy, Supreme | 9 |
| Pan Pizzas, average | 10 |
| Hand Tossed: Pepperoni Lover's | 11 |
| Ultimate Cheese Lover's | 10 |
| **Subway :** 6" Subs with standard toppings, no oil | |
| Black Forest Ham | 18 |
| Meatball Marinara | 21 |
| Spicy Italian | 20 |
| Subway Melt | 26 |
| Turkey Breast | 18 |
| **Taco Bell:** Bean Burrito | 14 |
| Cheesy Gordita Crunch | 20 |
| Chicken Quesadilla | 27 |
| Chicken/Steak Chalupas | 16 |
| Grilled Soft Steak Taco | 12 |
| Steak Burrito Supreme | 20 |
| **Wendy's:** | |
| Asiago Ranch Chicken Club | 38 |
| Dave's Double Cheeseburger | 49 |
| Jr Hamburger | 14 |

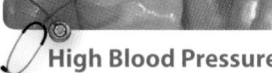

## High Blood Pressure

**Many American adults** have hypertension (high blood pressure), and are unaware of it. It is generally symptomless, so **have your blood pressure checked annually** – particularly if it runs in the family.

**Untreated hypertension** overworks the heart, damages arteries and promotes atherosclerosis. This in turn greatly increases the risk of heart disease, stroke, blindness, kidney disease and impotence. The earlier hypertension is detected, the sooner it can be brought under control.

### BLOOD PRESSURE CLASSIFICATION

*For Adults Age 18 & Older ~ Not Acutely ill or on Medication (American Heart Association)*

| | DIASTOLIC | | SYSTOLIC |
|---|---|---|---|
| Normal ➤ | Below 80 | and | Below 120 |
| Prehypertension ➤ | 80-89 | or | 120-139 |
| **Hypertension:** | | | |
| Stage 1 ➤ | 90-99 | or | 140-159 |
| Stage 2 ➤ | 100 or more | or | 160 or more |

### Treating Hypertension

**Prehypertension** (in the chart above) means you don't have high blood pressure now but are likely to develop it in the future.

**You can take steps to lessen the risk by adopting healthy lifestyle habits such as:**
- reducing sodium intake
- eating adequate fruit and vegetables
- losing weight if overweight
- limiting alcohol to 2 drinks or less daily
- quitting smoking
- exercising regularly, managing stress.

**Stage 1 hypertension** can often be treated with the above lifestyle changes.

**Stage 2 hypertension** usually requires drug therapy. However, salt restriction, abstaining from alcohol, and the above lifestyle changes will improve the success of drug therapy, and enable smaller drug doses to be prescribed.

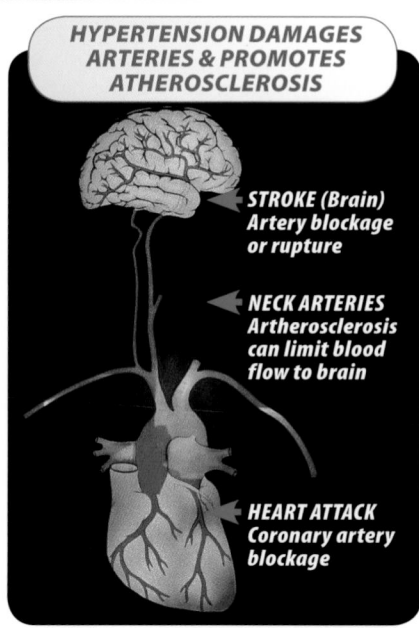

**HYPERTENSION DAMAGES ARTERIES & PROMOTES ATHEROSCLEROSIS**

*STROKE (Brain)*
*Artery blockage*
*or rupture*

*NECK ARTERIES*
*Artherosclerosis*
*can limit blood*
*flow to brain*

*HEART ATTACK*
*Coronary artery*
*blockage*

### STROKE
**KNOW THE WARNING SIGNS**

**Stroke is a medical emergency!**
**If you notice one or more of these signs, call 9-1-1 or your doctor immediately.**

These signs may be signalling a possible stroke or transient ischemic attack:

- **Sudden weakness** or numbness in your face, arm, or leg on one side of your body.

- **Sudden confusion,** trouble speaking or understanding. Slurred speech.

- **Sudden trouble seeing,** in one or both eyes

- **Sudden trouble walking,** dizziness, loss of balance or coordination.

- **Sudden severe headache** - 'a bolt out of the blue' – with no apparent cause.

***Extra Info: www.stroke.org***

# Salt & Sodium Guide

## Salt & Sodium

- **Sodium is a mineral element** most commonly found in salt (sodium chloride). It also occurs naturally in much smaller amounts in animal and plant foods, and water – normally sufficient for our needs without having to add salt to our diet.

- **Sodium is required** for nerve and muscle function, as well as to balance the amount of fluid in our tissues and blood. Sodium acts like a sponge to attract and hold fluids in body tissues.

- **Excess sodium** can cause water retention, and increase the risk of developing hypertension. Very high salt intake may also increase the risk of stomach cancer.

- **Too little sodium** may cause low blood pressure (hypotension), and decrease blood flow to the heart, brain and kidneys – especially during exercise. (A certain blood volume is required to sustain the blood pressure needed for adequate blood flow in the capillaries).

## Salt-Sensitive Persons

- **Normally, our kidneys** excrete excess dietary sodium. The thirst we feel after a salty meal is the body calling for water to dilute the sodium, and enable the kidneys to flush out excess sodium.

- **However, 'salt - sensitive'** persons (up to 70% of adults) tend to retain excess sodium (above approximately 3000mg daily) instead of excreting it. Such persons are more likely to develop hypertension and would benefit most from sodium restriction. Assume you are susceptible if there is a family history of hypertension.

- **Although not everyone will benefit, all Americans are being asked to moderate their salt and sodium intake** as a public health measure – particularly because so many do not know whether or not they have hypertension, and also because we do not know just who is salt-sensitive.

### FINDING HIDDEN SODIUM

On average, **less than one third of our sodium intake comes from the salt shaker.** The rest is hidden in processed foods that have salt added during manufacture.

Sodium compounds added to food or medicinals can also contribute significant sodium.

**Sodium bicarbonate** in particular is widely used in antacid tablets (such as *Alka Seltzer*) and powders. Sodium bicarbonate contains 27% sodium by weight. Each gram has 270mg of sodium. Large amounts of sodium can be unwittingly consumed – up to 600mg per tablet. (See Antacids ~ Page 280)

**Example:** 2 *Alka-Seltzer* Tablets = 1000mg sodium

**Other sodium compounds** include monosodium glutamate (MSG), sodium ascorbate, sodium nitrite, and sodium citrate.

### POTASSIUM BALANCES SODIUM

Potassium helps to balance sodium by helping the kidneys to excrete excess sodium. Fruit and vegetables are rich sources of potassium - another reason to ensure you have your 5-7 servings every day.

Nuts also provide potassium as well as magnesium and other heart-healthy nutrients and anti-oxidants. Eat them unsalted.

*Note: This info is only for people with normal kidney function. Also not for persons on potassium-sparing diuretics.*

### ALCOHOL DANGER

*Excessive alcohol intake contributes to hypertension. Susceptible persons should avoid or limit alcohol intake to 1-2 drinks per day.*

# Salt Sodium Guide

Sodium accounts for only 40% of the weight of salt (sodium chloride). Examples:

**1 gram (1000mg) Salt** has 400mg Sodium
**1 teaspoon (5g) Salt** has 2000mg Sodium

## HINTS TO REDUCE SODIUM

- **Cut down use of the salt shaker.** Start with an easy 50% cut in sodium by using Lite Salt (*Morton*) or *Cardia* Salt. Then gradually cut back until you can leave the salt shaker off the table. Sea salt is still high in sodium.

- **Use fresh herbs,** and salt-free seasonings to add flavor to food.

- **Choose low-sodium,** sodium-free, and reduced-sodium products in place of regular, salted products.

- **Check food labels for sodium levels.** FDA Guidelines for sodium descriptors are:
  - **Reduced Sodium:** At least 25% less sodium than the original product
  - **Low Sodium:** 140 mg or less/serving
  - **Very Low Sodium:** 35mg or less/serving
  - **Sodium Free:** Less than 5mg/serving
  - **No Salt Added:** Made without the salt normally added, but still contains the sodium that is a natural part of the food

- **Use reduced-sodium breads,** butter and margarine. Regular varieties are considered high in sodium in view of their significant contribution to our diet.

- **Go easy on salty condiments and sauces** such as ketchup, mustard, soy sauce, spaghetti sauces, and salad dressings. Use low-sodium varieties.

- **Limit pizzas and salty fast-foods.** Check the *CalorieKing.com* food database.

- **Avoid salty snack foods** such as potato chips, corn chips, salted nuts, pretzels and cheesy-flavored snacks. **Choose unsalted** popcorn, nuts or seeds. Eat more fruit.

- **Don't salt children's food** to your taste.

- **Avoid antacids with** sodium bicarbonate (such as *Alka-Seltzer*). They are high in sodium. Look for low-sodium alternatives.

## FOODS HIGH IN SODIUM

- Bread (4 slices/day), Bagels, Biscuits
- Cheese, Butter, Margarine
- Pickles, Sauerkraut, Olives
- Condiments, Sauces
- Salad Dressings
- Canned vegetables/salads/beans
- Deli Salads (with dressing)
- Frozen/Packaged Meals/Entrees
- Soups: Canned/dry; bouillon cubes
- Meats: Ham, bacon, sausage, luncheon meats, smoked meats
- Canned Fish (in brine/salt)
- Sea Salt, Garlic/Celery Salt
- Snack Foods (potato chips, pretzels)
- Tomato Juice (Canned), V8 Vegetable Juice
- Fast Foods: Pizza, Burgers, Chicken
- *Alka-Seltzer* Antacid

## MODERATE SODIUM

- Meat, Fish, Poultry - Unprocessed
- Milk, Yogurt, Soy Drinks, Eggs
- Peanut Butter
- Breakfast Cereals (less than 200mg/serving)
- Chocolate Candy, Fruit/Nut Bars
- *Reduced Sodium & Low Sodium* Products

## FOODS LOW IN SODIUM

- Products labelled *Very Low Sodium*, or *Sodium Free*
- Bread (No Salt Added)
- Fresh fruits and vegetables
- Canned and Dried Fruits
- Potatoes, Rice, Pasta
- Dried Beans & Lentils, Tofu
- Nuts & Seeds (unsalted)
- Corn & Popcorn (unsalted)
- Pepper, Spices, Herbs
- Jam, Honey, Syrup
- Candy, Gum
- Hard & Jelly Candy
- Coffee, Tea, Alcohol
- Fresh Fruit Juices, Water

# Sodium Counter

The American Heart Association recommends a sodium intake of less than 1500mg/day

## Milk & Dairy Products

| | Sodium |
|---|---|
| **Milk:** Whole/lowfat/skim, average | |
| 1 glass, 8 fl.oz | 120 |
| Whole, low sodium, 1 cup | 5 |
| **Choc Milk,** 1 cup | 130 |
| **Soy Milk,** 8 fl.oz | 30 |
| **Buttermilk,** cultured, 8 fl.oz | 250 |
| **Dry/Powder,** skim, 1/4 cup, 1 oz | 110 |
| **Yogurt,** with fruit average, 8 oz | 130 |
| **Cheese:** Bleu, 1 oz | 330 |
| Cottage Cheese, Creamed, 1/2 cup, 4 oz | 450 |
| **Kraft:** American, 2% milk, 1 sl., 0.7 oz | 230 |
| Philadelphia Cream Cheese Brick, Orig.,1 oz | 105 |
| Parmesan, 1 oz | 425 |
| Process Cheese., average,1 oz | 430 |
| Ricotta Cheese, 1/2 cup, 4 oz | 110 |
| Swiss, Deli Deluxe, 1 slice | 40 |

## Ice Cream, Frozen Yogurt

| | |
|---|---|
| Icecream, average, 1/2 cup | 50 |
| Frozen Yogurt, 1/2 cup | 50 |

## Fats/Oils

| | |
|---|---|
| **Butter/Margarine:** | |
| Regular, 2 Tbsp, 1 oz | 230 |
| Unsalted, reg., 2 Tbsp, 1 oz | 5 |
| **Mayonnaise,** avg., 2 Tbsp, 1 oz | 160 |
| **Oils/Lard/Drippings** | 0 |
| **Cream,** average, 1 Tbsp | 5 |
| *Coffee-Mate:* Powdered, 1 tsp | 2 |
| Liquid, 1 Tbsp | 5 |

## Eggs

| | |
|---|---|
| **Whole,** 1 large | 70 |
| **Omelet: 2 egg,** plain | 220 |
| With 1 oz Cheddar Cheese | 400 |
| ***Egg Beaters:*** Original, 3 Tbsp | 90 |
| Flavors, average, 3 Tbsp | 140 |

## Meats

| | |
|---|---|
| **Meat,** average all types, cooked | |
| Beef/Lamb/Veal/Pork, 4 oz | 80 |
| **Corned Beef,** cooked, 3 oz | 800 |
| **Bacon,** cooked, 2 slices, 0.5 oz | 270 |
| **Ham,** 3 oz | 1100 |

## Meat Substitutes (Vegan)

| | |
|---|---|
| ***Beyond Meat:*** Beef/Burger, 4 oz | 400 |
| Sausage, 1 link | 500 |
| ***Impossible,*** 4 oz patty | 370 |

**Sodium ~ Sodium (mg)**

## Sausages & Deli Meats

| | Sodium |
|---|---|
| Bologna, 1 oz | 280 |
| Frankfurter, 2 oz | 640 |
| Ham, chopped, 0.8 oz slice | 290 |
| Liverwurst (Braunschweiger), 1 oz | 320 |
| Pepperoni, 5 slices, 1 oz | 570 |
| Salami: Cooked, 1 oz | 350 |
| dry/hard, 1 oz | 600 |
| Sausage, 1 oz link | 220 |
| Pork, 2 oz patty | 260 |
| **Spam:** Classic, 2 oz | 790 |
| 25% Less Sodium, 2 oz | 580 |
| Turkey Roll, 1 oz | 160 |

## Chicken & Turkey

| | |
|---|---|
| **Chicken/Turkey,** cooked, unsalted, 4 oz | 80 |
| **Stuffing Mixes,** average., 1/2 cup | 500 |

## Fish:

| | |
|---|---|
| **Fresh Fish:** average, plain | |
| Cooked, 4 oz, without bone | 60 |
| Broiled w. butter, 4 oz | 150 |
| Breaded & fried, 4 oz | 320 |
| Fish fillets, batter-dipped 3 oz | 350 |
| Fish sticks, 1 oz stick | 160 |
| Gefilte Fish, with broth, 1 pce, 1.5 oz | 220 |
| Herring, pickled, 2 pces, 1 oz | 260 |
| Lobster, meat only, 4 oz | 180 |
| Oysters, fresh, 6 med., 3 oz | 95 |
| **Salmon:** Canned, 3 oz | 460 |
| No Salt Added, 3 oz | 65 |
| **Smoked fish,** average, 3 oz | 650 |
| **Tuna:** Canned, drained, 3 oz | 160 |
| Light, drained, 3 oz | 200 |
| No Added Salt, 3 oz | 40 |
| Spicy Flavored, 5 oz | 260 |

## Entrees & Meals

| | |
|---|---|
| **Frozen Meals,** average | 600-1300 |
| ***Lean Cuisine,*** average | 700 |
| ***Stouffer's,*** For One, Beef Pot Roast | 1570 |
| **Dinners,** average | 900-1200 |
| **Side Dishes,** average | 400-600 |
| **Pizza,** frozen, 1/4 large, 6 oz | 800-1200 |
| **Microwave,** Cup Meals | 900-1200 |
| **Cup O'Noodles,** average | 1500 |

**More Sodium Counts:**
**www.CalorieKing.com**

# Sodium Counter

## Soups

| | Sodium |
|---|---|
| **Condensed:** Average, 1 cup, 8 oz | 800-1000 |
| Low Sodium, average | 70 |
| **Chicken Noodle,** average, 1 cup | 900 |
| **Bouillon Cube,** average | 950 |
| **Ramen Noodle Soup,** av., 3 oz pkg | 1500 |
| **Soup Cups,** average | 850 |
| **Soup Mixes,** average, 1 cup | 900 |

## Condiments, Sauces, Dressings

| | |
|---|---|
| **A-1 Sauce,** 1 Tbsp | 280 |
| **Barbecue Sauce,** 1 Tbsp | 130 |
| **Bragg's Liquid Aminos,** 1 tsp | 220 |
| **Chili Sauce,** 1 Tbsp | 230 |
| **Ketchup:** Tomato, 1 Tbsp | 180 |
| Low Sodium, 1 Tbsp | 20 |
| **Mayonnaise,** 1 Tbsp | 80 |
| **Mustard,** 1 tsp | 70 |
| **Pizza Sauce,** 1/2 cup | 700 |
| **Salad Dressings,** 2 Tbsp, 1 oz | 160-400 |
| **Spaghetti Sauce,** 1/2 cup | 500 |
| **Soy Sauce:** 1 Tbsp | 900 |
| Lite, 1 Tbsp | 600 |
| **Sweet & Sour,** 1/2 cup | 250 |
| **Tabasco,** 1 tsp | 25 |
| **Vinegar,** Lemon Juice | 0 |
| **Worcestershire,** 1 Tbsp | 65 |
| **Tomato:** Sauce, 1 cup | 1200 |
| Paste/Puree (salted), 1/2 cup | 1000 |
| No Salt Added, 1/2 cup | 75 |

## Salt & Salt Substitutes

| | |
|---|---|
| **Table Salt:** 1 teaspoon, 6g | 2400 |
| Single Serve package, 1 g | 400 |
| *Cardia Salt,* 1 teaspoon | 1080 |
| **Lite Salt,** 1 teaspoon, 6g | 1200 |
| *Morton,* No Salt Substitute, 1 tsp | 5 |
| **Garlic/Onion/Seasoned Salt,** 1 tsp, 4g | 1350 |
| **Garlic/Seasoned Salt** 1 teaspoon, 4g | 1300 |
| **Sea Salt,** 1 teaspoon, 5g | 2250 |

## Seasonings, Herbs & Spices

| | |
|---|---|
| Baking Powder, 1 tsp, 3g | 340 |
| Baking Soda (Sodium bicarb), 1 tsp, 3g | 810 |
| *Accent,* Flavor Enhancer, 1 tsp | 680 |
| Chili Powder, 1 tsp, 3g | 25 |
| Curry Powder | 0 |
| Lemon Pepper 1 tsp | 340 |
| Meat Tenderizer, 1 tsp, 5g | 1750 |
| MSG (Monosodium Glutamate), 5g | 500 |
| *Mrs Dash,* Blends/Marinades | 0 |
| *Old Bay:* Seasoning, 1 tsp, 2.4 oz | 640 |
| Seasoning, Less Sodium, 1 tsp, 2.4 oz | 380 |
| Pepper, Mustard (dry), 1 tsp | 1 |
| Yeast, Nutritional, 1 Tbsp | 10 |

## Breakfast Cereals

| | Sodium |
|---|---|
| *Kellogg's:* | |
| All-Bran, Original, 1/2 cup, 1 oz | 80 |
| Special K, Original, 1¼ cups, 1.4 oz | 270 |
| Corn Flakes, 1 cup, 1 oz | 200 |
| Raisin Bran, 1 cup, 2 oz | 200 |
| *Quaker:* | |
| Corn Crunch, 1 cup, 1.3 oz | 220 |
| Multigrain Flakes, av., ¾ c., 2.2 oz | 40 |
| Puffed Rice/Wheat, 2 cups, 1 oz | 0 |
| Simply Granola, average, 1/2 cup | 30 |
| *General Mills,* Total, 3/4 cup, 1 oz | 140 |
| **Oatmeal:** Regular, 3/4 cup | 1 |
| *Quaker,* Instant Maple & Brown Sugar (1 pkt) | 260 |

## Breads, Bagels, Crackers

| | |
|---|---|
| **Bread:** Thin Slice, average 1 oz | 140 |
| Thick Slice, 1.5 oz | 210 |
| Low Sodium, 1 oz | 10 |
| **Bagels:** Plain, medium, 2 oz | 200 |
| Large, take-out, average, 4 oz | 550 |
| *Panera Bread,* 3.8 oz | 460 |
| **Biscuits,** average, 1 oz | 180 |
| **Bun/Roll:** 1 medium, 1.5 oz | 200 |
| Large, 4 oz | 560 |
| **Crackers:** Saltine, 2 crackers | 70 |
| Low Salt, 2 | 25 |
| Graham, 2 regular | 50 |
| **Croissant,** Plain, average, 2 oz | 280 |
| **Rice Cakes,** average | 25 |
| *Ritz Crackers,* Hint of Salt, 1 oz | 60 |
| *Ry-Krisp,* Crispbread, Sesame, 0.7 oz | 70 |

## Cookies, Cakes, Desserts

| | |
|---|---|
| **Cookies:** Average, 2-3 cookies, 1 oz | 100 |
| Average, 1 cookie, 2.5 oz | 180 |
| **Baked Custard,** 1/2 cup | 100 |
| **Brownie,** 1.5 oz | 130 |
| **Carrot Cake,** 8 oz | 650 |
| **Cheesecake,** 7 oz | 350 |
| **Cinnamon Sweet Roll,** 2 oz | 250 |
| **Danish,** Apple/Fruit | 250 |
| **Donut,** average | 150 |
| **Muffins:** 1 medium, 2 oz | 150 |
| 1 extra large, 4 oz | 300 |
| **Pancakes,** (4"), x 3 | 360 |
| **Fruit Pies,** average, 7 oz | 600 |
| **Pudding:** Average, 1/2 cup | 160 |
| *Jell-O* Instant Pudding Mix, 1/4 pkg | 360 |
| **Waffles:** Home-made, 7", 2.5 oz | 350 |
| Frozen: Average, 1.2 oz | 260 |
| *Aunt Jemima,* Homestyle, av., 2.5 oz | 480 |

# Sodium Counter

## Fruit & Juices
| | Sodium |
|---|---|
| **Fresh Fruit,** average all types, 1 serving | 1 |
| **Dried/Canned Fruit,** 1/2 cup | 1 |
| **Fruit Juice:** Fresh, squeezed, 6 fl.oz | 1 |
| Commercial, aver., 6 fl.oz | 20 |
| **Tomato Juice** *(Campbell's)*, 8 fl.oz | 680 |
| Low Sodium (No Salt Added), 8 fl.oz | 140 |
| **V8 Vegetable** *(Campbell's)*: | |
| 11.5 fl.oz bottle | 880 |
| Low Sodium, 5.5 fl.oz can | 80 |

## Vegetables
**Fresh/Frozen (No Salt Added):** Per 1/2 Cup
| | |
|---|---|
| Asparagus, Bean Sprouts, Corn | 3 |
| Beets, Carrots, Celery, 1/2 cup | 40 |
| Broccoli, Cabbage, Cauliflower | 10 |
| Cucumber, Green Beans, Mushroom, Okra | 3 |
| Onions, Peas, Potato, Pumpkin, Squash | 3 |
| Peppers, Hot Chili, raw, each | 3 |
| Spinach, Turnips, 1/2 cup, cooked | 40 |
| Tomato, 1 medium, 5 oz | 10 |
| **Canned:** Asparagus, 4 spears | 300 |
| Beans, baked in tomato sauce | 450 |
| Beets, 1/2 cup, 3 oz | 240 |
| Corn Kernels, 1/2 cup, 3 oz | 190 |
| Creamed, 1/2 cup, 4.5 oz | 330 |
| Mushrooms w. butter sce, 2oz | 550 |
| Peas, 1/2 cup, 3 oz | 250 |
| Sauerkraut, 1/2 cup, 4 oz | 750 |

## Pickles, Olives
| | |
|---|---|
| **Olives:** pickled: Green, 1 large | 90 |
| Ripe/black, 1 large | 40 |
| **Pickles:** Bread & Butter, 4 slices, 1 oz | 200 |
| Dill, 1 pickle, 2.5oz | 900 |
| Sweet, 1 gherkin, 0.5 oz | 130 |

## Soybean Products
| | |
|---|---|
| **Miso (Soy Paste),** 1/4 c., 2.5 oz | 2500 |
| **Soybean Protein Isolate,** 1 oz | 280 |
| **Tempeh,** Natural, 1/2 cup, 3 oz | 5 |
| **Tofu,** average, 1/2 cup, 4 oz | 5 |

## Jam, Honey, Syrups
| | |
|---|---|
| **Jam/Jelly,** 1 Tbsp | 2 |
| **Honey/Maple Syrup,** 1 Tbsp | 1 |
| *Log Cabin,* Syrup, 1 fl.oz | 35 |
| Lite, 1 fl.oz | 90 |

## Peanut Butter
| | |
|---|---|
| **Peanut Butter:** Regular, 2 Tbsp, 0.5 oz | 190 |
| *Jif,* Low Sodium, 2 Tbsp | 65 |
| *Trader Joe's,* Unsalted, 2 Tbsp | 5 |

## Snacks, Nuts
| | Sodium |
|---|---|
| **Cheese Balls/Curls,** 1 oz | 280 |
| **Cheetos,** 1 oz | 290 |
| **Corn/Tortilla Chips:** average, 1 oz | 220 |
| *Fritos,* Lightly Salted, 1 oz | 80 |
| **Granola bars,** average, 1 bar | 80 |
| **Nuts:** Plain, unsalted, 1 oz | 1 |
| Lightly salted, 1 oz | 80 |
| Salted or Honey Roasted, 1 oz | 160 |
| **Popcorn:** Plain (unsalted), 1 cup | 1 |
| Flavored, average, 1 cup | 60 |
| Salt added, 1 cup | 180 |
| **Potato Chips:** Plain, 1 oz | 160 |
| *Lay's,* Lightly Salted, 1 oz | 85 |
| Flavored, average, 1 oz | 200 |
| **Pretzels:** Regular, 3, 1 oz | 450 |
| Soft, salted, large | 1000 |

## Candy, Chocolate
| | |
|---|---|
| **Chocolate,** milk, 1 oz | 30 |
| **Fudge,** chocolate, 1 oz | 55 |
| **Candy Bars,** average, 1.5 oz | 60 |
| **Hard Candy,** 1 oz | 10 |
| **Licorice,** 1 oz | 30 |

## Beverages, Alcohol
| | |
|---|---|
| **Coffee or Tea,** 1 cup | 1 |
| **Cocoa:** Dry, plain, 1 Tbsp | 0 |
| Mix, average, 1 envelope | 120 |
| **Quik,** 2 tsp | 35 |
| **Soft Drinks,** average, 8 fl.oz | 20 |
| **Mineral Water:** Perrier, 8 fl.oz | 5 |
| *Gatorade,* Thirst Quencher, 8 fl.oz | 110 |
| *Red Bull:* 8.4 fl.oz can | 105 |
| Sugar Free, 8.4 fl.oz | 200 |
| **Water,** 1 cup, 8 fl.oz | 5 |
| **Alcohol:** Beer, average, 12 fl.oz | 15 |
| Wines, average, 4 fl.oz | 10 |
| Spirits (distilled), 1.5 fl.oz | 1 |

## Antacids ~ Alka-Seltzer
| | Sodium |
|---|---|
| Alka-Seltzer: *Per Tablet* | |
| Original; Heartburn | 570 |
| Extra Strength | 590 |
| Lemon Lime | 500 |
| Gold | 310 |
| *Alka-Mints,* chewable | 0 |
| *Bromo Seltzer,* 3/4 capful | 760 |
| *Picot,* 1 packet, 5g | 670 |
| *Rolaids,* All types | 0 |
| *Tums,* Regular/Extra Strength | 0 |

## Cold & Flu ~ Alka-Seltzer Plus
| | |
|---|---|
| Effervescents, average, 1 tablet | 480 |
| Fast Crystal Packs; Liquid Gels | 0 |

# Sodium Counter

## Fast-Foods & Restaurants

**Sodium**

### Burger King:

| | |
|---|---|
| **Bacon Double Cheeseburger** | 740 |
| **Cheeseburger** | 560 |
| **Hamburger** | 380 |
| **Triple Stacker King** | 2300 |
| **Whoppers:** Original | 980 |
| With Cheese | 1340 |
| Whopper Jr. | 390 |
| Impossible Whopper | 1080 |
| **Chicken Sandwich,** Original | 1170 |
| **Sides:** French Fries, medium, salted | 570 |
| Onion Rings, medium | 1080 |
| **Breakfast,** Ham, Egg & Cheese Croissan'wich | 1030 |

### Carl's Jr.:

| | |
|---|---|
| **Burgers:** Famous Star w/ Cheese | 1210 |
| Beyond Famous Star w/ Cheese | 1550 |
| The Big Carl | 1380 |

### Denny's:

| | |
|---|---|
| **Burgers:** Bacon Avocado Cheeseburger | 1830 |
| Spicy Sriracha | 2210 |
| **Sandwiches:** Club | 2180 |
| Prime Rib Philly Melt | 2340 |
| **Dinner:** Brooklyn Spaghetti & M'balls w/ Bread | 2480 |
| Sirloin Steak, with Bread | 1260 |
| Sides: Broccoli | 20 |
| French Fries, salted, 6 oz | 110 |
| Red-Skinned Potatoes | 590 |
| **Soup:** Loaded Baked Potato, 12 oz bowl | 1770 |
| Vegetable Beef, 12 oz bowl | 3420 |
| **Breakfast:** Buttermilk Pancakes (2), w/ Marg. | 1390 |
| Moons Over My Hammy Omelette, w/ Hash | 2560 |
| Supreme Skillet, 10 oz | 1180 |
| Sides: Hash Browns, 1 serving | 360 |
| Hearty Breakfast Sausage | 840 |

### Jack In The Box:

| | |
|---|---|
| **Burgers:** Bacon Ultimate Cheeseburger | 1590 |
| Hamburger | 570 |
| Jumbo Jack Cheeseburger | 990 |
| Sandwiches: H'style Ranch Chicken Club | 1880 |
| Sourdough Grilled Chicken Club | 1500 |

### KFC:

| | |
|---|---|
| **Chicken Breast:** Original | 1190 |
| Extra Crispy | 1150 |
| Georgia Gold, Grilled | 760 |
| **Popcorn Nuggets,** Large | 1820 |
| **Sandwich,** Crispy Twister | 1260 |
| **Tenders,** Extra Crispy Tenders, each | 610 |
| **Wings,** HBBQ Hot (1) | 160 |
| **Sides:** Macaroni & Cheese | 660 |
| Mashed Potatoes with Gravy | 510 |
| Potato Wedges | 700 |

## Fast-Foods & Restaurants

**Sodium**

### McDonalds:

| | |
|---|---|
| **Burgers:** Big Mac | 940 |
| Cheeseburger | 680 |
| Double | 1040 |
| Hamburger | 480 |
| Quarter Pounder with Cheese | 1120 |
| **Chicken McNuggets:** 4 pieces | 340 |
| Spicy Buffalo Sauce, 1 package, 0.8 oz | 510 |
| **McChicken,** Sandwich | 600 |
| **French Fries:** Small, 2.6 oz | 160 |
| Medium, 3.9 oz | 230 |
| Large, 5.9 oz | 350 |
| Ketchup, 1 package, 10g | 90 |
| **Breakfast:** Egg McMuffin | 730 |
| Big Breakfast, reg. size Biscuit | 1490 |
| Hash Browns, 2 oz | 320 |
| Hotcakes, with Syrup & Whipped Margarine | 610 |
| Sausage McGriddle | 990 |
| Southern Style Chicken Biscuit, regular | 1140 |
| **Desserts/Shakes:** Hot Fudge Sundae | 170 |
| Strawberry McCafe Shake, medium | 230 |

### Pizza Hut:

| | |
|---|---|
| **Original Pan Pizza:** *Per Slice, Medium 12"* | |
| Meat Lovers | 660 |
| Cheese | 440 |
| Pepperoni Lover's | 600 |
| Supreme | 500 |

### Subway: *On 9 Grain Wheat Bread*

| | |
|---|---|
| **6" Sandwiches:** *With Set Menu Toppings, no oil* | |
| Chicken Bacon Ranch Melt | 1290 |
| Meatball Marinara | 1000 |
| Spicy Italian | 1490 |
| **6" Breakfast S'wich:** *With Set Menu Toppings,no oil* | |
| Bacon, Egg & Cheese Omelet | 1310 |
| BMT Egg & Cheese Omelet | 1630 |
| Mega Melt Egg White & Cheese Omelet | 1830 |
| Sausage, Egg & Cheese Omelet | 1400 |

### Taco Bell:

| | |
|---|---|
| **Burritos:** Beefy 5-Layer | 1000 |
| Supreme, Chicken | 1110 |
| **Chalupa Supreme**, Chicken/Steak, av | 515 |
| **Gordita Supreme**, Steak | 550 |
| **Nachos**: BellGrande | 1310 |
| Supreme | 850 |
| **Specialties,** Cheese Quesadillas | 980 |
| **Tacos:** Soft Chicken | 450 |
| Crunchy Supreme | 340 |

## Symbols
3-Bean Salad 141
3-Layer Cakes 64
3 Musketeers 68, 74
5th Avenue 70
7-Eleven 236
7-UP 52
100 Calorie Cake 63
100 Grand 68

## A
A-1 144
  Marinades 144
  Steak Sauce 144
Abalone 95
Abba Zabba 68
Acorns 130
AdvantEDGE 31
Advocaat 29
After Dinner Mints 68
Agave 157
Ahi Tuna 95
Alcoholic Drinks with
  Alcohol Counts 24
Alfalfa Seeds 131
Alfalfa Sprouts 158
Alizé 29
All-Bran 59
Alligator 168
Almond Breeze 49
Almond Clusters 68
Almond Croissant 62
Almond Joy 68
Almond Milk 49
Almond Paste 30
Almond Roca 68
Almond Royal 73
Almonds 130
Almond Supremes 68
Aloe Vera Juice 41, 156
Alpha Bits 61
Altoids 68
Amaranth Flour 98
Amaretto 29
Amazake 49
Angostura Bitters 29
Animal Fats/Lards 94
Animalitos 82
Antacids 156
Antiox. Super Tea 53
Ants 174
Ants Eggs/Larvae 174
Applebees 176
Apple Blasts 59
Apple Danish 62
Apple & Fruit Sauces 102
Apple Jacks 59
Apple Juice 41
Apple Pie Filling 30
Apple Raspb. Turnover 64
Apples 99
Apple Sauce 80, 102
Apple Tapioca 90
Apricots 99
Aquafaba 30

## B
Arby's 177
Arcoiris Marshmallow 82
Arrowroot Flour 98
Asian Dishes 168
Asian Pear 99, 100
Asparagus 158
Atkins 31
Atlanta Bread Co 178
Atomic Fireball 68
Attune Bars 31
Au Bon Pain 179
Auntie Anne's 179
Avocado 99
A&W 176

B52 28
Baba Ghanoush 79
Babybel 76
Baby Ruth 68
Bacardi 27
Bacardi & Coke 28
Baci 68
Back Yard Burgers 179
Bacon 92, 126
Bagel Chips 56
Bagel Crisps 56
Bagel Dogs 128
Bagels 56, 165
Bagel Spreads 56
Bagel Thins 56
Baguette 54
Baileys Irish Cream 29
Baja Fresh 180
Baking Ingredients 30
Baklava 62
Bamboo Shoots 158
Banana 99
Banana Bread 63
Banana Cake 62
Banana Walnut Cake 62
Barbecue Sauce 80
Barley 98
Barnum's Animals 85
Barracuda 95
Bars ~ Brands 31
Basa 95, 97
Baskin Robbins 180
Bass 95
Batter Mix 30
Bawls Guarana 38
Bazooka 75
Bean Dip 79
Beans 158
Bear Claw 62
Bearnaise Sauce 80
Beef Ribs 124
Beef Tallow 94
Bee Maggots 174
Bee Pollen Granules 57
Beer 24
  Amstel 24
  Asahi 24
  Beck's 24
  Bud 24

Busch 24
King Cobra 25
Light Beer 24
Lone Star 25
Non-Alc. Brews 24
Red Dog 25
Regular Beer 24
Beerwurst 128
Bellini 28
BelVita 82
Benecol 93
Benedictine 29
Ben & Jerry's 104
Better Than Milk 49, 50
Beverages:
  Cocoa & Hot Choc. 35
  Coffee 35
  Energy, Protein,
    Diet Shakes 38
  Milk & Flav., Mixes 47
  Tea & Iced Tea 53
Beyond Meat 124
Big Apple Bagels 181
Biggby Coffee 181
Bimbo Bread 55
Biscotti 86
Biscuits, Bread Rolls &
  Buns 55
Biscuit Scrambles 92
BJ's Restaurant 182
Blackberries 99
Blackeye Peas 158
Black Forest Cake 62
Blancmange 90
Blimpie 182
Blintzes 171
Bliss 68
Blood Sausage 128
Bloody Mary 28
Blow Pops 68
Blueberries 99
Blue Tequila 28
Bob Evans 183
Boiled Egg 91
Bojangles 184
Bok Choy 158
Bologna 128
Bon Bons 68
Borscht 171
Boston Cream Pie 64
Boston Market 184
Boston Pizza 184
Bottled Teas 53
Bouillon Cubes 152
Bourbon & Soda 28
Boysenberries 99
Bran Flakes 58
Bratwurst 128
Braunschweiger 128
Brazil Nuts 130
Bread & Bagels 54

Bread & Butter Pickles 80
Bread Crumbs 55
Breadfruit 99
Bread Pudding 90
Breadsticks 55
Breakfast Biscuits 82
Breakfast Cereals 57
Breakfast Patties 127
Breakfast Sausages 127
Breath Savers 68
Brie 76
Brisket 124
Broadbeans 158
Broccoli 158
Brownie 62
Brownie Mix 65
Brown Rice 140
Bruegger's 185
Brussels Sprouts 158
Bubble Milk Tea 53
Bubble Yum 75
Buckwheat 98
Buckwheat Groats 57
Budweiser 24
Buffalo Steak 126
Buffalo Wing Sauce 80
Bulgur 57, 98
Bulls Eyes 68
Bundt Cakes 62
Bunny Grahams 81
Burger King 186
Burgerville 185
Burnt Peanuts 68
Butter & Blends 93
Butterfinger 69
Buttermilk 47
Butterscotch: 69
Butterscotch Chews 73
Butter Substitutes 93
Buttery Rounds 83

## C
Cabbage 158
Cabbage Rolls 171
Cacao Butter 30
Cacao Powder 30
Cactus Fruit 99
Cactus Leaf 158
Cactus Water 41
Caesar Salad 141
Cafeteria-Style Foods 165
Caffeine Guide &
  Counter 37
Caffe Latté 36
Cajun & Creole 168
Cake Frostings 62
Cakes ~ Mixes 64, 65
Cakes, Buns, Donuts,
  Muffins, Pastries,
  Frostings 62
Calamari 95

Camembert 76
Canadian Food 168
Candied Apple 167
Candied/Glazed Fruit 102
Candy 68
Candy Apple 69
Candy Cane 69
Candy, Chocolate, Gum 68
Candy-Coated Eggs 71
Canned Fruit 102
Canned & Dried Milk 47
Canned/Packaged:
  Fish 97
  Meals 111
Cantaloupe 99
Cape Gooseberries 99
Cappuccino 36
Captain D's Seafood 187
Caramel DeLites 82
Caramel Egg 69
Caramello Bar 69
Caramel Medallions 74
Caramel Popcorn 69
Caramels 69
Caribou Coffee 187
Carlsberg 24
Carl's Jr. 187
Carob Candy 75
Carob Flour 30, 98
Carrot Cake 62
Carrot Juice 41
Carrots 158
Carr's Crackers 82
Carvel 188
Cashews 130
Caterpillars 174
Catfish 95
Cauliflower 158
Caviar 95, 174
Cereal Drinks 49
Chai Tea 53
Challah 54
Champagne 26
Chapati 54
Charley's Grilled Subs 188
Charms 69
Cheddar Bunnies 81
Cheese 76
  Almond 76
  American 76
  Blue/Bleu 76
  Cheddar 76
  Cheshire 76
  Mexican 77
  Port Wine 78
  Romano 78
  String 78

**FAST-FOODS INDEX**
**~ PAGE 175 ~**

| | | | | | | | |
|---|---|---|---|---|---|---|---|
| Cheese Balls | 150 | Churros | 62 | Coffee | 36 | Corn Flakes | 58, 60 |
| Cheesecake | 62 | Chutney | 80 | Coffee Cake | 62 | Corn Flour | 98 |
| Cheesecake Factory | 188 | Ciabatta | 54 | Coffee Creamers | 89 | Corn Grits | 98 |
| Cheese & Dips | 76 | Cici's Pizza | 190 | Coffee Extras | 36 | Corn Kernels | 98 |
| Cheese Crackers | 81 | Cider: Alcoholic/Hard | 26 | Coffee Liqueur | 29 | Cornmeal | 98 |
| Cheese Nips | 85 | Cinnabon | 59, 190 | Coffee-Mate | 89 | Corn Nuts | 150 |
| Cheese Sauce | 80 | Cinnamon Muffin | | Coffee Milk | 37 | Cornstarch | 30, 98 |
| Cheese Whiz | 76 | Squares | 61 | Coffee Shops | 36 | Corn & Tortilla Chips | 149 |
| Cheetos | 151 | Cinn. Raisin Bagel | 56 | Cafe Au Lait | 36 | Corona | 24 |
| Cheez-It Snack | 87 | Cinnamon Rolls | 62 | Cafe Mocha | 36 | Cosmopolitan | 28 |
| Cherimoya | 99 | Cinnamon Streusel | 63 | Caffe Latté | 36 | Costco Food Court | 191 |
| Cherries | 99 | Circus Peanuts | 69 | Cappuccino | 36 | Cote d'Or | 69 |
| Cherry Brandy | 29 | Claim Jumper | 191 | Coffee | 36 | Cottage Cheese | 76 |
| Chestnuts | 130 | Clams | 95 | Frappuccino | 36 | Cotton Candy, | 69 |
| Chex | 59 | Clementine | 99 | Iced Latte | 36 | Cough/Cold Syrups | 156 |
| Chia Seeds | 131 | Clif | | Mocha | 36 | Cough Drops | 75, 156 |
| Chicken | 138 | Builder's | 31 | Coffee Substitute | 36 | Cough & Pharma | 156 |
| Chicken Eggs | 91 | Kid | 31 | Cointreau | 29 | Couscous | 98 |
| Chicken In Water | 139 | Mojo | 31 | Cola | 51 | Cousins Subs | 191 |
| Chicken Offal & | | Original | 31 | Colby | 76 | Cow's Milk | 47 |
| Stuffing | 138 | Club Soda | 51 | Colby-Jack | 76 | Fat Free/Skim | 47 |
| Chick-fil-A | 189 | Clusters | 61 | Cold Cereals | 58 | Light/Low-Fat | 47 |
| Chickpeas | 158 | Cocktail Mixers, | | Cold Stone Creamery | 191 | Reduced-Fat | 47 |
| Chicory | 35 | Non-Alcoholic | 28 | Concha | 62, 173 | Whole | 47 |
| Chili Powder | 147 | Cocktails | 28 | Condensed Milk | 47 | Crab | 95 |
| Chili's | 189 | Cocktail Sauce | 80 | Condiments, Salsa, | | Crabapples | 99 |
| Chili Sauce | 80 | Cocoa - Choc. Mixes | 35 | Pickles, Sauces | 80 | Crab Cakes | 95 |
| Chinook | 96 | Cocoa & Hot Choc. | 35 | Conversation Hearts | 69 | Crackers | 81 |
| Chipotle | 190 | Cocoa Powder | 30 | Cooked Cereals | 57 | Cranberries | 99 |
| Chips Ahoy! | 85 | Coconut | 99, 130 | Cooked Eggs | 91 | Cranberry Juice | 41 |
| Choc Chip Cookies | 151 | Coconut Cream/Milk | 89 | Cookie ~ Mixes | 87 | Cranberry Sauce | 80 |
| Choc Coated Peanuts | 73 | Coconut, dried | 30 | Cookie Cakes | 63 | Crayfish | 95 |
| Choc Lava Cake | 64 | Coconut Flour | 98 | Cookies, Crackers | 81 | Cream | 89 |
| Chocolate | 68 | Coconut Manna | 30 | Cooking Sprays/ | | Cream Cheese | 77 |
| Choc. Baking Bars | 30 | Coconut Milk Drinks | 50 | Squeezes | 94 | Cream & Creamers | 89 |
| Choc. Baking Chips | 30 | Silk | 50 | Cooking Wines | 26 | Creamers (Non-Dairy) | 89 |
| Chocolate Cake | 62 | So Delicious | 50 | Coolers & Premix | | Cream Horn | 62 |
| Choc. Chip Cookies | 81 | Trader Joes | 50 | Cocktails | 27 | Cream of Rice | 57 |
| Chocolate Croissant | 62 | Coconut Palm Sugar | 157 | Bartles & Jaymes | 27 | Cream of Wheat | 57 |
| Chocolate Cup Cake | 63 | Coconut Water | 41, 89 | Captain Morgan's | 27 | Cream Puff | 62 |
| Chocolate Eclair | 62 | Cod | 95 | Skinnygirl | 27 | Cream Soda | 51 |
| Chocolate Milk | 48 | Cod Liver Oil | 156 | TGI Friday's | 27 | Crème Brûlée | 90 |
| Chocolate Orange | 74 | | | Cool Whip | 89 | Creme de Cacao | 29 |
| Choc-O-Lunch | 84 | | | Coors | 24 | Creme de Menthe | 29 |
| Chuck Blade | 124 | | | Core Power | 38 | Creme Savers | 69 |
| Chuck E. Cheese | 190 | | | Corn | 158 | Cremora | 89 |
| Chunky Bar | 69 | | | Cornbread | 54 | Crispbread | 81, 82 |
| Chupa Chups, | 69 | | | Corn Dogs | 128 | Crispbreads | 88 |
| Chupa Naranjas | 28 | | | Corned Beef | 128 | Crispbreads, Matzo | 88 |
| Church's Chicken | 190 | | | Corn Flake Crumbs | 55 | Croissant-Donuts | 66 |

| | |
|---|---|
| Croissants | 134, 165 |
| Croutons | 55 |
| Cucumber | 158 |
| Culver's | 192 |
| Cup-a-Soup | 154 |
| Cupcakes | 62 |
| Curry Powder | 147 |
| Curves, Protein Drink | 38 |
| Custard Mix | 90 |
| Custards | 90 |
| Cuttlefish | 95 |

**D**

| | |
|---|---|
| Dairy Queen | 192 |
| D'Angelo's | 192 |
| Danish Pastries | 62 |
| Daphne's Greek Cafe | 193 |
| Dates | 99 |
| Davanni's | 193 |
| Deli Salads | 141 |
| Del Taco | 194 |
| Denny's | 194 |
| Dentyne | 75 |
| Desserts | 90 |
| Dessert Wines | 26 |
| Detour | 31 |
| Deviled Egg | 91 |
| Dextrose | 157 |
| Diabetic Tussin | 75 |
| Diabetisield | 39 |
| Diet Pepsi | 52 |
| Dill Pickles | 80 |
| Ding Dongs | 63 |
| Dippin' Dots | 196 |
| Dips/Spreads | 79 |
| Dolphinfish | 96 |
| Domino's | 196 |
| Donatos Pizza | 196 |
| Donut Holes | 66 |
| Donuts | 66 |
| Dos Equis XX | 24 |
| dotBAR/STICK | 31 |
| Double Dippers | 68 |
| Double Doozies | 83 |
| Double Peanut Bar | 73 |
| Dove | 69 |
| Dark Choc | 69 |
| Milk Choc | 69 |
| Sugar Free | 69 |
| Dragon Fruit | 99 |

# Index D - J

Drambuie 29
Dream Whip 89
Dried Egg Powder 91
Dried Fruit 102
Dried Milk 47
Drippings 94
Drumstick 109
Duck 139
Duck Egg 91
Dunkin' 66, 197
Durian 99

**E**

Easy Cheese 77
Eating Out:
  Cafeteria, S'wiches 165
  Fair/Carnival/
    Stadium Foods 166
  Restaurant &
    International 168
Eat 'N Park 198
Edam 77
Edamame 158
Edo Japan 199
Eel 95
Egg Custard 90
Egg Nog 91
Eggs 91
Eggs Benedict 91
Eggs Florentine 91
Egg Substitutes 91
Einstein Bros 199
Elderberries 99
El Pollo Loco 200
Empanadas 173
Enchilada Sauce 146
Ener-G: Bread 55
  Cookies 82
Energy Meal Shake 40
Energy/Protein Drinks 38
English Muffins 56
English Toffee 70
English Toffee Squares 74
Eskimo Pie 109
Espresso 36
Espresso con Panna 36
Espresso Macchiato 36
Evaporated Milk 47

**F**

Fair & Carnival Foods 166
Falafel 166
Farina 57, 98
Fast Break 70
Fatburger 200
Fat Free Puddings 90
Fats, Butter, Spreads,
  Oils, Mayonnaise 93

Fats & Cholesterol
  Guide 259, 263
Fazoli's 200
Feijoa 100
Ferrero Rocher 70
Feta 77
Fiber One 59
Fifty 50 Snack Bars 70
Fig Bars 62, 81
Fig Newman's 86
Figs 100
Filet Mignon 123
Firehouse Subs 201
Fish Oil Capsules 156
Fish Oils 94
Fish & Shellfish 95
Five Guys 201
Flame Broiler 201
Flavor Aid 52
Flav. Butter/Spreads 93
Flav. Coffee Mixes 35
Flavored Milk 48
Flavored Spirits 27
Flavor Extracts 30
Flaxseed 98
Flaxseeds 131
Flax Seeds 131
Flounder 95
Flourless Choc. Cake 64
Flours & Grains 98
Foccacia 54
Fosters 24
Franks & Weiners 127
Frappuccino 36
French Foods 169
French Onion Dip 79
French Stick 54
French Toast 54
Fresh Eggs 91
Freshens 201
Fresh Fish 95
Fresh Salad Packs 141
Fried Egg 91
Frog Legs 174
Froot Loops 60
Frosted Flakes 58
Frozen Custard 103
Frozen Egg Breakfasts 92
Frozen Egg Rolls 92
Frozen Pizzas 136
Frozen Vegetables 160
Frozen Yogurt 103
Fructose 157
Fruit Blends 41
Fruit Cake 62
Fruit Drops 70
Fruit 99
Fruit Leather Rolls 102
Fruit Leathers 70
Fruit Nectars 41

Fruit Pastilles 70
Fruit Pectin 30
Fruit Pies 134
Fruit Roll-Ups 70
Fruit Snack Cups 102
Fudge 70
Fudge Bar 109
Fudge Shoppe 83
Fuze 38

**G**

Galliano 29
Game & Other Meats 126
Garbanzo 98
Garlic 159
Garlic Bread 54
Garlic Butter 93
Garlic Powder 147
Gatorade 38
Gefilte Fish Balls 171
Gelatin 30
Gelatin Dessert Mix 90
Gelato 103
Gem Donuts 66
German Foods 169
Ghee (Clarified Butter) 93
Gherkins 80
Ghirardelli 70
Ginger 159
Ginger Ale 51, 52
Gingerbread 62
Ginkgo Nuts 130
Glucerna 32
  Crispy Delights 32
  Mini Snack Bar 32
Gluten Free Cake Mix 65
Gluten Free Flour 98
Gluten Free Puddings 90
Goat's Milk 47
Goat's Milk Cheese 77
Godfather's Pizza 202
Godiva 70
Golden Corral 202
Golden Puffs 60
Goldfish 86
Gold Star Chili 202
Goobers Peanuts 70
Goose 139
Gooseberries 100
Goose Egg 91
Gorgonzola 77
Gouda 77
Grahams 81

Granadilla 100
Grand Marnier 29
Granola 58, 59
Grapefruit 100
Grapefruit Juice 41
Grape Juice 41
Grape-Nuts 61
Grapes 100
Gravy 124, 144
Great American
  Bagel Co 203
Great Steak 203
Greek Foods 169
Green Burrito 203
Green Chiles 80
Grenadine 29
Grolsch 24
Ground Beef 124
Gruyere 77
Guacamole 79
Guanabana 100
Guava 100
Guinness 24
Gum 75
Gummi Bears 68
Guylian 70

**H**

Haagen-Dazs 204
Haddock 96
Haggis 174
Half & Half Cream 36, 89
Halibut 96
Hallah 171
Ham 92, 126
Hardee's 204
Hard Lemonade & Tea 27
Half & Half 27
Harvey Wallbanger 28
Hash Brown 92
Havarti 77
Hawaiian Foods 169
Hawaiian Sweet Bread 54
Hazelnuts 130
Heineken 24
Hemp Bread 54
Hemp Flour 98
Hemp Seeds 131
Herring 96
Hershey's 70
  Cookies 'n' Creme 70
Highball 28
Hissho Sushi 205
Ho Hos 63
Homemade Puddings 90
Home Pride Bread 55
Hominy Grits 57
Honey 157
Honey Bun, 62
Honey Bunches of Oats 61

Honey Butter 93
Honeycomb 71
Honeydew 100
Honey Murcots 100
Honey Mustard 80
Honey Smacks 60
Horchata Rice Drink 49
Horseradish 80
Hot Dog on a Stick 205
Hot Dogs 128
Hot Dog Toppings 128
Hot Pockets 115
Hot Tamales 71
Hot Toddy 29
Hubba Bubba 75
Hungry Howie's Pizza 206

**I**

I Can't Believe
  It's Not Butter! 93
Ice Breakers 75
Ice Cream 103
Ice Cream:
  Cones & Cups 103
  & Frozen Yogurt 103
  Toppings 157
Iced Mocha 36
Iced Tea 53
Ices 103
IHOP 206
Impossible Whopper
  (Vegan) 186
Indian & Pakistani 170
In-N-Out Burger 206
Instant Coffee 35
Instant Grits 57
Irish & Liqueur Coffees 36
Italian Bread 54
Italian Dishes 170

**J**

Jaboticaba 100
Jack Daniels 27
Jackfruit 100
Jack in the Box 207
Jack's 207
Jalapeno Relish 80
Jalapenos 80
Jam 157
Jamba Juice 208
Japanese Foods 171
Jarlsberg 77
Jawbreakers 71
Jell-O 90
Jelly Beans 71
Jelly Belly 71
Jellyfish 96
Jelly Roll 62

Jersey Mike's Subs 208
Jimmy John's 209
Johnny Rockets 209
Jolly Rancher 71
Jolt Gum 75
Juice 41
Jujubes 71
Junior Caramels 71
Junior Mints 71

**K**

Kahlua 29
Kahlua Mudslide 28
Kale 159
Kalettes 159
Kashi 32
Kefir 47
Ketchup 80
Key Lime Pie 62
KFC 210
Kidneys 126
Kikkoman 146
Kimchee 172
Kind Bars 32
Kinder Joy 71
Kirsch 29
Kisses 71
Kit Kat 71
Kiwifruit 100
Kix 59
Knish 171
Knockwurst 128
Kombucha Tea 53
Korean Food 172
Kosher/Deli Foods 171
Kozy Shack 90
Krave 60
Kringles 62
Krispy Kreme 211
Krystal 211
Kugel 171

**L**

Labneh 77
Labrada 32
Lean Body Prot. Bar 32
Lactose Free Milk 47
Lady Finger 62
Lamb 125
Larabar 32
LaRosa's Pizzeria 212
La Salsa Mexican 212
Latkes 171
Lean Pockets 117
Lebanese/Mid. East 172
Lecithin Granules 57, 156

Leek 159
Lemonade 51, 52
Lemon Cake 62
Lemon Drops 68, 71
Lemon/Lime Juice 41
Lemon/Orange Peel 30
Lemons 100
Lentils 159
Lettuce 159
Licorice 71
Lifesavers 71
Light & Reduced Fat
  Spreads 93
Lik-m-aid 72
Limes 100
Lindora Bars 32
Lindora Prot. Shakes 39
Lindt 72
Ling 96
Liqueur Coffee 36
Liqueurs/Cordials 29
Little Caesars 213
Liver 126
Liverwurst 128
Lobster 96
Locusts 174
Lollipops 72
Long Island Iced Tea 28
Long John Silver's 213
Loquats 100
Lorna Doone 85
Lower Carb Bread 54
Lox 96
Lucky Charms 59
Luna Bars 32
Lunchables 117
Lunch Meats 128
Lychees 100

**M**

Macadamia Nuts 130
Macaroni & Cheese 133
Macaroni Grill 214
Mackerel 96
Madeira 26
Mahi-Mahi 96
Mai Tai 28
Mallomars 85
Mamba Sours 72
Mamey Apple 100
Mandarin Orange 100
Mango 100
Manhattan 28
Manhattan Bagel 214
Maraschino Cherry 29

Marathon 32
  Energy 32
  Protein 32
Margarita 27, 28
Marias 82
Marie Callender's 215
Marinades 144
Marsala 26
Marshmallow Egg 72
Marshmallows 72
Martini 28
Marzipan 72
Masa 98
Mascarpone 77
Matzo 81, 88
Matzo Balls 171
Matzo Ball Soup 171
Matzo Meal 98
Matzos 88
Max & Erma's 215
Mayonnaise 94
McAlister's Deli 216
McDonald's 216
Meat Alternatives
  (Vegan) 124
Meats:
  Lunch/Deli & Spam 128
  Sausages, Franks &
    Hot Dogs 123, 127
Meat Spreads 129
Mega Mass 2000 40
Melba Toast 81
Mellow Mushroom 216
Mentos 72
Meringue Classiques 84
Meringues 90
Metamucil 156
Met-Rx, Big 100 33
Mexican Food 172
Mexican Hats 72
Michelob 25
Microwave Popcorn 148
Midori 29
Milk 47
  Flavored Milk 48
Milk Choc. Cherries 69
Milk Chocolate 68
Milk Duds 72
Milk Molasses Chips 73
Milky Way 72
Miller 25
Millet 57, 98

Millet Bread 54
Mimi's Cafe 218
Mineral Water 51
Mini-Wheats 60
Mississippi Mud Pie 62
M & M's 72
Mocha 36
Mojito 28
Molasses 157
Mole 80
Mon Cheri 72
Monkfish 96
Monster 39
Monterey Jack 77
Mortadella 128
Mounds 72
Mozzarella 77
Mr Goodbar 72
Mr. Goodcents 218
Mr. Hero 218
Mrs Fields Cookies 219
Mud Cake 62
Muenster 77
Muffin Mixes 67
Muffins 67
  Ready-To-Eat 67
Mulled Wine 26, 29
Mullet 96
MultiGrain Bread 54
Munch Bar 72
Muscle Milk 33
Mushrooms 159
Mushroom Sauce 80
Mussels 96
Mustard 80
My Favorite Muffin 219

**N**

Naan Flatbread 54
Nabisco Cookies 85
Nabisco Crackers 85
Nashi Fruit 100
Nathan's Famous 219
Nature's Path 33
Nature Valley 33
Nestle, Crunch 72
Newtons 85, 150
New York/Club Steak 123
Nilla Wafers 85
Ninety Nine 219
Nips 72
No Bake Cheesecake 65
Noni Juice 41

Noodles 133
Noodles & Company 220
Not Your Father's
  Root Beer 27
Nougat 72
N-Rich 89
NuGo 33
Nut Bread 54
Nut Drinks 49
Nutella 131
Nutrageous Bar 72
NutriSystem 33
Nuts 130
Nut & Seed Butters 131
Nuts, Seeds, Butter 130
N.Y. Style Cheesecake 64

**O**

Oat Bran 57, 98
Oat Bran Cereal 58
Oatmeal 57
Oats 98
Oats & O's 61
Ocean Perch 96
O'Charley's 220
Octopus 96
Oh Henry! 72
Oh Yeah! 33
Okra 159
Old Milwaukee 25
Old Spaghetti Factory 221
Olestra (Olean) 94
Olive Garden 221
Olives 100
Omelets 91
Onions 159
On the Border 221
Ooey Gooey
  Butter Cake 64
Orange 51
Orange Juice 41
Orange Julius 221
Orange Roughy 96
Oranges 100
Orchard Grape Soda 52
Oreo 85
Oreo Cookies 150
Outback Steakhouse 222
Ouzo 29
Oysters 96

**FAST-FOODS INDEX**
**~ PAGE 175 ~**

# Index P - S

**P**

Pabst 25
Pad Thai 174
Palm Sugar 157
Pancakes 132
Pancakes & Waffles 132
Panda Express 222
Pan Dulce 173
Panera Bread 223
Papa Gino's 223
Papa John's 224
Papa Murphy's 224
Papaya 100
Papaya/Peach Nectar 41
Parmesan 78
Parsnip 159
Passionfruit 100
Passion Fruit Juice 41
Pasta & Noodles 133
Pasta Sauces 144
Pastrami 129
Pastry & Pie Crust 134
Paté 129
PayDay Bar 72
Peaches 100
Peanut Brittle 72
Peanut Brittle Bar 73
Peanut Butter 131
Peanut Butter Cup 73
Peanut Butter Patties 82
Peanut Cluster 68
Peanuts 130
Pear Nectar 41
Pears 100
Peas 159
Pecan Crowns 74
Pecans 130
Pecan Shortbread 83
Pecan Twirls 62
Pei Wei Asian Diner 224
Pepper 147
Peppermint Pattie 75
Peppermints 73
Pepperoni, 129
Peppers 80, 159
Pepsi 52
Pepsi True 52
Performance Energy 33
Perkins 225
Pernod 29
Pesto Sauce 80
Peter Piper Pizza 226
P.F. Chang's 226
Philadelphia
  Cream Cheese 78
Pickled Cocktail On. 80
Pickled Egg 91
Pickled Red Cabbage 80
Pickles & Relish 80
Pie Fillings 134

Piels 25
Pies (Fruit) Pie &
  Pastry Crusts 134
Pike 96
Pillsbury Cookies 88
Pineapple 101
Pineapple Juice 41
Pine Nuts 130
Pink Lemonade 52
Pink Salmon 97
Pistachios 130
Pita 54
Pizza: Ready-To-Eat 135
  Frozen 136
Pizza Four Cheese 78
Pizza Hut 227
Pizza Ranch 228
Pizza Sauce 80
Plaintain 101
Plum Pudding 90
Plums 101
Poached Egg 91
Polish Food 173
Pollock 96
Pomegranate 101
Pomegranate Juice 41
Pompano 96
Popcorn 148
Popeye's 228
Popovers 54
Pop Rocks 73
Pork 125
Pork Cracklins 126
Port 26
Port de Salut 78
Porterhouse Steak 123
Port of Subs 228
Potato Chips/Crisps 149
Potatoes 159
Potato Flour 98
Potato Salad 141
Poultry, Chicken,
  Turkey, Duck, Goose 138
Pound Cakes 62
Powdered Sugar 157
Powerade 40
PowerBar 33
Pret A Manger 229
Pretzelmaker 230
Pretzels 149
Probiotics 164
Promax 34
Pro Perform. Powder 39
Prot. & Fiber Crunch 61
Protein Guide &
  Counter 270, 274
Provolone 78
Prune Juice 41
Psyllium Husks 57, 98
Puddings 90

Puddings & Mousse 90
Puffed Rice 58
Puffed Wheat 58
Pumpernickel 54
Pumpkin 160
Pumpkin Seeds 131

**Q**

Qdoba 230
Quail 139
Quail Eggs 91
Quaker Bars 34
Quark 78
Quinoa 98
Quiznos Subs 230, 231
Quorn 124

**R**

Rabbit 126
Radishes 160
Raisin Bran 58, 60
Raisin Bread 54
Raisinets 73
Rally's/Checkers 231
Rambutan 101
Ranch One 231
Raspberries 101
Ready To Drink Coffee 37
Ready-To-Eat Cereal 58
Red Bull 40
Red Bull & Vodka 28
Redd's: Ale 25
  Wicked 27
Red Hot & Blue 231
Red Lobster 231
Red Robin 232
Red Salmon 97
Reduced Calorie
  Puddings 90
Red Vines 71
Reese's 73
Relishes 80
Rennin 30
Rhubarb 160
Rice-A-Roni 119
Rice Bran 57, 98
Rice Cakes 56
Rice Crisps 58
Rice Dishes 140
Rice Drinks 49
Rice Flour 98
Rice Krispies 60
Rice Polish 98
Rice & Rice Dishes 140
Ricotta Cheese 78
Ring Cakes 63

Ritz 86
  Originals 86
  Crackers 'n Cheez Dip 77
Roast Beef 124, 129
Rockstar 40
Rocky Road 73
Roe 96
Rolaids 75
Rolo 73
Roly Poly 233
Root Beer: Hard 27
  Soft 51
Root Beer Barrels 73
Roquefort 78
Round Table Pizza 233
Rubio's Coastal Grill 234
Ruby Tuesday 234
Rum & Coke 28
Runza 235
Russell Stover Candy 73
Rye Bread 54
Rye Flour 98

**S**

Sablefish 96
Sake 26
Salad Dressings 142
Salads 141
Salad Toppings 141
Saladworks 236
Salami 129
Salmon 96
Salmon Cake 96
Salsa 80
Salt 147
Saltines 81
Salt/Sodium Counter
  with High Blood
  Pressure Guide 275, 281
Salt Water Taffy 73
Sambuca 29
Samuel Adams 25
Sandella's 237
Sandies Cookies 83
Sandwich Crackers 151
Sandwich Cremes 82
Sandwiches 165
Sandwich Pockets 54
Sangria 26, 28
Sardines 97
Sarku Japan 237
Sashimi 171
Satay Chicken 174
Sathers 75
Sauces & Gravy 144
Sauerkraut 80, 160

Sausages 92, 127
Savannah Smiles 82
Scallops 97
Schlotzsky's 237
Schnapps 29
Scone 62
Scotch Egg 91
Scrambled Eggs 91
Screwdriver 28
Seafood Cocktail Sce 80
Seashells 73
Seasonings & Spices 147
Seaweed 156, 160
See's Candies 73
Semolina Flour 98
Sesame Seeds 131
Sex On The Beach 28
Shakes 48
Shake Shack 238
Shakey's 238
Shallots 160
Shari's 239
Shark 97
Sheaf 25
Sheep's Milk 47
Sheetz 239
Sherry 26
Shooters 28
  Blue Tequila 28
  Kamikaze 28
  Orgasm 28
Shredded Wheat 58, 61
Shrimp 97
Silk 50
Silkworms 174
Sirloin 123
Sizzler 240
Skittles 73
Skratch Labs 40
Skyline Chili 240
Slim-Fast 40
Smarties 73
Smirnoff 27
Smoked Cheddar 78
Smoked Sausages 127
Smoothie King 241
Smoothies 48
Snackimals 81
Snack Pack Puddings 90
Snacks 148, 150
Snails in garlic butter 174
Snake 174
Snapper 97
Snappy Tomato 241
Snickers 74
Sockeye 96

**FAST-FOODS INDEX**
**~ PAGE 175 ~**

| | | | | | | | |
|---|---|---|---|---|---|---|---|
| Soda Crackers | 81 | Strawberries | 101 | TCBY | 250 | Turkish/Mid. Eastern | 54 |
| Sodium | 281 | Strawb./Raspb. Juice | 41 | Tea | 53 | Turnovers | 62, 64 |
| Sol | 25 | Strongbow Cider | 26 | Herbal | 53 | Turtle Egg | 91 |
| Sole | 95, 97 | Stuffing | 55 | Regular | 53 | Twix | 74 |
| Sonic Drive-In | 241 | Subway | 245 | Teff Seed Flour | 98 | Twizzlers | 74 |
| Sopapillas | 173 | Succotash | 160 | Tempura | 171 | Tybo | 78 |
| Sorghum | 98 | Sugar | 157 | Tequila | 27 | Tylenol | 156 |
| Soul Food | 173 | Sugar Babies | 74 | Tequila Sunrise | 28 | Tzatziki | 79 |
| Souplantation | 242 | Sugar Candy | 68 | Teriyaki | 171 | | |
| Soups | 152 | Sugar Cane | 101 | Beef | 171 | **U** | |
| Sour Cream | 89 | Sugar-coated Almonds | 68 | Chicken | 171 | U-No Bar | 74 |
| Sourdough | 54 | Sugar Coated Peanuts | 74 | Salmon | 171 | Uno Pizzeria & Grill | 253 |
| Sour Patch | 74 | Sugar Substitutes | 157 | Teriyaki Sauce | 80 | | |
| Southern Comfort | 29 | Sugar, Sweeteners, | | TGI Friday's | 251 | **V** | |
| Southern Tsunami | 242 | Honey, Jam | 157 | Thai Foods | 174 | Vanilla | 29 |
| Soybean Products | 156 | Sugar Wafers | 82 | Thundercloud Subs | 251 | Veal | 125 |
| Soybeans | 160 | Sundaes | 103 | Tic Tac | 74 | Vega: | |
| Soy Cheese | 78 | Sundried Tomatoes | 144 | Tiger's Milk | 34 | Protein Bars | 34 |
| Soy Dream | 50 | Sunflower Kernels | 131 | Tilapia | 97 | Protein Shake | 40 |
| Soy Flour | 98 | Supplements | 156 | Tilsit | 78 | Vegetable Juice | 41 |
| Soy Meal | 98 | Surimi | 97 | Tim Hortons | 252 | Vegetable Oils | 94 |
| Soy Milk | 49 | Sushi | 171 | Tiramisu | 62 | Vegetables: | |
| Soy Nuts | 130 | Sweetbreads | 126 | Tiramisu Torte | 64 | Canned/Bottled | 161 |
| Soy Powder Mix | 50 | Sweet Cream Butter | 93 | T.J. Cinnamons | 251 | Frozen | 160 |
| Soy Protein Isolate | 50 | Sweet Potatoes | 160 | Toast | 92 | Veg. Shortening | 94 |
| Soy Sauce | 80 | Sweet Rolls & Buns | 67 | Toast Crunch | 59 | Vegetables & | |
| Soy, Tofu | 156 | Sweet & Sour Sauce | 80 | Toaster Scrambles | 92 | Legumes | 158 |
| Spag. & Meatballs | 170 | Swiss Chalet | 246 | Toblerone | 74 | Vegetarian Patties | 127 |
| Spaghetti/Pasta | 133 | Swiss Chard | 160 | Tofu | 156 | Veggie Crisps | 151 |
| SPAM | 129 | Swiss Milk Choc. Bars | 72 | Togo's | 252 | Velveeta | 78 |
| Spanish Foods | 174 | Swiss Rolls | 62 | Tomatoes | 101, 160 | Vending Machine | 151 |
| Sparks | 25 | Swordfish | 97 | Tomato Juice | 41 | Vermouth | 26 |
| Spearmint Leaves | 74 | Symphony Milk Choc. | 74 | Tomato Ketchup | 144 | Vienna Fingers | 83 |
| Special K | 40, 60 | Syrups, Dessert | | Tomato Paste | 144 | Vietnamese Foods | 174 |
| Chewy Snack Bars | 34 | Toppings | 157 | Tomato Puree | 144 | Villa Fresh Italian | 254 |
| Protein Shakes | 40 | | | Tomato Sauce | 144 | Vinegar | 30, 80 |
| Spelt Bread | 54 | **T** | | Tongue | 126 | Vocelli Pizza | 254 |
| Spelt Flour | 98 | TAB | 52 | Tonic Water | 29, 52 | Vodka | 27 |
| Spices & Herbs | 147 | Tabasco Sauce | 80 | Tootsie Roll | 74 | Vodka Tonic | 28 |
| Spinach | 160 | Table Wines | | Tortilla Flour Mix | 98 | Voortman | 87 |
| Spirits/Liquors | 27 | Non-Alcoholic Wine | 26 | Tortillas & Shells | 56 | | |
| Spirulina | 156 | Red. Alcohol Wine | 26 | Trader Joe's | 50 | **W** | |
| Sponge Cake | 62 | Taco Bell | 247 | Bars | 34 | Wafers | 83 |
| Sponge Pudding | 90 | Taco Cabana | 248 | Soy Milk | 50 | Wahoo's Fish Taco | 254 |
| Sprinkles | 30 | Taco Del Mar | 248 | Trader Jose | 25 | Walnut Brownie | 63 |
| Sprite | 52 | Taco John's | 249 | Trail Mix | 130 | Walnuts | 130 |
| Spritzer | 28 | Taco Mayo | 249 | Trident | 75 | Water Cracker | 81 |
| Squash | 160 | Taco Sauce | 80, 146 | Trifle | 90 | Watermelon | 101 |
| Squaw Bread | 54 | Taco Time | 250 | Tri-O-Plex | 34 | WAWA | 254 |
| Stadium Foods | 167 | Taffy | 74 | Tripe | 126 | Wendy's | 255 |
| Starbucks | 243 | Take 5 | 74 | Triticale | 98 | Werther's | 75 |
| Starbucks, Bottled | | Tam Tams | 84 | Trix | 75 | WestSoy | 49, 50 |
| Coffees | 37 | Tang | 52 | Trop.Smoothie Cafe | 253 | Whataburger | 256 |
| Starburst | 74 | Tang-a-Roos | 74 | Trout | 97 | Wheat | 57 |
| Steak | 123 | Tangerine Juice | 41 | Tubby's | 253 | Wheat Bran | 98 |
| Steak Escape | 244 | Tapioca Cream | 90 | Tumeric | 147 | Wheat Crackers | 81 |
| Steak 'n Shake | 245 | Tapioca Pearl | 98 | Tuna | 97 | Wheat Flakes | 58 |
| Steak Sauce | 80 | Tartar Sauce | 80 | Turkey | 139 | Wheat Flour | 98 |
| Steaz | 40 | Tarts | 64 | Turkey Egg | 91 | Wheat-Free Breads | 54 |
| Stilton | 78 | T-Bone Steak | 123 | Turkey Jerky | 151 | Wheat Germ | 57, 98 |

| | |
|---|---|
| Wheat Grass Juice | 41 |
| Wheaties | 59 |
| Whey | 30 |
| Whipped Toppings | 89 |
| Whipping Cream | 89 |
| Whipps | 73 |
| Whiskey | 27 |
| Whiskey Sour | 28 |
| White Castle | 256 |
| Whitefish | 97 |
| White Rice | 140 |
| White Russian | 28 |
| White Sauce | 80 |
| Whiting | 97 |
| Whitman's Chocolate | 75 |
| Whoopie Pie | 64 |
| Whoppers | 75 |
| Wicked | 27 |
| Wickedly Prime Bars | 34 |
| Wienerschnitzel | 257 |
| Winchell's | 257 |
| WingStreet | 257 |
| Wintergreen | |
| Lozenges | 75 |
| Wonka | 75 |
| Won Ton Wrappers | 133 |
| Woodchuck Cider | 26 |
| Woody's Bar-B-Q | 257 |
| Worcestershire Sce | 80 |
| Wraps & Roll-Ups | 165 |
| Wrigley's | 75 |
| Wyder's Cider | 26 |
| | |
| **Y** | |
| Yakatori | 171 |
| Yams | 160 |
| Yard House | 258 |
| Yeast | 30 |
| Yellowtail | 97 |
| Yogurt | 162 |
| Yogurt ~ Brands | 162 |
| Yogurt Candy | 75 |
| Yogurt Drinks & | |
| Probiotics | 164 |
| Yogurt Raisins | 151 |
| Yoshinoya | 258 |
| | |
| **Z** | |
| Zaxby's | 258 |
| Zebra Cake | 63 |
| ZeigenBock | 25 |
| Zingers | 63 |
| Zola Acai | 40 |
| Zucchini | 160 |
| Zumbida Mango | 27 |

# Notes